AUDITORY-VERBAL THERAPY

For Young Children with Hearing Loss and Their Families, and the Practitioners Who Guide Them

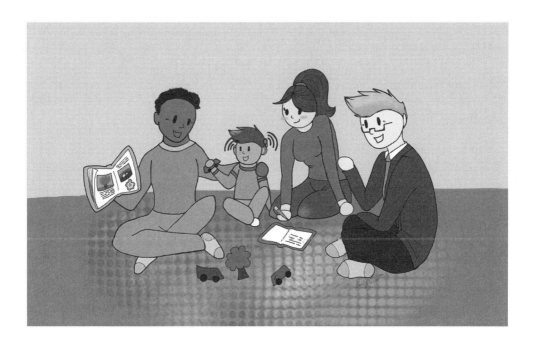

AUDITORY-VERBAL THERAPY

For Young Children with Hearing Loss and Their Families, and the Practitioners Who Guide Them

Warren Estabrooks,
M.Ed., Dip. Ed. Deaf, LSLS Cert. AVT

Karen MacIver-Lux
MA, Aud(C),
Reg.CASLPO, LSLS Cert. AVT

Ellen A. Rhoades
EdS, LSLS Cert. AVT

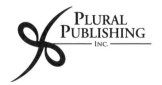

PLURAL
PUBLISHING
INC.

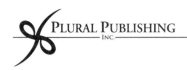

5521 Ruffin Road
San Diego, CA 92123

e-mail: info@pluralpublishing.com
Website: http://www.pluralpublishing.com

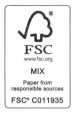

Typeset in 10½/13 Garamond by Flanagan's Publishing Services, Inc.
Printed in the United States of America by McNaughton & Gunn, Inc.
18 19 17 16   2 3 4 5

Cover: SoundIntuition/Stephen Owen
Inside diagrams: SoundIntuition
Therapy session artwork: Emily Lux

Library of Congress Cataloging-in-Publication Data

Names: Estabrooks, Warren, editor. | MacIver-Lux, Karen, editor. | Rhoades,
  Ellen A., editor.
Title: Auditory-verbal therapy for young children with hearing loss and their
  families and the practitioners who guide them / [edited by] Warren
  Estabrooks, Karen MacIver-Lux, Ellen A. Rhoades.
Description: San Diego, CA : Plural Publishing, [2016] | Includes
  bibliographical references and index.
Identifiers: LCCN 2016004229| ISBN 9781597568883 (alk. paper) | ISBN
  1597568880 (alk. paper)
Subjects: | MESH: Hearing Loss—rehabilitation | Language Therapy—methods |
  Speech Therapy—methods | Early Intervention (Education)—methods |
  Auditory Perception | Child
Classification: LCC RF291.5.C45 | NLM WV 270 | DDC 617.80083—dc23
LC record available at http://lccn.loc.gov/2016004229

CONTENTS

PREFACE

In the 21st century, Auditory-Verbal Therapy (AVT) continues to develop along with advances in newborn hearing screening, sophisticated hearing technologies, systems of family-centered intervention, creative service delivery models, the enhancement of continuous professional improvement, and the prevalence of evidence-based information.

Auditory-Verbal Therapy is now more widely accepted than ever and promoted around the world by many practitioners and parents of children with hearing loss, all who share the same desired outcomes. Today, many children with hearing loss can acquire unprecedented listening skills and spoken language equivalent to the quality and quantity of their peers with typical hearing, interact more easily in their communities, achieve higher levels of academic performance, realize an extensive range of careers and greater employment security, and experience fewer limitations in the personal and social aspects of their lives.

The charted course of the pioneers of Auditory-Verbal Therapy continues in *Auditory-Verbal Therapy for Young Children with Hearing Loss and Their Families, and the Practitioners Who Guide Them* as the contributors share comprehensive knowledge, skills, and collaborative work with those who are willing to listen anywhere, anytime.

Auditory-Verbal Therapy for Young Children with Hearing Loss and Their Families, and the Practitioners Who Guide Them is relevant to a broad range of practitioners worldwide: auditory-verbal practitioners, administrators, teachers of children with hearing loss, special educators, teachers in typical schools, audiologists, speech-language pathologists, physical therapists, occupational therapists, psychologists, physicians, surgeons, and university students. Likewise, the content is applicable across most settings where young children with hearing loss are learning to listen and talk and taking their place in a variety of environments, including early intervention programs, preschools, community speech and hearing centers, hospitals, private practices, and family homes. By applying the theories, strategies, and practices discussed in these pages, we anticipate that any practitioner will be better prepared to coach and guide families at any point on the listening and spoken language journey of their children.

Families of young children with hearing loss who embrace Auditory-Verbal Therapy need to be well informed about its principles, expectations, and evidence of expected outcomes. We anticipate that many parents around the world will find this book to be a source of comfort, inspiration, and hope. Through coaching and guided practice, parents and caregivers, the consumers of Auditory-Verbal Therapy, become engaged as their child's first and most enduring teachers of listening and spoken language. Following an evidence-based and evidence-informed framework, *Auditory-Verbal Therapy for Children with Hearing Loss and Their Families, and the Practitioners Who Guide Them* demonstrates how auditory-verbal practitioners work in partnership with the family and a number of interdisciplinary teams, to integrate listening and spoken language into the child's everyday life.

This book supports the belief that all children with hearing loss deserve the opportunity to acquire spoken language if that is the desired outcome of the family. For this to happen, purposeful plans need to be developed, implemented, adjusted, readjusted, and evaluated throughout the family's lifelong journey. At the heart of it all is the partnership between the parents and the practitioners—one that is built on shared knowledge, trust, mutual commitment, and respect.

Auditory-Verbal Therapy for Young Children with Hearing Loss and Their Families, and the Practitioners Who Guide Them is a comprehensive exploration of Auditory-Verbal Therapy where the reader will find the most current research relevant to Auditory-Verbal Therapy and associated themes, including the power of hearing, listening, and the brain; the application and support of audiology; hearing aids, implantable hearing technologies, assistive hearing and access technologies; stages of development; to encourage listening, talking, and thinking strategies in coaching and guiding parents; a blueprint for typical sessions; detailed session plans; children with complex hearing needs; inclusion at school; powerful partnerships; and family journeys from around the world.

In 2015, the World Health Organization estimated that 360 million people worldwide had moderate to profound hearing loss in both ears, and 80% of those lived in low- and middle-income countries. So, even though a great deal of progress has been made, there is still much to do. We hope that in the near future, all bar-riers to equitable services for young children with hearing loss will disappear, and that *Auditory-Verbal Therapy for Young Children with Hearing Loss and Their Families, and the Practitioners Who Guide Them* will play a pivotal role in building a worldwide community of parents and practitioners that will bring the gifts of listening and spoken language to young children with hearing loss and their families everywhere.

ACKNOWLEDGMENTS

The editors would like to express their gratitude to the parents whom we are honored to serve, to colleagues around the world with whom we are privileged to collaborate, and especially to those who worked along with us to bring this labor of love to life.

Alice Eriks-Brophy

Andrea Schopper

Angela Beard

Angie Singh

Anita Grover

Ariella Samson

Barbara Streicher

Becky Clem

Carol Flexer

Carolyne Edwards

Claire Campbell

Clari Denham

Claudia Ferreyra

Dale Atkins

Dave Sindrey

David Pisoni

David Quilico

Denise Wray

Don MacIver

Elaine Tel Al

Elizabeth Walker

Ellen Yack

Emily Lux

Gayla Hutsell Guignard

Glynnis Dubois

Hillary Ganek

Ivy Chan

Jace Wolfe

Janet Jamieson

Jennifer Sansom

Joanna Smith

K. Todd Houston

Katrin Kral

Kristy Gardner-Berry

Laurie Monsebraaten

Linda Daniel

Louise Honck

Lyn Robertson

Margit Pukonen

Martin Lux

Megan Carter

Miguel Angel Sanchez Cervera

Mila de Melo

Monica Cuartas

Nevin Yung

Nicole Bowman

Pam Steacie

Pierre-Roch Cote

Pradnya Yogesh

Rebecca Siomra

Rosie Quayle

Ruth Michnick Golinkoff

Ryan McCreery

Sally Tannenbaum-Katsaggelos,

Sam Atcherson

Sandra Medina

Sara Kelly Hull

Sara Neumann

Sarah Kennett

Sarah Little

Shefali Shah

Sheila MacIver

SoundIntuition

Stacey Lim

Stephen Owen

Tanya Goldsmith

Team at Plural Publishing

Tina Childress

Tina Olmstead

Valerie Johns

Walter Gazzoni

Wendy Visser

WE Listen International Inc.

EDITORS

Warren Estabrooks, M. Ed., Dip. Ed. Deaf, LSLS Cert. AVT, is President and CEO of *WE Listen International Inc.*, a global consulting company in Toronto, Canada. He and his team provide professional education, training, and development in Auditory-Verbal Therapy for practitioners who work with children with hearing loss and their families around the world. For many years, he was Director of the Auditory Learning Centre of the Learning to Listen Foundation at North York General Hospital in Toronto. He was also a Founding Director of Auditory-Verbal International and a Founding Director of the AG Bell Academy for Listening and Spoken Language. He is the Honored Patron of the Warren Estabrooks Centre in Sri Lanka. He is a Canadian of Distinction, recipient of numerous professional and humanitarian awards, and has made significant contributions to the literature.

Karen MacIver-Lux, MA, Aud(C), Reg. CASLPO, LSLS Cert. AVT, is President and CEO of *SoundIntuition*, a company that provides continuing education opportunities, training, and consulting for professionals who work with children who have communication disorders. She is also Director of MacIver-Lux Auditory Learning Services in Toronto, and a proud consultant of *WE Listen International Inc.* Formerly, she was Coordinator of Clinical Services at the Learning to Listen Foundation, of which she is a graduate. She has had a cochlear implant since 2009 after which she received auditory skills training. Karen was director of the Board of Auditory-Verbal International Inc., and was honored by Maclean's magazine as one of the top 100 young Canadians.

Ellen A. Rhoades, EdS, LSLS Cert AVTT An international consultant, mentor, and speaker, Ellen established and directed several Auditory-Verbal centers and programs. She was a Founding Director of Auditory-Verbal International and served on AG Bell Association's Board of Directors. She is Associate Editor of *The Volta Review* and Review Editor for other professional journals. She has authored many papers, chapters, and books including, *Aural (Re)Habilitation for Adolescents with Hearing Loss* and *Auditory-Verbal Practice: Toward a Family-Centered Approach, 2nd ed.* Her awards include Professional of the Year (AVI), Program of the Year (AG Bell), and Nitchie Award in Human Communication (League for the Hard of Hearing). She has a congenital bilateral profound hearing loss.

CONTRIBUTORS

Samuel R. Atcherson, PhD, is Associate Professor of Audiology in the Department of Audiology and Speech Pathology at the University of Arkansas at Little Rock/University of Arkansas for Medical Sciences. He is a prolific author and speaker in the areas of auditory rehabilitation, assistive and mobile technology, clinical electrophysiology, age-related hearing loss, auditory processing disorders, and health literacy. He has hearing loss from childhood and is a user of bilateral cochlear implants.

Dale V. Atkins, PhD, is a licensed psychologist, relationship expert, educator, media commentator, and author. For 45 years she has focused on children's issues, family relationships, adaptation to childhood or adult hearing loss, aging well, and handling transitions and stress while maintaining a balanced life. Her chapters on working effectively with families appear in premier audiology, parenting, and psychology texts. A commentator in the media, she also contributes articles in popular and professional journals.

Tina Childress, MA, CCC-A, is an educational audiologist in the mainstream and residential school settings, technology and social media aficionado, late-deafened adult and bilateral cochlear implant recipient. With her unique perspective and passion for sharing information through social media, she is a sought-out presenter and adjunct lecturer to families and professionals on a variety of topics but especially Hearing Assistive Technology, apps, cochlear implants, advocacy, and effective strategies for coping with hearing loss.

Becky Crow Clem, MA, CCC-SLP, LSLS Cert. AVT, is the Rehabilitation Services Education Coordinator at Cook Children's Medical Center in Fort Worth, Texas. Passionate about working with children with hearing loss and their families, family-centered care and health literacy, her extensive experience includes mentoring and coaching professionals in Auditory-Verbal Therapy, teaching and giving professional presentations in state, national, and international programs. She has contributed to the literature in *The Volta Review*, *ASHAsphere*, and *ASHA Perspectives*.

Glynnis DuBois RN, BScN, BA, MHSc, Dip AV Studies, S-LP Reg CASLPO, is a Master's student in the Childhood Hearing Loss Lab at the University of Toronto. She is a clinician both in the community and in a hospital setting. She has undergraduate degrees in Nursing and Psychology and a Master's degree in Health Sciences from the University of Toronto. She also completed a postgraduate diploma in Auditory-Verbal Studies at the University of Ottawa.

Carolyne Edwards, MClSc, MBA, is Director of Auditory Management Services, a private educational audiology practice that provides consultation in auditory management of children with hearing loss in school districts across southwestern Ontario. She is the author of a number of publications in the area of educational audiology and counseling and lectures throughout North America. She is also a registered psychotherapist and Executive Director and Senior Faculty at the Gestalt Institute of Toronto, in Toronto, Canada.

Maria Emilia (Mila) de Melo, S-LP, Aud(C), Reg. CASLPO, LSLS Cert. AVT, has been providing family-centered therapy services to children with hearing loss and their families, giving professional consultations, and organizing workshops for parents, caregivers, and practitioners since 1992. She has been working with the Infant Hearing Program, Toronto Public Health, since 2007. She has contributed to literature in publications such as *Auditory-Verbal Therapy and Practice* (2006) and *101 FAQ About Auditory-Verbal Practice* (2012).

Alice Eriks-Brophy, BA, BEd, MSc(A), MSc, PhD, is associate professor in the Department of Speech-Language Pathology at the University of Toronto where she teaches courses in aural rehabilitation, articulation, and speech disorders. Her research investigates culturally appropriate service provision for minority children and the impact of family involvement on AVT outcomes. She was previously an itinerant teacher at the Montreal Oral School for the Deaf and a classroom teacher on several Canadian First Nations reserves.

Carol Flexer, PhD, CCC-A, LSLS Cert. AVT, received her doctorate in Audiology from Kent State University in 1982. She is a Distinguished Professor Emeritus of Audiology, The University

of Akron. An international lecturer in pediatric and educational audiology and author of more than 155 publications including 14 books, she is a past president of the Educational Audiology Association, the American Academy of Audiology, and the AG Bell Academy for Listening and Spoken Language.

Hillary Ganek, MA, CCC-SLP, LSLS Cert. AVT, is a doctoral candidate in the Childhood Hearing Loss Lab at the University of Toronto. She worked clinically at the Cora Barclay Centre in South Australia and at Johns Hopkins in Baltimore. Hillary also volunteers with the Global Foundation for Children with Hearing Loss. She holds a bachelor's degree in linguistics from McGill University in Montreal and a master's degree in speech-language pathology from Northwestern University in Chicago.

Louise Hönck, Cert. MRCSLT, PG DipAVT, LSLS Cert. AVT, is the senior AV practitioner at Auditory Verbal[UK] She's involved in multiple outreach programs across the United Kingdom and the Republic of Ireland, combining clinical work and training. She advises on rehabilitation in joint audiology and cochlear implant clinics. She delivers training in various AV[UK] programs for groups including professionals. Additionally, she mentors practitioners toward AV certification. Her particular interests are collaborative work, theory of mind, and purposeful play.

Lisa Katz, MHSc, SLP(C), Reg. CASLPO, LSLS Cert. AVT, works for the Toronto Infant Hearing Program. Previously, she worked as an AV Practitioner and Coordinator of Professional Education at the Learning to Listen Foundation. She also worked in the Cochlear Implant Program at the Hospital for Sick Children and as Consultant to WE Listen International, Inc. Lisa has trained and mentored professionals nationally and internationally, presented at many conferences and made numerous contributions to the literature.

Sarah Warren Kennett, AuD, PhD Candidate, is a clinical audiologist and researcher at Arkansas Children's Hospital who works with pediatric hearing aid users and cochlear implant users of all ages. She is also an adjunct instructor at UAMS/UALR, where she takes great pride inspiring future audiologists in advancing the field. Her clinical and research experience drives her passion for evidence-based practice in recommending, fitting, optimizing, and innovating technology for individuals with hearing loss.

Stacey R. Lim, AuD, PhD, CCC-A is an Assistant Professor of Audiology at Central Michigan University, where she teaches graduate-level audiology courses and supervises in the Audiology Clinic. Her research and clinical areas of expertise are cochlear implants, pediatric and educational audiology, and aural rehabilitation of children and adults. She was born with bilateral, profound, sensory/neural hearing loss and currently wears a cochlear implant and a hearing aid and attended Auditory-Verbal Therapy.

Ryan W. McCreery, PhD, is Director of the Center for Audiology, Boys Town National Research Hospital. He has the privilege of leading a large group of audiologists who provide care for

individuals with hearing and balance problems across the life span. He is also a scientist. His laboratory explores the factors that support speech recognition in children who wear hearing aids. The goal of this research is to optimize developmental outcomes for all children with hearing loss.

Sara Neumann, AuD, is a pediatric and cochlear implant audiologist and deaf education consultant at Hearts for Hearing in Oklahoma City, Oklahoma. Prior to that, she was an educator of the deaf. She has coauthored several textbook chapters on pediatric amplification and cochlear implants. She has a B.S. in Deaf Education (2003) from Northern Illinois University and Doctorate in Audiology (2012) from Illinois State University. Her special interests include cochlear implants, electrophysiology, and teleaudiology.

Rosie Quayle, Cert. MRCSLT, PGDip-AVT, LSLS CertAVT, Churchill Fellow, is Clinical Lead Auditory Verbal Practitioner at Auditory Verbal[UK] in England where she leads the clinical team across AV[UK]'s centers, trains practitioners and ensures high-quality service. She has developed courses for practitioners who are seeking certification in the United Kingdom and Europe. She is particularly interested in working with parents who have varying learning styles as they help their children learn to listen and talk through play.

Lyn Robertson, PhD, emerita professor of Education, Denison University, Granville, Ohio, received her Ph.D. in Reading from the Ohio State University. She has authored *Literacy Learning for Children Who Are Deaf or*

Hard of Hearing (Alexander Graham Bell, 2000), and *Literacy and Deafness* (Plural, 2009; 2014, 2nd ed.), as well as articles about listening, language, and reading. She has served as board president of the Alexander Graham Bell Association Academy for Listening and Spoken Language.

Ariella Blum Samson, MA, is a parent and grandparent of children with hearing loss. She has contributed to the literature in publications such as *Do You Hear That?*, *Auditory-Verbal Therapy for Parents and Professionals*, and *Auditory-Verbal Therapy and Practice*. She also contributed to the video *Jacob's Journey* and to one of the earliest books about auditory learning called *Learning to Listen*. She has written a family memoir titled *A Letter from My Father*. She currently resides in Toronto.

Jennifer K. Sansom, PT, MPT, MS, PhD, is an Assistant Professor at Central Michigan University within the Doctor of Physical Therapy program. During her career as a physical therapist, she has had the opportunity to work in diverse settings with patient populations ranging from children with developmental disabilities to adults following stroke. Currently, her research examines neural control during movement and the impact of environmental influences on motor performance for populations across the life span.

David Sindrey, MClSc, LSLS Cert. AVT, is an AV practitioner and the author/illustrator of many activities designed for promoting listening and spoken language. His online resources include *the ListeningRoom* at Advanced Bion-

ics, *Listeningtree*, and *Actividades de Audición* for Phonak PIP in Spain. His materials have been translated into six different languages. Sindrey is now completing a combined Masters of Audiology degree and a PhD in Hearing Science at the University of Western Ontario, Canada.

Rebecca A. Siomra, MSc, SLP(C), Reg. CASLPO, is a Speech-Language Pathologist with Markham Stouffville Hospital's Child Development Programs in Ontario, Canada. Since completing her master's degree at the University of Western Ontario in 2001, she has dedicated her clinical work to early intervention programs for children 0–6 years of age with and without hearing loss and their families. She enjoys taking on new professional challenges and is currently pursuing her studies toward the LSLS Cert. AVT.

Pamela Steacie, DipEd, MSc, LSLS Cert. AVT, obtained a Master's degree in aural habilitation from McGill University in 1980. She has worked for most of the last 35 years with preschool-aged children with hearing loss, in the Audiology service of the Children's Hospital of Eastern Ontario. She has also taught and mentored students, presented at conferences, participated in research, and contributed to several publications about auditory-verbal practice in both English and French.

Sally Tannenbaum-Katsaggelos, MEd, DTH, LSLS Cert. AVT, is Co-Director of the Pediatric Hearing Loss Program at the University of Chicago Medicine. Having worked with children with hearing loss for over 35 years, she recently participated in Project ASPIRE, a parent-directed intervention initiative for children with hearing loss from low socioeconomic environments. She received the Helen Beebe Award for Outstanding Auditory-Verbal Clinician, was a founding director of Auditory-Verbal International, Inc. She consults and lectures worldwide.

Wendy D. Visser, MEd, Dipl. AV Studies, is an itinerant teacher of children with hearing loss at the Ottawa District School Board, in Ontario, Canada. She has been a teacher for 18 years and her career has involved being a classroom teacher, itinerant resource teacher, teacher of children with autism, and her current role. Visser has provided workshops and specialized Ministry of Education training through the Special Education Department at the Ottawa Catholic School Board.

Elizabeth A. Walker, PhD, CCC-A/SLP, is an assistant professor in the Department of Communication Sciences and Disorders at the University of Iowa, Iowa City, Iowa. Her area of research is aural habilitation, specifically examining factors that influence individual differences in speech perception and language outcomes for children with hearing loss. She is an investigator on several NIH-funded research grants focusing on children with hearing loss, and has published many peer-reviewed articles related to pediatric audiology.

Jace Wolfe, PhD is the Director of Audiology and research at Hearts for Hearing. He is also an Adjunct Assis-

tant Professor at the University of Oklahoma Health Sciences Center and Salus University, and he teaches courses in the AuD programs at several other universities. He is the coauthor of the book, *Programming Cochlear Implants* (2nd ed.), and he has authored numerous chapters, peer-reviewed articles, and the "Tot Ten," a monthly column on pediatric hearing health care.

Denise Wray, PhD, CCC-SLP, LSLS Cert. AVT, is a Professor Emeritus in the School of Speech-Language Pathology and Audiology at the University of Akron. She has c-directed the Auditory-Verbal Clinic in the University's Audiology and Speech Center for more than two decades. She has coauthored over 25 articles in literacy and codirected two grants including the Auditory-Options Project with the Ohio Department of Health and a training grant with the U.S. Department of Special Education.

Ellen Yack, MEd, BSc, OT, is an occupational therapist and director of Ellen Yack and Associates Pediatric Therapy Services, a private agency providing occupational therapy and speech and language pathology services in Toronto. Her areas of expertise include sensory processing disorders, autism spectrum disorders, attention deficit disorders, and disorders of self-regulation. Ellen conducts a variety of workshops and coauthored *Building Bridges through Sensory Integration: Occupational Therapy for Children with Autism and other Pervasive Developmental Disorders.*

1

AUDITORY-VERBAL THERAPY: AN OVERVIEW

Warren Estabrooks, Karen MacIver-Lux,
Ellen A. Rhoades, and Stacey R. Lim

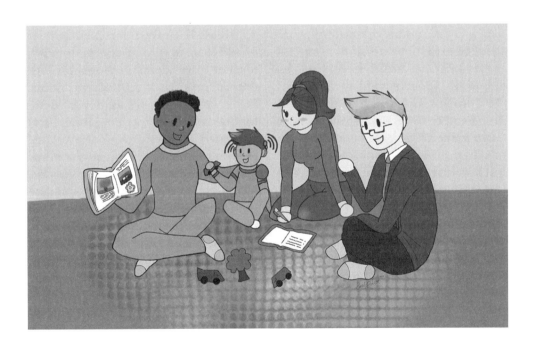

INTRODUCTION

Children who are born with hearing loss, or who acquire hearing loss in early childhood, have unprecedented potential, like never before, to develop listening skills, develop intelligible spoken language, and enjoy the social and academic standards commensurate with peers with typical hearing. To foster this potential, most parents make an educated choice from a variety of communication approaches, to help their young children, to satisfy their family goals, and to embrace their culture. Auditory-Verbal Therapy (AVT), a listening and spoken language (LSL) approach, is one such choice; AVT follows specific principles of practice (Appendix 1–A) and a stringent code of ethics (Appendix 1–B) and uses evidence-based and evidence-informed strategies to develop and grow the child's brain toward the preferred listening and spoken language outcomes.

Through AVT, many of these children learn to *listen* to their own voices, *listen* to the voices of others, and *listen* to the other exciting sounds of life. By learning to *listen*, they learn to *talk*. By learning to *talk*, they learn to engage in *meaningful spoken conversations* with their parents, siblings, and friends. While the children learn to *listen and talk*, the auditory and language centers of the brain expand to support the infrastructure for reading, writing, and use of electronic media. Consequently, many of the children can be fully included in regular preschools and grow up enjoying the abundance of social and academic freedoms of life in the 21st century.

HISTORY OF AUDITORY-VERBAL THERAPY

In the late 1930s, three pioneering practitioners (Helen. H. Beebe, Ciwa Griffiths, and Doreen Pollack) began providing services that were the precursors to AVT as it is practiced today. Independently of each other, these pioneers implemented strategies that emphasized the use of hearing devices and the development of listening skills and spoken language through family-based nonprofit programs. These AV practitioners, all working in different parts of the United States, were strongly influenced by Max Goldstein, an American otologist who proposed an *acoustic method* so children with hearing loss could learn through the auditory sense (Duncan & Rhoades, 2010).

Helen H. Beebe trained as a *teacher of the deaf* and as a speech reading teacher in residential schools for children across the northeastern United States. When *Beebe*, as her students fondly called her, met Emil Froeschels, an Austrian physician, in New York, he became her lifelong mentor and encouraged her to establish a very different type of program for children with hearing loss and their families. So Beebe developed the *Unisensory Approach* that she offered through her private practice in Pennsylvania. Beebe felt that practitioners and parents needed to avoid speech reading as much as possible, so that children would rely on their amplified residual hearing rather than depend on the subtle speech cues offered by watching the speaker's lips. Parents always *observed* or participated in Beebe's therapy sessions, taking notes so that they could facilitate their child's listening and spoken language at home (Beebe, 1953).

Ciwa Griffiths trained as an audiologist and educator and provided her services across the state of California. Similarly, in the late 1930s, Griffiths realized that children with severe-to-profound hearing loss could learn to listen with high-powered hearing aids and could be mainstreamed in regular preschool classrooms. Like Beebe, Griffiths felt that parents needed to be involved as much as possible in both the *listening sessions* and in mainstream education. Her ideas, known as the *Auditory Approach*, were implemented in California and also in a federally funded model program in New York City (Griffiths, 1967). Like Beebe, she established a nonprofit program for families. Until the early 1940s, children with hearing loss were typically not fitted with hearing aids until they were ready for elementary school. Griffiths realized this was too late, so she began aggressively promoting early identification and early use of amplification technology for children with hearing loss. Consequently, as early as 1946, some babies and toddlers started wearing hearing aids and were learning to listen and talk (Fiedler, 1952). Griffiths developed the blueprint for California's first statewide newborn hearing screening (Wilson & Rhoades, 2004).

Doreen Pollack, a speech therapist and audiologist, was strongly influenced by Henk Huizing, a Dutch otologist. She first worked in a hospital in New York City with Huizing as her mentor. During that time, she was instrumental in the development and implementation of many strategies that were designed to facilitate listening and spoken language by children with hearing loss who used effective amplification devices, and the parents were always present in her sessions. Upon relocating to Colorado, she refined her strategies, and referred to her work as *Acoupedic* (a combination of the words "acoustic" and "pediatric") (Pollack, 1993). It is widely accepted that Pollack was most responsible for the prolific dissemination of knowledge in the initiation of AVT across the USA and Canada. Her seminal work, *Educational Audiology for the Limited Hearing Infant and Preschooler* (Pollack, 1970) set the foundation for the work that AV practitioners embrace today.

Elsewhere, practitioners such as Edith Whetnall in England and Petar Guberina in Yugoslavia had similar understandings to those of the pioneers and provided great support for auditory learning (Northern & Downs, 2002).

From the late 1950s and throughout the 1960s, a small group of practitioners followed the groundbreaking work of Beebe, Griffiths, and Pollack. Most notably, they were Antoinette Goffredo and Marion Ernst in the United States, Louise Crawford in Canada, Daniel Ling and Agnes Ling Philips in both the United Kingdom and Canada, and Susann Schmid-Giovannini in Austria and Switzerland and throughout other parts of Europe. However, it was not until the 1970s that the number of practitioners following and promoting AVT began to significantly increase due to the influence of training courses and internships offered by Pollack and Beebe. More teachers, audiologists, and speech-language pathologists were beginning to use the intervention strategies, as the pioneers themselves were *spreading the word* that children with hearing loss could learn to listen and talk.

In 1972 and 1977, Griffiths organized two international conferences about the *Auditory Approach* in Pasadena, California. At the conference in 1972 , Griffiths, Beebe, and Pollack met for the first time. Subsequently, with an attendance of more than 500 people at the conference of 1977, great attempts were made to bring the work of these pioneering practitioners together in one well-defined approach. Then, in 1978, at the invitation of the Alexander Graham Bell Association for the Deaf in Washington, DC, a coalition was formed of AV practitioners, and this group embraced the basic components of Acoupedics as defined by Huizing (Pollack, 1993). At that same meeting, Daniel Ling suggested that the term *auditory-verbal* replace Acoupedics, Unisensory, and Auditory Approach (Ling, 1993). Subsequently, the *International Committee on Auditory-Verbal Communication* (ICAVC) was created, and the principles of Acoupedics were transferred to ICAVC.

Initially established as an independent group of clinical practitioners and parents of children benefiting from AVT, ICAVC shortly evolved into a special committee of the AG Bell Association for the Deaf (Ling, 1993).

In 1987, after many years of collaboration with various clinical practitioners around the world, committee members of ICAVC agreed to establish Auditory-Verbal International (AVI) as an independent nonprofit organization. The primary goal of AVI was to ensure that children with hearing loss had access to a worldwide professionally recognized, standardized, and integrated system of habilitation based on AV principles. AVI concentrated primarily on promoting AVT and became responsible for certifying practitioners as Certified Auditory-Verbal Therapists with the first examination in 1994. In 2005, after 18 years of incorporation and ongoing financial challenges, AVI members dissolved the organization and transferred its assets to the AG Bell Association for the Deaf and Hard of Hearing, where an affiliate, the AG Bell Academy for Listening and Spoken Language (The Academy) was incorporated as a nonprofit entity in Washington, DC. Today, The Academy is responsible for the ongoing certification of Listening and Spoken Language professionals, including the Certified Auditory-Verbal Therapists (LSLS Cert. AVT).

PRINCIPLES OF AUDITORY-VERBAL THERAPY

Today, AVT is viewed as a holistic early intervention model for children with hearing loss and their families in which social interactions are essential for the development of independent cognitive and linguistic functioning. In essence, AVT is the application and management of the most current hearing technologies, in conjunction with specific strategies that foster listening and spoken conversations through artful coaching of the child's parents.

Parents who choose AVT are regarded as the *key stakeholders*, the *primary clients*, and become the most significant *agents of change* in the life of their child. Over time, they form a partnership of trust and respect as they work in tandem with highly qualified auditory-verbal (AV) practitioners. AV practitioners use their expertise to integrate nine domains of knowledge that represent core competencies: hearing and hearing technology; auditory functioning; spoken language communication; child development; parent guidance; education and support; strategies for listening and spoken language development; history, philosophy, and professionals issues; education; and emergent literacy, as they coach and guide parents of children with hearing loss following *Ten Principles of Auditory-Verbal Therapy.*

1. Promote early diagnosis of hearing loss in newborns, infants, toddlers, and young children, followed by immediate audiologic management and AVT.

We hear with the brain; the ears are the *doorway* to the brain for auditory information. Consequently, hearing loss is primarily a brain issue—not an ear issue. Auditory-verbal practitioners, therefore, advocate diagnosis of hearing loss as early in life as possible, followed by consistent use of appropriately programmed hearing technology and weekly sessions of AVT in order to develop the baby's auditory brain centers. Children who are identified with hearing loss by 3 months of age and enrolled in family-centered intervention programs by 6 months of age can have similar language development as children with typical hearing (Fulcher, Purchell, Baker, & Munro, 2012). They can also achieve better reading skills, educational outcomes (Yoshinago-Itano, 2003), and social-emotional growth over time when auditory neural connections are developed in early childhood (Langereis & Vermeulen, 2015).

For various reasons, some children who pass the newborn hearing screening acquire hearing loss during the preschool years (Chen, Fu, Luo, Zhang, & Yang, 2013). It is imperative, therefore, that hearing screening be provided as early as possible during those years followed by AVT to ensure continued development of listening and spoken language.

2. Recommend immediate assessment and use of appropriate, state-of-the-art hearing technology to obtain maximum benefits of auditory stimulation.

Once hearing loss is identified, immediate assessment and consistent use of appropriately programmed hearing technology are essential. The purpose of hearing technology is to get auditory information through the doorway to the brain. There is no other purpose. Consistent use of hearing technology provides auditory stimulation/information that facilitates the development of new neural connections in the brain; these neural connections provide the foundation for spoken language, reading, and academics (Cole & Flexer, 2015). If access to hearing technology is delayed, particularly during developmentally sensitive periods, cortical reorganization will occur (Sharma, Dorman, & Kral, 2005). With early access to amplification and its consistent use, children with hearing loss demonstrate significantly higher scores on vocabulary, grammar, and phonological awareness (Walker et al., 2015). In addition, early and consistent access to electrical stimulation/information as provided by a cochlear implant promotes spoken communication outcomes (Geers & Nicolas, 2013).

3. Guide and coach parents to help their child use hearing as the primary sensory modality in developing listening and spoken language.

Competency in spoken language, social-emotional development, and literacy skills is highly dependent on brain access of auditory information and the subsequent development of listening skills. Parents who choose AVT make a commitment to provide abundant meaningful listening and spoken language learning opportunities. Consequently, the child learns to listen during all waking hours and eventually *listens to learn* as his or her brain is activated by auditory information. As parents take advantage of opportunities to help their child develop confidence in listening, and later, in becoming independent managers of their hearing technology, children learn to navigate difficult listening environments and to repair communication breakdowns due to mishearing.

4. Guide and coach parents to become the primary facilitators of their child's listening and spoken language development through active consistent participation in individualized AVT.

Parents are their child's first and most enduring teachers and the *primary agents of change* in their child's listening and spoken language development . The quantity and quality of spoken language they provide to their child's brain using technologies such as hearing aids or cochlear implants can have a profound impact on the child's linguistic development, educational attainment, and cognitive outcomes (Suskind, 2015).

AV practitioners provide individualized one-on-one auditory-verbal sessions where they demonstrate strategies that promote development in audition, speech, language, cognition, and communication. By practicing in the session, parents learn how to augment their child's listening and language development, to enhance their responsiveness to all the child's communication attempts, and to evaluate progress.

5. Guide and coach parents to create environments that support listening for the acquisition of spoken language throughout the child's daily activities.

In order to reach the child's brain, auditory information must pass through an environment. The young child's daily environment is noisy and presents listening challenges for *all* children. Full maturation of the central auditory nervous system (CANS) is not achieved until children reach late adolescence (Bellis, 2011). Therefore, immature auditory processing skills, coupled with poor acoustics in the home, nursery school, and classroom, can cause children to have difficulty attending to the voices of their peers and caregivers. Children with hearing loss need to expend more energy to understand spoken language and this increases the likelihood that information will be missed. Consequently, many children with hearing loss, during the early stages of listening and spoken language development, will require effective practitioner-demonstrated strategies, and modifications such as FM systems or wireless remote microphones coupled to the child's hearing aids and/or cochlear implants, that help in providing the most acoustically friendly environment.

6. Guide and coach parents to help their child integrate listening and spoken language into all aspects of the child's life.

The brain requires a great deal of focused auditory practice in order to cement neural connections and to develop the necessary "data files" of knowledge. Therefore, a key predictor of a child's linguistic, social-emotional, literacy, and academic competencies is the parents' ability to provide an environment that is rich in meaningful and complex spoken language experiences (Leffel & Suskind, 2013; Suskind, 2015). The AV practitioner gets only a snapshot of the family's daily routines, so it is critical that he or she devises a plan *in partnership with the family* to take advantage of all opportunities for listening and spoken language development. Once parents learn to provide and/or take advantage of auditory experiences during the child's daily life, they come to view their youngster as *a child who hears and actively listens.* Subsequently, the child learns to value hearing and listening and begins to view himself/herself similarly *and actively listens to learn.*

7. Guide and coach parents to use natural developmental patterns of audition, speech, language, cognition, and communication.

The writing, delivery, and evaluation of individualized AVT plans that are consistent with the developmental stages of children with typical hearing are standard procedures of AV practitioners. During AV sessions, the AV practitioner and parent jointly observe and evaluate the child's current skills and identify skills that the child has not yet attained but could learn with an adult's help (Vygotsky, 1978, zone of proximal development). This process enables the AV practitioner and parent to select appropriate short-term objectives and long-term goals. The aim is to close the listening and spoken language gap between the child's hearing age and chronological age as quickly as possible by developing and cementing neural connections through the provision of auditory information.

8. Guide and coach parents to help their child self-monitor spoken language through listening.

Children speak what and how they hear. Auditory feedback of one's own speech is of great importance for the attainment of auditory goals and the acquisition of fluent spoken language (Perkell, 2008). Effective listening and voice modulation prepare the child for independent verbal communication with minimal need for clarification or interpretation. During the early stages of development, AV practitioners encourage parents to imitate their child's vocalizations. These imitations set the stage for vocal turn-taking. As the child learns to listen with his or her hearing technology, spoken language and communication skills begin to develop. As children gain more sophisticated listening and linguistic competence, they use listening to self-monitor their speech and language and self-correct whenever necessary. The ability to self-monitor spoken language is a lifelong skill that is valuable for facilitating clear communication with others, managing and repairing communication breakdowns, learning new languages, and integrating into their society of choice.

9. Administer ongoing formal and informal diagnostic assessments to develop individualized auditory-verbal treatment plans, to monitor progress, and to evaluate the effectiveness of the plans for the child and family.

Parents and AV practitioners create an auditory neural infrastructure in their child's brain upon which they scaffold the higher-level linguistic skills of reading and writing. Thus, every therapy session is diagnostic in order to monitor the development of the infrastructure. The child's auditory functioning and use of communication in meaningful contexts are recorded to assist the AV practitioner in finding the child's zone of proximal development and planning the next steps. In addition to informal observations, once every 3 to 6 months, the AV practitioner administers a battery of tests standardized on children with typical hearing. In conjunction with audiological assessments, tests are used to assess articulation, receptive and expressive vocabulary, receptive and expressive language, and auditory skills. Such assessments assist the AV practitioner and parent in making certain that AVT meets the needs of the child and the family by evaluating progress.

10. Promote education in regular schools with peers who have typical hearing and with appropriate services from early childhood onward.

Children with hearing loss who are identified early, fitted with hearing technology, and enrolled in early intervention programs are able to achieve excellent levels of listening, speech perception, language, social-emotional development, and education, because consistent and meaningful auditory information has been made available to their brain from infancy (Langereis & Vermeulen, 2015; Yoshinago-Itano, 2003). AV practitioners *help parents help their child* attain the requisite school-entry skills in linguistic competence, social cognition, and preliteracy.

Inclusion in school may require the support services of a hearing resource teacher, educational audiologist, speech-language pathologist, and/or other school personnel who need to work as a team. This collaboration creates a *safety net* that promotes full brain access to educational opportunities and helps in fostering self-advocacy skills and facilitating self-actualization.

THE NATURE OF AVT SESSIONS

AVT sessions are *individualized, tailored to the specific needs of the child and family, and enhanced by the family's culture*. AVT integrates the development of listening and talking into all aspects of the child's social, emotional, cognitive, and cultural experiences, so that listening becomes an integral part of his or her life. AVT activities are designed to help each child achieve the general long-term goals of listening and spoken language. This means that monthly and quarterly goals are flexible and malleable, influenced by the needs of child and family. AVT is not a prescription of exercises, and it is *not* conducted with a group of children and/or parents.

Generally speaking, AV practitioners provide weekly therapy sessions, lasting for an hour or an hour and a half each. This is in keeping with the position statement on pediatric habilitation following cochlear implantation (ACIA, 2015) in which the recommendation is for one to two (1) hour habilitation sessions per week (Dettman, Wall, Constantinescu, & Dowell, 2013). One can extrapolate that the same recommendation applies to children wearing hearing aids. In each of these 50–100 hour-long sessions per year, parents learn to apply the short-term objectives of each session into natural language experiential contexts in the child's daily life in ways that promote curiosity and flexible thinking. Parents then acquire the confidence to implement practitioner-coached strategies to help their child attain these objectives that are consistent with typical developmental milestones achieved by children with typical hearing.

The AV practitioner provides an ongoing assessment of the child's progress in all AV sessions and the AV practitioner and parents focus on *listening* and the development of discrete auditory skills rather than watching, so that the auditory and language centers of the brain become the architectural foundation for verbal communication. The AV practitioner leads the parent through various strategies that help the child maximize his or her auditory perception of spoken language. These strategies are presented through games, books, and guided, purposeful play activities. Following the practitioner's model, parents practice using strategies with their child, and then engage in discussions with the AV practitioner about the effectiveness of those strategies.

Based on outcomes, they jointly establish or revise long-term and short-term goals in listening, expressive and receptive language, cognition, and general communication development. Finally, through the guidance of the AV practitioner, parents generate additional strategies and activities that facilitate incorporation of these goals into the everyday life of the family. The progress of children and their parents toward the desired outcomes of AVT are supported by a number of variables including

- *age at diagnosis* (an earlier age of identification is associated with better language outcomes) (JCIH, 2007; Kennedy et al., 2006; Yoshinaga-Itano, 2003);
- *cause of hearing loss* (how the auditory and neural structures are affected can influence the decisions for amplification or cochlear implantation) (JCIH, 2007);
- *degree of hearing loss* (can affect the identification of hearing loss and the decision to pursue amplification quickly that has a direct correlation to positive spoken language outcomes) (Harrison, Roush, & Wallace, 2003);
- *effectiveness of amplification device(s) or cochlear implant(s)* (appropriate settings of hearing aids and programming/mapping of the CI, can provide greater access to all speech frequencies) (Nicholas & Geers, 2006; Waltzman & Roland, 2005);
- *effectiveness of audiological management* (timely audiological assessments, fittings, and so on, with regular monitoring of auditory progress) (JCIH, 2007);

- *hearing potential of the child* (provided by the neural plasticity of the brain) (Sharma et al., 2005);
- *health of the child* (poorer health can negatively affect educational outcomes) (Fransoo et al., 2008);
- *emotional state of the family* (where the family is in terms of grieving can affect its ability to be a partner in the child's auditory-verbal development) (Yoshinaga-Itano, 2003; Young & Tattersall, 2007);
- *level of participation of the family* (higher levels of family participation positively influence the child's language and social growth) (Leffel & Suskind, 2013; Moeller, 2000; Suskind, 2015);
- *skills of the AV practitioner* (paramount in guiding parents to become the primary facilitators, by using evidence-based practice and knowledge) (Graham, Rodger, & Ziviani, 2009; Kaiser & Hancock, 2003; Rush, M'Lisa, & Hanft, 2003);
- *skills of the parents or caregiver* (parent-implemented intervention leads to better outcomes) (Roberts & Kaiser, 2011);
- *child's learning style* (all sessions may require creating or modifying the session plan to best suit the child's learning (Tomlinson et al., 2003); and
- *child's intelligence* (children with significant cognitive delays may develop listening and spoken language slowly and/or require an alternative approach) (Yoshinaga-Itano, 2003).

AVT can take place in a hospital, a clinic, a private practice, and/or in the home. Actually, AVT can take place in the park, at the zoo, in the supermarket, or on the playground. It is always a *team effort* as the family and the AV practitioner work in close collaboration with the audiologist, educators and school personnel, and allied health professionals.

Open, reliable, and consistently cooperative communication among and between team members ensures that the child's overall development is maximized as efficiently as possible. This collaborative communication helps to assure that AVT is appropriate for a child and his or her family. This communication also assists in determining the various diagnostic assessments required to identify the child's specific strengths and learning needs. In turn, this can provide the AV practitioner with information needed for referring the family to another intervention model, if necessary. Considering all aspects of progress, AV practitioners either continue to provide AVT services or initiate a transitional plan, assisting in its implementation as smoothly as possible.

CURRENT STATUS AND REQUIREMENTS OF AUDITORY-VERBAL PRACTITIONERS

Auditory-verbal practitioners (therapists) originate from the professions of audiology, speech-language pathology, and/or teaching (education of children with hearing loss) and are certified by the AG Bell Academy for Listening and Spoken Language (the Academy), which "is an independently governed subsidiary corporation of the Alexander

Graham Bell Association for the Deaf and Hard of Hearing and was established in 2005. It envisions a future where individuals and families will have qualified listening and spoken language professionals available in their immediate geographic area" (http://www.agbellacademy.org).

As a 501(c)(6) nonprofit organization in the United States with the mission of "advancing listening and talking through standards of excellence and international certification of professionals," the Academy offers two certifications: Listening and Spoken Language Specialist, Certified Auditory-Verbal Therapist, (LSLS Cert. AVT) and Listening and Spoken Language Specialist, Certified Auditory-Verbal Educator (LSLS Cert. AVEd). These two professions have commonalities and differences that are reflected in the Principles of Practice for each designation. For the purposes of *Auditory-Verbal Therapy for Children with Hearing Loss and Their Families and the Practitioners Who Guide Them*, the focus is on the Principles of Practice specific to AVT and the designation of LSLS Cert. AVT. An extensive explanation of requisites for this designation can be found at http://www.agebellacademy.org.

OUTCOMES ON THE CURRENT STATE OF AUDITORY-VERBAL THERAPY—A SURVEY

In the past decade, there has been a significant shift in the evolution of AVT and knowledge about hearing loss, hearing technology, and best practices in audiology and AVT. This paradigm shift can be observed in the responses to an informal questionnaire administered to LSLS professionals. This survey was administered to AV practitioners in a closed social media group to determine what kinds of changes have been observed in AV practice over the last 10 years. One simple question was asked: "How has AVT changed in the last 10 years?" Based on personal perspectives, thirty-five AV practitioners provided responses that are divided into four categories: clients, practitioner development, therapy practices, and other.

Clients

The respondents stated the following:

- Children in AVT seem to be younger than ever before and are discharged earlier.
- The public seems to be much more aware of AVT and this is often viewed as a "first option."
- There has been a dramatic increase in the use of cochlear implants with young children.
- More children with additional challenges seem to be enrolling in AVT programs.
- AVT has seemingly embraced bilingualism and multiethnic services.
- Parents seem better informed due to the Internet and social media.
- More fathers seem to be actively involved.
- Parental expectations seem to have increased.
- More children seem to be transitioning from other intervention models to AVT.

Practitioner Development

The respondents stated the following:

- Many practitioners seemingly want to become "certified" and more are needed.
- More assessment outcomes on children's progress are seemingly being collected by practitioners.
- More practitioner training programs are available and more seem to be needed.

Therapy Practices

The respondents stated the following:

- AVT seems to be less formal and more parent focused.
- Parents and practitioners seem to be talking more at natural distances from the children.
- Purposeful play seems to be much more the norm.
- Cross-professional collaboration seems to be increasing.
- Application of AVT strategies for children with multiple challenges seems to be increasing.
- Practitioner expectations seem to be shifting.
- AV practitioners seem to listen more to what children say and how they say it.
- Practitioners and parents seem to embrace a developmental model rather than a remedial model.
- Full inclusion in regular schools seems to be more common.

Other

The respondents stated the following:

- AV children seem to learn language more informally than ever before.
- There seems to be greater focus on family-based intervention with the AV practitioner serving as a guide.
- The degree of hearing loss (without use of hearing technology) no longer seems to be a factor in AVT outcomes.
- AVT and cochlear implants seem to "go together."
- The audiologist seems more widely recognized as being critical to ensuring that the child has auditory access to conversational speech.
- Children who receive AVT appear to be enrolled in regular preschool programs before the first grade.
- Acoustic accessibility to intelligible speech seems to be more widely understood as being essential for brain growth.
- Advances in (hearing) technology have made spoken language easier to learn.

Given the existing body of knowledge about the benefits of early identification of hearing loss and early intervention (JCIH, 2007), it is not surprising that there has been a tremendous shift in the knowledge and delivery of AVT. Rapid advances in hearing technology have given children with hearing loss more access than ever to a greater quantity and quality of spoken language

(Chapters 3, 4, 5, and 6). Interprofessional collaborations are essential to AVT (Chapter 16), and active parental engagement is at the core of *auditory-verbal work* (Chapters 11 and 17). Over time, the role of the AV practitioner has undergone a remarkable evolution.

CULTURAL CONSIDERATIONS IN AUDITORY-VERBAL THERAPY

Culture, as a broad construct, involves ethnicity, religion, language, skin color, socioeconomic status, age, gender orientation, and wholeness/disability status as well as family structure and dynamics. Across all nations, families are changing, and diversity is becoming the norm. For example, in many parts of Anglo-Western countries, *minority groups* are collectively becoming the *majority*. AV practitioners need to demonstrate multicultural competence and embrace such trends (Rhoades, 2013).

There are data, unfortunately, to indicate that insufficient cultural responsiveness remains a barrier to optimal outcomes for early identified children with hearing loss (Fulcher et al., 2015). The current need is for AV practitioners to demonstrate interest, understanding, and respect for each family's culture, including their behavior and interactional styles. Prior to implementing AVT, practitioners seek information from each child's family by way of an informal interview or by a tool such as the *Caregiver Intake Interview*, which is accessible online via the Academy's website (http://www.listeningandspokenlanguage.org) (Rhoades, 2013).

AVT sessions need to reflect culturally responsive practices in order to facilitate increased family engagement (Paul & Roth, 2011) and promote optimal learning opportunities and outcomes for the child (Han & Thomas, 2010). In general, the most challenging cultural issues facing many AV practitioners are race, language, and poverty.

First, AV practitioners need to acknowledge the existence of racism and to consciously avoid all racist behaviors. AV practitioners strive to learn about each family's culture and preferred ways of interacting, and to ensure that persons of different ethnicities are embraced across all AVT activities (Hagiwara, Kashy, & Cesario, 2012). Books, toys, and games that reflect as many cultures as possible need to be in every practitioner's collection (Rhoades, 2013).

Second, most AV practitioners speak only English (Rhoades, 2013). With a limited number of well-trained interpreters to meet the demands of families who speak other languages, practitioners must often depend on friends of families in order to effectively communicate with the child's caregivers. Although challenging, the AV practitioner arranges for parents to receive coaching, whenever possible, in their native language.

Third, practitioners develop sensitivities to the issues of families who are challenged financially. Children from financially disadvantaged families have generally less language input and growth compared to children who are from families who are have a higher socioeconomic status (Hart & Risley, 1995; Leffler & Suskind, 2013). Across all ethnicities, single-parent families are more likely to be among the poorest;

hence, children tend to face daily stressors that can negatively influence development (Evans & Kim, 2013; Hirschl & Rank, 2015). However, with guidance from professionals, parents who are economically disadvantaged can develop the skills and techniques to foster language growth in their children (Leffel & Suskind, 2013; Suskind, 2015). For these families, AV practitioners often need to provide more intensive parent coaching and to enlist an expanded, supportive social network of friends and other service providers in the family's community.

Demonstrating empathy and unconditional positive regard for each family is a requisite for all AV practitioners (Joint Committee on Infant Hearing, 2013). Nonjudgmental listening and engaging in positive strategies are essential for establishing an ongoing effective alliance with each family (Rhoades, 2010). Effective AV practitioners become culture brokers who embrace family differences.

AUDITORY-VERBAL THERAPY IN THE FUTURE

Today, AV practitioners are working in tandem with parents to prepare their children with hearing loss to lead abundant lives well beyond the year 2030. We are also working in the spirit of community with partners across the planet. This involves the use of telecommunications technology (telepractice). We are in a unique position to harness this synergy to increase the health, wellness, and opportunities for all children with hearing loss and their families. As hearing technology and neuroscience continue to intersect and provide high-quality sound accessibility for children with hearing aids, cochlear implants, and other implantable devices, we are focusing our energy in bringing needed AVT to all children and their families who desire it. Throughout the world, audiologists, speech-language pathologists, and teachers of children with hearing loss are seeking certification as auditory-verbal practitioners, so that they can meet the desires of many families.

We are committed to uniting agencies, manufacturers, hearing health and rehabilitation practitioners, scientists, researchers, and families, to optimize hearing, listening, thinking, and spoken language for children with hearing loss across all countries and all cultures. We look forward to a global commitment to the provision of high-quality AVT by building an exceptional community of success that embraces literacy and educational standards for all children with hearing loss.

As AVT continues to transform the lives of children whose parents commit to the demands of being the primary agents of change, more evidence-based information about AVT, and more immediate and direct access to programs based on best practices will be needed.

In the spirit of community, we advance the work of AVT to help make all barriers to equitable services disappear.

REFERENCES

AG Bell Academy for Listening and Spoken Language. (2015). *LSLS certification handbook.* Retrieved from http://listeningandspokenlanguage.org/Academy Document

American Cochlear Implant Alliance. (2015). Position paper. Retrieved from http:// www.acialliance.org

Beebe, H. (1953). *A guide to help the severely hard of hearing child*. New York, NY: Karger.

Bellis, T. J. (2011). *Assessment and management of central auditory processing disorders in the educational setting: From science to practice*. Clifton Park, NY: Delmar Learning.

Chen, G., Fu, S., Luo, S., Zhang, W., & Yang, G. (2013). Screening of delayed-onset hearing loss in preschool children in the mid-south of China. *International Journal of Audiology*, *52*(8), 568–571.

Cole, E. B., & Flexer, C. A. (2015). *Children with hearing loss: Developing listening and talking birth to six* (3rd ed.). San Diego, CA: Plural.

Dettman, S., Wall, E., Constantinescu, G., & Dowell, R. (2013). Communication outcomes for groups of children enrolled in auditory-verbal, aural-oral and bilingual-bicultural early intervention programs. *Otology and Neurotology*, *34*, 451–459.

Duncan. J. & Rhoades, E.A. (2010). Introduction to auditory-verbal practice. In E. A. Rhoades & J. Duncan [Eds.], *Auditory-verbal practice: Toward a family-centered approach* (pp. 5–22). Springfield, IL: Charles C. Thomas.

Evans, G. W., & Kim, P. (2013). Childhood poverty, chronic stress, self-regulation, and coping. *Child Development Perspectives*, 7, 43–48.

Fiedler, M. F. (1952). *Deaf children in a hearing world*. New York, NY: The Ronald Press.

Fransoo, R. R., Roos, N. P., Martens, P. J., Heaman, M., Levin, B., & Chateau, D. (2008). How health status affects progress and performance in school: A population-based study. *Canadian Journal of Public Health/Revue Canadienne de Sante'e Publique*, *99*(4), 344–349.

Fulcher, A., Purchell, A. A., Baker, E., & Munro, N. (2012). Listen up: Children with early identified hearing loss achieve age-appropriate speech/language outcomes by 3 years of age. *International Journal of Pediatric Otorhinolaryngology*, *76*(12), 1785–1794.

Geers, A. E., & Nicholas, J. G. (2013). Enduring Advantages of Early Cochlear Implantation for Spoken Language Development. *Journal of Speech, Language, and Hearing Research*, *56*(2), 643–655. http://doi .org/10.1044/1092-4388(2012/11-0347)

Graham, F., Rodger, S., & Ziviani, J. (2009). Coaching parents to enable children's participation: An approach for working with parents and their children. *Australian Occupational Therapy Journal*, *56*(1), 16–23.

Griffiths, C. (1967). *Conquering childhood deafness*. New York, NY: Exposition Press.

Hagiwara, N., Kashy, D. A., & Cesario, J. (2012). Independent effects of skin tone and facial features on Whites' affective reactions to Blacks. *Journal of Experimental Social Psychology*, *48*, 892–898.

Han, H. S., & Thomas, S. (2010). No child misunderstood: Enhancing early childhood teachers' multicultural responsiveness to the social competence of diverse children. *Early Childhood Education Journal*, *37*(6), 469–476.

Harrison, M., Roush, J., & Wallace, J. (2003). Trends in age of identification and intervention in infants with hearing loss. *Ear and Hearing*, *24*(1), 89–95.

Hart, B., & Risley, T. R. (1995). *Meaningful differences in the everyday experience of young American children*. Baltimore, MD: Paul H. Brookes.

Hirschl, T. A., & Rank, M. R. (2015). The life course dynamics of affluence. *PLOS ONE*, *10*(1), e0116370. doi:10.1371/jour nal.pone.0116370

Joint Committee on Infant Hearing. (2007). Year 2007 position statement: Principles and guidelines for early hearing detection and intervention programs. *Pediatrics*, *120*(4), 898–921.

Kaiser, A. P., & Hancock, T. B. (2003). Teaching parents new skills to support their young children's development. *Infants and Young Children*, *16*(1), 9–21.

Kennedy, C. R., McCann, D. C., Campbell, M. J., Law, C. M., Mullee, M., Petrou, S., . . . Stevenson, J. (2006). Language ability after early detection of permanent childhood hearing impairment. *New England Journal of Medicine, 354*(20), 2131–2141.

Langereis, M., & Vermeulen, A. (2015). School performance and well-being of children with CI in different communicative-educational environments. *International Journal of Pediatric Otorhinolaryngology, 79*(6): 834–839.

Leffel, B. S., & Suskind, D. (2013). Parent-directed approaches to enrich the early language environments of children living in poverty. *Seminars in Speech and Language, 34*(4), 267–277.

Ling, D. (1993). Auditory-verbal options for children with hearing impairment: Helping to pioneer an applied science. *The Volta Review, 95,* 187–196.

Moeller, M. P. (2000). Early intervention and language development in children who are deaf and hard of hearing. *Pediatrics, 106*(3), 1–9.

Nicholas, J. G., & Geers, A. E. (2006). Effects of early auditory experience on the spoken language of deaf children at 3 years of age. *Ear and Hearing, 27*(3), 286–298.

Northern, J., & Downs, M. (2002). *Hearing in children* (5th ed.). Philadelphia, PA: Lippincott Williams & Wilkins.

Paul, D., & Roth, F. P. (2011). Guiding principles and clinical applications for speech-language pathology practice in early intervention. *Language, Speech, and Hearing Services in Schools, 42,* 320–330.

Perkell, J. S. (2008, June 29). *Auditory feedback and speech production in cochlear implant users and speakers with typical hearing.* Paper presented at 2008 Research Symposium of the AG Bell Association International Convention, Milwaukee, WI.

Pollack, D. (1970). *Educational audiology for the limited hearing infant.* Springfield, IL: Charles C. Thomas.

Pollack, D. (1993). Reflections of a pioneer. *The Volta Review, 95,* 197–204.

Rhoades, E. A. (2013). An international perspective on audiologic rehabilitation. In E. Fitzpatrick and S. Doucet (Eds.), *Pediatric audiologic rehabilitation: From infancy to adolescence* (pp. 184–185). New York, NY: Thieme.

Roberts, M. Y., & Kaiser, A. P. (2011). The effectiveness of parent-implemented language interventions: A meta-analysis. *American Journal of Speech-Language Pathology, 20*(3), 180–199.

Rush, D. D., M'Lisa, L. S., & Hanft, B. E. (2003). Coaching families and colleagues: A process for collaboration in natural settings. *Infants and Young Children, 16*(1), 33–47.

Sharma, A., Dorman, M. F., & Kral, A. (2005). The influence of a sensitive period on central auditory development in children with unilateral and bilateral cochlear implants. *Hearing Research, 203*(1), 134–143.

Suskind, D. (2015). *Thirty million words: Building a child's brain.* New York, NY: Dutton.

Tomlinson, C. A., Brighton, C., Hertberg, H., Callahan, C. M., Moon, T. R., Brimijoin, K., & Reynolds, T. (2003). Differentiating instruction in response to student readiness, interest, and learning profile in academically diverse classrooms: A review of literature. *Journal for the Education of the Gifted, 27*(2–3), 119–145.

Vygotsky, L. (1978). *Mind in society: Development of higher psychological processes.* Cambridge, MA: Harvard University Press.

Walker, E. A., Holte, L., McCreery, R. W., Spratfor, M., Page, T., & Moeller, M. P. (2015). The influence of hearing aid use on outcomes of children with mild hearing loss. *Journal of Language and Hearing Research, 58*(5), 1611–1625.

Waltzman, S. B., & Roland, J. T. (2005). Cochlear implantation in children younger than 12 months. *Pediatrics, 116*(4), e487–e493.

Whitehurst, G., Falco, F. L., Lonigan, C. J., Fischel, J. E., DeBaryshe, B. D., Valdez-Menchaca, M. C., Caufield, M. (1988). Accelerating language development through picture book reading. *Developmental Psychology, 24,* 552–559.

Wilson, J., & Rhoades, E. (2004). Ciwa Griffiths: A celebration of a pioneer (1911–2003). *Volta Voices, 11*(3), 34–35.

Yoshinaga-Itano, C. (2003). From screening to early identification and interventions: Discovering predictors to successful outcomes for children with significant hearing loss. *Journal of Deaf Studies and Deaf Education, 8,* 11–30.

Young, A., & Tattersall, H. (2007). Universal newborn hearing screening and early identification of deafness: Parents' responses to knowing early and their expectations of child communication development. *Journal of Deaf Studies and Deaf Education, 12*(2), 209–220.

Appendix 1–A

PRINCIPLES OF AUDITORY-VERBAL THERAPY[1]

1. Promote early diagnosis of hearing loss in newborns, infants, toddlers, and young children, followed by immediate audiologic management and Auditory-Verbal therapy.

2. Recommend immediate assessment and use of appropriate, state-of-the-art hearing technology to obtain maximum benefits of auditory stimulation.

3. **Guide and coach parents** to help their child use hearing as the primary sensory modality in developing listening and spoken language.

4. **Guide and coach parents** to become the primary facilitators of their child's listening and spoken language development through active consistent participation in individualized Auditory-Verbal therapy.

5. **Guide and coach parents** to create environments that support listening for the acquisition of spoken language throughout the child's daily activities.

6. **Guide and coach parents** to help their child integrate listening and spoken language into all aspects of the child's life.

7. **Guide and coach parents** to use natural developmental patterns of audition, speech, language, cognition, and communication.

8. **Guide and coach parents** to help their child self monitor spoken language through listening.

9. Administer ongoing formal and informal diagnostic assessments to develop individualized Auditory-Verbal treatment plans, to monitor progress and to evaluate the effectiveness of the plans for the child and family.

10. Promote education in regular schools with peers who have typical hearing and with appropriate services from early childhood onwards.

Note. The term "parents" also includes grandparents, relatives, guardians, and any caregivers who interact with the child.

Appendix 1-B

PROFESSIONAL CODE OF ETHICS[1]

The AG Bell Academy for Listening and Spoken Language® (Academy) is dedicated to the purpose of ensuring that all children with hearing impairment who have the potential to develop speech and language through the optimal use of amplified residual hearing have the opportunity to do so. Establishing the highest standards of professional integrity based on accepted ethical principles and practice is vital to the fulfillment of this purpose.

This **Professional Code of Ethics** applies to those members who are responsible for the proper delivery of (re)habilitative services to such clients. The **Professional Code of Ethics** also seeks to protect persons served and to ensure the integrity of recognized auditory-verbal practices. Professional conduct of a member that is in violation of the spirit and purpose of this Code shall be considered unethical. Failure to specify any particular responsibility or practice in this Code should not be construed as denial of the existence of such responsibilities or practices. Professional members are hereinafter referred to as "individuals."

The fundamentals of ethical conduct are described by **Principles of Ethics and Rules of Ethics** as they relate to responsibility to persons served, to the public, and to the professions engaged in the provision of auditory-verbal services.

Principles of Ethics, aspirational and inspirational in nature, form the underlying moral bases for the **Professional Code of Ethics**. Individuals shall observe these principles as affirmative obligations under all conditions of professional activity. **Rules of Ethics** are specific statements of minimally acceptable professional conduct or of prohibitions and are applicable to all individuals.

PRINCIPLE I

Individuals shall agree with the purpose, philosophy and working principles of the Academy. Individuals shall honor their responsibility to make fully available to all children with hearing impairment those aspects of auditory-verbal practice that encourage habitual and maximal use of amplified residual hearing, and are known to have positive effects upon the human auditory system and the subsequent development of verbal communication.

Rules

- ▪ Individuals shall support programs for the early detection and identification of hearing impairment and the auditory management of infants, toddlers and children so identified.
- ▪ Individuals shall seek to provide the earliest possible use of the

---

[1]Reprinted with permission from the AG Bell Academy for Listening and Spoken Language®.

most appropriate technology in order that their clients obtain the maximum auditory benefits possible.

- Individuals shall seek to instruct primary caregivers in ways to provide optimal acoustic stimulation within meaningful contexts and support the development of the most favorable auditory learning environments for the acquisition of spoken language.
- Individuals shall seek to integrate listening into the child's total personality.
- Individuals shall support the view that communication is a social act and seek to improve verbal (spoken) interaction within the typical social dyad of infant/child and primary caregiver(s). Parents are viewed as the primary models for the development of a child's spoken language with the provision that one-to-one teaching is critical to communication development.
- Individuals shall work to ensure that the child's emerging speech will be self-monitored through audition to the greatest possible extent.
- Individuals shall use natural sequential patterns of auditory, perceptual, linguistic and cognitive stimulation to encourage the emergence of listening, speech and language abilities.
- Individuals shall make ongoing evaluation and prognosis of the development of listening skills an integral part of the (re) habilitative process.
- Individuals shall support mainstreaming/integration of children with hearing impairment into

regular education classes with appropriate support services and to the fullest extent possible.

PRINCIPLE II

Individuals shall honor their responsibility to hold paramount the welfare of persons served professionally.

Rules

- Individuals shall maintain high standards of professional competence in rendering services, providing only those professional services for which they are qualified by education and experience.
- Individuals shall provide professional services with honesty and compassion and shall respect the dignity, worth, and rights of those served.
- Individuals shall use every resource, including referral when appropriate, to ensure that the highest quality service is provided.
- Individuals shall not discriminate in the delivery of professional services on the basis of race, sex, religion, national origin, or sexual orientation.
- Individuals shall provide accurate information about the nature and management of hearing impairment and about the services and products offered.
- Individuals shall evaluate the effectiveness of services rendered and of products dispensed and shall provide

services or dispense products only when benefit can reasonably be expected.

■ Individuals shall maintain adequate records of professional services rendered and products dispensed and shall allow access to these records when appropriately authorized.

■ Individuals shall not reveal, without authorization, any professional or personal information about the person served professionally, unless required by law to do so.

■ Individuals may make a statement of prognosis, but shall not guarantee results, mislead, or misinform families or person served.

■ Individuals shall recognize the right of parents to select the type of (re)habilitative, communicative or educational system or program they wish for their child.

■ Individuals shall charge only for services rendered. They shall not misrepresent, in any fashion, services rendered or products dispensed.

PRINCIPLE III

Individuals shall honor their responsibility to achieve and maintain the highest level or professional competence.

Rules

■ Individuals engaging in any aspect of the professions shall

perform within the scope of their competence, education, training and experience.

■ Individuals shall maintain professional competence, including participation in continuing education.

■ Individuals shall provide appropriate supervision and assume full responsibility for services delegated to their staff.

■ Individuals shall ensure that all equipment used in the provision of services is in proper working order and is properly calibrated.

PRINCIPLE IV

Individuals shall honor their responsibilities to the public through providing information and education and the development of services for unmet needs.

Rules

■ Individuals shall not misrepresent their credentials, competence, education, training or experience.

■ Individuals shall not participate in professional activities that constitute a conflict of interest.

■ Individuals shall not misrepresent diagnostic information, services rendered, or products dispensed or engage in any scheme or artifice to defraud in connection with obtaining payment or reimbursement for such services or products.

2

HEARING, LISTENING, THE BRAIN, AND AUDITORY-VERBAL THERAPY

Carol Flexer and Ellen A. Rhoades

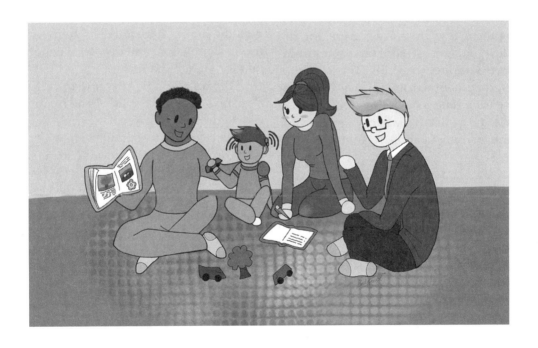

INTRODUCTION

Historically, conversations about hearing loss have focused on the ear. But, due to neurobiological research, today's conversations about sensory input focus on the brain. For example, we see with the brain; the eyes are the entryway to the brain for visual information. We smell with the brain; the nose is the pathway to the brain for olfactory stimuli. We hear with the brain; the ears are the *doorway* to the brain for auditory information. Consequently, hearing loss is primarily a brain issue—not an ear issue (Figure 2–1).

Anytime the word *hearing* is used, we need to think about "auditory brain development." Acoustic accessibility of *intelligible* speech is essential for brain growth because auditory brain development is a first-order event for the development of spoken communication and literacy skills. There is substantial neurobiological evidence that hearing (auditory brain stimulation) is the most effective sensory modality for the learning of spoken language, read-

ing, and cognitive skills that create the foundation for tomorrow's workforce (Robertson, 2014; Werker, 2012; Zupan & Sussman, 2009).

The purpose of this chapter, therefore, is to present the scientific basis of hearing and listening, including basic terminology, and a motivational outlook for Auditory-Verbal Therapy (AVT).

HEARING

Hearing, the most universal of all senses, is acoustic access of auditory information to the brain. Quantitatively speaking, hearing is the *fastest* sense; as such, it enables the brain to be attuned to the environment more rapidly than any other sense (Horowitz, 2012). The organic design of human beings triggers the neural imperative of auditory input, stimulation, and development of auditory neural pathways.

Human beings are organically designed without "ear lids." The brains of children with typical hearing are exposed to auditory stimuli 24 hr every day. The brains of children with hearing loss have access to sound only when they are wearing their hearing devices —far less than 24 hr. Unfortunately, none of our current hearing devices, including cochlear implants and hearing aids, are engineered for 24-hr use. Yet, our brains are organically designed for continuous auditory stimulation, even during sleep. Parents often report that their children with hearing loss request to keep their hearing devices on when sleeping.

Further organic evidence of the power of hearing is that the inner ear is fully developed by the fifth month

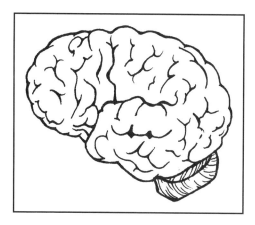

Figure 2–1. The human brain: the "Real Ear."

of gestation. Therefore, a typically developing human fetus potentially has 4 months of *in utero* auditory brain stimulation (Simmons, 2003). At approximately 1 year of age, after 16 months of meaningful and interactive listening (including before-birth listening), a child with typical hearing begins to produce words. The key point is that 'listening time' cannot be skipped, and a child who misses months of brain access to auditory input needs to make up for it (Golinkoff, 2013). The brain requires extensive listening experience to properly organize itself around the speech signal. Importantly, infants also must hear their own vocalizations, creating an auditory feedback loop that is critical for motivating frequent early vocalizations (Fagan, 2014).

HEARING LOSS

The ear is the "doorway to the brain" for sound (Cole & Flexer, 2016). Hearing loss, then, is a *doorway* problem. Hearing loss obstructs that doorway in various ways and to varying degrees, preventing auditory input from reaching the brain. Hearing devices break through the doorway to allow access, stimulation, and development of auditory neural pathways with auditory information, including spoken language. The purpose of hearing technology is to get auditory information through the doorway to the brain. There is no other purpose. The child's listening and spoken language outcomes, therefore, are not determined by 16,000 (or likely much fewer) hair cells, or by 30,000 auditory nerve fibers, but by 100 billion neurons in the brain, processing 100 trillion instructions per second (Pakkenberg, & Gundersen, 1997).

For children with hearing loss, lack of high-fidelity acoustic information to the brain is the biggest challenge worldwide. It is imperative to have very high expectations for today's hearing technology in order to make soft sounds available to the brain at a distance and in the presence of noise. Children must use hearing technology that enables them to overhear conversations and to benefit from incidental learning in order to maximize auditory exposure for social and cognitive development.

SOUND

Sound is *an event* rather than a name or label. For example, you can "see mommy" but you cannot "hear mommy" if she is motionless. You hear mommy walking, talking, typing on a computer, cooking, and so on. You hear mommy engaged in an event, an activity, or an action. An event creates vibrations. Vibrations are picked up by the "ear doorway" and are sent to the brain as energy for coding, and for perception as information. Sound is a temporal event, not a spatial label (Boothroyd, 2014).

LISTENING

Listening is purposeful attention to auditory information as evidenced by activation of the prefrontal cortex (Musiek, 2009). There is a distinction between hearing and listening. Hearing is acoustic access of auditory information to the brain. For children with hearing loss, hearing includes improving the signal-to-noise ratio by managing the environment and utilizing hearing technologies. Listening, on the other hand, is when the individual attends to acoustic events with intentionality. *Hearing* must be made available before *listening* can be taught or learned. In AVT, parents and auditory-verbal (AV) practitioners focus on using intervention strategies to develop and enhance the child's listening, spoken language, and cognitive skills after the audiologist channels acoustic information to the brain by fitting and programming hearing devices.

How do we create a hearing brain, and then teach it to be a listening brain? In order to change the prefrontal cortex of the brain, auditory attention and working memory must be fostered (see Chapter 9 for more information on these critical cognitive capacities), and training needs to commence in acoustically favorable conditions (Doidge, 2007). Extensive auditory practice creates the neurobiological foundation not only for spoken language and literacy skills, but also for age-appropriate social and cognitive skills.

The child has to learn to attend to auditory information. This process, called "auditory attentional focus," can be viewed as a controlled act, referred to as either "active hearing" or "listening" (Moore, 2007). Initially, listening requires effortful attention to a particular sound while hearing other sounds; therefore, the listening process voluntarily occurs on a conscious level. This auditory attentional focus can typically be observed during mid-infancy (Newman, Morini, & Chatterjee, 2013). The more focused the attention of the child needs to be, the more effort he or she needs to expend in listening.

THE INVISIBLE ACOUSTIC FILTER EFFECT OF THE DOORWAY PROBLEM

Hearing loss of any type or degree that occurs in infancy or childhood can hinder the development of a child's spoken language, reading and writing skills, and academic performance (Madell & Flexer, 2014). That is, a doorway problem (hearing loss) functions as an *invisible acoustic filter* that distorts, smears, or eliminates incoming sounds to the brain, especially auditory information from even a short distance away. The negative effects of a hearing loss may be apparent, but the hearing loss itself is unseen and easily discounted.

Human beings are neurobiologically "wired" to develop spoken language and reading skills through the central *auditory* system. For example, most people think that reading is a visual skill, but recent research on brain mapping shows that primary reading centers of the brain are located in the auditory cortex—in the auditory areas of the brain (Chermak & Musiek, 2014; Pugh, Sandak, Frost, Moore, & Menci, 2006). That is why many children who are born with hearing loss and who do not have brain access to auditory information when they are very young (through hearing devices and auditory learning) tend to have a great deal of difficulty reading, yet their vision is fine (Robertson, 2014). Therefore, the earlier and more efficiently a child's brain has access to meaningful sound followed by direction of the child's attention to auditory information, the better opportunity the child will have to develop spoken language, literacy, and academic skills. With the technology and early auditory intervention available today, a child with a "doorway problem" *can* have the same opportunity as a child with typical hearing to develop spoken language, reading, and academic skills even though the child has atypical hearing.

AUDITORY NEURAL DEVELOPMENT

Brain imaging procedures, currently used by neurobiologists to study the brain and nervous system, have dramatically influenced our understanding of hearing and learning how to listen. These procedures provide us with data-driven insights into the neural structures and pathways underlying our sensory and thinking processes.

Neuroplasticity

Neuroplasticity refers to the brain's availability and malleability to grow, develop, and alter its structure as a function of external stimulation (Chermak & Musiek, 2014; Kilgard, Vasquez, Engineer, & Pandya, 2007). Neuroplasticity is greatest during the first three and a half years of life (Sharma, 2013; Sharma, Nash & Dorman, 2009). The younger the infant, the more neuroplasticity the child has (Sharma, 2013; Sharma, Dorman, & Kral, 2005). Rapid infant brain growth requires prompt intervention, typically including amplification and/or a cochlear implant and a comprehensive intervention program to promote the development of auditory skills. In the absence of sound, the brain reorganizes itself to receive input

from other senses, primarily vision; this process is called *cross-modal reorganization,* and it reduces auditory neural capacity (Sharma, Campbell, & Cardon, 2015). Early amplification or cochlear implantation stimulates a brain that is in the initial process of organizing itself and is therefore more receptive to auditory information, resulting in greater auditory capacities (Sharma & Nash, 2009). Therefore, identification of newborn hearing loss and other hearing differences should be considered a neurodevelopmental emergency.

As a result of brain modifiability, today's young children born with hearing loss of any degree have incredible possibilities for achieving higher levels of spoken language, reading skills, and academic competencies that were not available to most children in previous generations (Gifford, 2014; Nicholas & Geers, 2006; Yoshinaga-Itano, 2004). We are experiencing a new population of babies, toddlers, and preschoolers with hearing differences—a population that some of us have never experienced.

Critical Stages of Auditory Neural Development

Auditory neural development is a complex and lengthy process. While the cochlea (organ of hearing outside of the brain) is mature at birth, and frequency resolution is mature by 6 months of age, peak synaptic density within the auditory cortex in children with typical hearing, occurs between 2 and 4 years of age. Thereafter, synaptic counts decrease, and unused synapses are eliminated (Kral & O'Donoghue, 2010). Temporal processing likely remains in flux until adolescence (Kraus &

White-Schwoch, 2015). Therefore, stages of auditory neural development are layered and nuanced; they are not discrete.

The cortex of the brain also matures in stages, and the level of maturity depends on the richness of exposure and experience (Merzenich, 2010). Level one of cortical development probably matures by 12 months. This first stage, the "setup" stage for the cortex, has the brain being "always-on." In this period, all it takes to develop auditory pathways is exposure to sound. The brain's task is to create a model of the culture into which it has been born. The baby learns how to control the actions required for surviving and thriving in that world (Merzenich, 2010).

The second stage of cortical development has the brain now controlling its own plasticity as the child masters skill after skill. These are learning-driven changes and they are huge. The higher levels of the cortex continue to mature up to age 17 to 19 years (Giedd, 2008). Neural organization is bottom-up maturation. The quality of this lower level of maturation, stimulation, and practice influences the potential quality of higher-level neural maturation.

The auditory cortex is composed of a number of functionally and structurally discrete Brodmann's areas. These areas are firmly interrelated and together characterize one functional unit. Lower-order areas activate higher-order areas showing bottom-up interactions, and higher-order areas modulate those below demonstrating top-down interactions (Kral & O'Donoghue 2010). Anything we can do to access and "program" those critical and powerful auditory centers of the brain with acoustic detail will expand children's abilities to lis-ten, learn spoken language, and read. As Robbins and colleagues (2004) contend, early and ongoing auditory intervention is essential.

A Forward-Thinking Brain

The neocortex, a part of the cerebral cortex and the crowning feature of evolution, is goal directed and primed to think ahead to the future (Rakic, 2009). Due to its plasticity, children who experience positive outcomes integral to AVT are likely to develop neural pathways wired for success. This gives rise to hope and optimism. Hope, based on motivation, sustains progress in goal pursuit (Snyder, Lopez, & Pedrotti, 2009). Optimism, a learned belief system, affects thought processes enabling a positive approach to life (Carver & Scheier, 2014; Seligman, Ernst, Gillham, Reivich, & Linkins, 2009). While optimism and hope are separate psychological constructs reflecting positive expectations about the future, they both influence how the brain is wired and the manner in which the brain thinks about the future (Alarcon, Bowling, & Khazon, 2013).

Expectations Influence Outcomes

An expectation is a specific belief about a person's capabilities. As reviewed by Rhoades (2010), the science of expectations is rooted in psychological research. It informs us that the perceptions or expectations of both the AV practitioner and the parent can affect the child's performance (Hyde, Punch,

& Grimbeek, 2011; Patterson & Vakili, 2014). Expectations of others toward a child affect how they behave with the child. In turn, expectations can become truths, thus becoming self-fulfilling prophecies. AV practitioners and parents are known to have high expectations (Wu & Brown, 2004). The forward-thinking brain, when influenced by high expectations, hope, and optimism, is a powerful brain for children with hearing loss who have learned to listen.

AUDITORY DOMINANCE

Information from all senses competes for attention. More attention is given to the information that is either most meaningful or relevant to the task. Thus, competition between sensory modalities typically leads to one modality dominating both attention and perception. Sensory dominance is influenced by the demands of the task, how quickly the information is processed, and practice.

For young children with typical hearing, hearing is the preferred sense, hence the term *auditory dominance.* Indeed, auditory input has a "privileged processing status" for infants and preschoolers, across all their language learning years (Nava & Pavani, 2013; Robinson & Sloutsky, 2004). This overall auditory preference even applies to children with hearing loss, provided they have learned to listen (Zupan & Sussman, 2009).

Some children, due to their impoverished hearing sense (doorway problems that have not been addressed),

learn to compensate by depending on their visual modality. A prevailing assumption about children with hearing loss (lack of auditory information through the doorway to the brain) is that they compensate for their hearing loss by becoming visual learners. However, there is insufficient evidence to support this assumption, regardless of whether the children use signed or spoken language (Marschark et al., 2015).

Interestingly, later, when auditory information reaches a child's auditory brain during the most sensitive period of growth, neuroimaging methods show that the brain begins to change. This demonstrates brain plasticity (Kral & O'Donoghue, 2010). Brain plasticity is most pronounced during the child's critical early learning years (Hernandez & Li, 2007). It is important that auditory information be restored to the child's brain as soon as possible, especially for facilitating access to soft conversational sound.

There are considerable advantages to having auditory dominance (Sandhu & Dyson, 2012). These include improvements in auditory attention that lead to improved behavioral performances, such as faster reaction times and increased accuracy of speech perception (Cohen, Cavanagh, Chun, & Nakayama, 2012). Auditory dominance enables auditory perceptual learning to occur (Finneran, Francis, & Leonard, 2009; Gomes, Molhom, Christodoulou, Ritter, Cowan, 2000). Other benefits to demonstrating auditory dominance include much-improved listening skills and academic performance (Moore, Ferguson, Halliday, & Riley, 2008). Consequently, the importance of an intervention model such as AVT cannot be underestimated.

Important Definitions

Sensory Deprivation

This refers to the systematic prevention of information from reaching one or more senses. Early deprivation or alteration of sensory input leads to impaired sensory perception (Hernandez & Li, 2007). For example, congenital profound deafness without the use of hearing devices causes absence of auditory attention.

Sensory Compensation

This refers to improvement in the remaining senses after the loss of one sensory system in order to counteract the lost capabilities (Hoover, Harris, & Steeves, 2012). Attention is focused on the remaining senses.

Sensory Competition

Information from all senses competes for attention. More attention is paid to the information that is most meaningful. Attentional learning allows us to focus more on specific information and to suppress other information (Schwartz et al., 2005). Attentional learning facilitates sensory bias.

Sensory Dominance

When two or more senses are stimulated at the same time, this refers to which sensory modality prevails over the others (Nava & Pavani, 2013). Sensory dominance depends on attentional focus and attentional selection. Attentional learning facilitates a bias for one sense over another (Vidnyánszky & Sohn, 2003).

THE BRAIN BASIS OF AVT

The amazing truth is that AV practitioners have always followed brain-based principles, even before those principles were substantiated by hard scientific data. Current neurobiological findings confirm the following principles of AV practice: (a) human beings are "wired" to listen and talk; (b) the brain requires a great deal of focused auditory stimulation in order to cement neural connections and to develop the necessary "data files" of knowledge; (c) when the brain is stimulated early with auditory information, the baby's motor speech centers are activated; (d) parents and AV practitioners create an auditory neural infrastructure on which they scaffold the higher-level linguistic skills of reading and writing; and (e) AVT is an important and viable intervention model. And now, due to ongoing scientific data, practitioners offer brain-based reasons for AVT strategies. AVT is informed by brain research.

AVT, therefore, epitomizes the power of hearing, listening, and the brain.

REFERENCES

Alarcon, G. M., Bowling, N. S., & Khazon, S. (2013). Great expectations: A meta-analytic examination of optimism and hope. *Personality and Individual Differences, 54,* 821–827.

Boothroyd, A. (2014). The acoustic speech signal. In J. R. Madell & C. Flexer (Eds.),

Pediatric audiology: Diagnosis, technology, and management (2nd ed., pp. 201–208). New York, NY: Thieme.

Carver, C. S., & Scheier, M. F. (2014). Dispositional optimism. *Trends in Cognitive Science, 18,* 293–299.

Chermak, G. D., & Musiek, F. E. (Eds.). (2014). *Handbook of central auditory processing disorder: Comprehensive intervention* (Vol. II). San Diego, CA: Plural.

Cohen, M. A., Cavanagh, P., Chun, M. M., & Nakayama, K. (2012). The attentional requirements of consciousness. *Trends in Cognitive Sciences, 16,* 411–417.

Cole, E., & Flexer, C. (2016). *Children with hearing loss: Developing listening and talking birth to six* (3rd ed.). San Diego, CA: Plural.

Doidge, N. (2007). *The BRAIN that changes itself.* London, UK: Penguin Books.

Fagan, M. K. (2014). Frequency of vocalization before and after cochlear implantation: Dynamic effect of auditory feedback on infant behavior. *Journal of Experimental Child Psychology, 126,* 328–338.

Finneran, D. A., Francis, A. L., & Leonard, L. B. (2009). Sustained attention in children with specific language impairment (SLI). *Journal of Speech, Language, and Hearing Research, 52,* 915–929.

Gifford, R. H. (2014). Cochlear implants for infants and children. In J. R. Madell & C. Flexer (Eds.), *Pediatric audiology: Diagnosis, technology, and management* (2nd ed., pp. 238–254). New York, NY: Thieme.

Giedd, J. N. (2008). The teen brain: Insights from neuroimaging. *Journal of Adolescent Health, 42,* 335–343.

Golinkoff, R. (2013, April). *Development of infant language.* Session presented at the American Academy of Audiology 2013 Conference, Anaheim, CA.

Gomes, H., Molholm, S., Christodoulou, C., Ritter, W., & Cowan, N. (2000). The development of auditory attention in children. *Frontiers in Bioscience, 5,* 107–120.

Hernandez, A. E., & Li, P. (2007). Age of acquisition: Its neural and computational mechanisms. *Psychological Bulletin, 133,* 638–650.

Hoover, A. E., Harris, L. R., & Steeves, J. K. (2012). Sensory compensation in sound localization in people with one eye. *Experimental Brain Research, 216,* 565–574.

Horowitz, S. S. (2012). *The universal sense: How hearing shapes the mind.* New York, NY: Bloomsbury.

Hupp, J. M., & Sloutsky, V. M. (2011). Learning to learn: From within-modality to cross-modality transfer during infancy. *Journal of Experimental Child Psychology, 110,* 408–421.

Hyde, M., Punch, R., & Grimbeek, P. (2011). Factors predicting functional outcomes of cochlear implants in children. *Cochlear Implants International, 12,* 94–104.

Kilgard, M. P., Vazquez, J. L., Engineer, N. D., & Pandya, P. K. (2007). Experience dependent plasticity alters cortical synchronization. *Hearing Research, 229,* 171–179.

Kral, A., & O'Donoghue, G. M. (2010). Profound deafness in childhood. *The New England Journal of Medicine, 363,* 1438–1450.

Kraus, N., & White-Schwoch, T. (2015). Auditory brainstem development: More than meets the ear. *Hearing Journal, 68*(7), 30–32.

Madell, J. R., & Flexer, C. (2014). *Pediatric audiology: Diagnosis, technology and management* (2nd ed.). New York, NY: Thieme.

Marschark, M., Spencer, L. J., Durkin, A., Borgna, G., Convertino, C., Machmer, E., . . . & Trani, A. (2015). Understanding language, hearing status, and visual-spatial skills. *Journal of Deaf Studies and Deaf Education, 20*(4), 310–330.

Merzenich, M. M. (2010, April). *Brain plasticity-based therapeutics in an audiology practice.* Learning Lab presented at the American Academy of Audiology National Conference, San Diego, CA.

Moore, D. (2007). Auditory cortex 2006— The listening brain. *Hearing Research, 229,* 1–2.

Moore, D. R., Ferguson, M. A., Halliday, L. F., & Riley, A. (2008). Frequency discrimination in children: Perception, learning and attention. *Hearing Research*, *238*, 147–154.

Musiek, F. E. (2009). The human auditory cortex: Interesting anatomical and clinical perspectives. *Audiology Today*, *21*(4), 26–37.

Nava, E., & Pavani, F. (2013). Changes in sensory dominance during childhood: Converging evidence from the Colavita effect and the sound-induced flash illusion. *Child Development*, *84*, 604–616.

Newman, R. S., Morini, G., & Chatterjee, M. (2013). Infants' name recognition in on- and off-channel noise. *Journal of Acoustical Society of America*, *133*, 377–383.

Nicholas, J. G., & Geers, A. E. (2006). Effects of early auditory experience on the spoken language of deaf children at 3 years of age. *Ear and Hearing*, *27*, 286–298.

Pakkenberg, B., & Gundersen, H. J. G. (1997). Neocortical neuron number in humans: Effect of sex and age. *Journal of Comparative Neurology*, *384*, 312–320.

Patterson, J. E., & Vakili, S. (2014). Relationships, environment, and the brain: How emerging research is changing what we know about the impact of families on human development. *Family Process*, *53*, 22–32.

Pugh, K. R., Sandak, R., Frost, S. J., Moore, D. L., & Menci, W. E. (2006). Neurobiological investigations of skilled and impaired reading. In D. Dickinson & S. Neuman (Eds.), *Handbook of early literacy research* (Vol. 2, pp. 64–76). New York, NY: Guilford.

Rakic, P. (2009). Evolution of the neocortex: Perspective from developmental biology. *Nature Reviews Neuroscience*, *10*, 724–735.

Rhoades, E. A. (2010). Evidence-based auditory-verbal practice. In E. A. Rhoades & J. Duncan (Eds.), *Auditory-verbal practice: Toward a family-centered approach* (pp. 23–52). Springfield IL: Charles C. Thomas.

Robbins, A. M., Koch, D. B., Osberger, M. J., Zimmerman-Philips, S., & Kishon-Rabin, L. (2004). Effect of age at cochlear implantation on auditory skill development in infants and toddlers. *Archives of Otolaryngology-Head and Neck Surgery*, *130*, 570–574.

Robertson, L. (2014). *Literacy and deafness: Listening and spoken language* (2nd ed.). San Diego, CA: Plural.

Robinson, C. W., & Sloutsky, V. M. (2004). Auditory dominance and its change in the course of development. *Child Development*, *75*, 1387–1401.

Sandhu, R., & Dyson, B. J. (2012). Re-evaluating visual and auditory dominance through modality switching costs and congruency analyses. *Acta Psychologica*, *140*, 111–118.

Schwartz, S., Vuilleumier, P., Hutton, C., Maravita, A., Dolan, R. J., & Driver, J. (2005). Attentional load and sensory competition in human vision: Modulation of fMRI responses by load at fixation during task-irrelevant stimulation in the peripheral visual field. *Cerebral Cortex*, *15*, 770–786.

Seligman, M. E. P., Ernst, R. M., Gillham, J., Reivich, K., & Linkins, M. (2009). Positive education: Positive psychology and classroom interventions. *Oxford Review of Education*, *35*, 293–311.

Sharma, A. (2013, May). *Post-implantation developmental neuroplasticity.* Plenary session presented at the 11th European Symposium on Paediatric Cochlear Implantation (ESPCI 2013), Istanbul, Turkey.

Sharma, A., Campbell, J., & Cardon, G. (2015). Developmental and cross-modal plasticity in deafness: Evidence from the P1 and N1 event-related potentials in cochlear implanted children. *International Journal of Psychophysiology*, *95*(2), 135–144.

Sharma, A., Dorman, M. F., & Kral, A. (2005). The influence of a sensitive period on central auditory development in children with unilateral and bilateral cochlear implants. *Hearing Research*, *203*, 134–143.

Sharma, A., Nash, A. A., & Dorman, M. (2009). Cochlear development, plasticity and re-organization in children with cochlear implants. *Journal of Communication Disorders, 42,* 272–279.

Simmons, D. D. (2003). The ear in utero: An engineering masterpiece. *Hearing Health, 19*(2), 10–14.

Snyder, C. R., Lopez, S. J., & Pedrotti, J. T. (2009). *Positive psychology: The scientific and practical exploration of human strengths.* Thousand Oaks, CA: Sage.

Vidnyánszky, Z., & Sohn, W. (2003). Attentional learning: Learning to bias sensory competition. *Journal of Vision, 3,* 1741–1746.

Werker, J. (2012). Perceptual foundations of bilingual acquisition in infancy. *Annals of the New York Academy of Sciences, 125,* 50–61.

Wu, C-j. D., & Brown, P. M. (2004). Parents' and teachers' expectations of auditory-verbal therapy. *The Volta Review, 104,* 5–20.

Yoshinaga-Itano, C. (2004, September). *Issues and outcomes of early intervention.* Presentation at the Consensus Conference on Early Intervention, Washington, DC.

Zupan, B., & Sussman, J. E. (2009). Auditory preferences of young children with and without hearing loss for meaningful auditory—Visual compound stimuli. *Journal of Communication Disorders, 42,* 381–396.

3

EVALUATING THE RESEARCH AND EXAMINING OUTCOMES OF AUDITORY-VERBAL THERAPY

Moving From Evidence-Based to Evidence-Informed Practice

Alice Eriks-Brophy, Hillary Ganek,
and Glynnis DuBois

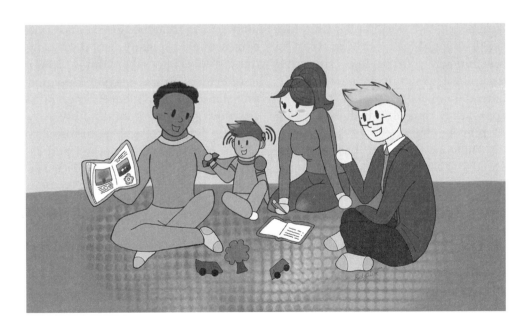

INTRODUCTION

Evidence-based practice (EBP) is defined as the "conscientious, explicit, and judicious use of current best evidence in making decisions about the care of individual patients" (Sackett, 1997, p. 3). The goal of EBP is to enhance our knowledge of the effectiveness of existing clinical practices by gathering outcome data related to specific clinical intervention approaches (Dollaghan, 2004). The primary benefits of EBP are that it permits practitioners to effectively plan for intervention activities, and to develop new and improved intervention and service delivery strategies based on solid evidence supporting their decisions. Practitioners turn to research findings to inform their daily practice. Constant upgrading of current practices in light of compelling research evidence is expected to lead to improved outcomes for families and their children with hearing loss. EBP also allows auditory-verbal (AV) practitioners to demonstrate to other practitioners that AVT works and is therefore worth doing. Finally, EBP enables AV practitioners to make links with other disciplines, resulting in new applications of knowledge and new treatment approaches, thus continually advancing AV practice.

The concept of EBP has long governed and directed audiology, speech-language pathology, and other disciplines in medicine and rehabilitation. An earlier version of this chapter (Eriks-Brophy, 2006) as well as an article published in *The Volta Review* (Eriks-Brophy, 2004) explored the existing state of knowledge of EBP as it applied to Auditory-Verbal Therapy (AVT). How-ever, in the years since that chapter was originally published, a number of considerations related to EBP in the context of rehabilitation generally and related to AVT specifically have arisen. In particular, the requirement that only the most scientifically rigorous research generating the highest levels of research evidence should be considered in order to support any given treatment approach has been called into question (Nevo & Slonim-Nevo, 2011). AV practitioners have an obligation to not only consider the existing evidence that AV intervention works, but also to find the flexibility to support all families based on an informed understanding of listening and spoken language intervention and practice. AV practice must be individualized to best accommodate the needs of each family (AG Bell, 2007). This basic principle of AVT leads AV practitioners to regularly adjust or modify existing AV strategies to fit the needs of individual families. However, a strict EBP approach limits the consideration and value given to studies investigating the ways in which unique cases influence intervention outcomes, often disregarding or dismissing these studies altogether (Rubin, 2007). Furthermore, it has become apparent that the level of evidence assigned to an intervention outcome study may obscure issues related to the quality of the research methodology and its reported results, as will be discussed in more detail below (Strauss, Glasziou, Richardson, & Haynes, 2011).

Practitioners and researchers alike have therefore begun to move away from strict definitions of EBP, recognizing the importance of considering all levels of evidence for an intervention approach as the basis upon which to identify and evaluate the best possible treatment strategies for clinical caseloads. As a result, the term *evidence informed practice* (EIP) has recently come into wider usage. EIP uses both scientific research outcomes and insights from practitioners and clients to form the basis for decisions regarding AVT. At the same time, a critical stance toward the evidence provided from each source of data is maintained, resulting in a more comprehensive and inclusive approach to the evaluation of therapy outcomes (Nevo & Slonim-Nevo, 2011). Nevo and Slonim-Nevo (2011, p. 1178) define EIP as research based but with room for "constructive and imaginative judgment and knowledge of practitioners and clients." They state that research findings alone should not override, take precedence over, or negate clinical experience or the experiences, knowledge, and values of the clients we serve. In particular, the EIP philosophy challenges the current dependency and priority given to randomized controlled trials (RCTs) in existing frameworks of EBP and argues that the currently undervalued lower levels of evidence should be considered alongside higher level evidence in some cases (Clarke, Gillies, Illari, Russo, & Williamson, 2013; Howick, 2011). In an RCT, participants are randomly assigned to a study or a control group and either receive or do not receive a specific experimental intervention or treatment. Clarke and colleagues (2013) go so far as to argue that strong evidence obtained through studies at lower levels of the evidence hierarchy may sometimes override evidence obtained through statistically controlled studies that are higher up in the hierarchy, including RCTs.

As its name implies, EIP allows for a more flexible method of assessing practice through the inclusion of complementary converging evidence at all levels of the hierarchy, including the clinical experience of practitioners and the needs and wishes of clients, to add to the support base for a particular practice. Although EIP is still research supported, it does not rely exclusively on a defined hierarchy or framework for assessing outcomes. Instead, EIP includes all available outcome data in order to better inform decision making (Nevo & Slonim-Nevo, 2011). Encouraging practitioners to take a broad yet critical view of available information in light of their own experience and that of their clients ultimately allows for a greater number of alternatives to be generated that might be used to inform clinical practice. According to Nevo and Slonim-Nevo (2011, p. 1178), "practice is as much art as it is science, and as much a dialogue as it is an application of empirical findings to clients' unique characteristics and context". Critically evaluating research outcomes obtained from diverse sources of evidence is an important part of clinical practice; however, developing the skill set to be able to synthesize many ideas and techniques into a well-supported set of therapeutic practices can be challenging as well as time consuming. An AV practitioner must use his or her clinical expertise in order to quickly identify available research, evaluate its utility in a particular situation and with a particular client, and then apply this information to determine an appropriate course of action (Gambrill, 2007). Stated succinctly, "(e)vidence-informed practice describes a philosophy and an evolving process designed to help practitioners gain needed information and to become lifelong learners. The uncertainty in making decisions is highlighted, efforts to decrease it are made, and clients are involved as informed participants" (Gambrill, 2007, p. 458).

NEW OUTCOME EVIDENCE IN SUPPORT OF AVT

The current chapter sought to investigate and evaluate new research that has documented outcomes in AVT over the last 15 years. The revision of this chapter has been guided by three primary objectives. The first was to incorporate an EIP perspective into the review of the existing evidence base supporting AVT outcomes. The second was to locate any new research articles on the topic of outcomes of AVT that had been published in peer-reviewed journals since the time the original chapter had been published. The third was to update the evaluative framework on the basis of which the scientific merits of these new articles could be judged. The framework used in the original article was no longer current, and a more recent and transparent framework was required.

Meeting each of these objectives required methodological decisions in order to reach a consensus among the authors both on which articles to include in the review and on the level of evidence each of these articles represented. Although the search strategy did not adhere to the strict standards that systematic reviews are held to, a transparent search methodology was devised to ensure that as much of the currently published research as possible would be located.

The authors began by compiling a list of key words from several AV-related outcome studies that were located previously. After the list was shortened to better serve the research objectives for this chapter, these search terms were used to look for new articles. The list of search terms used in the review is presented in Table 3–1.

The most relevant databases were chosen in order to maximize the chances of capturing publications in both medical and education-related journals. These databases were Medline, Psych INFO, ERIC, and Google Scholar. In order to be included in the review, all articles were required to meet the following criteria:

- a publication date after 2001 unless not reported in the previous version of this chapter;
- an explicit statement that the children received AVT, as opposed to other forms of auditory-oral therapy; and
- documented outcomes in the domains of speech, language, listening, literacy, and/or social-emotional development.

Studies were excluded if the children receiving different types of intervention were grouped together as part of a single cohort; for example, studies where children with hearing loss who received AVT and children who received sign language intervention were grouped together. No qualitative studies examining parent outcomes were included in this review.

Twenty-seven new articles were retrieved following this protocol. They were divided among the three authors, who each independently extracted study information and evaluated the

Table 3-1. List of Search Terms Used in Locating AVT Outcomes Research

Search Terms	
Speech	Intervention
Speech perception	Early intervention (support)
Speech production measurement	Preschool
Speech recognition assessment	Auditory-oral
Comprehension	Treatment/long-term/clinical outcomes
Vocabulary	
Language	Verbal learning
Language development	Infants
Language development disorders—rehabilitation speech and language	Children and youth/toddler, preschool
(Spoken) language outcomes	Parents and parenting
Hearing impairments/hearing impaired	Reading comprehension
Deaf/deafness—rehabilitation	AVT
Prelingual deafness	Listening
Hearing aids	Speech therapy
Hearing	Speech-language pathology
Pediatric cochlear implants	Language therapy
Acoustic analysis	Audition
Auditory-verbal (therapy)	Communication methods

study design and the quality of the research methodology. Following this, the three authors met to ensure their judgments were aligned and accurate. The studies were then grouped according to their level of evidence following the definitions contained in the Oxford Centre for Evidence-Based Medicine 2011 Levels of Evidence (Oxford Center for Evidence-Based Medicine, 2011), an internationally accepted frame of reference for the evaluation of clinical research evidence. During discussions among the three authors, decisions

were made regarding how to rank the studies reviewed in order to maintain consistency. A consensus was reached for all included studies. Research in which all children received AVT, but AV treatment effects were not the specific focus of investigation, were separated into an independent category.

The Oxford Centre for Evidence-Based Medicine 2011 (OCEBM, 2011) Levels of Evidence uses the methodology from an individual study to determine its place on the hierarchy, with further rankings possible based on the overall quality of the research. There are five levels or steps of evidence, with specific methodological parameters provided for ranking the scientific rigor of research at each level. In order to aid in decision making, a glossary is also available defining each of these research methodologies. The levels of evidence available through the OCEBM 2011 vary depending on the specific question the research review is attempting to answer. Thus, levels of evidence for ranking studies examining questions related to prognosis or diagnosis differ somewhat from those used in examining treatment outcomes. The five levels of evidence from the OCEBM 2011 are summarized in Table 3–2, with Level 1 being considered the strongest evidence supporting a particular research question and Level 5 being considered the weakest evidence. For the purposes of this review, the evidence levels associated with the evaluation of treatment outcomes formulated in the hierarchy as, "Does this intervention help?" were used in organizing and representing relevant research articles.

In the case of treatment studies, **Level 1 evidence** consists of either a systematic review or an N-of-1 study. These two research methodologies are considered to constitute the highest level of evidence in assessing treatment efficacy. N-of-1 studies are single-subject research paradigms in which an experimental and a control treatment are applied and then withdrawn using random allocation and a carefully implemented multiple baseline design in order to demonstrate treatment efficacy. Ideally, both the child and the practitioner should be blinded to the control versus the experimental conditions while outcomes are moni-

tored. Treatment periods continue until evidence demonstrating that the treatment outcomes associated with the two conditions are or are not different is generated (Center for Evidence-Based Medicine, 2014). An aggregated series of N-of-1 studies can also be used to prospectively document the effectiveness of a specific treatment. Systematic reviews examine peer-reviewed publications about a well-defined health-related question using a rigorous, standardized, and transparent methodology for determining which articles to include in the review. Researchers conducting systematic reviews perform extensive orderly database searches with specific search terms to ensure no relevant study is overlooked. The individual studies are then critically appraised and synthesized, often providing a quantitative summary of the results through the application of a complex statistical procedure known as a meta-analysis (Center for Evidence-Based Medicine, 2014; Strauss et al., 2011). This process minimizes the bias and random error found in individual studies (Strauss et al., 2011). In many cases, only studies that consist of RCTs are included in systematic reviews. The synthesized results from a specific field of study obtained through a systematic review are perceived as contributing the highest level of evidence to justify interventions and treatment decisions.

Level 2 evidence in treatment studies consists of RCTs or less well-controlled observational studies with very large effect sizes. As described above, in an RCT participants are randomly assigned to either an experimental or a control group and either receive or do not receive the specific intervention or treatment under investigation.

Table 3–2. Table Oxford Centre for Evidence-Based Medicine 2011 Levels of Evidence

Question	Step 1 (Level 1*)	Step 2 (Level 2*)	Step 3 (Level 3*)	Step 4 (Level 4*)	Step 5 (Level 5)
How common is the problem?	Local and current random sample surveys (or censuses)	Systematic review of surveys that allow matching to local circumstances**	Local non-random sample**	Case-series**	n/a
Is this diagnostic or monitoring test accurate? (Diagnosis)	Systematic review of cross sectional studies with consistently applied reference standard and blinding	Individual cross-sectional studies with consistently applied reference standard and blinding	Non-consecutive studies, or studies without consistently applied reference standards**	Case-control studies, or "poor or non-independent reference standard**	Mechanism-based reasoning
What will happen if we do not add a therapy? (Prognosis)	Systematic review of inception cohort studies	Inception cohort studies	Cohort study or control arm of randomized trial*	Case-series or case-control studies, or poor quality prognostic cohort study**	n/a
Does this intervention help? (Treatment Benefits)	Systematic review of randomized trials or n-of-1 trials	Randomized trial or observational study with dramatic effect	Non-randomized controlled cohort/follow-up study**	Case-series, case-control studies, or historically controlled studies**	Mechanism-based reasoning

continues

Table 3-2. *continued*

Question	Step 1 (Level 1*)	Step 2 (Level 2*)	Step 3 (Level 3*)	Step 4 (Level 4*)	Step 5 (Level 5)
What are the COMMON harms? (Treatment Harms)	Systematic review of randomized trials, systematic review of nested case-control studies, *n*-of-1 trial with the patient you are raising the question about, or observational study with dramatic effect	Individual randomized trial or (exceptionally) observational study with dramatic effect	Non-randomized controlled cohort/follow-up study (post-marketing surveillance) provided there are sufficient numbers to rule out a common harm. (For long-term harms the duration of follow-up must be sufficient.)**	Case-series, case-control, or historically controlled studies**	Mechanism-based reasoning
What are the RARE harms? (Treatment Harms)	Systematic review of randomized trials or *n*-of-1 trial	Randomized trial or (exceptionally) observational study with dramatic effect			
Is this (early detection) test worthwhile? (Screening)	Systematic review of randomized trials	Randomized trial	Non-randomized controlled cohort/follow-up study**	Case-series, case-control, or historically controlled studies**	Mechanism-based reasoning

Note. *Level may be graded down on the basis of study quality, imprecision, indirectness (study PICO does not match questions PICO), because of inconsistency between studies, or because the absolute effect size is very small. Level may be graded up if there is a large or very large effect size.

Note. **As always, a systematic review is generally better than an individual study.

Source: OCEBM Levels of Evidence Working Group*. "The Oxford 2011 Levels of Evidence." Oxford Centre for Evidence-Based Medicine. http://www.cebm.net/index.aspx?o=5653

*OCEBM Table of Evidence Working Group = Jeremy Howick, Iain Chalmers (James Lind Library), Paul Glasziou, Trish Greenhalgh, Carl Heneghan, Alessandro Liberati, Ivan Moschetti, Bob Phillips, Hazel Thornton, Olive Goddard, and Mary Hodgkinson.

Again, ideally, both the participants and the practitioners administering treatment should be blinded to the control versus the experimental conditions. Rigorous statistical comparisons between the outcomes of the two groups, which are often matched on certain variables, demonstrate the effectiveness or ineffectiveness of the applied treatment. Also included in this level of evidence are observational studies with large effect sizes. These are studies that were not well controlled methodologically but nevertheless yielded a significant enough performance difference between the control and experimental groups that it cannot be ignored.

Effect size is a way of quantifying the size of the difference between two groups and is particularly useful in evaluating the effectiveness of a specific intervention relative to a comparison. It allows us to evaluate how well a treatment works in a specific context rather than simply asking whether or not a treatment works. Effect size complements statistical hypothesis testing by emphasizing the size of the difference between groups independently from sample size (Ellis, 2010).

Level 3 evidence in treatment studies consists of non-randomized cohort studies in which subsets of a predefined population are, have been, or in the future may or may not be exposed, or be exposed in different degrees, to an intervention that is hypothesized to influence the probability of achieving a certain outcome. Cohort studies typically conduct observations of large numbers of participants over a long period of time, often many years. Outcomes across participant groups are compared as a function of differences in exposure levels to a specific

treatment (Center for Evidence-Based Medicine, 2014). A non-random sample is a population that has been defined through a non-random method where some members of the overall population have no chance of being selected to participate in the study. For the purposes of this review, a non-randomized controlled cohort study was defined as a study that included a comparison group but lacked randomization in the selection of participants. Any studies that did not contain a comparison group were ranked as case series studies (Level 4 evidence) as this glossary definition was deemed to be best suited to their methodology.

Level 4 evidence in treatment studies consists of case series, case-control studies, or historically controlled studies. A case series is defined as consisting of a series of case reports involving children who were exposed to a similar treatment. Such case series reports typically contain detailed information about individual participants including demographic information such as age, gender, ethnic origin, as well as information on diagnosis, treatment, response to treatment, and follow-up after treatment (Center for Evidence-Based Medicine, 2014). A case-control study compares children who have a hearing loss or outcome of interest (cases) with children who do not have a hearing loss or outcome (controls). This type of study uses retrospective observations in order to determine the relationship between any given factor and the child's hearing status (Center for Evidence-Based Medicine, 2014). In a historically controlled study, data are collected from a control group of children who were recruited prior to the beginning of the study, and data from the experimental group are collected prospectively (Center for Evidence-Based Medicine, 2014).

Level 5 evidence in treatment studies consists of mechanism-based reasoning, a form of inferential thinking through which a logical chain or link is made between a specific intervention and a treatment outcome through relevant mechanisms (Howick, 2011). Illari and Williamson (2012) define a mechanism as consisting of "entities and activities organized in such a way that they are responsible for the phenomenon" (p. 120). This form of reasoning involves an inferential chain that links the intervention (such as AVT) with a clinical outcome (such age-appropriate communication outcomes). Evidence of mechanisms is typically obtained through laboratory or statistical studies and relies on clinical expertise and observation in the linking of an intervention to client outcomes. For example, prior to direct studies examining the impact of early identification of hearing loss, AVTs frequently claimed that early identification allowed children to receive hearing technology earlier, thus reducing the period of sensory deprivation, which, in turn, improved speech perception abilities leading to better overall language outcomes (Pollack, Goldberg, & Caleffe-Schenck, 1997). By linking this evidence together, AV practitioners claimed that early identification led to higher language performance scores. AV practitioners along with many other medical and rehabilitation professionals have used mechanism-based reasoning to defend their methodology for many years.

Demographic information from the 27 articles retained for inclusion in this review along with their evidence-level ranking from the OCEBM 2011 is provided in Table 3–3 (pp. 52–67). This information was synthesized based on a thorough analysis of the methodology and outcomes of each of the included articles. The authors ranked one study as representing Level 1 evidence related to AVT; no studies were ranked as contributing Level 2 evidence; eight studies were found to represent Level 3 evidence; and nine studies were classified as Level 4 studies. No studies representing Level 5 evidence were located for inclusion in the review; however, there were nine articles that were categorized as non-AVT treatment studies that were considered to be of interest to this review and have therefore been included in a separate section.

In light of the considerations around EIP previously discussed, the OCEBM 2011 Levels of Evidence were used in organizing and synthesizing the most recent AV research rather than as a strict evaluative tool for classifying the quality of the existing research in AVT. As discussed above, lower levels of evidence may still provide important support in favor of an intervention approach as long as the quality of the research receives appropriate critical appraisal and any areas of potential bias are clearly identified. The importance of evaluating not only the level of evidence a study provides but also the quality of this evidence is discussed in further detail below.

Level 1 Evidence

One systematic review that examined the effectiveness of AVT following the guidelines set out by the Cochrane Collaboration was identified as part of the chapter update. The Cochrane Collaboration is a nonprofit organization dedicated to conducting and transmitting the results of systematic reviews, compiling medical research evidence in many domains to aid health workers in their clinical decision making. In this systematic review, Brennan-Jones, White, Rush, and Law (2014) searched 18 databases and reviewed reference lists in other AVT articles using a comprehensive set of search terms. The investigation yielded 2,233 titles. The authors screened all of the titles and abstracts and found only 13 that were potentially relevant to their systematic review. These articles were then reviewed for inclusion based on the following criteria: (a) the study had to consist of a RCT, (b) the children with bilateral moderate to profound hearing loss had to be enrolled in AVT that was provided by a LSLS Cert. AVT, and (c) language level or rate of language growth had to be the primary outcome measure. As none of the 13 identified studies were RCTs, they were all excluded, resulting in an empty review (Brennan-Jones et al., 2014).

Due to the lack of well-controlled, randomized, and blinded studies reviewed as part of their systematic review, the authors were unable to draw any conclusions about the potential effects of AVT intervention. This rejection of all of the articles from the systematic review highlights the risk of bias within the current body of AV literature. Without randomization, studies may fall victim to selection bias. For example, an investigator may ask a family to participate because they are familiar with the child's language abilities and believe the child's results will impact outcomes in a particular direction. Brennan-Jones and his team also noted that the reviewed studies did not use blinded assessors. Consciously or unconsciously, a professional administering an assessment who is familiar with the child's therapy history could influence outcomes. Finally, using a comparison group of typically developing children, rather than children with hearing loss, could also skew results toward a possible positive outcome (Brennan-Jones et al., 2014).

In a follow-up article, White and Brennan-Jones (2014) reiterated the importance of research generally and RCTs specifically within communication interventions for families of children with hearing loss. They stated that AVT was well suited for higher levels of investigation in part because of the clarity with which AVT is defined (see Principles of AVT in Chapter 1). White and Brennan-Jones (2014) propose a large-scale multicenter RCT investigation of AVT as the next step toward proving AV efficacy. However, many factors make it difficult to execute an RCT in AV practice. First and most importantly, since AV practice is dependent on parental choice and involvement, assigning a family to a treatment method rather than allowing them to make their own informed decisions concerning their child's intervention goes against the basic principles of AVT. Furthermore, it would be near to impossible to blind a family or a practitioner to the type of treatment they were receiving or providing. Parent involvement is key to AVT, thus it would be equally difficult to disguise most caregiver-focused AV strategies (see Chapter 11). Additionally, AV researchers have not yet come to any consensus about which outcomes to measure and how to best accomplish this. Deciding whether speech, language, or socioemotional factors or some combination of these are the best measure of AV outcomes and those assessment tools that might best represent such outcomes is also a point of continuing debate. In addition, an individual child's access to acoustic information is a critical yet unique variable in examining child outcomes in AVT, making subject matching particularly difficult. Confounds regarding consistency in the type of hearing device(s) and the use of unilateral versus bilateral hearing aids or cochlear implants further complicate questions regarding how best to match children when examining AVT outcomes. Finally, and perhaps most importantly, randomly assigning children to a treatment or a nontreatment control group could potentially delay or limit access to intervention for children in the control group, which might have a significant disruptive effect on their listening and spoken language development (Stewart-Brown et al., 2011).

Level 2 Evidence

No published articles representing this level of evidence were identified in the review. The reasons for this are analogous to the arguments presented above regarding the difficulties associated with random assignment of children to AVT and non-AVT treatment groups. Furthermore, as none of the retrieved studies reported effect size, no observational research could be included at this evidence level.

Level 3 Evidence

Eight studies located through the review were ranked as providing Level 3 evidence in favor of AVT. These studies

are presented in Table 3–4 (pp. 68–73). All of the studies were ranked as representing non-randomized control studies as defined above. Sample size ranged from 12 to 60 participants, with some studies attempting to match the control and the experimental groups, in some cases retrospectively. In most cases, the control groups consisted of children with typical hearing. The majority of studies involved the administration of various standardized measures of articulation and language to both groups of children, comparing their performance using statistical analyses that ranged from descriptive statistics to mixed model analyses. Some of the studies were based on retrospective data obtained from the children's case files, while others were longitudinal in nature. In most studies, a convenience sample of children enrolled in AVT at a specific treatment center providing AVT intervention formed the experimental group; only a few of the identified studies recruited children enrolled in AVT from diverse treatment centers. A complete list of the test measures (in alphabetical order according to test acronym) and their authors is provided in Appendix 3–A.

Level 4 Evidence

Of the research evaluated in this review, nine articles were ranked as representing Level 4 evidence in favor of AVT. These articles are summarized in Table 3–5 (pp. 74–79). Samples size ranged from 1 to 47, with several of the studies representing small case studies of individual children. None of the studies had a control group and most consisted of convenience samples of children enrolled in AVT at various treatment centers. In many of the studies, children were administered standardized tests and their performance was compared to the test norms using chronological and/or hearing age. Some studies had no statistical analyses, and others reported *t*-tests, ANOVAs, and correlational findings. A number of the studies were retrospective in nature.

Level 5 Evidence

No studies at this evidence level were identified in this review. Historically, however, AV practitioners have frequently used this form of evidence to support their practice. Such studies should continue to be cited as contributing to the research evidence in favor of AVT outcomes.

Non-AVT Outcome Research

Nine articles that utilized children enrolled in AVT as an inclusion criterion to examine outcomes not directly related to AVT were identified in this review. These articles are summarized in Table 3–6 (pp. 80–85), as the findings are of considerable interest to the field, although they do not specifically constitute AVT outcome research. The included studies examined variables such as age of diagnosis and age of cochlear implantation, speech perception and coarticulation abilities, gender differences, the impact of educational placement on speech and language outcomes, and the impact of concomitant disorders in addition to hearing loss on various domains of communication outcome. Some of the studies represented

relatively high levels of evidence, including one multiple baseline across subjects research design with each participant serving as his or her own control, although there was no randomization to control or treatment groups in that study. In other cases, random assignment to treatment groups was possible as the focus of the studies was not AVT *per se*. Statistical analyses varied, ranging from descriptive to linear regressions and mixed model analyses.

EVALUATING RESEARCH QUALITY

Rankings of research evidence levels as described above provide important information to evaluate the scientific rigor of research findings, but a number of other important variables should also be taken into account when determining the quality of research contributing to the understanding of treatment efficacy. Although two studies may be ranked as representing the same evidence level, their overall quality may nevertheless differ considerably. Gradations in the overall quality of the evidence provided by the studies ranked at Levels 3 and 4 of the hierarchy can be determined by asking ourselves a series of questions related to the finer points of the methodological approaches and analyses used in a particular study. Such questions provide important information to practitioners when making evidence informed practice decisions. These questions consist of the following:

■ Is the study design prospective or retrospective? Prospective designs are generally considered higher in quality than retrospective designs, as retrospective designs often rely on information obtained through file reviews as opposed to the direct administration of a selected outcome measure to a participant group.

- Are participants randomly assigned to treatment groups? Although this variable is an essential one in deciding the level of evidence attributable to any study, it is also a quality indicator, as random assignment is a central component in avoiding bias. As has been discussed previously, however, randomly assigning participants to interventions such as AVT is not feasible.

- Were participants, practitioners, and those professionals administering the outcome measures blinded to which children were contained in the treatment versus the experimental group? Unblinded studies have a much larger chance of introducing bias both into the treatment itself as well as into the analysis of results.

- Do the participants represent a convenience sample or were they specifically recruited for the study? A recruited sample is generally considered to contain less bias than a convenience sample.

- If the study involves a comparison group, were the participants matched on relevant variables? Matched group designs are considered to contain less bias than unmatched group designs.

- If the study involves a comparison group, were both groups treated equally as part of the study design with respect to all study elements other than the treatment itself? Studies that provide equivalent exposure to all participants and that document differences in performance post-treatment provide higher-quality evidence in support of the intervention under review.

- What is the sample size used in the research? Studies involving larger numbers of participants are generally viewed as being less biased and more generalizable than studies with a small numbers of participants.

- How complete is the demographic information provided about the participant groups? Does this information contribute to understanding any group differences in the results reported in the study? Providing adequate demographic information about participant groups can be essential to explaining differences in group performance following treatment in many cases.

- What outcome measures were used in documenting treatment outcomes? Measures with well-known reliability and validity provide higher-quality evidence than nonstandardized assessment instruments.

- What types of outcome scores are reported? Are they standard scores obtained through the administration of a test measure, or are they observations or parent reports? Outcomes reported as standard scores on a test measure are considered to be more reliable indicators of outcome than informal test measures and are also more readily analyzed using higher-level statistical analyses.

▪ What level of statistical analysis was performed on the outcome data? Is effect size reported, and, if so, what is the magnitude of the effect size? Higher-level statistical analyses that show significant differences in performance between the sample participants or achieve high effect sizes are considered to be of substantially higher quality than descriptive observations of performance.

▪ Was the treatment provided for a long enough period of time to illustrate a difference between treatment groups? The potential benefits of a particular treatment may be masked if the intervention period is too short for any effect to be demonstrated.

▪ Were any of the participants lost to follow-up or did any participants drop out of the study as it was being conducted? Is the participant dropout rate reported and discussed? Studies with many participants lost over the course of the study raise questions about possible underlying reasons why participants might chose to leave a particular study.

Areas for Improvement in Conducting and Reporting AVT Outcome Research

Since the original publication of this chapter (Eriks-Brophy, 2006), an impressive amount of new research has been carried out examining the outcomes of AVT for children with hearing loss in a variety of domains including auditory, speech, language, and social-emotional development. The existing research base has become increasingly international and has examined outcomes for children who speak languages other than English and/or who are being raised to be bilingual. The evidence levels as well as the overall quality of the existing research have increased, indicative of important advances in the scientific rigor represented by current studies examining the outcomes of AVT. Clearly the call to action put forward in the previous version of this chapter as well as in the article in *The Volta Review* (Eriks-Brophy, 2005) has had an important influence on the formulation of recent research questions and their associated methodologies.

Nevertheless, certain obstacles to conducting research into the outcomes of AVT remain. First, as discussed previously, conducting research that would demonstrate a clear cause-effect relationship between AVT and children's communication outcomes through RCTs remains problematic primarily due to issues associated with random group assignment to AVT and non-AVT interventions, as this circumvents some of the basic principles of AV practice. Fortunately the OCEMB 2011 now considers observational studies with large effect sizes as providing equally convincing evidence, offering AVT researchers alternative design options for generating high-level evidence. Nevertheless, systematic reviews and the RCT research they encompass are extremely important to evidence-based practice in AVT and are a gold standard toward which we should continue to strive. Through the lens of an EIP approach, however, we can use our critical appraisal skills to evaluate all the research we have access to, including the lower levels of evidence that the Cochrane systematic review was forced to disregard. This information can be used to inform our clinical treatment decisions and our conclusions regarding intervention outcomes, as well as to develop research questions appropriate for higher levels of evidence.

Second, the existing evidence base is difficult to integrate and summarize due to variations in the quality of evidence provided by the current studies. This point is well illustrated through the inconclusive results obtained by the systematic review on AVT conducted by Brennan-Jones et al. (2014) described previously. Third, some of the methodologies utilized in the studies reviewed do not permit sophisticated statistical analyses, which limits their potential contribution as supporting evidence for AVT outcomes. For example, none of the studies reviewed provided effect sizes for their results, a common current practice in reporting research findings, while only two studies had research designs that would allow for magnitude of effect size to be calculated. Fourth, the demographic information provided in the various studies differs widely, making comparisons across research studies difficult to carry out. This is illustrated in Table 3–3. It would be useful for researchers in AVT to come to a consensus on the demographic information to be reported for all participants in order to eventually be able to carry out systematic reviews leading to conclusive results. Consistency in reporting information including age at diagnosis, age at amplification/implantation, hearing age, length and amount of time using hearing technology, amount of time spent in AVT, language(s) used in the home, and socioeconomic status would permit greater generalization of findings across comparable groups. Socioeconomic status in particular has been identified as a potentially key variable influencing communication outcomes for children with and without communication disorders, and reporting this information in a consistent manner across studies would permit its impact to be examined more carefully. There continue to be a large number of studies that use convenience samples and do not include a control group, an important limitation to the existing evidence base. Furthermore, in those studies where a comparison group was included, participants were generally poorly matched. Very few studies compared outcomes for different groups of children with hearing loss, thus preventing a rigorous analysis of treatment effect.

Although this chapter has argued that all levels of evidence are informative and acceptable in the context of EIP, including mechanism-based reasoning, it is nevertheless incumbent on researchers in AVT to conduct research of the highest possible quality. Advances in the evidence levels as well as the quality of the current research base supporting AVT outcomes illustrates that researchers are indeed taking up this challenge. Taking an EIP approach to the generation and interpretation of research studies examining the outcomes of AVT has great potential to improve clinical practices and decision making, resulting in enhanced outcomes for the children we serve and providing increased authority and credibility to the field of AVT as a whole.

Table 3-3. Demographic Information From Reviewed Articles

Level 3			
Authors	**Age Range**	**Gender**	**SES**
Dettman, S., Wall, E., Constantinescu, G., & Dowell, R. (2013). Communication outcomes for groups of children using cochlear implants enrolled in auditory-verbal, aural-oral, and bilingual-bicultural early intervention programs. *Otology and Neurotology, 34,* 451–459.	AV: 6.2 years AO: 4.9 years BB: 4.9 years	All male	Not reported
Dornan, D., Hickson, L., Murdoch, B., Houston, T., & Constantinescu, G. (2010). Is auditory-verbal therapy effective for children with hearing loss? *The Volta Review, 110*(3), 361–387.	AV: 96.26 months (SD = 15.32) TD: 87.84 months (SD = 16.68)	14 male 5 female in each group	HL: Professional: 14% Manager: 43% Trade: 29% TD: Professional: 65% Manager: 15% Trade: 5% Both groups had 18 parents with higher education
Dornan, D., Hickson, L, Murdoch, B., & Houston, T. (2009). Longitudinal study of speech perception, speech, and language for children with hearing loss in an auditory-verbal therapy program. *The Volta Review, 109*(2–3), 61–85.	AV: 68.4 months TD: 57.42 months	18 male 7 female in each group	High SES

Level 3				
Age at Dx	**Technology**	**Length of Time With Technology**	**Length of Time With AVT**	**Language**
Not reported	HAs followed by CIs	AV: 4.2 years AO: 3.3 years BB: 3.1 years	Not reported	Australian English and AUSLAN
22.29 months (SD = 11.82)	6 bilateral CI 1 unilateral CI 6 HA and CI 1 unilateral HA 5 bilateral HA	Not reported	70 months (SD = 16.34)	Australian English
24.6 months	2 CI only 12 HA and CI 1 unilateral HA 10 bilateral HA	Not reported	41 months (SD = 16.34)	Australian English

continues

Table 3–3. *continued*

Level 3			
Authors	**Age Range**	**Gender**	**SES**
Dornan, D., Hickson, L., Murdoch, B., & Houston, T. (2007). Outcomes of an auditory-verbal program for children with hearing loss: A comparative study with a matched group of children with normal hearing. *The Volta Review, 107*(1), 37–54.	AV: 3.79 years (SD = 1.25) TD: 2.97 years (SD = 13 months)	21 male 8 female in each group	High SES
Eriks-Brophy, A., Gibson, S., & Tucker. S. (2013). Articulatory error patterns and phonological process use of preschool children with and without hearing loss. *The Volta Review, 113*(2), 87–125.	HL: 52.3 months TD: 52.1 months	Not reported	Not reported but: HL: 17.8 years of education (SD = 2.3) TD: 18.11 years of education (SD = 2.5)
Hogan, S., Stokes, J., & Weller, I. (2010). Language outcomes for children of low-income families enrolled in auditory verbal therapy. *Deafness and Education International, 12*(4), 204–216.	28.33 months at entry (range: 5–42 months)	Not reported	Low income (less than 30,000 British pounds/ year)
Robertson, L., Dow, G., & Hainzinger, S. (2006). Story retelling patterns among children with and without hearing loss: Effects of repeated practice and parent-child attunement. *The Volta Review, 106*(2), 147–170.	HL: 4;9 months (range: 3–6 months) TD: 4;7 months (range: 3–5 months)	AV: 6 male 4 female TD: 6 male 5 female	Not reported

Level 3				
Age at Dx	**Technology**	**Length of Time With Technology**	**Length of Time With AVT**	**Language**
24.6 months	14 CI 15 HA (2 children with HAs received CIs during the study)	Not reported	20 months	Australian English
14 months (SD = 8.6)	15 unilateral CI 10 bilateral HA	30.1 months (SD = 13.9)	34.8 months (SD = 8.5)	Canadian English 25% of the participants spoke a second language
2.75 months (range 1–9 months)	4 bilateral CI 2 unilateral CI 1 HA followed by CI 6 HA	Not reported	At least 12 months	Not reported
Not reported	3 CI 7 HA	1.6–4.8 years	Not reported	Not reported

continues

Table 3–3. *continued*

Level 3			
Authors	**Age Range**	**Gender**	**SES**
Yanbay, E., Hickson, L., Scarinci, N., Constantinescu, G., & Dettman, S. (2014). Language outcomes for children with cochlear implants enrolled in different communication programs. *Cochlear Implants International,* *15*(3), 121–135.	AV: 3.64 years (SD = 1.16) AO: 4.6 years (SD = 1.47) SS: 4.31 (SD = 1.68)	AV: 8 male 10 female AO: 7 male 7 female SS: 4 male 6 female	AV: 8 low to mid 6 high AO: 8 low to mid 10 high SS: 7 low to mid 3 high

Level 4			
Authors	**Age Range**	**Gender**	**SES**
Eriks-Brophy, A., Durieux-Smith, A., Olds, J., Fitzpatrick, E., Duquette, C., & Whittingham, J. (2012). Communication, academic, and social skills of young adults with hearing loss. *The Volta Review, 112*(1), 5–35.	18.6 years (range: 14–30 years)	Not reported	Not reported but 73.9% of mothers had postsecondary educations
Fairgray, E., Purdy, S., & Smart, J. (2010). Effects of auditory-verbal therapy for school-aged children with hearing loss: An exploratory study. *The Volta Review, 110*(3), 407–433.	9.8 years (range: 5.5–17.7 years)	2 male 5 female	Not reported

Level 3				
Age at Dx	**Technology**	**Length of Time With Technology**	**Length of Time With AVT**	**Language**
AV: 0.34 years (SD = 0.44) AO: 0.42 years (SD = 0.38) SS: 0.68 years (SD = 0.67)	All CI	PPVT: AV: 3.66 years (SD = 0.95) AO: 3.70 years (SD = 1.13) SS: 3.14 years (SD = 1.08) PLS-4 AV: 2.59 years (SD = 0.97) AO: 3.55 years (SD = 1.34) SS: 2.72 years (SD = 1.59)	PPVT: 4.05 years (SD = 1.18) PLS-4 2.92 years (SD = 1.01)	Australian English
Level 4				
Age at DX	**Technology**	**Length of Time With Technology**	**Length of Time With AVT**	**Language**
Not reported	All HA	Not reported	25 months (SD = 6.9)	Canadian English
1.9 years (range: 11 months to 2.5 years)	2 bilateral CI 3 unilateral CI 2 bilateral HA	Not reported	Not reported	Not reported

continues

Table 3–3. *continued*

Level 4			
Authors	**Age Range**	**Gender**	**SES**
Harris, L. (2014). Social-emotional development in children with hearing loss. (Unpublished masters thesis). University of Kentucky: Lexington.	3–6.6 years	Children: 3 male 2 female Caregivers: 1 male 4 female	Not reported but caregiver education level: 1 high school diploma 3 bachelor's degree 1 master's degree
Hogan, S., Stokes, J., White, C., Tyszkiewicz, E., & Woolgar, A. (2008). An evaluation of auditory verbal therapy using the rate of early language development as an outcome measure. *Deafness and Education International, 10*(3), 143–167.	23 months at entry (range 5–56 months)	Not reported	Not reported
Sahli, A., & Belgin, E. (2011). Researching auditory perception performance of children using cochlear implants and being trained by an auditory-verbal therapy. *The Journal of International Advanced Otology, 7*(3), 385–390.	44 months (SD = 5.2)	9 male 6 female	Not reported

Level 4				
Age at Dx	Technology	Length of Time With Technology	Length of Time With AVT	Language
9.6 months (range: birth–24)	2 bilateral CI 2 bilateral HA 1 unilateral HA	Not reported	Not reported	Not reported
12 months (range: 1–47 months)	5 bilateral CI 18 unilateral CI 14 bilateral HA	Not reported	89% of participants received less than 3 years of AVT 62% of participants received less than 2 years of AVT (range: 13–60 months)	Not reported
14 months (SD = 5.4)	All CI	18 months (SD = 4.8)	15 months (SD = 3.7)	Not reported

continues

Table 3–3. *continued*

Level 4			
Authors	**Age Range**	**Gender**	**SES**
Von Muenster, K., & Baker, E. (2014). Oral communicating children using a cochlear implant: Good reading outcomes are linked to better language and phonological processing abilities. *International Journal of Pediatric Otorhinolaryngology*, *78*(3), 433–444.	At reading and phonological processing testing: 8.75 years (SD = 2.05) At speech perception, speech and language testing: 8.74 years (SD = 2.15)	23 male 24 female	Not reported
Warner-Czyz, A., Davis, B., & Morrison, H. (2005). Production accuracy in a young cochlear implant recipient. *The Volta Review*, *105*(1), 5–25.	One participant from 13–32 months	1 female	Not reported
Wong, S., Scarinci, N., Hickson, L., Rose, T., & Constantinescu, G. (2013). Bilateral cochlear implants in children: A preliminary study of language and speech perception outcomes. *The Australian and New Zealand Journal of Audiology*, *33*(1), 48–68.	9.9 years (SD = 3.8)	11 males 11 females	Not reported
Wood, Jackson, C., & Schatschneider, C. (2014). Rate of language growth in children with hearing loss in an auditory-verbal early intervention program. *American Annuals of the Deaf*, *158*(5), 539–554.	3 months– 6.5 years	12 male 12 female	Not reported

Level 4				
Age at Dx	Technology	Length of Time With Technology	Length of Time With AVT	Language
Not reported	All CI	5.37 years (SD = 1.93)	At least 6 to 12 months	Australian English
12 months of age	HA followed by CI	12 months with HA 8 months with CI	19 months	American English
At birth	All sequential bilateral CI	7.9 years from first CI (range: 2;2 to 14;2)	Not reported	Australian English
10.75 months (range birth–36 months)	11 CI 13 HA	Not reported	Not reported	American English

continues

Table 3-3. *continued*

NON-AVT			
Authors	**Age Range**	**Gender**	**SES**
Allegro, J., Papsin, B., Harrison, R., & Campisi, P. (2010). Acoustic analysis of voice in cochlear implant recipients with post-meningitic hearing loss. *Cochlear Implants International, 11*(2), 100–116.	7.2 years (range; 2.1–11.1 years)	3 male 7 female	Not reported
Bakhshaee, M., Ghasemi, M., Shakeri, M., Razmara, N., Tayarani, H., & Tale, M. (2007). Speech development in children after cochlear implantation. *Ear Archives of Otorhino-laryngology, 264,* 1263–1266.	Not reported	Not reported	Not reported
Easterbrooks, S., & O'Rourke, C. (2001). Gender differences in response to auditory-verbal intervention in children who are deaf or hard of hearing. *American Annals of the Deaf, 146*(4), 309–319.	Not reported	28 male 42 female	Affluent, highly educated mothers

NON-AVT				
Age at Dx	Technology	Length of Time With Technology	Length of Time With AVT	Language
18 months (range: 4 days to 5 years)	All unilateral CI	58 months (range: 21 to 95 months)	Not reported	Not reported
2.05 years (SD = 6.17)	All CI	5 years	Not reported	Not reported
Not reported	Not reported	Not reported	Males: 39 months (SD = 25.1) Females: 51.6 months (SD = 26.6)	Not reported

continues

Table 3–3. *continued*

NON-AVT			
Authors	**Age Range**	**Gender**	**SES**
Fulcher, A., Purcell, A., Baker, E., & Munro, N. (2012). Listen up: Children with early identified hearing loss achieve age-appropriate speech/language outcomes by 3 years-of-age. *International Journal of Pediatric Otorhinolaryngology, 76*, 1785–1794.	Assessed at 3, 4, and 5 years old	Early ID'd: 29 male; 16 female Late ID'd: 27 male 22 female	Early ID'd: 9 lower 32 middle 4 upper middle Late ID'd: 16 lower 32 middle 1 upper middle
Lew, J., Purcell, A., Doble, M., & Lim, L. (2014). Hear here: Children with hearing loss learn words by listening. *International Journal of Pediatric Otorhinolaryngology, 78*, 1716–1725.	2 years, 8 months (range: 2.6–3.1)	Not reported	Not reported
Moog, J. & Geers, A. (2010). Early educational placement and later language outcomes for children with cochlear implants. *Otology & Neurotology, 31*, 1315–1319.	5 years, 10 months (SD = 6 months)	Not reported	Not reported but the mean highest educational level completed by either parent was close to completion of a 4-year college program.

NON-AVT				
Age at Dx	Technology	Length of Time With Technology	Length of Time With AVT	Language
Early ID'd: Severe/ profound: 8.4 weeks (SD = 8.7) Mild/ moderate: 7.2 weeks (SD = 5.3) Late ID'd: Severe/ profound: 92.1 weeks (SD = 25.6) Mild/ moderate: 114.4 weeks (SD = 45.8)	Not reported	Not reported	Not reported	Not reported
Not reported	1 bilateral CI 2 bilateral HA	Not reported	Not reported	English but may have had some exposure to other languages
2 months (SD = 5)	All CI	3 years, 7 months (SD = 10 months)	Not reported	Not reported

continues

Table 3–3. *continued*

NON-AVT			
Authors	**Age Range**	**Gender**	**SES**
Morrison, H. (2011). Coariculation in early vocalizations by children with hearing loss: A locus perspective. *Clinical Linguistics & Phonetics, 26*(3), 288–309.	11–50 months longitudinally	2 male 1 female	Middle Class families with all adults having a university degree
Pundir, M., Nagarkar, A., & Panda, N. (2007). Intervention strategies in children with cochlear implants having attention deficit hyperactivity disorder. *International Journal of Pediatric Otorhinolaryngology, 71,* 985–988.	6 years. and 7 years	1 male 1 female	Not reported
Wolfe, J., Baker, S., Caraway, T., Kasulis, H., Mears, A., Smith, J., Swim, L., & Wood, M. (2007). 1-year postactivation results for sequentially implanted bilateral cochlear implant users. *Otology and Neurotology, 28*(5), 589–596.	Not reported	Not reported	Not reported

NON-AVT				
Age at Dx	Technology	Length of Time With Technology	Length of Time With AVT	Language
1.33 months (range: 1–2 months)	2 CI 1 HA	7–32 months longitudinally (corrected for cochlear implantation)	Not reported	American English
1.5 years	Both CI	Male: 4.5 years with HA 9 months with CI Female: 5 years with HA 9 months with CI	9 months	Not reported
Not reported	All bilateral CI	Not reported	Not reported	Not reported

Table 3–4. Quality of Evidence for Studies Ranked as Level 3 Evidence

Authors	N	Comparison Groups	Matching	Sample Pool
Dettman, S., Wall, E., Constantinescu, G., & Dowell, R. (2013). Communication outcomes for groups of children using cochlear implants enrolled in auditory-verbal, aural-oral, and bilingual-bicultural early intervention programs. *Otology and Neurotology, 34*, 451–459.	AV: 8 AO: 23 BB: 8	AV, AO, and BB Retrospective data	Retrospective matching Age at implant Age at hearing aid fitting test age device experience at the time of Ax	Multisite
Dornan, D., Hickson, L., Murdoch, B., Houston, T., & Constantinescu, G. (2010). Is auditory-verbal therapy effective for children with hearing loss? *The Volta Review, 110*(3), 361–387.	19 in each group	AV and TD	Total language age Receptive vocab Gender SES	1 site
Dornan, D., Hickson, L, Murdoch, B., & Houston, T. (2009). Longitudinal study of speech perception, speech, and language for children with hearing loss in an auditory-verbal therapy program. *The Volta Review, 109*(2–3), 61–85.	25 in each group	AV and TD	Total language age Receptive vocab Gender SES	1 site

Study Design	Tests	Stats	Findings
Prospective	PPVT, CNC, and BKB wordlists	ANOVA, correlations, and descriptive statistics	Three years post cochlear implantation, children in AVT and auditory-oral intervention programs outperformed children in bilingual-bicultural programs on speech perception and receptive vocabulary assessments.
Prospective	PLS-4, CELF-3, PPVT-3, GFTA-2, Reading Progress Test (RPT), I Can Do Maths, Progressive Achievement Tests in Mathematics, and Insight (self-esteem test: parent report)	Wilcoxon signed rank test, Mann Whitney Test, and descriptive statistics	Children in AVT for 50 months had speech, language and self-esteem levels similar to their typically developing peers and comparable reading and math scores.
Prospective	PLOTT Manchester junior words, PBK, CNC, BKB word list, PLS-4, CELF-3, PPVT-3, GFTA2, and CASALA	Wilcoxon signed rank test, t-test, ANOVA, descriptive statistics	Over 21 months, children in AVT improved their live-voice speech perception, language and speech scores significantly and similarly to typically developing peers. While both groups were in the normal range for receptive vocabulary development, the typically developing group did outperform the children in AVT.

continues

Table 3-4. *continued*

Authors	N	Comparison Groups	Matching	Sample Pool
Dornan, D., Hickson, L., Murdoch, B., & Houston, T. (2007). Outcomes of an auditory-verbal program for children with hearing loss: A comparative study with a matched group of children with normal hearing. *The Volta Review, 107*(1), 37–54.	29 in both groups	AV and TD	Total language age Receptive vocab Gender SES	1 site
Eriks-Brophy, A., Gibson, S., & Tucker. S. (2013). Articulatory error patterns and phonological process use of preschool children with and without hearing loss. *The Volta Review, 113*(2), 87–125.	AV: 25 TD: 35	AV and TD	Age, Family structure, Home language, Parental education	Multisite
Hogan, S., Stokes, J., & Weller, I. (2010). Language outcomes for children of low-income families enrolled in auditory verbal therapy. *Deafness and Education International, 12*(4), 204–216.	Low SES AV: 12 AV: 37 (collected in Hogan et al., 2008)	Low SES in AV and the subjects in Hogan et al., 2008	No matching	Multisite
Robertson, L., Dow, G., & Hainzinger, S. (2006). Story retelling patterns among children with and without hearing loss: Effects of repeated practice and parent-child attunement. *The Volta Review, 106*(2), 147–170.	AV: 10 TD: 11	AV and TD	No matching	1 site

Study Design	Tests	Stats	Findings
Prospective	PPVT-3, PLS-4 or CELF-3, and GFTA-2	*t*-test, mixed model analysis, and descriptive statistics	Children enrolled in AVT performed similarly to typically developing peers on speech and language assessments.
Prospective	GFTA-2 and KLPA-2	*t*-test, descriptive statistics, and correlation	Typically developing children outperformed children in AVT on articulation and phonologic processing assessments. However, the children in AVT did have phonologic processing systems that resembled their peers' and most demonstrated at least 12 months progress in 12 months' time.
Prospective	RLD (rate of language delivery) calculated using PLS-4 (UK) scores Ax done every 6 months	Mann, Whitney, *t*-test, and descriptive statistics	SES did not play a role in spoken language outcomes for children in AVT.
Prospective	PPVT-3 , transcripts coded for memory tasks	Descriptive statistics, *t*-test, ANCOVA	Children with hearing loss benefited from shared reading activities and memory for the text was improved when the parents were more directed to the child's listening needs.

continues

Table 3–4. *continued*

Authors	N	Comparison Groups	Matching	Sample Pool
Yanbay, E., Hickson, L., Scarinci, N., Constantinescu, G., & Dettman, S. (2014). Language outcomes for children with cochlear implants enrolled in different communication programs. *Cochlear Implants International*, *15*(3), 121–135.	AV: 18 AO: 14 SS: 10	AV, AO, SS Retrospective data	No matching	1 site

Study Design	Tests	Stats	Findings
Retrospective	PPVT, PLS4, FPRS (family participation rating scale)	ANCOVA, *t*-test, Pearson correlation	Regardless of communication option, children with hearing loss who were diagnosed early and had parents who are highly involved produced higher language scores than those who did not.

Table 3–5. Quality of Evidence for Studies Ranked as Level 4 Evidence

Authors	N	Comparison Groups	Matching	Sample Pool
Eriks-Brophy, A., Durieux-Smith, A., Olds, J., Fitzpatrick, E., Duquette, C., & Whittingham, J. (2012). Communication, academic, and social skills of young adults with hearing loss. *The Volta Review*, *112*(1), 5–35.	43 24 of those in phase 2	N/A	N/A	1 site
Fairgray, E., Purdy, S., & Smart, J. (2010). Effects of auditory-verbal therapy for school-aged children with hearing loss: An exploratory study. *The Volta Review*, *110*(3), 407–433.	7	N/A	N/A	Multisite
Harris, L. (2014). Social-emotional development in children with hearing loss. (Unpublished master's thesis). University of Kentucky: Lexington.	5	N/A	N/A	1 site

Study Design	Tests	Stats	Findings
Prospective	Questionnaire based on Goldberg & Flexer 1993, PPVT-R, CID SPINE, WIAT: academic function oral language skills and academic achievement, WRAT-3, and SDQ: Self perception	t-test, ANOVA, Chi^2, and descriptive statistics	People who received AVT in childhood and were supported throughout their school years were successful in mainstream environments. They also performed comparably to their typically hearing peers on communication and self-perception assessments as well as in academic achievement.
Prospective	Australian CELF-4, HAPP-3, NZAT, WIAT- II: Word Reading, Pseudo-word Decoding, and reading comprehension, and LNT speech in noise recorded with NZ female speaker	Wilcoxon Matched Pairs, descriptive statistics	After 20 weeks of AVT, children showed improvement in speech perception, speech production, and receptive language measures. There was less improvement shown in the area of reading.
Prospective	Penn Interactive Peer Play Scale (PIPPS) (McWayne, Sekino, Hampton, & Fantuzzo, 2007), the Social Competence and Preschool Edition (SCBE) (LaFreniere & Dumas, 1995), and the Behaviour Assessment System for Children–Second Edition (BASC-2) (Kamphaus & Reynolds, 2007) PPVT-4, EVT-2 and GFTA-2 scores taken retrospectively	N/A	Using psychosocial scales of social-emotional development, only one of the five participants appeared to demonstrate problems in this area.

continues

Table 3–5 *continued*

Authors	N	Comparison Groups	Matching	Sample Pool
Hogan, S., Stokes, J., White, C., Tyszkiewicz, E., & Woolgar, A. (2008). An evaluation of auditory verbal therapy using the rate of early language development as an outcome measure. *Deafness and Education International, 10*(3), 143–167.	37	N/A	N/A	1 site
Sahli, A. & Belgin, E. (2011). Researching auditory perception performance of children using cochlear implants and being trained by an auditory-verbal therapy. *The Journal of International Advanced Otology, 7*(3), 385–390.	15	N/A	N/A	1 site
Von Muenster, K., & Baker, E. (2014). Oral communicating children using a cochlear implant: Good reading outcomes are linked to better language and phonological processing abilities. *International Journal of Pediatric Otorhinolaryngology, 78*(3), 433–444.	47	N/A	N/A	1 site

Study Design	Tests	Stats	Findings
Prospective	RLD (rate of language delivery) calculated using PLS-3 (UK) scores	Kolmogorov-Smirnov tests, *t*-test, and descriptive statistics	AVT improved rate of language development regardless of the child's age or hearing technology.
Prospective	IT MAIS/MAIS, LIP, Ling 5 sound test, MTP	Mann-Whitney U-test, and descriptive statistics	A combination of cochlear implants and AVT improved auditory perception skills in children with hearing loss.
Prospective	Sight word reading–TOWRE Sight word reading of non-words–QUIL Passage reading–Neal-3 Reading comprehension–Neal-3 Words level–CNC Sentence level–BKB PPVT 3 Receptive/expressive language–CELF 3 or CELF preschool Production of mono, di, and polysyllabic words–ACAP-A Phonological awareness, Phonological working memory, Phonological retrieval–CTOPP	Pearson Product Moment Correlation and Principal Component Analysis	Children with hearing loss who had higher language and phonologic processing skills had better reading outcomes.

continues

Table 3-5 *continued*

Authors	N	Comparison Groups	Matching	Sample Pool
Warner-Czyz, A., Davis, B., & Morrison, H. (2005). Production accuracy in a young cochlear implant recipient. *The Volta Review, 105*(1), 5–25.	1	N/A	N/A	1 site
Wong, S., Scarinci, N., Hickson, L., Rose, T., & Constantinescu, G. (2013). Bilateral cochlear implants in children: A preliminary study of language and speech perception outcomes. *The Australian and New Zealand Journal of Audiology, 33*(1), 48–68.	21	N/A	N/A	1 site
Wood, Jackson, C., & Schatschneider, C. (2014). Rate of language growth in children with hearing loss in an auditory-verbal early intervention program. *American Annuals of the Deaf, 158*(5), 539–554.	24	N/A	N/A	1 site

Study Design	Tests	Stats	Findings
Prospective	Rosetti Infant Toddler Language Scale	Descriptive statistics	A child who received a cochlear implant at 24 months showed an increase in her phonetic inventory over a 4-month period.
Prospective	Plott battery tests, CNC test, Manchester Junior Words Test, BKB Sentences, PPVT-3, PLS-4, CELF-P, CELF-3, and CELF-4	Descriptive statistics, and Wilcoxon signed-rank test	Bilateral cochlear implantation did not seem to affect spoken language or receptive vocabulary scores but some of the children did improve in the area of speech perception.
Retrospective	PLS-4 (retrospectively)	Mixed Model Analysis (hierarchal linear modeling) and descriptive statistics	Over a 6-month period, children in AVT did not demonstrate an improvement in standard language scores. However, the longer the child had been enrolled in AVT, the better they performed; indicating the impact of AVT on language development.

Table 3-6. Quality of Evidence for Studies Ranked as Non-AVT Outcomes

Author	N	Comparison Groups	Matching	Sample Pool
Allegro, J., Papsin, B., Harrison, R., & Campisi, P. (2010). Acoustic analysis of voice in cochlear implant recipients with post-meningitic hearing loss. *Cochlear Implants International, 11*(2), 100–116.	10	N/A	N/A	1 site
Bakhshaee, M., Ghasemi, M., Shakeri, M., Razmara, N., Tayarani, H., & Tale, M. (2007). Speech development in children after cochlear implantation. *Ear Archives of Otorhinolaryngology, 264,* 1263–1266.	47	N/A	N/A	1 site
Easterbrooks, S., & O'Rourke, C. (2001). Gender differences in response to auditory-verbal intervention in children who are deaf or hard of hearing. *American Annals of the Deaf, 146*(4), 309–319.	70	N/A	N/A	1 site
Fulcher, A., Purcell, A., Baker, E., & Munro, N. (2012). Listen up: Children with early identified hearing loss achieve age-appropriate speech/language outcomes by 3 years-of-age. *International Journal of Pediatric Otorhinolaryngology, 76,* 1785–1794.	Early ID'd: 45 Late ID'd: 49	Early ID'd and Late ID'd	No matching	1 site

Study Design	Tests	Stats	Findings
Prospective	Multidimensional Voice program	Descriptive statistics and trend analysis	After meningitis, children who had aided residual hearing, received a cochlear implant, attended AVT, and did not have cochlear ossification had better long-term control of vocal frequency and amplitude.
Prospective	Speech Intelligibility Rating (SIR) test	Mann-Whitney U test	Subjective speech intelligibility rankings of children post cochlear implant increased significantly for three years and did not seem to plateau after five years.
Prospective/ retrospective	Parent Interview and Leiter International Performance Scale, revised	Descriptive statistics and *t*-test	Although both boys and girls had high language scores, the girls outperformed the boys. Parents were more likely to say that their sons behave well in AVT sessions.
Prospective/ retrospective	GFTA-2, PPVT-4, PLS-4	Independent *t*-tests, Cohen's d, ANOVA, Cohen's f, & Mann-Whitney U	Children who were early diagnosed, received amplification by 3 months, AVT by 6 months, and cochlear implants by 18 months, did not demonstrate a delay of speech and language skills by age 3.

continues

Table 3-6. *continued*

Author	N	Comparison Groups	Matching	Sample Pool
Lew, J., Purcell, A., Doble, M., & Lim, L. (2014). Hear here: Children with hearing loss learn words by listening. *International Journal of Pediatric Otorhinolaryngology*, 78, 1716–1725.	3	N/A	N/A	1 site
Moog, J., & Geers, A. (2010). Early educational placement and later language outcomes for children with cochlear implants. *Otology and Neurotology*, 31, 1315–1319.	141	N/A	N/A	Multisite
Morrison, H. (2011). Coariculation in early vocalizations by children with hearing loss: A locus perspective. *Clinical Linguistics and Phonetics*, 26(3), 288–309.	3	N/A	N/A	1 site
Pundir, M., Nagarkar, A., & Panda, N. (2007). Intervention strategies in children with cochlear implants having attention deficit hyperactivity disorder. *International Journal of Pediatric Otorhinolaryngology*, 71, 985–988.	2	N/A	N/A	1 site

Study Design	Tests	Stats	Findings
Prospective	ESP, SPEAK-probes, PPVT-4, 2500+ Words List, GFTA-2, & CASALA Analysis	*t*-test and descriptive statistics	Intervention directed at listening alone improves vocabulary and speech skills without having to focus on them as specific goals.
Prospective	PPVT, EOWPVT, and CELF-P, Wechsler preschool and primary scale of intelligence	Descriptive, ANOVA	Children with hearing loss benefit from cochlear implantation by age 1 and parent-focused spoken language intervention supplemented by an LSLS classroom by age 2.
Prospective	Rosetti, MCDI, acoustic analysis of speech segments based on production characteristics, Locus Equation Analyses	Descriptive statistics	Children who received hearing aids by 5 months had anticipatory coarticulation patterns similar to typically developing peers. Anticipatory coarticulation patterns were affected by whether or not the child had acquired that syllable before or after cochlear implantation.
Prospective	Integrated Scales of Language Development	None	Two children receiving AVT did not begin to show improvements in listening, speech, and language skills until their ADHD was controlled using medication.

continues

Table 3-6. *continued*

Author	N	Comparison Groups	Matching	Sample Pool
Wolfe, J., Baker, S., Caraway, T., Kasulis, H., Mears, A., Smith, J., Swim, L., & Wood, M. (2007). 1-year postactivation results for sequentially implanted bilateral cochlear implant users. *Otology and Neurotology, 28*(5), 589–596.	12	N/A	N/A	1 site

Study Design	Tests	Stats	Findings
Retrospective	MLNT (Multisyllabic Lexical Neighborhood Test) or ESP, speech recognition in noise	Linear, regression, correlation, and t-test	Sequential bilateral cochlear implantation improved children's ability to recognize speech in noise. Children who received their second cochlear implant before 4 years old did better than those who received theirs later.

REFERENCES

AG Bell Academy for Listening and Spoken Language. (2007). *Principles of LSLS*. Retrieved September 8, 2015, from http://www.listeningandspokenlanguage.org/AcademyDocument.aspx?id=563

Allegro, J., Papsin, B., Harrison, R., & Campisi, P. (2010). Acoustic analysis of voice in cochlear implant recipients with post-meningitic hearing loss. *Cochlear Implants International, 11*(2), 100–116.

Bakhshaee, M., Ghasemi, M., Shakeri, M., Razmara, N., Tayarani, H., & Tale, M. (2007). Speech development in children after cochlear implantation. *Ear Archives of Otorhinolaryngology, 264*, 1263–1266.

Bero, L. A., Grilli, R., Grimshaw, J. M., Harvey, E., Oxman, A. D., & Thomson, M. A. (1998). Closing the gap between research and practice: An overview of systematic reviews of interventions to promote the implementation of research findings. *British Medical Journal, 317*, 465–468.

Brennan-Jones, C., White, J., Rush, R., & Law, J. (2014). Auditory-verbal therapy for promoting spoken language development in children with permanent hearing impairments. *Cochrane Database of Systematic Reviews (3)*, CD010100. doi:10.1002/14651858.CD010100.pub2

Center for Evidence-Based Medicine. (2014). Glossary. Center for Evidence-Based Practice. Retrieved August 28, 2015, from http://www.cebm.net

Clarke, B., Gillies, D., Illari, P., Russo, F., & Williamson, J. (2013). The evidence that evidence-based medicine omits. *Preventive Medicine, 57*(6), 745–747.

Dettman, S., Wall, E., Constantinescu, G., & Dowell, R. (2013). Communication outcomes for groups of children using cochlear implants enrolled in auditory-verbal, aural-oral, and bilingual-bicultural early intervention programs. *Otology and Neurotology, 34*, 451–459.

Dollaghan, C. (2004). Evidence-based practice myths and realities. *ASHA Leader, 9*(7), 4–12.

Dornan, D., Hickson, L., Murdoch, B., & Houston, T. (2007). Outcomes of an auditory-verbal program for children with hearing loss: A comparative study with a matched group of children with normal hearing. *The Volta Review, 107*(1), 37–54.

Dornan, D., Hickson, L, Murdoch, B., & Houston, T. (2009). Longitudinal study of speech perception, speech, and language for children with hearing loss in an auditory-verbal therapy program. *The Volta Review, 109*(2–3), 61–85.

Dornan, D., Hickson, L., Murdoch, B., Houston, T., & Constantinescu, G. (2010). Is auditory-verbal therapy effective for children with hearing loss? *The Volta Review, 110*(3), 361–387.

Dunn, L., & Dunn, D. (2007). *Peabody Picture Vocabulary Test* (4th ed.). Circle Pines, MN: American Guidance Service.

Dunst, C., Trivette, C., & Cutspec, A. (2002). Toward an operational definition of evidence-based practices. *Centerscope, 1*(1), 1–10.

Easterbrooks, S., & O'Rourke, C. (2001). Gender differences in response to auditory-verbal intervention in children who are deaf or hard of hearing. *American Annals of the Deaf, 146*(4), 309–319.

Ellis, P. (2010). *The essential guide to effect sizes: statistical power, meta-analysis, and the interpretation of research results*. Cambridge, UK: Cambridge University Press.

Eriks-Brophy, A. (2004). Outcomes of Auditory-Verbal Therapy: A summary of the evidence and a call for action. *The Volta Review, 104*(1), 21–35.

Eriks-Brophy, A. (2006). Research in Auditory-Verbal Therapy. In W. Estabrooks (Ed.), *Auditory-Verbal Therapy* (2nd ed., pp. 273–289). Washington, DC: AG Bell.

Eriks-Brophy, A., Durieux-Smith, A., Olds, J., Fitzpatrick, E., Duquette, C., & Whittingham, J. (2012). Communication, academic, and social skills of young adults with hearing loss. *The Volta Review*, *112*(1), 5–35.

Eriks-Brophy, A., Gibson, S., & Tucker. S. (2013). Articulatory error patterns and phonological process use of preschool children with and without hearing loss. *The Volta Review*, *113*(2), 87–125.

Fairgray, E., Purdy, S., & Smart, J. (2010). Effects of auditory-verbal therapy for school-aged children with hearing loss: An exploratory study. *The Volta Review*, *110*(3), 407–433.

Fulcher, A., Purcell, A., Baker, E., & Munro, N. (2012). Listen up: Children with early identified hearing loss achieve age-appropriate speech/language outcomes by 3 years-of-age. *International Journal of Pediatric Otorhinolaryngology*, *76*, 1785–1794.

Gambrill, E. (2007). Views of evidence-based practice: Social workers' code of ethics and accreditation standards as guides for choice. *Journal of Social Work Education*, *43*(3), 447–462.

Hargrove, P. (2002). Evidence-based practice tutorial #3: Identifying the magnitude of the effect. *SIG 1 Perspectives on Language Learning and Education*, *9*(3), 34–36.

Harris, L. (2014). *Social-emotional development in children with hearing loss*. (Unpublished master's thesis). University of Kentucky, Lexington.

Higgins, J., & Green, S. (2008). *Cochrane handbook for systematic reviews of interventions*. Chichester, UK: Wiley-Blackwell.

Hogan, S., Stokes, J., & Weller, I. (2010). Language outcomes for children of low-income families enrolled in auditory verbal therapy. *Deafness and Education International*, *12*(4), 204–216.

Hogan, S., Stokes, J., White, C., Tyszkiewicz, E., & Woolgar, A. (2008). An evaluation of auditory verbal therapy using the rate of early language development as an outcome measure. *Deafness and Education International*, *10*(3), 143–167.

Howick, J. (2011). *The philosophy of evidence-based medicine*. Hoboken, NJ: Wiley-Blackwell BMJ.

Howick, J., Chalmers, I., Glasziou, P., Greenhalgh, T., Heneghan, C., Liberati, I., . . . Hodgkinson, M. (2011). *The Oxford 2011 Levels of Evidence*. Oxford Centre for Evidence-Based Medicine. Retrieved August 14, 2015, from http://www.cebm .net/index.aspx?o=5653

Howick, J., Glasziou, P., & Aronson, J. (2010). Evidence-based mechanistic reasoning. *Journal of the Royal Society of Medicine*, *103*, 433–441.

Illari, P., & Williamson, J. (2012). What is a mechanism? Thinking about mechanisms across the sciences. *European Journal of Philosophical Science*, *2*, 119–135.

Jackson, C., & Schatschneider, C. (2014). Rate of language growth in children with hearing loss in an auditory-verbal early intervention program. *American Annuals of the Deaf*, *158*(5), 539–554.

Lew, J., Purcell, A., Doble, M., & Lim, L. (2014). Hear here: Children with hearing loss learn words by listening. *International Journal of Pediatric Otorhinolaryngology*, *78*, 1716–1725.

Lomas, J. (1991). Words without action? The production, dissemination, and impact of consensus recommendations. *Annual Review of Public Health*, *12*, 41–65.

Moog, J., & Geers, A. (2010). Early educational placement and later language outcomes for children with cochlear implants. *Otology and Neurotology*, *31*, 1315–1319.

Morrison, H. (2011). Co-articulation in early vocalizations by children with hearing loss: A locus perspective. *Clinical Linguistics and Phonetics*, *26*(3), 288–309.

Nevo, I., & Slonim-Nevo, V. (2011). The myth of evidence-based practice: Towards evidence-informed practice. *British Journal of Social Work*, *41*(6), 1176–1197.

Oxford Center for Evidence-Based Medicine (OCEBM) Levels of Evidence Working Group. (2011). *The Oxford 2011 Levels of Evidence*. Oxford Centre for Evidence-Based Medicine. Retrieved September 8, 2015, from http://www.cebm.net/index.aspx?o=5653

Oxman, A., Thomson, M., Davis, D., & Haynes, R. (1995). No magic bullets: A systematic review of 102 trials of interventions to improve professional practice. *Canadian Medical Association Journal, 153*, 1423–1431.

Pollack, D., Goldberg, D., & Caleffe-Schenck, N. (1997). *Educational audiology for the limited-hearing infant and preschooler.* Springfield, IL: Charles C. Thomas.

Pundir, M., Nagarkar, A., & Panda, N. (2007). Intervention strategies in children with cochlear implants having attention deficit hyperactivity disorder. *International Journal of Pediatric Otorhinolaryngology, 71*, 985–988.

Robertson, L., Dow, G., & Hainzinger, S. (2006). Story retelling patterns among children with and without hearing loss: Effects of repeated practice and parent-child attunement. *The Volta Review, 106*(2), 147–170.

Rubin, A. (2007). Improving the teaching of evidence-based practice: Introduction to the special issue. *Research on Social Work Practice, 17*, 541–547.

Sackett, D. (1997). Evidence-based medicine. *Seminars in Perinatology, 21*(1), 3–5.

Sahil, A., & Belgin, E. (2011). Researching auditory perception performance of children using cochlear implants and being trained by an Auditory-Verbal Therapy. *Journal of International Advanced Otology, 7*(3), 385–390.

Stewart-Brown, S., Anthony, R., Wilson, L., Winstanley, S., Stallard, N., Snooks, H., & Simkiss, D. (2011). Should randomized controlled trials be the "gold standard" for research on preventive interventions for children? *Journal of Children's Services, 6*(4), 228–235.

Strauss, S., Glasziou, P., Richardson, W., & Haynes, R. (2011). *Evidence-based medicine: How to practice and teach it* (4th ed.). Toronto, Canada: Churchill Livingstone Elsevier.

Von Muenster, K., & Baker, E. (2014). Oral communicating children using a cochlear implant: Good reading outcomes are linked to better language and phonological processing abilities. *International Journal of Pediatric Otorhinolaryngology, 78*(3), 433–444.

Warner-Czyz, A., Davis, B., & Morrison, H. (2005). Production accuracy in a young cochlear implant recipient. *The Volta Review, 105*(1), 5–25.

White, J., & Brennan-Jones, C. (2014). Auditory-verbal therapy: Improving the evidence-base. *Deafness and Education International, 16*(3), 125–128.

Wolfe, J., Baker, S., Caraway, T., Kasulis, H., Mears, A., Smith, J., Swim, L., & Wood, M. (2007). 1-year postactivation results for sequentially implanted bilateral cochlear implant users. *Otology and Neurotology, 28*(5), 589–596.

Wong, S., Scarinci, N., Hickson, L., Rose, T., & Constantinescu, G. (2013). Bilateral cochlear implants in children: A preliminary study of language and speech perception outcomes. *Australian and New Zealand Journal of Audiology, 33*(1), 48–68.

Yanbay, E., Hickson, L., Scarinci, N., Constantinescu, G., & Dettman, S. (2014). Language outcomes for children with cochlear implants enrolled in different communication programs. *Cochlear Implants International, 15*(3), 121–135.

Appendix 3-A

A COMPLETE LIST OF TEST MEASURES (IN ALPHABETICAL ORDER ACCORDING TO TEST ACRONYM) AND THEIR AUTHORS

Test Acronym	Full Title	Reference
ACAP-A	Assessment of Children's Articulation and Phonology	James, D. (1995). *Assessment of children's articulation and phonology.* South Australia: Flinders University.
BASC-2	Behavioral and Emotional Screening System—Second Edition	Kamphaus, R., & Reynolds, C. (2007). *Behavioral and Emotional Screening System Manual.* Bloomington, MN: NCS Pearson.
BKB	Bamford-Kowal-Bench	Bench, J., & Bamford, J. (1979). *Speech-hearing tests and the spoken language of hearing-impaired children.* London, UK: Academic Press.
BKB/A	Bamford-Kowal-Bench/Australian	Bench, R., Doyle, J., & Greenwood, K. (1987). A standardization of the BKB/A sentence test for children in comparison with the NAL-CID sentence test and CAL-PBM word test. *Australian Journal of Audiology, 9,* 39–48.
CASALA	Computer Aided Speech and Language Analysis	Serry, A., Dorman, M., & Kral, A. (1997). Computer aided speech and language analysis. *Australian Communication Quarterly* (Spring), 27–28.
CELF-3	Clinical Evaluation of Language Fundamentals—Third Edition	Semel, E., Wiig., E., & Secord, W. (1995). *Clinical evaluation of language fundamentals—Third Edition.* San Antonio, TX: The Psychological Corporation.
CELF-4	Clinical Evaluation of Language Fundamentals—Fourth Edition	Semel, E., Wiig., E., & Secord, W. (2003). *Clinical evaluation of language fundamentals—Fourth Edition.* San Antonio, TX: The Psychological Corporation.

continues

Test Acronym	Full Title	Reference
CELF-P	Clinical Evaluation of Language Fundamentals—Preschool	Wiig, E., Secord, W., & Semel, E. (1992). *Clinical evaluation of language fundamentals—Preschool.* San Antonio, TX: The Psychological Corporation.
CNC	Consonant-nucleus-consonant word lists	Peterson, G., & Lehiste, I. (1962). Revised CNC word lists for auditory tests. JSHD, 27, 67Y70.
CTOPP	Comprehensive Test of Phonological Processing	Wagner, R., Torgesen, J., & Rashotte, C. (1999). *Comprehensive Test of Phonological Processing.* Texas: Pro-Ed.
EOWPVT	Expressive One-Word Picture Vocabulary Test	Gardner, M. (2000). *Expressive One-Word Picture Vocabulary Test.* Novato, CA: Academic Therapy.
ESP	Early Speech Perception	Moog, J., & Geers, A. (1990). *Early Speech Perception (ESP) Test.* St. Louis, MO: Central Institute for the Deaf.
EVT-2	Expressive Vocabulary Test	Williams, K. (2007). *Expressive Vocabulary Test Manual—Second Edition.* Minneapolis, MN: NCS Pearson.
FPRS	Family Participation Rating Scale	Moeller, M. (2000). Early intervention and language development in children who are deaf and hard of hearing. *Pediatrics, 106*(3), 1–9.
GFTA-2	Goldman-Fristoe Test of Articulation—Second Edition	Goldman, R., & Fristoe, M. (2001). *Goldman-Fristoe Test of Articulation—Second Edition.* Shoreview, MN: American Guidance Service.
HAPP-3	Hodson Assessment of Phonological Patterns—Third Edition	Hodson, B. (2004). *HAPP-3 Hodson Assessment of Phonological Patterns—Third Edition.* Austin, TX: Pro-Ed.
I Can Do Maths	I Can Do Maths	Doig, B., & de Lemnos, M. (2000). *I Can Do Maths.* Melbourne, Australia: ACER Press.

Test Acronym	Full Title	Reference
Insight	Insight	Morris, E. (2003). *Insight.* London, UK: NFER Nelson.
Integrated Scales of Language Development	Integrated Scales of Language Development	Cochlear Ltd. (2003). *Integrated Scales of Language Development.* Listen, Learn, & Talk. Sydney, AU: Cochlear Ltd.
IT-MAIS	Infant-Toddler Meaningful Auditory Integration Scale	Zimmerman-Phillips, S., Robbins, A., & Osberger, M. (2001). *Infant-Toddler Meaningful Auditory Integration Scale.* Sylmar, CA: Advanced Bionics Corp.
KLPA-2	Khan-Lewis Phonological Analysis —Second Edition	Kahn, L., & Lewis, N. (2002). *Khan-Lewis Phonological Analysis—Second Edition.* Circle Pines, MN: American Guidance Systems.
Ling 5	Ling 5	Ling D. (1989). *Foundations of Spoken Language for Hearing-Impaired Children.* Washington, DC: Alexander Graham Bell Association for the Deaf.
LIP	Listening Process Profile	Archbold, S. (1994). Monitoring progress in children at the preverbal stage. In McCormick B., et al. (Eds.), *Cochlear implants for young children* (pp. 197–213). London, UK: Whurr.
Leiter-R	Leiter International Performance Scale —Revised	Roid, G., & Miller, L. (1997). *Leiter-R Parent Rating Scale.* Wood Dale, IL: Stoelting.
LNT	Lexical Neighborhood Test	Kirk, K., Pisoni, D., & Osberger, M. (1995). Lexical effects on spoken word recognition by pediatric cochlear implant users. *Ear and Hearing, 16,* 470–481.
MAIS	Meaningful Auditory Integration Scale	Robbins, A., Renshaw, J., & Berry, S. (1991). Evaluating meaningful integration in profoundly hearing impaired children. *American Journal of Otolaryngology, 12*(Suppl.), 144–150.

continues

Test Acronym	Full Title	Reference
MCDI	MacArthur-Bates Communicative Inventories	Fenson, L., Dale, P., Reznick, J., Thal, D., Bates, E., Hartung, J., Pethick, S., & Reilly, J. (1993). *MacArthur Communicative Inventories: User's Guide and Technical Manual*. San Diego, CA: Singular.
MDVP	Multi-Dimensional Voice Program	Kay Elemetrics Corp. (1999). *Multi-Dimensional Voice Program Software* instruction manual.
MLNT	Multisyllabic Lexical Neighborhood Test	Kirk, K., Pisoni, D., & Osberger, M. (1995). Lexical effects on spoken word recognition by pediatric cochlear implant users. *Ear and Hearing, 16*, 470–481.
MTP	Monosyllable, Trochee and Polysyllabic Test	Erber, N., & Alencewicz, C. (1976). Audiological evaluation of deaf children. *Journal of Speech and Hearing Disorders, 41*, 256–267.
Neale-3	Neale Analysis of Reading Ability—Third Edition	Neale, M. (1999). *Neale Analysis of Reading Ability*. Melbourne, Vic: Australian Council of Educational Research Ltd.
NZAT	New Zealand Articulation Test	Moyle, J. (2005). The New Zealand Articulation Test Norms Project. *New Zealand Journal of Speech-Language Therapy, 60*, 61–75.
PAT Maths	Progressive Achievement Tests in Mathematics—Third Edition	Australian Council of Education Research. (2005). *Progressive Achievement Tests in Mathematics—Third Edition*. Melbourne, Australia: ACER Press.
PBK/ Manchester Junior Words	Phonetically Balanced Kindergarten Lists	Watson, T. (1957). Speech audiometry for children. In A.W.G. Ewing (Ed.), *Educational guidance and the deaf child* (pp. 278–296). Manchester, UK: The University Press.
PIPPS	Penn Interactive Peer Play Scale	McWayne, C., Sekino, Y., Hampton, G., & Fantuzzo, J. (2007). *Penn Interactive Peer Play Scale Manual*. Philadelphia, PA: John Fantuzzo.

Test Acronym	Full Title	Reference
Plott Test Battery	The PLOTT test	Plant, G., & Westcott, S. (1983). *The PLOTT test*. Chatswood, Australia: National Acoustic Laboratories.
PLS-3 (UK)	Preschool Language Scale—Third Edition (UK Adaptation)	Zimmerman, I., Steiner, V., Pond, R., Boucher, J., & Lewis, V. (1991). *Preschool Language Scales—Third Edition* (UK Adaptation). London, UK: The Psychological Corporation.
PLS-4	Preschool Language Scale—Fourth Edition	Zimmerman, I., Steiner, V., & Pond, R. (2002). *Preschool Language Scale—Fourth Edition*. San Antonio, TX: The Psychological Corporation.
PPVT-3	Peabody Picture Vocabulary Test—Third Edition	Dunn, L., & Dunn, D. (1997). *Peabody Picture Vocabulary Test—Third Edition*. Circle Pines, MN: American Guidance Service.
PPVT-4	Peabody Picture Vocabulary Test—Fourth Edition	Dunn, L., & Dunn, D. (2007). *Peabody Picture Vocabulary Test—Fourth Edition*. Circle Pines, MN: American Guidance Service.
QUIL	Queensland Inventory of Literacy	Dodd, B., Holm, S., Oerlemans, M., & McCormick, M. (1996). *Queensland Inventory of Literacy*. Queensland: University of Queensland.
Reading Progress Tests	Reading Progress Tests	Vincent, D., Crumpler, M., & Mare, M. (1997). *Reading Progress Tests*. Berkshire, UK: Nfer Nelson.
Rossetti Infant-Toddler Language Scale	Rossetti Infant-Toddler Language Scale	Rossetti, L. (1990). *The Rossetti Infant-Toddler Language Scale*. East Moline, IL: Linguisystems.
SCBE	Social Competence and Behavior Evaluation	LaFreniere, P., & Dumas, J. (1995). *Social Competence and Behavior Evaluation: Preschool Edition Manual*. Los Angeles, CA: Western Psychological Services.
SDQ-2	Self-Description Questionnaire—Second Edition	Marsh, H. (1990). *Self-Description Questionnaire II: Manual*. New South Wales, Australia: University of Western Sydney, Macarthur Faculty of Education Publication Unit.

continues

Test Acronym	Full Title	Reference
SDQ-3	Self-Description Questionnaire—Third Edition	Marsh, H. (1992). *Self-Description Questionnaire III: Manual.* New South Wales, Australia: University of Western Sydney, Macarthur Faculty of Education Publication Unit.
SIR	The Speech Intelligibility Rating	Cox, R., & McDaniel, D. (1989). Development of the Speech Intelligibility Rating (SIR) test for hearing aid comparisons. *Journal of Speech and Hearing Research, 32*(2), 347–352.
SPEAK-probes	Speech Perception Education and Assessment Kit—Probes	Boothroyd, A. (1978). Speech perception and sensorineural hearing loss, in: M. Ross & T. Giolas (Eds.). *Auditory management of hearing-impaired children* (pp. 117–144). Baltimore, MD: University Park Press.
SPINE	SPeech INtelligibility Evaluation	Monsen, R., Moog, J., & Geers, A. (1988). *CID Picture SPINE (SPeech INtelligibility Evaluation).* St. Louis, MO: Central Institute for the Deaf.
TOWRE	Test of Word Reading Efficiency	Wagner, R., Torgesen, J., & Rashotte, C. (1999). *Test of Word Reading Efficiency.* Texas: Pro-Ed.
Wechsler Preschool and Primary Scale of Intelligence	Wechsler Preschool and Primary Scale of Intelligence	Wechsler, D. (2002). *Wechsler Preschool and Primary Scale of Intelligence.* San Antonio, TX: Psychological Corporation.
WIAT-2	Wechsler Individual Achievement Test—Second Edition	Wechsler, D. (1992) *Wechsler Individual Achievement Test—Second Edition.* San Antonio, TX: Harcourt Assessment.
WIAT-2 (Australian)	Wechsler Individual Achievement Test—Second Edition (Australian Adaptation)	Pearson PsychCorp. (2007). *Wechsler Individual Achievement Test—Second Edition, Australian Standardised Edition.* Sydney, NSW: NCS Pearson.
WRAT-3	Wide Range Achievement Test—Third Edition	Jastak, J., & Wilkinson, G. (1993). *Wide Range Achievement Test—Third Edition.* Wilmington, DE: Wide Range.

4

AUDIOLOGY: IMPLICATIONS FOR AUDITORY-VERBAL THERAPY

Carolyne Edwards

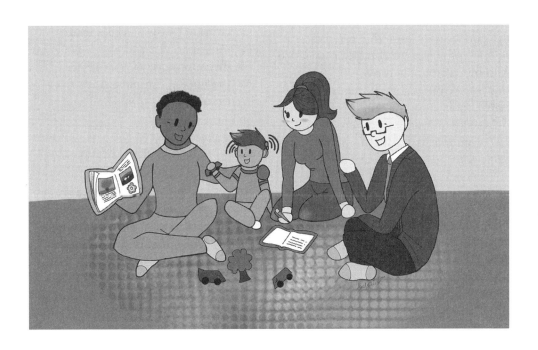

INTRODUCTION

Interpretation of the results of audio-logical assessment has long been the realm of audiologists alone. Yet the understanding and application of audiological information by the auditory-verbal practitioner and parents is crucial to the optimal development of listening, speech, and language skills in the child with hearing loss. Auditory threshold and discrimination measures have direct implications for speech perception and the subsequent development of speech production; it is the perception of speech which leads to recognition, comprehension, and ultimately language expression with family members and peers.

This chapter provides a basic description of conventional audiological procedures and the relevance of this information for the key players in Auditory-Verbal Therapy (AVT). In addition, descriptions of a number of qualitative tools now available for hearing professionals to assess different aspects of communicative functioning for children with hearing loss are outlined.

THE OVERALL PICTURE

Audiological assessment addresses a broad spectrum of auditory issues. Although the pure tone audiogram often attracts more attention than other audiological procedures, it is only one part of the audiological picture. A comprehensive audiological assessment in a clinical setting will evaluate the following areas.

Nature of Hearing Loss and Auditory Potential

- provision of information about auditory function
- description of current hearing levels
- description of the child's auditory potential for perception of speech, and auditory monitoring of the environment
- evaluation of electroacoustical functioning of amplification

Listening Skills

- description of the child's current listening skills
- observation of the child's attitude toward listening, communication, and social interaction
- measurement of changes in the child's listening skills over time

Communication

- observation of the communication strategies the child is currently using and additional
- strategies that would enhance the child's comprehension of speech
- recommendation for alternate teaching/communication strategies when auditory limitations are present
- determination of the amplification strategies that will enhance the child's communication

Children and Parents/Family

- evaluation of the parents' and child's acceptance of the hearing loss and the child's overall sense of self-worth
- determination of the need for additional counseling

The AV practitioner and/or the parents may be interested in particular areas of assessment or a review of all of the areas noted above. The following review of audiological tests will provide common ground for both to discuss results with the audiologist.

Implications

- Inform the audiologist of any areas in which you have a particular interest, based on your observations or current concerns.

Ask the Audiologist

- Which areas have you focused on today?
- How will today's information affect the child's programming?

NATURE OF HEARING LOSS AND AUDITORY POTENTIAL

The Pure Tone Audiogram

The pure tone audiogram (Figure 4–1) is a graph indicating the softest level in each ear at which the child can hear a range of pitches that are important for comprehension of speech. The purpose of the audiogram is to compare the child's results to a graph of normal hearing to determine the

- presence or absence of hearing loss,
- type of hearing loss,
- degree of hearing loss,
- shape of hearing loss, and
- auditory differences between ears.

The type of sound used in testing varies with the means of presentation. Using insert earphones or headphones, pure tone stimuli are presented at octave frequencies of 250, 500, 1000, 2000, 4000, and 8000 Hz in each ear. Narrowband noise or warble tone stimuli at 250 to 6000 Hz are used during sound-field testing in unaided or aided condition.

A threshold is the softest level at which a child hears a sound 50% of the time. Thresholds are measured in decibels (dB), the unit of sound intensity. On the audiogram, intensities range from the softest level (–10 dB) to the loudest level (120 dB). Zero dB does not imply the absence of sound; rather it represents the softest level that the average young adult with normal hearing can detect sound, although some individuals are able to detect sound at levels of –5 or –10 dB HL.

Thresholds are typically measured at frequencies between 125 and 8000 Hz and plotted on the pure tone audiogram. Hearing levels can differ from one frequency to the next, resulting in an audiogram with a flat, rising, falling, trough, or cookie bite configuration from the low to the high frequencies. The shape of the hearing loss can

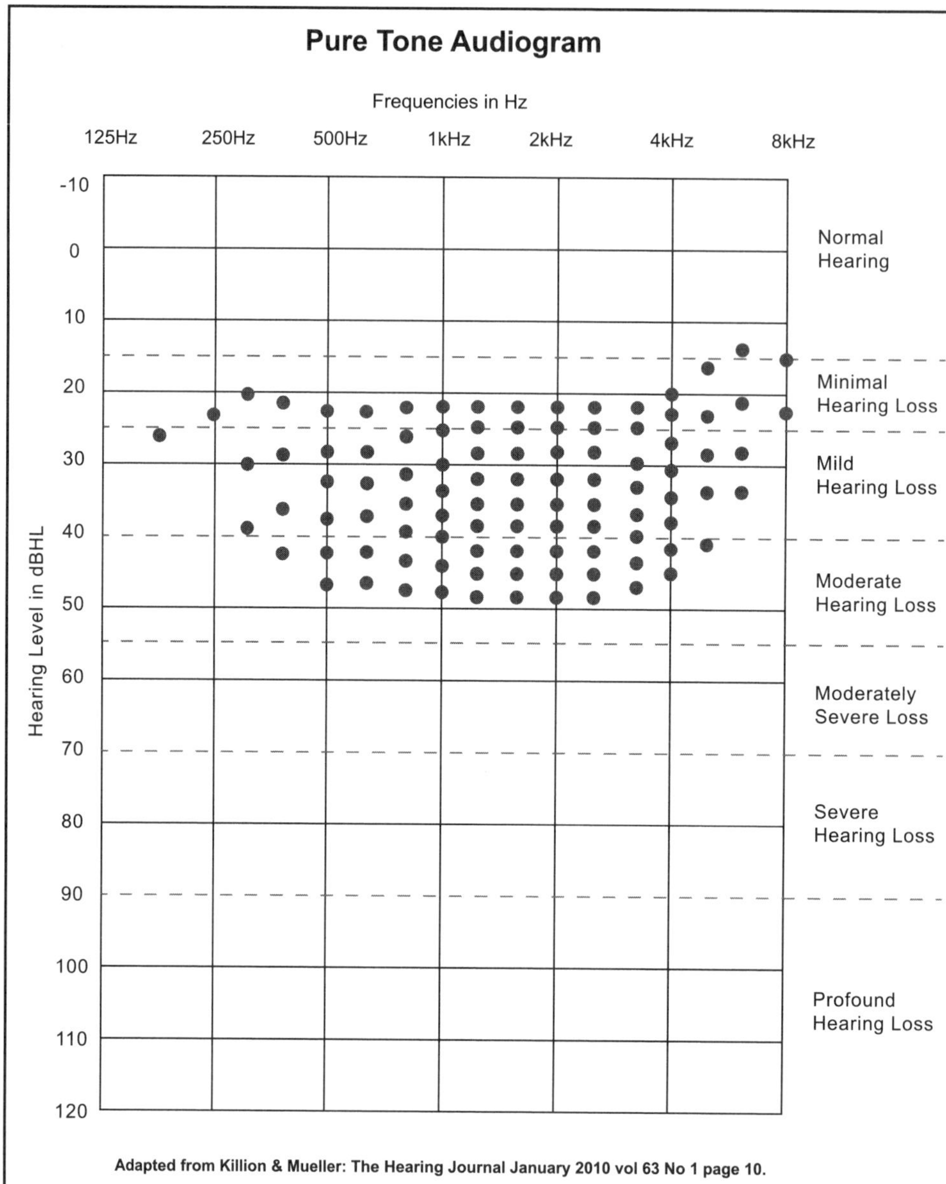

Pure Tone Audiogram

Frequencies in Hz

Figure 4-1. Pure tone audiogram—Count the Dot audiogram and degrees of hearing loss.

suggest some of the auditory perceptual difficulties that the child might experience.

Frequencies at 500, 1000, and 2000 Hz are called the *speech frequencies* because the majority of all vowel

and consonant energy is concentrated in this region. The one hundred dots from Killion and Mead's Count the Dot audiogram (2010) shown in Figure 4–1 reflect the range of the speech spectrum and the importance of the different frequencies and intensities for the perception of speech. The greater the number of dots at a frequency, the more important it is for speech perception. Note that there are also more *audible dots* above 4 kHz in the speech spectrum than was reported in earlier literature.

The pure tone average, which represents the overall hearing level for each ear, is also calculated as the average of the thresholds at 500, 1000, and 2000 Hz. The degree of hearing loss is based on the interpretation of the pure tone average for each ear. For example, a pure tone average of 25 dB represents a minimal hearing loss. There is a danger however in looking only at the pure tone average to describe hearing loss. The PTA cannot accurately estimate the effect of the hearing loss on speech recognition when the audiogram configuration is steeply sloping, and there can be a varying relationship between PTA and word recognition ability for children with severe and profound hearing loss.

Example:

Two children were seen for audiological assessment. The first child had a PTA of 95 dB in both ears and a word discrimination score of 72%. The second child had a PTA of 95 dB and a word discrimination score of 24%. Both children had a profound hearing loss and yet had very different speech recognition abilities.

Testing is completed by air conduction or bone conduction. Sound presented through headphones or insert phones is conducted by air to the eardrum, whose motion then stimulates the ossicular chain, the oval window, the fluid within the cochlea (inner ear), and subsequently the hair cells in the inner ear. Bone-conducted sound occurs when a vibrator is placed on the mastoid bone behind the ear, and the sound vibrates the skull which in turn vibrates the fluid in the cochlea, stimulating the hair cells within the inner ear. Thus, bone-conducted sound bypasses any obstruction or damage to the outer or middle ear. Comparison of the results of thresholds obtained by air and bone conduction testing differentiates among conductive, sensorineural, or mixed hearing loss.

A *conductive hearing loss* is caused by damage or obstruction in the outer or middle ear. Bone conduction thresholds are within normal limits, and a gap of 15 dB or more exists between air and bone conduction thresholds.

A *sensorineural hearing loss* is caused by damage or obstruction to the inner ear or auditory nerve. Bone conduction thresholds are poorer than 15 dB, and there is no gap between air and bone conduction thresholds.

A *mixed hearing loss* is caused by a combination of damage or obstruction in the outer/middle ear and the inner ear/auditory nerve. In this case, bone conduction thresholds are poorer than 15 dB, and there is a gap of 15 dB or more between air and bone conduction thresholds. A *fluctuating* mixed hearing loss can result when a child experiences recurrent otitis media in conjunction with a sensorineural hearing loss.

Auditory neuropathy spectrum disorder (ANSD), a more recently diagnosed auditory disorder, presents with considerable variability in auditory capacity from normal hearing to profound sensorineural hearing loss, and is distinguished by particular patterns on electrophysiological testing and disproportionately poor speech recognition abilities for the degree of loss. Recent definitions of ANSD include either present otoacoustic emissions or a present cochlear microphonic, in combination with either markedly abnormal or absent auditory brainstem response (ABR).

Implications

■ Infants and very young children may not respond at threshold levels during audiologic testing. Instead their responses may be described as minimal response levels (MRLs), suggesting that hearing levels may be better at a later date, than those indicated on the audiogram.

■ Although there is variability within each category of hearing loss, the degree of loss conveys information about potential auditory, speech, and language difficulties. (See Anderson 2007 for extensive handouts on the relationship between different degrees of hearing loss and listening and learning needs.)

■ The type of hearing loss also has implications for AVT. The child who has congenital conductive hearing loss will not experience the auditory perceptual distortion of speech sounds that the child with mixed or sensorineural hearing loss does, and thus listening *training* needs to be adjusted accordingly.

■ The child with ANSD may not derive the same benefits from amplification as those children with sensorineural hearing loss.

Ask the Audiologist

■ What is the child's overall degree and type of hearing loss?
■ Does the child hear better at some frequencies than others? If so, which frequencies?
■ Which frequencies is the child unable to hear, if any?
■ Which ear has more hearing? At what frequencies?
■ Is there any indication of middle ear dysfunction on today's testing?
■ Do today's results reflect the child's optimal hearing levels?
■ Has there been any change in hearing levels since the last assessment?

Auditory Brainstem Response (ABR)

Auditory brainstem response (ABR) is an electrophysiological test to evaluate auditory function. It is used to assess hearing acuity when measurements from behavioural audiological procedures cannot be reliably obtained. Sound is presented through earphones or through a bone conduction oscillator. Electrodes attached to the scalp and at the earlobe measure the electrical activity generated by the neurons in the auditory (eighth) nerve and brainstem for the first 10 milliseconds after a sound is presented. Clicks centered around the frequency region of 2000 to 4000 Hz or brief frequency-specific tone bursts are presented many times, and the responses at each stimulus intensity are recorded. A computer averages the electrical response over numerous presentations. The ABR threshold is the lowest level at which the response is visible.

Unlike the pure tone audiogram which provides information at frequencies from 250 to 8000 Hz, results of ABR testing reflect primarily responses for a few frequencies. The maximum intensity level used in ABR is typically less than the maximum level used in behavioral testing with headphones. Thus, it is also possible to indicate no response on ABR testing and show thresholds at 105 to 120 dB at the higher frequencies on the pure tone audiogram. Whereas pure tone thresholds are obtained using 5 dB intervals, ABR is usually obtained using 20 dB changes in presentation level. Thus, results of ABR testing provide the degree of hearing loss at selected frequencies but do not have the specificity of pure tone thresholds.

Implications

■ ABR provides information on the degree of hearing loss in each ear, and the presence or absence of a conductive component, and does so without the active participation of the child.
■ ABR provides less specific information regarding frequency sensitivity and thresholds than behavioral audiometry, and therefore is not a substitute for behavioral testing.
■ No response on ABR does not mean no measurable hearing. It means no measurable hearing at the maximum intensity tested in that frequency region.

■ ABR is a diagnostic test completed at the initial assessment; it is not used to monitor hearing levels unless behavioral testing is not possible.

Ask the Audiologist

■ Do behavioral observations agree with the ABR findings?
■ Are there any discrepancies between the results of ABR and other audiological tests?
■ What is the type and degree of hearing loss?
■ What is the difference in hearing levels between ears?

Otoacoustic Emissions

Evoked otoacoustic emissions (EOAE) are another electrophysiological measure of hearing sensitivity. Otoacoustic emissions are low-level sounds generated in the cochlea that can be recorded in the external ear canal using a sensitive microphone. EOAEs occur following acoustic stimulation with clicks or short-duration tones. A microphone is inserted into a soft rubber or foam tip and placed in the child's ear canal. Sounds are presented through miniature earphones, and response tracings are averaged and recorded.

The main types of EOAE are transient-evoked otoacoustic emissions (TEOAE) and distortion product otoacoustic emissions (DPOAE), and both can be used to evaluate the status of the cochlea. Like the ABR, TEOAE and DPOAE testing do not require the child's cooperation. In fact, because it is noninvasive, there is minimal preparation required of the child. However, middle ear function must be normal in order to obtain an accurate test. OAEs are an essential part of a diagnostic test battery to identify auditory neuropathy (ANSD).

Implications

- As a diagnostic measure, EOAE testing permits the audiologist to differentiate between sensory and neural hearing loss. Reduction in otoacoustic emissions reflects sensory loss due to damage to the cochlea, and abnormal evoked potentials on ABR reflect neural loss due to damage to the auditory nerve and brainstem.
- EOAE testing is used as a hearing screening measure in newborn screening protocols.

Ask the Audiologist

- (Screening tool) Is there evidence of hearing loss?
- (Diagnostic tool) What is the nature of the sensory/neural hearing loss?

Impedance Audiometry

Impedance audiometry is a test battery consisting of *tympanometry, static compliance*, and *acoustic reflex tests*. *Tympanometry* is an objective test used to determine normal or abnormal middle ear function based on measurement of middle ear pressure and tympanic mobility. Of the three subtests within impedance audiometry, tympanometry is the test of most ongoing interest to the AV practitioner and the parents.

A tone is introduced through a probe tip placed in the child's ear canal. The measurement of the intensity of the sound reflected back from the eardrum as air pressure in the ear canal is varied, provides information on the status of the middle ear. The following terms are used to describe middle ear dysfunction:

- *Negative middle ear pressure and normal tympanic mobility* reflect retraction of the eardrum and yet normal mobility within the middle ear system; the physical sensation is similar to the pressure experienced during airplane takeoff and landing. This dysfunction is often seen when young children have congestion.
- *Negative middle ear pressure and reduced tympanic mobility* reflect a stiff middle ear system due to conditions commonly seen in young children such as wax buildup, extreme negative middle ear pressure, or fluid buildup in the middle ear.
- *Extremely high tympanic mobility* reflects a highly mobile middle ear system due to conditions such as ossicular discontinuity or flaccid eardrum.

The transient nature of fluid buildup in the middle ear space plays havoc with auditory learning for children with hearing loss. Hearing levels can decrease by 5 to 40 dB, in the presence of temporary middle ear dysfunction. The need to listen more intently due to a temporary decrease in hearing levels, and the resulting fatigue, are rarely discussed.

Parents and the AV practitioner need to be sensitive to the child's need for auditory *rest* during periods of middle ear dysfunction and put less auditory demands on the child. In addition, the audiologist may suggest increasing the volume of the child's hearing devices in response to depressed hearing levels.

Implications

- For children with sensory/neural hearing loss, the additional presence of a fluctuating loss due to middle ear dysfunction can be devastating. AV practitioners and parents need to be aware that significant interruptions in auditory learning can occur during episodes of fluid buildup in the middle ear.
- The majority of episodes of middle ear dysfunction are symptom free, other than a decrease in hearing levels. Therefore it is important for the parents and therapist to be alert to any changes in hearing sensitivity.
- Children with chronic histories of middle ear dysfunction need to have routine tympanometry, preferably every 3 months, to monitor both the status of the middle ear and hearing levels, and any concerns need to be relayed to the therapist and the child's teachers.

Example:

A child with a profound sensorineural hearing loss arrives at the clinic. The parent has been concerned about the child's poorer responses to sound at home during the past week. The parent wonders if the child's hearing has shifted, if the hearing device is working properly, if the child has fluid buildup, or if it is simply an "off" week. Results of tympanometry show a flat tympanogram in both ears, and a resulting decrease in hearing levels of about 15 dB. For this child, this decrease is enough to lose audibility of normal conversational speech at 2000 and 4000 Hz, thus losing ability to monitor all of the mid and high frequencies in their speech. The parent's only clue of the change in hearing levels in the past week was increased feedback (whistling) from the hearing aids despite no change in volume setting. Increased acoustic feedback can occur in the presence of decreased tympanic mobility and fluid buildup.

Ask the Audiologist

- Is there any indication of middle ear dysfunction today that would affect hearing levels?
- How chronic is the middle ear dysfunction?
- When should the child return for a recheck of middle ear function?
- Should the volume setting on the hearing aid be adjusted during periods of middle dysfunction?
- For children with programmable hearing aids and chronic middle ear dysfunction, can another program be designated for those periods when hearing levels are depressed by middle ear dysfunction?

Electroacoustical Evaluation

Once hearing aids have been selected for a child, the electroacoustical characteristics must be assessed routinely to ensure satisfactory functioning. The audiologist evaluates

- the gain (intensity across various frequencies);
- the frequency response (the bass, mid, and treble response);
- the saturation sound pressure level (the maximum intensity produced by the hearing aid at various frequencies);
- the equivalent input noise level (the internal noise produced by the hearing aid); and
- the distortion levels (the clarity of the sound produced by the hearing aid).

With very young children, it is desirable to obtain electroacoustical evaluation every 3 to 6 months, *or any time there is a decrease in auditory responsiveness or clarity of speech*. When a child is using an FM system in combination with personal hearing devices, the electroacoustical response of the combined system should be tested to ensure compatibility and optimal response.

Ask the Audiologist

- Is the personal hearing device and/or FM system working appropriately?
- Are there any modifications to amplification or earmold characteristics that would enhance audibility and perception of speech?

- Do the hearing aid settings need to be adjusted when coupled to the FM system?
- Has the FM system been adjusted to match the hearing aid response when they are coupled together?
- Which FM accessories would enhance the child's audibility of speech in various listening environments (e.g., use of boom microphone, use of pass-around microphone, or use of patch cords to audio or audiovisual equipment)?

Real-Ear or Simulated Real-Ear Measurement

Acoustic performance of the hearing aid fitting can also be measured in the child's ear canal using real-ear measurement or for infants and very young children, using a simulated real-ear or coupler approach to verification of hearing aid characteristics.

The real-ear instrumentation uses an external microphone sitting outside the ear, connected to a soft silicone tube which is inserted into the ear canal to measure the difference in acoustic response between the unaided and aided condition. A loudspeaker generates a known intensity across a number of frequencies. The external microphone measures the changes in intensity detected through the tube sitting in the ear canal close to the eardrum, first without and then with the hearing aid.

Real ear or simulated real-ear measurement is used to determine

- audibility of various speech features with the child's

amplification, specifically the gain, frequency response, and saturation sound pressure level of the hearing aid in the child's ear;

■ effects of altering the volume setting or other settings;

■ the effect of the shape of the child's ear canal on the hearing aid response; and

■ effects of various earmold modifications on the hearing aid response.

Hearing aid fitting protocols using real-ear or simulated real-ear measurement provide a means of selecting and fitting hearing aids for children that is more reliable, provides more comprehensive and reliable data across frequencies, and requires less cooperation from the child than traditional aided sound-field testing.

The following guidelines summarize predictions for auditory potential based on audibility of various speech features measured through real-ear or simulated real-ear testing. The goal of fitting hearing devices is for the child to have sufficient audibility at each frequency to detect and identify speech features. It is beyond the scope of this chapter to review the principles of speech science; the reader can refer to Ling (1976, 1989) for detailed information. Only through ongoing assessment of auditory perceptual skills will the therapist determine the child's capacity to utilize acoustic cues at various frequencies.

Audibility within the speech spectrum at 250 to 4000 Hz suggests the following auditory potential:

■ detection of all suprasegmentals (duration, loudness, and pitch characteristics of speech) and segmentals (vowel and consonant characteristics);

■ identification of all suprasegmental features;

■ identification of all vowels;

■ recognition of voicing, manner, and place characteristics of consonants;

■ identification of selected consonants (*depends on the degree of hearing loss); and

■ detection and identification of most environmental sounds.

Note. Children with severe and profound sensory/neural hearing loss will show greater variability in the recognition of segmental characteristics.

When audibility within the speech spectrum is limited to frequencies from 250 to 2000 Hz, the child may experience difficulty with

■ identification of front vowels;

■ detection of high-frequency consonants such as /s/, /f/, voiceless th (θ); and

■ identification of place characteristics of consonants.

When audibility within the speech spectrum is limited to frequencies from 250 to 1000 Hz, the child may experience difficulty with

■ identification of mid and front vowels;

■ detection of mid- and high-frequency consonants;

■ identification of some manner characteristics of consonants;

■ identification of place characteristics of consonants; and

■ identification of some environmental sounds.

Audible hearing within the speech spectrum at 250 and 500 Hz only will create difficulties with

- detection of some back and mid vowels;
- identification of back, mid, or front vowels;
- detection of the mid- and high-frequency consonants;
- categorization of voicing, manner, or place of consonant production;
- detection of some environmental sounds; and
- identification of environmental sounds.

Implications

- Audibility throughout the speech spectrum is measured through real-ear or simulated real-ear measures. These measures are essential to ensure that optimal audibility is obtained and maintained.
- An alteration in the gain or frequency response, either electroacoustically or acoustically through a modification in the earmold, can affect speech perception and production.
- Any deterioration in the child's responses to sound or speech quality needs to be followed with an immediate check of the hearing device.

Example:

The parents of a young preschooler who had a sloping severe to borderline profound sensorineural hearing loss had tracked their child's auditory and speech development carefully over the past year in AVT. Their child was able to identify all of the vowel sounds and produce the vowels accurately in everyday speech. One day, the parents noticed the child was not able to recognize the difference between /u/ and /i/ ("oo" and "ee"). After the child's sound confusion persisted for several days, they called their audiologist. Electroacoustical and real-ear measurement of aided function showed that the shape of the canal of the new earmold had reduced the high-frequency information sufficiently that the child was unable to hear the second formant of /i/, and thus discrimination between /u/ and /i/ was impossible. Modifications to the new earmold restored the child's high-frequency perception, and speech production returned to previous levels.

Ask the Audiologist

- Does the child have the ability to detect and identify supra-segmental features (duration, loudness, and pitch)?
- Which vowel sounds does the child have the auditory potential to detect?
- Which vowels does the child have the auditory potential to recognize?
- Which vowels might sound the same to the child, and thus need visual clues to distinguish one from the other?
- Which consonant sounds does the child have the auditory ability to detect?

- Which consonant sounds would be difficult to detect in isolation?
- Which consonant features (voicing, manner, place) does the child have the potential to recognize?

LISTENING SKILLS

Audiological assessment measures a variety of listening skills ranging from detection, discrimination, recognition, through to comprehension. The assessment tools are presented here in increasing range of complexity on this hierarchy in order to track the auditory development of the child from the outset.

DETECTION

Detection is the ability to respond to the presence of absence of sound. Thus, the child learns to respond to sound, to pay attention to sound, and not to respond when there is no sound. The child's thresholds on the pure tone audiogram provide the first formal evidence of auditory detection.

Speech Awareness Threshold (SAT)

The speech awareness threshold, sometimes called the speech detection threshold (SDT), is the softest level at which one can detect the presence of speech 50% of the time. It provides a measure of the minimum loudness level necessary for the child to detect speech, and suggests the loudness level necessary for detection and possible identification of speech features. For detection of the full intensity range of speech sounds from the quietest consonant (voiceless "th" or /θ/ to the loudest vowel ("ah" or /a/), speech must be delivered 30 dB above threshold (Ling 1989). As in other threshold measures, the preschool child may be conditioned through visual or conditioned play audiometry, or at a later age, simply instructed to raise his or her hand when the sound is heard.

Implications

- The SAT is the gauge for the loudness levels that can be detected in training—whispered (30 dB), quiet (40 dB), normal (50 dB), and loud voice (65 dB).
- Note that these dB levels are approximations.
- The SAT is also an indicator of potential audibility of the speech spectrum. The range between the softest consonant and the loudest vowel is 30 dB. Thus, the speech signal needs to be 30 dB louder than the SAT in order to obtain complete audibility. Particularly for children who have a severe or profound hearing loss where audibility is most compromised, use of an FM system can enhance the perception of low-intensity speech sounds.
- The SAT reflects the optimal level that the child detects speech, under ideal, one-to-one, quiet listening conditions where the child anticipates a sound. The child's response level in noisier environments will necessarily be reduced.

Example:

A child establishes an SAT of 40 dB. In ideal listening situations, the child can detect quiet, normal, and loud conversational speech. If listening in less than optimal situations (at a distance, in background noise), the child may only detect normal or loud speech levels. The child may only respond to speech spontaneously when presented at loud conversational levels. The SAT does not confirm audibility at all frequencies but simply evidence of sufficient intensity at one or more frequencies to detect speech.

Ask the Audiologist

- What is the intensity level of speech that the child is just beginning to detect?
- What loudness level would the child be able to detect in a lesson situation?
- What level of voice would the child find difficult or impossible to detect in a lesson situation?
- What level of voice would the child detect spontaneously in the everyday environment?

Ling's Six-Sound Test

The Six-Sound Test (Ling, 2002) is a detection task of six speech sounds: m, oo, a(r), ee, sh, and s (/m/, /u/, /a/, /i/, /ʃ/, /s/) presented at normal conversational level when the child is using his or her hearing devices. Each of these sounds represents critical information in a different frequency range of the speech spectrum. The results can be used in a variety of ways:

- Predict the ability to recognize various speech features.
- Monitor changes in hearing due to middle ear dysfunction.
- Measure any changes in aided performance from day to day.
- Measure effects of distance from the speaker on the audibility of various speech features (from 6 inches to 15 feet away).
- Observe increases in audibility when an FM system is used in combination with personal amplification.
- Observe differences in audibility with different FM microphones. Comparisons can be made between omnidirectional, directional, boom, and/or pass-around microphones. Each of these microphones has different auditory characteristics and uses; consult with the audiologist to select the appropriate microphone(s) for the FM transmitter.

The Glendonald Auditory Screening Procedure: Test 1 (GASP 1)

The Glendonald Auditory Screening Procedure: Test 1 (GASP 1) is an expansion of the Six-Sound Test (Erber, 1982). The speech sounds in the detection task include 10 vowels and 12 consonants (nasals, laterals, voiced and unvoiced fricatives) presented at normal conversational level. Erber describes several additional purposes for this test, including

- evaluation of audibility of speech spectrum of therapist's and parents' voice, by having the therapist and parent present the speech sounds to the child; and

▪ evaluation of any strategies to enhance audibility of the phoneme tested, such as talking closer to the microphone of the child's hearing device, using an FM system, or intentionally distorting the speech sound by directing the breath-stream directly across the microphone opening.

Note that the Six-Sound Test and the GASP 1 can also both be used as identification tasks if the child's auditory skills are more advanced, and then the child is asked to repeat the sound heard.

Implications

▪ If the child detects the sounds tested, she or he has the potential to detect the full range of the speech spectrum.

▪ If the child detects /m, a, u, i, and ʃ/, auditory potential is similar to audibility within the speech spectrum at 250 to 2000 Hz.

▪ Detection of the three vowels and /m/ suggests potential similar to audibility thresholds within the speech spectrum at 250 to 1000 Hz.

Ask the Audiologist

▪ Which speech sounds can the child detect?

▪ Does the child have the auditory potential to
  ▪ detect all of the vowels;
  ▪ identify the back, central, and/or front vowels;

▪ detect all of the consonants; and
▪ identify voicing, manner, and/or place features for consonants?

▪ Which speech sounds would be most sensitive to changes in middle ear function?

▪ At what distance does the child lose audibility of a specific speech sound?

▪ What acoustic or electroacoustic strategies are recommended to enhance audibility of particular speech sounds?

Detection of sound is the obvious and essential first step in learning to listen. When the child is first fitted with his or her hearing devices, the initial indicators of aided benefit are usually a change in conditioned or spontaneous alerting responses, and increased vocalization when the devices are worn. It is critical that parents and the AV practitioner are cognizant of unaided and aided responses obtained by the child in the audiological assessment. This information, a prerequisite for comprehensive AVT, is a valuable predictor of the child's ability to detect, identify, and comprehend auditory stimuli. Although it is important to experiment with detection of a variety of sounds, children need not be frustrated by perseveration with listening activities that continue to focus on sounds they are unable to detect.

Spontaneous Alerting Response for Babies and Young Children

A variety of spontaneous behaviors that indicate detection of sound may be observed in response to sound with infants, including searching for the sound, turning eyes or head toward the sound, cessation of activity, quieting, startling, or vocalizing, and this is the focus of behavioral observation for babies and toddlers.

In AVT, the parent or AV practitioner can spontaneously present various speech sounds or environmental sounds, such as a musical clock, during the auditory-verbal session. If spontaneous alerting does not occur, the adult needs to encourage the child to search for the sound. This is a natural activity in which to engage the child and progresses in step with cognitive development. The parents and caregivers are encouraged to create similar experiences at home using sounds relevant to the child's environment. When the child begins to demonstrate some spontaneous responses to sound, it is a good indication that the child has attached meaning to sound, an essential step in listening development. Spontaneous alerting in the everyday environment will continue to be a listening goal at all ages.

Conditioned Play Response

Most children are cognitively ready to perform a conditioned play response only around the age of 2 years and above, although a few master the task at 18 to 24 months.

The conditioned play response used in pediatric audiological assessment protocols requires the child to perform an action upon hearing a sound. The action might include placing a block in a bucket, stacking rings on a pole, or any other similarly repetitive play

response. The activity is first demonstrated for the child. A sound is presented; the audiologist leads the child's hand through the action and praises the child at the finish. After six to 10 randomly timed presentations of the sound in which the audiologist helps the child to respond, the child is encouraged to perform the action alone.

The AV practitioner and parents may teach the child a conditioned play response in preparation for audiological testing. This serves two purposes: to consolidate the child's conditioned response to sound and to observe changes in the child's responsiveness to detection tasks. The practitioner and/or parent can use the sounds from the Ling Six-Sound Test—m, oo, ah, ee, sh, and s (/m/, /u/, /a/, /i/, /ʃ/, and /s/) —for teaching and monitoring detection skills. Note that sounds need to be presented at random intervals to ensure that the child does not develop a timed response to the task.

Once a stable response to sound is established, the AV practitioner will have a tool for detection of possible middle ear dysfunction and associated temporary decrease in hearing levels, hearing device malfunctions, or changes in the acoustic properties of the earmold. Occasionally, changes in responsiveness may signal permanent changes in hearing levels due to progressive hearing loss.

Overhearing is an essential auditory skill utilized by children in the development of spoken language; in fact considerable language learning occurs incidentally through overhearing others' conversation. Therefore, developing the awareness of *all* sounds in the child's environment is the critical first step.

There are a variety of evaluation tools that audiologists or AV practitioners may share with the parents to record the child's alerting to various sounds in their environment. The Early Listening Function (ELF), designed for children from 5 months to 3 years, teaches families to observe how children respond in 12 listening situations at different distances and then suggests activities to stimulate alerting responses in their young child (Anderson, 2002). The Infant Toddler Meaningful Auditory Integration Scale (IT- MAIS) provides 10 questions that evaluate the meaningful use of sound in everyday situations, from vocal behavior, to use of hearing instrument, to ability to alert to sound to ability to attach meaning to sound (Zimmerman-Phillips , Osberger, & Robbins, 1997).

DISCRIMINATION

Discrimination is the ability to perceive similarities and differences between two or more sounds. The child learns to attend to differences among sounds, or to respond differently to different sounds.

Same-Different Test: Minimal Auditory Capabilities (MAC) Test

This is the only formal test that assesses the child's ability to perceive differences between two sounds although being unable to identify the sounds. This subtest from the (MAC) battery (Owens, Kesssler, Telleen, & Schubert, 1981) assessed the child's ability to discriminate differences between pairs of spondees (two syllable words with equal stress on both syllables). Two words are presented, and the child is asked if the word pairs are the same two words, or two different words. This is primarily a vowel discrimination task. It is useful to assess this skill when a child is able to differentiate among stress patterns on the GASP 2 but not yet able to identify vowel differences when given a speech reception threshold (SRT).

Informal Testing

Simple informal tests using the same format can be administered by the audiologist or the AV practitioner to determine when the child has difficulty discerning any auditory difference between two speech sounds. For example, two vowel sounds such as /ɪ/ and /i/ or consonants such as 'sh' and 's' might sound identical to the child when presented in same or different pairings.

Discrimination activities involving same-different tasks are used primarily for clarification of identification or comprehension errors, rather than as a developmental step between detection and identification. The practitioner may present the pairs *dog–dog, dog–dogs, dogs–dogs* and ask the child to tell whether the words are the same or different. Or she/he may say *dog–dog–dog–dogs–dog* and ask the child to signal when the sound was different. If the child is unable to determine whether the word pairs are the same or different, or when the different sound occurred, and the /s/ is within the audible range for the child, then the AV practitioner may return to specific discrimination tasks to further develop the child's auditory skills. Other strategies used in AVT may also be helpful here. (See Chapter 11.)

Ask the Audiologist

▥ Can the child discriminate differences between the speech spectrum of two words?

IDENTIFICATION OR RECOGNITION

Identification or recognition is the ability to reproduce a speech stimuli or environmental sound by naming or identifying through pointing to an object or picture, by writing the word, or by repeating the word or sound heard.

Suprasegmentals

The importance of suprasegmental features for identification and comprehension of speech and for enhancement of speech intelligibility is paramount, and the auditory channel provides the most complete information on duration, loudness, and pitch. Suprasegmental information obtained through visual or tactile input is often ambiguous or entirely absent. The cues for identification of high versus low pitch, for example, occur primarily through hearing. Visual cues cannot help to differentiate varying pitch levels, although tension in the vocal cords may provide some limited tactile/kinesthetic cues.

All children with minimal to severe sensorineural hearing loss, and most with profound sensorineural hearing loss who use hearing aids, have the auditory potential to detect and identify

suprasegmental features (Ling, 1989). Children with profound loss who use cochlear implants typically have no difficulty discriminating and recognizing suprasegmental features.

Although the child first recognizes suprasegmental characteristics of speech before identifying specific speech sounds, there are few audiological tests that measure the growth in the ability to identify differences in duration, loudness, and pitch, so this is an area of assessment that falls back on the AV practitioner to determine the child's current skills.

AV practitioners need to assess the child's ability to discern the differences between different durations of sounds, loud and soft sounds and high- and low-pitch sounds. The features of loudness and pitch are often confused by children with severe and profound sensorineural hearing loss at the outset of therapy. (For example, "high" may suggest "loud"; "low" is confused with "soft.") It is important for children to acquire sound vocabulary to better describe and classify what they hear. Teaching the classification of loudness and pitch separately (high pitch–low pitch or loud–soft) followed by differentiation of paired loudness-pitch characteristics, such as loud-high versus loud-low voice creates opportunities for those distinctions to develop. If a preschool child finds simple labeling of voice patterns uninteresting after a short time, activities may be created using puppets in which one puppet has a high-pitched voice and the other has a low-pitched voice. The AV practitioner may then alter the loudness of each of the puppets' voices to create paired voice characteristics, and the child selects the correct puppet and identifies the voice as loud or soft.

Later the child can be asked to attach meaning to changes in loudness, duration, and pitch characteristics in voices. Instead of labeling a voice as high-loud or low-soft, the child learns to label the emotional content of a person's voice as angry (high-loud or low-loud) or sad (low-soft).

Pitch differences determine the identification of male and female voices. Differentiation among the average fundamental frequency of a male voice (125 Hz), a female voice (250 Hz), and a child's voice (325 Hz) is possible for most children with profound sensorineural hearing loss who have audibility within the speech spectrum at 250 to 1000 Hz. Most children with hearing loss appear to acquire this auditory distinction naturally without additional training.

Description of Environmental Sounds: Onomatopoeic Words or "Sound" Vocabulary

This activity does not appear to be part of auditory curricula, and yet comprehension of onomatopoeic words is important to the child's understanding in reading. The child with hearing loss often has not experienced vocabulary words such as *jingling, tinkling, clanging, rustling,* and *crackling;* these words are not often learned through meaningful experience. Yet comprehension of these words gives the child a rich vocabulary with which to classify and categorize sounds in the everyday environment and in literature. The AV practitioner can present a variety of environmental stimuli when the child first learns the specific vocabulary; later the child can be asked to describe or contrast various sounds. The child may then write sentences, poems, or stories using the sound vocabulary.

Segmentals

Identification of segmentals (vowels and consonants) requires more functional hearing than the identification of suprasegmental information. Children with greater degrees of hearing loss who are highly successful in auditory identification of suprasegmentals may rely more heavily on visual cues for identification of segmentals in everyday situations.

There is a wide variety of speech tests used in audiological assessment with young children that assess recognition of segmentals of speech. The following list, while not intended to be exhaustive, provides a sampling of the diversity of test tools now available.

Glendonald Auditory Screening Test 2 (GASP 2)

The Glendonald Auditory Screening Test 2 (GASP 2) is a recognition test that assesses the child's ability to identify words based on differences in stress patterns among familiar one-, two-, and three-syllable words, and based on vowel and consonant differences (Erber, 1982). A closed set of words is presented, and the child is asked to point to a picture of the word heard.

Implications

This test is an intermediate step between the SAT and the SRT, and *the ability to recognize some words on the GASP 2 is often a signal of emerging word recognition skills.*

The Early Speech Perception Battery

The Early Speech Perception Battery (Moog & Geers, 1990) for young children incorporated a pattern perception and/or simple word identification task, using objects rather than picture stimuli. The AV practitioner can easily create a similar informal test using familiar objects in the child's environment. There are different levels of difficulty, ranging from contrasting one- and two-syllable words, contrasting one-, two-, and three-syllable words, and finally contrasts between two-syllable words with different stress patterns.

Ask the Audiologist

- Is the child able to recognize differences among stress patterns of one-, two-, and three-syllable words? If not, are there any stress patterns that they identify correctly?
- Are there any words that the child identifies correctly within each stress pattern category?

Speech Reception Threshold

The speech reception threshold (SRT), sometimes called the spondee threshold (ST), is the softest level at which the child can familiar two-syllable words (spondees) or point to pictures or objects representing them 50% of the time. Spondees are words with equal stress on both syllables such as hot dog, ice cream, or baseball. The SRT provides a reliability check on the pure tone thresholds. If the child is respond-

ing accurately, one would expect to see agreement between the SRT and the pure tone average.

Implications

- *The first indication of the child's emerging ability to identify speech sounds and words on formal testing is the child's ability to establish an SRT.*
- *The ability to establish an SRT is primarily based on the child's ability to differentiate vowels.* A child with poor consonant identification skills will often have little or no difficulty establishing an SRT.
- The SRT will typically be about 5 to 10 dB greater than the SAT. A listener requires more intensity to identify words than to simply detect the presence of speech.
- Similar to the SAT, the SRT will provide an indication of the optimal level for the identification of speech. For example, listeners with normal hearing require speech at approximately 30 dB above the SRT in order to achieve 100% discrimination scores.

Ask the Audiologist

- Can the child understand familiar words through hearing only?
- What is the softest level at which the child can identify words?
- In the everyday environment where background noise is present, what is the softest level at which the child can identify a small group of words?

- What is the optimal listening level for recognition of speech for this child?
- Can we achieve this optimal level with his or her current amplification—at what distance?
- Can we achieve this optimal level with the use of an FM system coupled to the child's amplification?

Word Discrimination Tests

Word discrimination tests are a measure of the child's ability to recognize monosyllabic words under ideal and typical listening conditions. Ideal conditions include listening at intensity levels of 25 to 30 dB above the SRT without any background noise. Typical conditions may include presenting speech at quiet or normal conversational levels with and without background noise. The child is asked to repeat a list of 25 or 50 words, and the word discrimination score (WDS) is calculated as a percentage reflecting the number of words correct (Example: 16/25 = 64%). The words may be presented in quiet or in noise, and with or without speech reading cues.

A picture word discrimination task such as the NUCHIPS or the WIPI is designed for children of 3 years and above. Four or six words are pictured on each page of a 25- or 50-page booklet, and the child is asked to point to one of the pictures on each page. Because the words on each page use the same vowel but vary the intial and/or final consonant, *this is actually a consonant recognition task from a closed set or mutiple choice format. Word discrimination ability will improve during the*

preschool and early school years, and then stabilize as the child reaches his or her maximum auditory potential.

Word lists such as the PBK or NU-6 are used as the child gets older and refer to open set word repetition tasks where the child has no contextual clues—that is, the words are totally unrelated. The child is required to identify both the vowel and consonant sounds in each word in order to obtain a correct word score. An alternate way of scoring these word lists is by phoneme scoring where each sound in the word is scored (three sounds per word). This provides a better estimate of the child's degree of difficulty with specific speech sounds, especially for children with high-frequency hearing losses.

There are varying interpretations for the WDS. For example, a score of 90% to 100% may be described as excellent word discrimination ability and 50% to 60% as poor word discrimination ability. (See WDS at the end of the chapter.) It is important to remember that the score reflects discrimination ability for a specific task, single words without context, which is the most difficult recognition task possible. If the child was asked to repeat sentence material, the child's word score would increase significantly due to the increased contextual and syntactic clues inherent in sentence material.

Implications

- Closed and open set discrimination test scores cannot be directly compared. Closed set tasks are typically easier than open set tasks. It is therefore important to know which discrimination test has been administered in order to interpret the results. A child receiving 60% on a closed set test does not necessarily have the same auditory capacity as a child receiving 60% on an open set test.

- Word discrimination scores can underestimate the child's recognition of speech, particularly for those with high-frequency precipitous or steeply sloping hearing loss. In these cases, sentence recognition tests provide additional information.
- Speech perception and speech production are integrally linked. The auditory channel is the most natural route through which to learn to talk, and thus listening skills are vital to the development of accurate speech production of vowels and consonants (Ling, 1989). Thus, inclusion of auditory detection and identification exercises for segmental contrasts in learning speech production is highly beneficial.

Ask the Audiologist

- Are there any speech sounds that the child cannot hear?
- What is the child's ability to recognize single words?
  - from a multiple choice format
  - from an open set
- What types of identification errors did the child make?
  - vowels
  - consonant voicing
  - manner of consonant production

- place of consonant production
- Which modalities does the child rely on most for identification of words under ideal conditions?
  - listening only
  - speechreading only
  - combined listening and speechreading
- What effect does the presence of background noise have on the child's identification of words?

Connected Speech

The purpose of using connected speech, such as phrase or sentence repetition tasks, is to assess the child's ability to use contextual clues for identification of speech. Although single word repetition is the most commonly used speech recognition task, it does not reflect the auditory challenges presented in the child's everyday environment, which are recognition and comprehension of a series of sentences. As with word testing, testing can be presented by listening only, by listening and speechreading, by speechreading alone, and in quiet or in noise.

A wide variety of sentence tests are available. The child's task is to repeat the entire sentence as in the BKB Sentences (Bench, Kowal & Bamford, 1979) or the HINT test (Nisson, Soli, & Sullivan, 1994) or the last word in the sentence, as in the Speech Perception in Noise (SPIN) test (Kalikow, Stevens, & Elliott, 1977). The SPIN test adds an additional testing feature by creating sentences with high predictability and low predictability, in order to assess the child's ability to use context.

Ask the Audiologist

- How well is the child able to identify phrase or sentence material, and with what level of complexity (short, medium, or long sentences)?
- Does the addition of speechreading cues improve his or her recognition of sentence material significantly?
- What is the child's ability to recognize sentence material presented in background noise?

COMPREHENSION

Comprehension is the ability to understand the meaning of speech by a variety of responses such as answering questions, following instructions, paraphrasing, or participating in a conversation. By definition, the child's response must be qualitatively different from the stimulus presented (Erber, 1982).

In practice, comprehension activities for very young children are a natural part of communication. Parents are encouraged to develop simple comprehension activities concurrently with identification activities.

The AV practitioner may elicit the first measures of comprehension long before this is tested by the audiologist, through work on following directions, sequencing two or three directions, answering questions about a story first from a closed set and then from an open set, and later as the child gets older, work on single or multiple classroom instructions. Paraphrasing, another type of comprehension task, is essential to

train for clarification of a speaker's message. Paraphrasing is a more sophisticated listening function, blending cognitive, linguistic, and auditory skills, a higher-level activity in AVT, and an essential skill for the classroom.

Standardized Audiological Tests

There are very few formal audiological tests at the comprehension level. The Test of Auditory Comprehension (TAC) is no longer widely used but continues to have value in assessing different levels of phrase complexity and comprehension tasks from a closed set. Subtests 7 through 10 are the only standardized tests of comprehension, and more closely represent the auditory demands of the classroom. However, due to the ease created by the multiple choice answer format and picture cues, they create only a beginning measure of comprehension performance. More sophisticated standardized measures are still needed in an open set context.

Descriptive Measures

Some of the most instructive measures of comprehension are qualitative questionnaires completed by the parent in the preschool years, or the teacher and then the child in the elementary and secondary years. The Children's Home Inventory for Listening Difficulties (CHILD) (Anderson & Smaldino, 2000) is designed for children between 3 and 12 years of age. It is completed by the parent and at later ages by the parent and the child, where the parents assess their child's abilities for 15 different listening situations in the home/family environment. The Listening Inventory for Education-Revised (LIFE-R) (Anderson, Smaldino, & Spangler, 2011) is designed for teachers and children from 6 years and older and looks at challenging listening situations in the classroom. There are additional self-assessment tools for the adolescent with hearing loss that are outside the scope of this chapter. Readers are referred to the Self Assessment of Communication (SAC-A) and the Significant Other Assessment of Communication (SOAC-A) (Crowell, English, McCarthy, & Elkayam, 2005) for this age group.

Results of these descriptive tools provide excellent information for discussion with parents and the child, and provide additional directions for listening practice and support for the child.

Ask the Audiologist

- Is the child able to recognize words and phrases from a closed set of responses?
- Can the child comprehend a short or a long story and answer questions about the story?
- Can the child comprehend a story presented in background noise?

Listening in Noise and Overhearing

Classroom listening conditions vary considerably depending on the grade level, the classroom activity, the number of students in the class, the location of the student in the classroom and proximity to the teacher, and the acoustical conditions of the classroom.

Testing with a variety of speech materials at speech to noise ratios of +5 dB or 0 dB will best replicate the challenging acoustic conditions in most classrooms when the child is not using a classroom amplification system (Crandell & Smaldino, 2005; Hetu, Truchon-Gagnon, & Bilodeau, 1990).

The presence of background noise interferes with comprehension of speech for all children with hearing loss. The extent to which it affects a child depends on the type and degree of the hearing loss and the individual child. Comprehension activities presented in background noise can provide the child an opportunity to practice listening under progressively more difficult listening situations. In this manner, the AV practitioner and the parents can provide successful listening experiences that can change the child's attitude toward noise. The child may become more willing to persevere listening under difficult conditions for a longer time as a result of positive listening experiences.

In order to create listening experiences in noise that range in difficulty, the AV practitioner can use the following guidelines. The least interfering noise conditions are steady-state environmental noises such as fan-type noise, the noise of an overhead projector motor, or the steam from a boiling kettle. Moderately interfering noises include random environmental noises with less predictability, such as cafeteria noise or traffic. The most interfering *noise* is speech from other talkers at the same language level as the listener. (For example, a preschool child would find a familiar fairytale in the background more interfering than a news report on the radio.) Finally, a few speakers talking in the background is more interfering for the listener than many speakers talking at once. (The latter condition more closely resembles random environmental noise.)

Any of the comprehension activities presented in quiet can be reintroduced in noise, beginning with the easiest and moving to more difficult noise conditions if and when the child is ready. This is the most challenging and the most tiring listening activity. The child will be the guide and will indicate, either verbally or nonverbally, when it is time to start and stop.

The Paradox

We define background "noise" as sounds that interfere with the primary signal. But what if the secondary signal also has value? Language research now clearly indicates that overhearing supports language growth in children with normal hearing (Moeller, 2007). It is paradoxical to our earlier approaches in listening skills training where the focus has been to help children to attend only to the primary signal. We now need to incorporate overhearing in AVT by helping children to learn to "listen in" on conversations that are not their own as a tool to their language development. And we need to create assessment tools to evaluate how well children extract information from overhearing.

Content Versus Affect

Much of the audiological data are focused on the content—what did the child hear, what were the optimal thresholds for audibility, or what were the scores under a variety of conditions.

But equally important is how the child approached the task—was the child encouraged or discouraged by the listening tasks, was the child curious about ways to enhance his or her listening, was the child creative in finding new strategies to cope with difficult situations, how does the child engage with others, and how does the child express his or her concerns or challenges? That will determine the directions for discussion, coaching, and counseling. The question that must be asked is how best can we as audiologists and AV practitioners empower the child and the family so they can make these steps with confidence. As practitioners we need to continue to expand our repertoire of skills in co-empowerment to support and enhance the family's journey.

SUMMARY

When the child and family walk through the door to see the audiologist, a myriad of auditory skills can be explored. Often lack of familiarity with audiological terminology and assessment procedures can distance parents and practitioners from the audiologist. (See Appendix 4–A for a list of selected audiological terminology and Appendix 4–B for symbols on the audiogram.) In AVT, however, it is imperative that the practitioner works in tandem with the audiologist. The audiologist and the AV practitioner share the same goals of early identification and management of children with hearing loss, supporting parents to become the primary teachers and providers of an auditory environment, the optimal development of speech and listening skills through the habilitation process, and the integration of auditory skills into everyday living. The information and questions for the audiologist listed in this chapter provide parents and AV practitioners with the basis for mutual sharing of concerns. Areas of mutual exploration can then be identified so that all the key players on the team can contribute to the directions and the outcome of the audiological assessment and ongoing auditory management.

REFERENCES

Anderson, K. L. (2002). *ELF: Early listening function.* Tampa, FL: Educational Audiology Association.

Anderson, K. (2007). *Relationship of hearing loss to listening and learning needs.* Retrieved from http://www.successfor kidswithhearingloss.com

Anderson, K. L., & Smaldino, J. J. (2000). *Children's Home Inventory of Listening Difficulties (CHILD).* Tampa, FL: Educational Audiology Association.

Anderson, K., Smaldino, J., & Spangler, C. (2011). *Listening inventory for education-revised (LIFE-R).* Retrieved from http://www.successforkidswithhearing loss.com

Bench, J., Kowal, A., & Bamford, J. (1979). The BKB (Bamford-Koval-Bench) sentence lists for partially-hearing children. *British Journal of Audiology, 13,* 108–112.

Crandell, C., & Smaldino, J. (2005). Classroom acoustics. In C. Crandell, J. Smaldino, & C. Flexer (Eds.), *Sound field FM amplification: Applications to speech perception and classroom acoustics* (2nd ed., pp. 69–82). New York, NY: Thomson Delmar Learning.

Crowell, R., English, K., McCarthy, P., & Elkayam, J. (2005). Use of a self-assessment technique in counseling adolescents with hearing loss. *Journal of Educational Audiology, 12,* 86–99.

Erber, N. (1982). *Auditory training.* Washington, DC: AG Bell Association for the Deaf and Hard of Hearing.

Hetu, R., Truchon-Gagnon, C., & Bilodeau, S. (1990). Problems of noise in school settings: A review of the literature and the results of an exploratory study. *Journal of Speech Language Pathology and Audiology/Revue d´Orthophonie et d´Audiologie, 14*(3), 31–39.

Kalikow, D., Stevens, K., & Elliott, L. (1977). Development of a test of speech intelligibility in noise with sentence materials using controlled word predictability. *Journal of the Acoustical Society of America, 61,* 1337–1351.

Killion, M., & Mueller, H. (2010). Twenty years later: A new count the dot method. *Hearing Journal, 63*(1), 10.

Ling, D. (1976). *Speech and the hearing-impaired child.* Washington, DC: AG Bell Association for the Deaf and Hard of Hearing.

Ling, D. (1989). *Foundations of spoken language for hearing-impaired children.* Washington, DC: AG Bell Association for the Deaf and Hard of Hearing.

Ling, D. (2002). *Speech and the hearing-impaired child* (2nd ed.). Washington, DC: AG Bell Association for the Deaf and Hard of Hearing.

Moeller, M. P. (2007). What's in a word? In R. Seewald & J. Bamford (Eds.), *A sound foundation through early amplification 2007: Proceedings of the fourth international conference* (pp. 19–31). Switzerland: Phonak AG.

Moog, J. S., & Geers, A. E. (1990). *Early speech perception test for profoundly hearing-impaired children.* St. Louis, MO: Central Institute for the Deaf.

Nisson, M., Soli, S., & Sullivan, J. (1994). Development of the Hearing in Noise Test for the measurement of speech reception thresholds in quiet and in noise. *Journal of the Acoustical Society of America, 95,* 1085–1099.

Office of the Los Angeles County Superintendent of Schools. (1976). *Test of Auditory Comprehension*. North Hollywood, CA: Foreworks.

Owens, E., Kessler, D., Telleen, C., & Schubert, E. (1981). *The Minimal Auditory Capabilities Battery*. St. Louis, MO: Auditec.

Zimmerman-Phillips, S., Osberger, M. F., & Robbins, A. M. (1997). *Infant-Toddler: Meaningful Auditory Integration Scale (IT-MAIS)*. Sylmar, CA: Advanced Bionics Corp.

Appendix 4–A

SELECTED AUDIOLOGICAL TERMINOLOGY

Table 4A-1. Summary Chart of Standard Audiological Tests

Assessment Technique	Measurement of	Determines
Pure tone audiogram	Hearing sensitivity	• Degree of hearing loss • Type of hearing loss • Shape of hearing loss • Ear differences
Impedance audiometry	Middle ear function	• Need for medical intervention • Possible reason for a temporary shift in hearing levels • Need to adjust volume setting of amplification
Speech Awareness Threshold (SAT)	Hearing sensitivity for speech	• Minimal audibility for speech detection • Prediction of optimal intensity for speech
Six-Sound Test GASP 1	Hearing sensitivity using amplification	• Potential for detection and recognition of speech features and environmental sounds • Benefit of amplification
Speech Reception Threshold (SRT)	Hearing sensitivity for speech recognition	• Ability to recognize vowels within words • Minimal audibility and prediction of optimal listening levels for speech recognition
Word discrimination scores (WDS)	Identification of speech	• Ability to recognize vowels and consonants • Differences in word recognition ability between ears

Amplification: refers to hearing aids

BOA: behavioral observation audiometry
method of assessment used with young children; sound is presented and the child's behavioral responses to sound are observed.

CNA: could not average
person did not have measurable hearing at one or more frequencies used to calculate the pure tone average (PTA)

CNT: could not test

CPA: conditioned play audiometry
method of assessment used with children with cognitive age of 2–5 years of age; sound is presented and child is taught to perform some play activity each time he or she heard the sound

DNT: did not test

Hearing Device: refers to hearing aids and other implantable devices

Hearing Technology: refers to hearing aids, other implantable devices, and assistive listening devices

MCL: most comfortable level

NBN: narrow-band noise
noise bands centered at frequencies of 250 through 8000 Hz; used in masking, unaided and aided sound-field testing

NR: no response
no measurable hearing when signal presented at the limits of the audiometer

PTA: pure tone average
average of the pure tone thresholds at 500, 1000, and 2000 Hz in each ear

PTA = −10 to 15 dB: normal hearing

PTA = 16 to 25 dB: minimal hearing loss

PTA = 26 to 40 dB: mild hearing loss

PTA = 41 to 55 dB: moderate hearing loss

PTA = 56 to 70 dB: moderately severe hearing loss

PTA = 71 to 90 dB: severe hearing loss

PTA = 91 dB +: profound hearing loss

SAT: speech awareness threshold, sometimes called speech detection threshold
the faintest level at which the child can detect the presence of speech 50% of the time

SDS: speech discrimination scores
         refers to percentage scores obtained using words, phrases, or sentences

SF: sound field
         refers to the way sound is presented to the child; sound is presented
         through loudspeakers in a soundproof suite; used in unaided and aided
         testing; results always reflect hearing in the better ear

SRT: speech reception threshold
         the faintest level at which the child can repeat or point to pictures of a
         small group of familiar two-syllable words 50% of the time

UCL: uncomfortable loudness level

VRA: visual reinforcement audiometry
         method of assessment where the child is conditioned to look at a toy
         each time he or she hears the sound; used with children with cognitive
         ages of 6–8 months to 3 years.

WDS: word discrimination score
         percentage score obtained by repeating unrelated one-syllable words (or
         pointing to pictures of them); in a 25- or 50-item list; there are varying
         interpretations of the scores such as the following:

         90%–100%:   excellent word discrimination ability

         75%–89%:   slight difficulty

         60%–74%:   moderate difficulty

         50%–59%:   poor word discrimination ability

         Below 50%: very poor word discrimination ability

WT: warble tone
         frequency-modulated pure tones used in unaided and aided sound-field
         testing; used as an alternative stimuli to narrow-band noise stimuli.

Appendix 4-B

SYMBOLS ON THE AUDIOGRAM

○   Pure tone threshold for the right ear

✕   Pure tone thresholds for the left ear

△   Masked pure tone thresholds for the right ear

□   Masked pure tone thresholds for the left ear

< > Bone conduction thresholds for right and left ears

[ ]   Masked bone conduction threshold for right and left ears

S   Unaided thresholds in sound field

MRL Minimal response level

A   Aided thresholds in sound field

5

HEARING AIDS AND AUDITORY-VERBAL THERAPY

Ryan W. McCreery and Elizabeth A. Walker

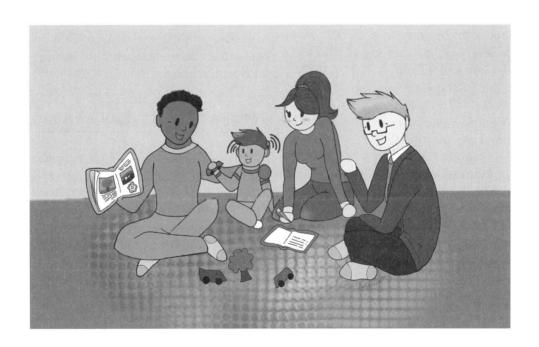

INTRODUCTION

Hearing aids are the most frequently used technology to help improve auditory access for children who have hearing loss. Without amplification, children with hearing loss will experience reduced access to a wide range of sounds, including those that are needed to develop speech and language. As a result, optimizing amplification and promoting consistent hearing aid use are essential for promoting listening and spoken language skills. Parents, audiologists, and auditory-verbal (AV) practitioners all play important roles in maximizing auditory access for children who wear hearing aids.

Here the authors provide a detailed overview of how hearing aids support listening and spoken language in children with hearing loss for AV practitioners, parents, and others who serve children with hearing loss. Hearing aids are a fundamental component of the process of providing Auditory-Verbal Therapy (AVT). Because speech and language are among the most important sounds that children can hear, the importance of making those sounds audible is a key theme. The basic function of hearing aids will be discussed including the latest advances in how hearing aids process sound. Demonstrating the benefits of hearing aids for supporting AVT is important for parents and practitioners. Hearing aids cannot be beneficial if they are not worn, so strategies for promoting consistent hearing aid use across a wide range of listening situations are presented. Children with mild hearing loss and children with auditory neuropathy spectrum disorder are two groups where amplification benefits have been debated and are included at the end of the chapter.

HOW DO HEARING AIDS SUPPORT THE GOALS OF AUDITORY-VERBAL THERAPY?

One key feature of AVT is the emphasis on using the child's listening and auditory skills as the foundation for promoting the development of spoken language and literacy. This emphasis on listening and auditory skills means that hearing aids and cochlear implants (see Chapter 6) are fundamental to AVT. Hearing aids enhance the child's access to sound by increasing its intensity and by processing the sound in specific ways that are discussed later. For now, we will focus broadly on how hearing aids support the goals of AVT.

Maximizing Residual Hearing

The use of auditory skills requires the enhancement of every child's remaining auditory abilities. Children who are born with profound or complete hearing losses that eliminate the child's access to sound may only receive auditory access through cochlear implantation. However, most children with hearing have some amount of hearing, even without amplification. The remaining hearing that is present for children with hearing loss is known as *residual hearing*. In order for children to learn to develop listening skills and spoken language, hearing aids must be used to amplify sounds to maximize the child's ability to use this residual hearing. The range of residual hearing can also be defined as the *dynamic range of hearing*. The dynamic range is the difference between the softest sounds we can hear (hearing thresholds) and the loudest sounds we can tolerate without experiencing discomfort. Hearing thresholds increase with hearing loss, but the listener's ability to tolerate loud sounds does not increase. Sometimes, the ability to tolerate loud sounds decreases with hearing loss. As a result residual hearing decreases as degree of hearing loss gets worse, as illustrated by the two panels in Figure 5–1.

Amplified sound that is above threshold and within the child's dynamic range is considered to be audible to the child. The dynamic range of hearing may be large for children with mild and moderate hearing losses, which makes amplification of speech sounds rela-tively easy to accomplish. The dynamic range becomes narrow for children with severe or profound hearing losses. Hearing aids make speech and other sounds audible to maximize the resid-ual hearing of each child and increase the dynamic range. The amount of amplification, also known as *gain*, pro-vided by a hearing aid is customized based on the child's residual hearing. The individual prescription of amplifi-cation is crucial to providing auditory access and maximizing audibility.

Making Speech and Other Environmental Sounds Audible

Children are exposed to a wide range of sounds in their everyday listening environments. One focus of AVT is on increasing the child's access to the

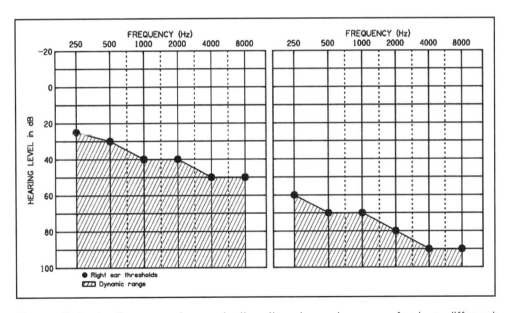

Figure 5-1. Audiograms demonstrating the dynamic range for two different degrees of hearing loss. Actual dynamic ranges for two individuals with these audiograms may vary.

sounds. The amount of access that a child has to sound with their residual hearing is known as *audibility*. Audibility is often defined in reference to how well a listener can hear the sounds that make up speech. The audibility for speech can be quantified using metrics like the Speech Intelligibility Index (SII; ANSI S3.5:1997 R2007), which is a number between 0 and 1 that describes the amount of the speech spectrum that is audible. Higher numbers mean that more of the speech spectrum is audible to the listener. However, environmental sounds also serve important purposes for learning, awareness of sound, and safety. Children often encounter listening situations with multiple talkers and different sources of background noise where these sound sources can change in terms of location or intensity. For example, in school classrooms, a child may need to attend to the teacher and other students during a classroom discussion, while also hearing steady background noise from the air-conditioner and intermittent noise from students in the hallways outside the classroom. In social situations, children may listen to multiple friends with background noise that includes different people talking. These situations require the child to pay attention to the specific talker of interest and to know which talkers are part of the background. Hearing aids can help in these complex listening situations by increasing audibility for speech and environmental sounds. In environments with high levels of background noise, additional hearing assistance technology, such as remote-microphone frequency or digital modulation (FM or DM, respectively) systems may be used to enhance the child's access to a specific talker of interest,

such as the teacher (see Chapter 7). The improved audibility provided by hearing aids provides the best auditory access in a wide range of listening situations that will support learning, socialization, and greater opportunities for social participation with hearing peers.

Increasing Auditory Stimulation to Promote Linguistic and Cognitive Development

Hearing aids increase a child's access to the acoustic cues needed to support listening and learning. More recently, the positive impact of auditory stimulation on brain development in children with hearing loss has been reported in the literature. Limited auditory exposure has been linked to lack of development of the auditory areas of the brain (e.g., Sharma, Dorman, & Spahr, 2002). Auditory stimulation from hearing aids and cochlear implants is likely to promote development of these areas (e.g., Sharma, Dorman, & Kral, 2005). Research suggests that there are two mechanisms by which auditory stimulation provided by hearing aids can support development. Children with better auditory access will have higher performance on a wide range of auditory tasks because the hearing aids provide immediate access to the cues needed to perform the task. Additionally, there is a cumulative impact of increasing auditory access on the development of linguistic and cognitive abilities over time (Pisoni, 2000; Tomblin et al., 2015). The cumulative effect of auditory stimulation is that children with greater auditory experience will develop stronger cognitive and linguistic skills that will enhance their ability to listen, speak, and learn over time.

Consider two hypothetical children who wear hearing aids and are entering primary school. Jimmy has good audibility for speech through his hearing aids and has worn his hearing aids during all waking hours since early childhood. Timmy has good audibility for speech through his hearing aids but has experienced long periods of time without amplification during infancy and early childhood. Both Jimmy and Timmy have the same immediate auditory access to speech from their teacher and classmates. Jimmy is also more likely to have the cumulative benefits of auditory experience because of greater hearing aid use. When access to the acoustic cues that are needed to understand speech are reduced, listeners must rely on top-down processing to help them understand the message. Top-down processing skills are cognitive and linguistic skills that enable a listener to understand and process incoming information. As a result of enhanced cumulative auditory experience, Jimmy may have better cognitive and linguistic skills to support speech recognition when audibility is reduced by background noise. Timmy may lag behind due to limited device use. This comparison highlights the importance of promoting consistent early auditory experience, not only for immediate access to sounds in the environment, but also for increasing the cumulative auditory stimulation needed to support the development of auditory, linguistic, and cognitive abilities that enhance listening in everyday situations.

AN INTRODUCTION TO HEARING AIDS

A deep understanding of how hearing aids work is essential to AV practitioners and parents. Examples of two types of behind-the-ear hearing aids are displayed in Figure 5–2.

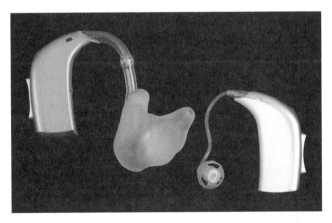

Figure 5–2. A behind-the-ear hearing aid coupled to an earmold (*left*) and a behind-the-ear hearing aid coupled to a receiver-in-the-ear with a comfort dome.

Hearing aids receive sounds from the environment through a microphone. The acoustic energy from the environment is converted to an electrical signal. In most modern hearing aids, the electrical signal from the microphone is converted to a digital signal. Digital hearing aids contain a small microprocessor (a computer) that changes the digital signal based on the listener's hearing needs. After processing, the digital signal is converted back to an electrical signal and sent to a speaker, known as the receiver. The receiver changes the electrical signal back into amplified sound that is sent to the ear. The entire amplification process must happen in less than 10 thousandths of a second or the listener may notice that the amplified sound is delayed compared to the visual cues in the environment. For most children with hearing loss, the hearing aid produces sound that is routed into the ear canal using air conduction. In some cases, children may be born without an ear canal or with physical differences that prevent sound from being routed through the ear canal with air conduction. Using bone conduction, amplified sound can also be converted to mechanical vibra-

tions by the hearing aid, which can be transmitted to the skull using a hard or soft headband or surgical implant. Different bone conduction hearing aid devices are shown in Figure 5–3.

Who Should Wear Hearing Aids?

Generally, hearing loss of any degree can have a negative impact on a child's development of spoken language. Therefore, organizations such as the American Academy of Audiology (American Academy of Audiology, 2013) and Australian Hearing (King, 2010) recommend that every child with hearing loss be considered a candidate for hearing aids. Figure 5–4 shows the range of hearing thresholds that are usually recommended for hearing aids in children.

Hearing aids are typically recommended for children with mild to severe hearing losses. Children in the severe or profound hearing loss range are often considered to be candidates for cochlear implants and will use hearing aids prior to receiving cochlear implantation to provide auditory stimulation and awareness of sound.

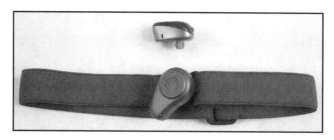

Figure 5–3. A Cochlear Baha bone conduction sound processor (*top*) and an Oticon Ponto bone conduction sound processor coupled to a soft headband. Both devices take incoming acoustic energy and convert it to vibrations for conduction to the inner ear.

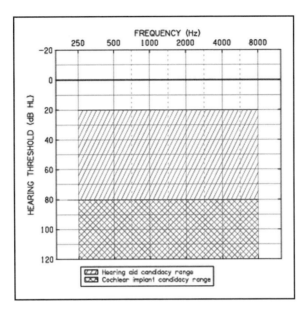

Figure 5-4. The typical candidacy range for hearing aids (*hatched area*) and for cochlear implants (*cross-hatched area*). Other factors beyond the audiogram are also important for determining cochlear implant candidacy, including the child's development, aided audibility, and speech recognition ability in older children.

When Should Hearing Aids Be Fit?

Although babies often do not say their first words until around 12 months of age, auditory experience during infancy is crucial for promoting the development of spoken language (Kuhl, Conboy, Padden, Nelson, & Pruitt, 2005). For example, an infant's ability to hear the difference between two vowel sounds at 6 months of age is a strong predictor of his or her spoken language development up to 2 years of age (Tsao, Liu, & Kuhl, 2004). Therefore, early provision of amplification for children with hearing loss can ensure that the process of neural maturation and awareness of speech sounds begins as soon as possible. A shift toward early identification of hearing loss and fitting of amplification has occurred rapidly over the past two decades. In a paper by Moeller in 2000, for example, the average age of diagnosis for children with hearing loss was around 2½ years of age. More recently, studies have shown the median age of diagnosis is around 3 to 4 months with a median age of hearing aid fitting around 6 to 7 months of age (Holte et al., 2012). Generally, children with hearing loss should be fit with amplification as soon as possible after hearing loss has been diagnosed to minimize the amount of time where auditory stimulation is limited, consistent with the core tenets of AVT. The timing of amplification may be affected by a wide range of factors, including inconclusive diagnostic results, waiting time for audiology appointments, the presence of middle ear fluid or other general health concerns, and children who are lost during the follow-up process (Walker et al., 2014). Many of these factors that could delay amplification are preventable, and audiologists and others who serve children with hearing loss should strive to minimize delays in fitting amplification.

THE HEARING AID FITTING PROCESS

Fitting children with hearing aids is not a single, one-time event. Rather, it is an ongoing process that occurs regularly throughout the child's development and involves the audiologist, parents, AV practitioners, and others. The hearing aid fitting process is initiated with the confirmation of permanent hearing loss with a diagnostic hearing evaluation by an audiologist. Based on the results and input from the parents, the audiologist selects the appropriate hearing aids and signal processing technologies for the child. The hearing aids are then programmed and fit on the child, and the audibility provided by the hearing aids is verified. The parents and other professionals involved in the use of hearing aids are oriented as to the care, maintenance, and function of the devices by the audiologist. Finally, the benefits of hearing aids must be assessed by parents, AV practitioners, and/or audiologists during the outcome validation phase of the process. Each of these steps is repeated as

necessary based on the child's progress and development.

Diagnostic Assessment

In order to know whether or not a hearing aid is needed and how much amplification should be provided, a diagnostic assessment of hearing (discussed more specifically in Chapter 3) is an important first step in the process of providing hearing aids to infants and young children. Hearing thresholds in each ear are measured using either behavioral audiometry or estimates of behavioral hearing based on electrophysiological measures, such as the auditory brainstem response (ABR) or auditory steady-state response (ASSR). Unlike adults, where the entire audiogram may be measured in both ears in a single test, both electrophysiological and behavioral tests may provide less information in children because the child may wake up or lose interest during the test. Other tests, such as tympanometry and otoacoustic emissions, may provide supplemental information about the status of the middle ear and inner ear organ of hearing (cochlea) but do not measure frequency-specific hearing thresholds that are needed to fit hearing aids. After a diagnosis of hearing loss is made based on the diagnostic hearing evaluation, the audiologist should refer the family to an ear, nose, and throat (ENT or otolaryngologist) physician for medical evaluation and clearance for hearing aids. This process helps to ensure that any underlying medical concerns related to the hearing loss are identified. Additionally, referrals to ophthalmology and medical genetics may also be recommended to assess the child's vision and potential genetic causes of hearing loss, respectively.

Earmolds

Earmolds are molds of the child's ear that are used to connect a behind-the-ear hearing aid to the child's ear canal for air-conduction hearing aids. Impressions of the ear for earmolds are often taken at the diagnostic evaluation if permanent hearing loss is confirmed. Taking ear impressions early in the process allows time for fabrication prior to the fitting and avoids delays in the amplification fitting. The earmold is not simply a conduit for sound to reach the child's ear canal from the hearing aid but can be manufactured to alter the sound that passes through it. Dampers or filters can be used to enhance or minimize specific frequencies. Increasing or decreasing the diameter of the tubing can affect the amount of amplification at specific frequencies. Even with digital hearing aid signal processing that allows precise manipulation of the amount of gain provided by the hearing aid, selecting earmolds with specific features to enhance the frequency response of the hearing aid can be useful. The audiologist will select the earmold characteristics that are appropriate for the child's ear and degree of hearing loss. For young children, audiologists are likely to select a soft earmold material that is easy to modify, such as silicone or vinyl. Older children may transition to harder acrylic material depending on their preference. Parents and children can select from a wide range of earmold colors from clear or skin color, to bright neon colors or mixtures of colors.

Earmolds have a limited life span and should be regularly replaced to ensure consistent coupling with the ear canal. An earmold that provides a good connection with the ear canal ensures the amount of gain provided by the hearing aid is consistent as the child's ear canal grows. The length of time that each earmold lasts depends on the age of the child, the earmold material, and the care and maintenance of the earmold. Infants and younger children usually experience significant ear canal growth, particularly during the first year of life, which means that a new earmold may be needed as often as every 3 months. As children get older, their ear canals continue to grow, but the rate of growth is much slower, and earmolds can provide a good fit of the ear canal for over a year in some cases. Hard earmold materials, such as vinyl and acrylic, tend to last longer than softer materials, such as silicone.

Selection of Amplification

After the diagnostic assessment indicates the presence of permanent hearing loss, the audiologist, in consultation with the family, must select the hearing aid and signal processing characteristics that will provide the child with the best auditory access. The audiologist may be selecting a hearing aid for an infant but should select a device that can adapt to the child's needs over as long as 5 years. Although the child's earmold will be replaced numerous times as the child's ear grows, replacement of hearing aids can be cost prohibitive.

As a result, behind-the-ear (BTE) hearing aids are most frequently recommended for use with infants and young children. Another consideration when selecting a BTE hearing aid is the color of the case, which can be selected by the family. Bright colors are easier to find if the hearing aid is misplaced compared to beige or other neutral colors. Additional advantages of BTE hearing aids over other styles of hearing aids for children are summarized in Table 5–1.

Levels of Technology

Most hearing aid manufacturers offer at least three different levels or tiers of technology. The cost of the hearing aid increases as the level of technology increases. Higher cost often leads to the conclusion that higher (and more expensive) levels of technology might lead to better hearing and developmental outcomes. There is little evidence, however, to suggest that higher levels of technology create better outcomes in terms of speech recognition or language development. If an audiologist recommends a higher level of technology, the parents need to ask for research to support the recommendation. Parents and AV practitioners also can ask the dispensing audiologist for hearing aid specifications for the specific makes and models of hearing aids being recommended. Fortunately, audibility for speech can be achieved at all levels of technology. Selecting a less expensive hearing aid may allow the family to purchase additional hearing assistance technology or other devices that support connectivity.

Selection of Hearing Aid Signal Processing

As part of the selection process, the dispensing audiologist must determine what specific signal processing features in the hearing aid will be activated for each child. Nearly all modern digital hearing aids include a wide range of signal processing features that can be activated by the audiologist through programming. The audiologist needs to use a pediatric, evidence-based rationale for activating specific features. Preferably, the research used to justify the activation of specific signal processing features should be based on data obtained from children who wear hearing aids. This research evidence is increasing but is still extremely limited. Following is a brief review of the major types of hearing aid signal processing and considerations for parents and AV practitioners for common features. A more complete review of hearing aid signal processing considerations for children and evidence-based systematic reviews are available on the topics of amplitude compression (McCreery et al., 2012a), frequency lowering (McCreery et al., 2012c), and digital noise reduction and direction microphones (McCreery et al., 2012b).

Amplitude Compression

As mentioned earlier, the sounds that comprise speech must be made audible with amplification without making those sounds uncomfortably loud. In order to provide audibility across a wide range of different sounds, nearly all hearing aids use a feature called *amplitude compression* to adjust the amount

Table 5–1. Advantages of Behind-the-Ear Hearing Aids for Children

1. **Durability**: Behind-the-ear (BTE) hearing aids are more resistant to moisture and debris than smaller in-the-ear (ITE) hearing aids. On average, the increased durability means that BTE hearing aids need fewer repairs and also last 2–3 years longer than ITE hearing aids.
2. **Growth**: As the child's ear grows, the earmold used with a BTE hearing aid can be replaced to improve the fit of the device. Replacing the shell on an ITE means that the entire device must be sent to the manufacturer to make a new shell. Time without amplification reduces auditory experience and access for children with hearing loss and should be minimized.
3. **Adaptability**: If the child experiences a change in hearing, the amount of amplification provided by a BTE hearing aid can be adjusted over a much larger range than with an ITE hearing aid. The ability to change the amount of gain provided by the hearing aid decreases the potential that new hearing aids will be needed if the child's hearing changes.
4. **Real-ear-to-coupler difference:** The acoustics of the child's earmold can be estimated using a real-ear-to-coupler difference measurement with a BTE hearing aid. Verification for ITE hearing aids must occur with all of the measurements in the child's ear canal, which may not be possible for many children.
5. **Connectivity**: BTE hearing aids are more likely to connect hearing aids to accessories via hard-wired, wireless, or Bluetooth connections than ITE hearing aids. The connectivity of BTE hearing aids can increase access to different listening environments and devices like computers and tablets that can be important educationally and socially.

of amplification or gain that sounds receive. Soft sounds receive the most gain, average sounds receive slightly less gain, and loud sounds receive little or no gain. In other words, as the input level of sound to the hearing aid increases, the amount of amplification provided by the hearing aid decreases. This strategy provides enough amplification to make soft sounds audible without making loud sounds uncomfortable. The amount of amplitude compression that is prescribed will depend on how much hearing loss the child has. Different amounts of amplitude compression can be used to accommodate two children with different amounts of residual hearing.

Guidance for the AV Practitioner

If the parent or AV practitioner notices that a child is having difficulty hearing soft sounds or is experiencing loudness discomfort, the audiologist should be notified to adjust the amplitude compression parameters of the hearing aid. Conversely, too much amplitude compression can reduce the contrast between speech sounds and make speech understanding more difficult. Providing specific information about the types of sounds that are inaudible or uncomfortable can help the audiologist pinpoint the specific areas of difficulty without compromising audibility for speech sounds. *The AV practitioner may ask the child's audiologist:* How is the amount of amplitude compression in the hearing aid fitting determined? How audible are soft sounds with and without the hearing aid? How does the hearing aid make the sounds of conversational speech more audible? How does the hearing aid process louder speech, compared to average or soft speech?

Feedback Suppression

The whistling sound that is produced by a hearing aid when it is held in the hand or not fully inserted is known as *acoustic feedback.* Feedback most commonly occurs when amplified sound from the hearing aid reaches the microphone and is amplified over and over again in a feedback loop. Children who wear hearing aids may not even hear feedback, but parents and practitioners may notice feedback when inserting the hearing aids or holding them in their hands. Most hearing aids contain some type of signal processing to minimize the likelihood of feedback. Feedback suppression systems in hearing aids may limit the gain of the hearing aid at high frequencies in an attempt to limit feedback. In some cases, it may be possible to preserve gain for high-frequency sounds by addressing feedback through new earmolds that better seal the child's ear canal. Feedback suppression needs to be activated for children at all ages, as long as it does not impose significant limitations on amplification for high-frequency sounds.

Guidance for the AV Practitioner

AV practitioners or parent(s) may be the first to notice that the fit of the earmold is insufficient. Signs to watch for include difficulty with keeping the earmold in the ear or excessive feedback. Gaps around the earmold may become larger as children's ears grow. Large gaps in the earmold might indicate that new earmolds may be needed. Feedback suppression makes changes to the sound coming out of the hearing aid, which can lead to distortion of sounds, particularly for listeners with severe or profound hearing loss. Prompt replacement of earmolds can help to minimize the unnecessary application of feedback suppression and distortion of speech. *The AV practitioner may ask the child's audiologist:* Does the feedback management system in this hearing aid limit the amount of high-frequency amplification? If so, is it possible to provide more amplification and better audibility with a new earmold? Does feedback suppression, when activated, change the quality of speech?

Frequency Lowering

High-frequency speech sounds, such as /s/ and /sh/, serve important functions for communication. The /s/ sound, for example, is the third most frequently occurring phoneme in English. Recent research suggests that even well-fit hearing aids may not provide enough amplification in the high frequencies to make /s/ audible (Kimlinger, McCreery, & Lewis, 2015)., and this, of course, will negatively affect speech and language development (Koehlinger, Van Horne, Oleson, McCreery, & Moeller, 2015;

Moeller et al., 2007). An alternative to amplifying high-frequency sounds is to process those sounds at lower frequencies, where the child's degree of hearing loss might be less and the amount of amplification provided by the hearing aid could be greater. Different hearing aid manufacturers use different approaches to frequency lowering, but most are in two categories. Frequency compression lowers high-frequency sounds by moving them to lower frequencies and compacting those sounds into a smaller range. Frequency transposition moves high-frequency information to lower frequencies using a "cut-and-paste" approach that places those sounds on top of speech sounds at lower frequencies. The type of approach used for a specific child may depend on the child's degree and configuration of hearing loss and some other factors, but the overall goal is to make high-frequency sounds more audible to promote auditory access.

Guidance for the AV Practitioner

AV practitioners need to be aware that without frequency lowering, many children will not be able to discriminate between /s/ and /sh/ sounds easily, because those sounds are not sufficiently amplified. Limited high-frequency amplification can be related to the child's degree of hearing loss, limited high-frequency gain in hearing aids, or a combination of these factors. Frequency lowering can increase audibility for high-frequency sounds for children with mild to moderate hearing losses (McCreery et al., 2014; Wolfe et al., 2011) and those with severe to profound hearing loss (Glista et al.,

2009). Audiologists may not always communicate that frequency lowering has been activated. In some cases, the initial setting for frequency lowering may not optimize audibility. Therefore, AV practitioners may need to inquire about the activation of frequency lowering, particularly in cases when children are not perceiving or producing high-frequency speech sounds. *The AV practitioner may want to ask the child's audiologist:* Is frequency lowering activated in the hearing aid? What type of frequency lowering is used? What speech sounds are likely to be lowered? How does frequency lowering affect vowel and consonant discrimination when appropriately used? What types of errors would be expected if frequency lowering needs settings need to be adjusted? If the speaker moves closer to the microphone of the hearing aid, will this affect frequency lowering?

Directional Microphones

Background noise is a persistent problem in most everyday listening environments, where children need to learn, socialize, and communicate. Although hearing assistance technologies, such as frequency-modulation (FM) systems, can be used in classrooms, these options may not be optimal for listening situations with more than one talker. Hearing aids often have multiple microphones that can be used to determine the location of sound relative to the listener and reduce the amount of gain provided to sounds that originate from the side or behind the listener. Omnidirectional microphones are equally sensitive to sounds from all directions. Directional microphones are more sensitive to sounds that arrive from a specific direction, usually in front of the listener, while providing less amplification for sounds that arrive from the sides and behind the listener. Intuitively, reducing sound from the sides and behind the listener will enhance listening for sounds that the listener is facing. However, children are not always facing the people with whom they are communicating. If the parent or other important speaker is to the side or behind the child, the audibility for those listeners may be reduced, although typically the amount of reduction is very small (1–3 dB; Ching et al., 2009). Overhearing is also an important mechanism to support vocabulary development in children (Akhtar, 2005), and there are concerns that overhearing may be reduced in children if they are using directional microphones. For this reason, directional microphones need to be used selectively in older children who are reliably able to orient toward the talker of interest. In some hearing aids, directionality can be activated automatically when the hearing aid detects that the listener is in a noisy environment.

Guidance for the AV Practitioner

AV practitioners need to know whether or not a child's hearing aid has directional microphones. If so, he or she can help the audiologist, child, and parents to determine the listening environments where directional microphones may be most beneficial (the child is facing the talker of interest with noise sources behind) and situations where the benefit of directional microphones may be limited (the speaker of interest may move around the child and/or where

sources of noise come from in front of the child). *The AV practitioner may ask the child's audiologist:* Does the hearing aid have directional microphones? How are the directional microphones activated (automatically or manually)? Who is responsible for switching the hearing aid to directional mode? If the directional microphone is used in therapy sessions, how can I help my child or client to listen if I need to sit facing him or her? Is there a way that the hearing aid can tell automatically whether omnidirectional or directional microphones should be activated?

Noise Reduction

In addition to directional microphones, many hearing aids include additional signal processing that reduces the amount of gain provided by the hearing aid when the hearing aid detects background noise. Noise reduction reduces the amount of gain provided by the hearing aid, but can also reduce the amount of audibility for speech sounds. Some hearing aids avoid this by reducing input only when steady-state noises, such as noise from ventilation systems or a computer fan, are detected by the hearing aid. The frequencies where gain is reduced can depend on the noise reduction system. In some cases, gain is reduced only in the low frequencies, whereas other systems may reduce gain across the entire speech frequency range. The reduction in gain also means that current noise reduction systems cannot improve speech understanding in noise. However, research suggests that noise reduction may improve the comfort of listening situations for children (Stelmachowicz et al., 2010). Because most digital noise reduction systems would be unlikely to have a negative or positive effect on speech understanding, noise reduction should be considered as a feature for children.

Guidance for the AV Practitioner

For children who experience loudness discomfort in background noise, the AV practitioner may ask if the audiologist would recommend that noise reduction be activated or the amount of noise reduction increased. *The AV practitioner may ask the child's audiologist:* Is noise reduction activated in the hearing aid? If so, how much reduction in gain or audibility occurs when the noise reduction is activated? What signs will be present if there is too much or not enough noise reduction? What methods does the audiologist could use to determine the benefits of noise reduction?

Hearing Aid Fitting and Verification

Following the selection of the device and which features will be activated, the child can be fit with the hearing aid. The primary goal at the hearing aid fitting is to verify that the hearing aid provides audibility for speech sounds and to orient the caregivers and the child to the device. Verification is a crucial step in making sure that the hearing aid is doing what it is supposed to do. Orientation helps to increase the comfort level of caregivers and children with managing amplification on a day-to-day basis, including insertion and removal of earmolds, care and maintenance of the hearing aids and earmolds, and establishing a schedule for hearing aid use.

Verification

Ear canal size varies across children and over time as they grow. Hearing aids deliver sound to the ear canal, but the amount of sound received depends on the size of the ear canal. A hearing aid set to provide a specific amount of gain in a large, adult ear canal will produce a much louder sound level in a smaller ear canal of a child because of how sound pressure increases in smaller spaces. The differences in ear canal size among children mean that the level of the hearing aid in the child's ear canal must be verified to ensure the levels are safe and that sounds are audible. Changes in ear canal size over time also will affect the sound level delivered by the hearing aid. Therefore, hearing aid verification needs to be repeated periodically. Generally, it is recommended that hearing aid verification be completed every 3 to 6 months in children less than 3 years of age and every year in children over 3 years of age. Verification also needs to happen any time the child receives a new earmold, because a new earmold can change the sound level delivered to the ear canal.

Hearing aid verification is completed using a probe microphone system. A small, flexible tube, known as a probe tube, is placed into the child's ear canal. The probe tube is connected to a microphone that typically hangs over the child's ear. The probe microphone compares the sound delivered outside the ear to the sound level inside the ear canal to estimate the output of the hearing aid. There are two types of probe microphone measures that can be completed, depending on the age of the child. For older children, the output of the hearing aid in the ear canal is measured using multiple measures of speech at soft, average, and loud levels to ensure that the range of speech is audible. For infants and younger children who may not have the attention and patience to cooperate with multiple measurements in each ear canal, the audiologist can measure the acoustics of the child's ear canal with the earmold, which is called the real-ear-to-coupler difference (RECD). The RECD is actually a comparison of a soft sound presented through the child's earmold to the same sound measured in a coupler that is designed to mimic the volume of an adult ear canal. By taking an RECD measurement in the child's ear, the child's individual ear canal acoustics can be incorporated into hearing aid measurements completed in the coupler. This requires only a single measurement in the child's ear. Age-related average RECD values are available but are not as accurate as RECD values from individual children.

Once the aided levels of speech have been measured in the child's ear canal or in the coupler using the RECD, the audibility of each level can be calculated. The aided level of speech measured in the child's ear canal is compared to the child's hearing thresholds to determine how much of the aided speech energy is above the child's threshold. Most verification equipment provides an estimate of the aided audibility as the SII. Research has demonstrated that children who wear hearing aids who have better aided audibility have higher language abilities (Tomblin et al., 2015) and better speech recognition (McCreery et al., 2015) than children with poorer audibility. The audiologist may also measure a loud sound through the hearing aid in order to ensure that the hearing aid does not exceed a level that would be uncomfortably loud. The audiologist needs to report the aided audibility to the parents and the AV practitioner to monitor the audibility provided by hearing aids over time. Figure 5–5 includes two examples of children with different amounts of audibility provided by their hearing aid fittings. Verification needs to be repeated at the initial hearing aid fitting and also any time that there is a change in the audiogram, earmold, or hearing aid. Typically, hearing aid verification is repeated every 3 months for children under 1 year of age, every 6 months for children under 3 years of age, and annually for children over 3 years of age.

Guidance for the AV Practitioner

Verification measures can help the AV practitioner to set realistic goals and expectations for sound detection and speech recognition. For example, if probe microphone verification indicates that high-frequency (4000 Hz and above) audibility is limited, the child may not be able to discriminate between fricative speech sounds without frequency lowering. Results from verification can also help the AV practitioner to visualize the relative amounts of amplification for soft, average, and loud speech signals to determine if the speech spectrum is audible and how much compression is present. *The AV practitioner may ask the child's audiologist:* How audible are soft and average speech with and without the hearing aid? Is the amount of audibility within the expected range for this child's

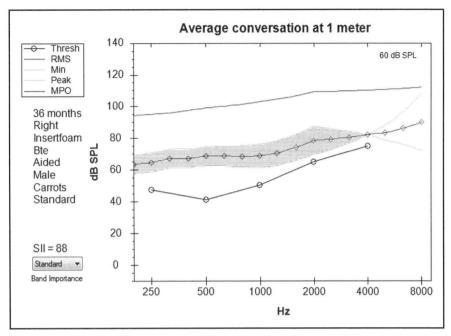

A

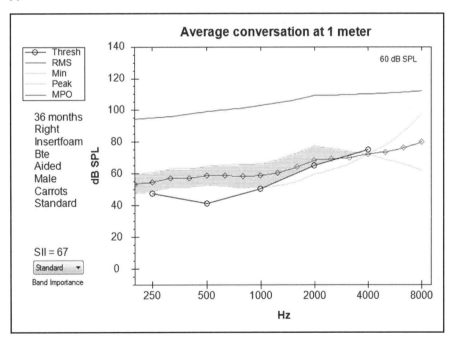

B

Figure 5-5. Audibility for the long-term average speech spectrum for a hearing aid fitted to optimize audibility (*Panel A*) and fitted at less than optimal audibility (*Panel B*). Note the lower Speech Intelligibility Index (SII) for the right panel, even though the audiogram is the same.

degree of hearing loss? Does the verification suggest that the speech spectrum is receiving too much or too little amplitude compression? How audible are high-frequency sounds?

Hearing Aid Validation

Verification ensures that the hearing aids provide audibility for speech, which is important for success in AVT. Therefore, the child's progress in listening and spoken language development needs to be documented through validation, in addition to other formal developmental assessments. Two types of validation are commonly recommended for children: parental questionnaires and aided speech perception assessment. Both types of assessments provide important information about the child's auditory development and are covered in greater detail in Chapter 3. Additionally, McCreery and colleagues (2015) have cited outcomes on parent questionnaires and aided speech recognition measures for a large group of children who use hearing aids.

Parent Questionnaires

Questionnaires about the child's progress in audition and spoken communication can provide valuable information about the parents' perspectives on a child's development. A large number of these are available that cover age ranges from infancy through adolescence. Most can be completed by parents independently, or through an interview. Many provide an age-equivalent score to give parents and the AV practitioner a perspective on the child's development of auditory skills. Question-

naires need to be appropriate for a child's developmental age, rather than chronological age, as parents may become frustrated if the questions discuss developmental milestones that the child has yet to achieve or if the child has advanced beyond the skills assessed by the questionnaire. Comparing questionnaire scores to normative data for children with typical hearing and repeated administrations of parent questionnaires can provide some evidence of progress, but this is not in lieu of standardized speech, language, and hearing assessments. Questionnaires can provide a useful framework for parents to understand what types of auditory skills and behaviors to watch for as their child develops. Specific examples are provided in Chapter 3.

Aided Speech Perception Assessment

In Chapter 3, the use of unaided speech recognition assessment was discussed. Similarly, aided speech recognition assessment provides valuable information about how the child uses the audibility provided by hearing aids to support listening and spoken language. Awareness of speech can be assessed during infancy. Starting at a developmental age of 18 to 24 months, most children can participate in some form of generative speech recognition assessment. Some tasks, such as the Ling Six-Sound Test (Ling, 1978), can be used to assess a child's detection or discrimination of isolated speech sounds with the hearing aids. The ability to recognize familiar words or sentences can also be assessed using speech materials that are appropriate for children. If children have limited expressive speech or language skills, speech recognition can also be assessed using toys or pictures that the child can point to. Once a child has achieved high levels of word or sentence recognition in quiet, speech recognition can also be tested with background noise to more closely approximate conditions in everyday listening situations.

Children who wear hearing aids have a wide range of auditory skills and abilities, which means that it can be difficult to determine whether or not a child with hearing loss is achieving an appropriate level of aided speech recognition. Even for the few speech recognition tests with normative data for children who wear hearing aids, the range of typical performance can be large. Poor speech recognition abilities in children who wear hearing aids can be due to a number of different factors. If a child with hearing aids has poorer speech recognition than would be expected, the audibility of the hearing aid can be verified to ensure that the speech signal is audible. Speech recognition is dependent on language and cognitive abilities, so children with deficits in these areas of development may have lower speech recognition than children with hearing loss who have stronger skills in these areas. Repeated speech recognition assessment over time can provide evidence for growth of auditory skills. Children should generally continue to improve in speech recognition abilities as they grow and develop.

Aided Pure Tone Thresholds or Functional Gain

Prior to the development of probe microphone systems that could be used for verification of audibility, audiologists would often measure a listener's audiometric thresholds through a loudspeaker to provide evidence that amplification was improving the detection of pure tones compared to their unaided thresholds. Although the approach of measuring the same pure tones used to assess unaided hearing with amplification may seem intuitive, the limitations of this approach are substantial. Pure tones may be affected by signal processing in hearing aids, leading to responses that are not reflective of audibility for speech. Even if a child can detect pure tones at very soft levels in a sound booth, aided pure tone thresholds provide limited information about how well the child can understand speech in realistic situations. Aided pure tone thresholds should only be completed when other measures of audibility are not possible, such as in children with bone-conduction devices and children with cochlear implants. Aided speech recognition assessment has greater validity for predicting speech recognition in everyday listening situations, because the stimulus is speech.

HEARING AID USE

The principles of AVT are closely tied to the issue of audibility. Unfortunately, the benefits of audibility are restricted by the amount of time hearing aids are worn throughout the day. Even the most optimally fit hearing aid cannot help with learning speech and language skills if the child is not wearing it. As anyone with a toddler or preschooler knows, it can be challenging to even get them to wear socks some days, let alone a device that goes in his or her ear and can be easily removed. The following describes strategies for maximizing hearing aid use, and ways that parents and AV practitioners can track this.

How to Measure Hearing Aid Use?

Our target goal for daily hearing aid use in infants and children is all waking hours (with the exception of bath time and other water activities). Parents and practitioners have several tools to determine how often hearing aids are being worn throughout the day. When parents just estimate the average number of hours the child wears hearing aids, it is difficult to estimate what an "average" day is. In a recent study (Walker et al., 2013), parents reported that consistency of their child's hearing aid use often depended on the situation; for example, infants and toddlers were less likely to wear hearing aids in unsupervised settings such as in the car or at day care. Parents also noted that it is difficult to get children to wear hearing aids during activities such as nursing the child, when there is loud background noise, or the child is tired, sick, or having a tantrum (Moeller, Hoover, Peterson, & Stelmachowicz, 2009). Thus, the amount of time a child is wearing his or her hearing aids is likely to depend on what's going on— if parents are running errands and the child is in his or her car seat, the hearing aids may not be worn because of concerns about losing them. If the family is home all day or the child is at school and is closely monitored, hearing aid use time may be higher. The busy, fluctuating schedules of typical families may make it difficult to estimate daily use time, even for the most attentive parents. Therefore, we may need to use other, more objective tools for determining daily use.

A relatively recent technology in hearing aids is data logging. Data logging is an automatic feature built into most current hearing aids (McCreery, 2013; Mueller, 2007), which reports on how often hearing aids are turned on (more specifically, how often the battery door is closed and the battery is activated). Audiologists can utilize the data logging function by connecting hearing aids to the programming software for that particular hearing aid manufacturer. It records the average amount of time a child is wearing each hearing aid per day, based on the most recent date that the hearing aid was hooked up to the software.

Investigators have just recently started using data logging to find out how often children are wearing hearing aids. Jones and Feilner (2013) examined a national database with anonymous data logging results from 6696 children with hearing loss, ranging in age from infancy to 18 years of age. Children wore hearing aids an average of 6.1 hr per day, based on data logging. Infants and toddlers averaged less, around 5.5 hr per day. For the whole sample of children, data logging showed that only 33% wore hearing aids more than 8 hr a day, which could be considered a low estimate for use time during all waking hours. Walker et al. (2015a) looked at data logging results from a longitudinal sample of 290 children, between the ages of 5 months and 9 years. Their findings indicated that all the children in the group were wearing hearing aids around 8.5 hr per day. Infants had an average use time of 4.5 hr per day, while preschoolers increased their usage to around 7.5 hr. Together, these articles indicate that some children are wearing hearing aids at less-than-optimal amounts, particularly at younger ages. Given the importance of early, consistent auditory exposure for later cognitive and language skills, AV practitioners and audiologists need to guide parents in helping their children achieve full-time use of their hearing aids (Eyes open, Ears on!). The principles of AVT strongly emphasize coaching parents to *integrate spoken language and listening into all aspects of their child's life.* The core principles of AVT cannot be achieved without consistent daily hearing aid use.

How Does Hearing Aid Use Affect Outcomes?

It may seem intuitive that children who wear hearing aids more hours will have better outcomes than children who wear them less often. Greater daily use of hearing aids provides better access to speech sounds, and subsequently more progress will happen in listening and spoken language. One of the principles of AVT concerning the recommendation of the use of amplification to obtain benefits of auditory stimulation is based on this notion. Until recently, however, there was not much research evidence to support it. Tomblin and his colleagues (2015) followed 317 preschool-age children with mild to severe hearing loss, over a period of up to 4 years. The researchers looked at performance on different outcome measures (articulation, vocabulary, grammar, social use of language). Of particular

interest was whether or not amount of hearing aid use made a difference in the outcomes of these children. In support of the principles of AVT, results from this study showed that hearing aid use does matter. Average daily hearing aid use was a significant predictor of better language outcomes, regardless of the degree of hearing loss of the children. In other words, children with milder hearing loss benefitted from more daily hearing aid use as well as children with moderate or severe hearing loss.

The same research group also looked at how daily hearing aid use affected growth of language skills. One expects a child who is typically developing to show steady growth in language skills over time, making 1 year of language growth over 12 months. Young children with hearing loss may start off with delays compared to children with typical hearing, so they have even more to do. Closing the gap can only really be done with consistent all day use of amplification and it is critical for success in the regular school (see Chapter 15). Therefore, research results that show a steeper growth trajectory are considered to be positive findings. As Figure 5–6 shows, amount of hearing aid use influenced the language growth trajectory; children who wore hearing aids more often throughout the day displayed steeper change in language skills over time, while children who wore hearing aids less often showed a flat trajectory (Tomblin et al., 2015).

More specifically, children who wore their hearing aids for less than 10 hr a day showed no change in their rate of language growth between 2 and 6 years of age (i.e., the gap between their language skills compared to average performance for same-age children

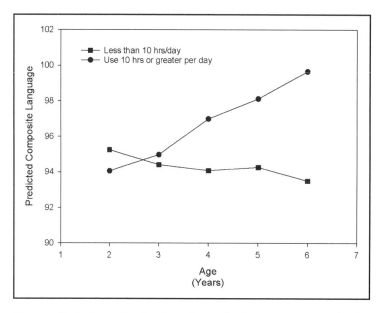

Figure 5-6. Longitudinal patterns in language growth for children who wore hearing aids more than 10 hr per week (*black circles*) and less than 10 hr per week (*black squares*). Modified from a figure in Tomblin et al. (2015).

with typical hearing remained the same over time). In contrast, children who wore hearing aids more than 10 hr a day made more than a year's worth of language gains in a year's time, effectively closing the language gap between themselves and children with typical hearing. These results provide strong evidence for the importance of consistent amplification use for achieving maximum benefits from auditory stimulation, particularly during important periods of early brain development.

Importance of Situational Assessment of Hearing Aid Use

So what can be done to improve the amount of time a child wears amplification, particularly in the case of noncom-

pliant toddlers? Consistent with the AVT principle of *administering formal and informal assessments for the purpose of developing treatment plans, monitoring progress, and evaluating the effectiveness of them,* AV practitioners and audiologists need to encourage parents and service providers to regularly monitor hearing aid use as part of treatment plans. Parents, AV practitioners, and other service providers need to work together: to identify situations of successful hearing aid use; to encourage families to be aware of situations that pose problems; and to take proactive steps to limit challenges. In doing so, the child's entire management team is able to implement the principles of AVT to *create environments that support listening for the acquisition of spoken language throughout the child's daily activities.*

An informal tool to monitor situational assessment of hearing aid use can be found in articles by Moeller et al. (2009) and Walker et al. (2013). Both studies used a parent-report measure in which families rated consistency of pediatric hearing aid use in specific situations, based on a 5-point scale of always, often, sometimes, rarely, or never. The situations included (a) riding in the car, (b) day care, (c) mealtimes, (d) playing with parents, (e) playing alone, (f) book sharing, (g) playing outside, and (h) in public (e.g., zoo, restaurant). Moeller and her colleagues completed telephone interviews using the rating scale with seven mothers of infants with hearing loss, starting when their children were around 10 months old. The mothers reported that certain situations were more challenging in achieving consistent hearing aid use than others, particularly riding in the car, outdoor play, and going out in public. This was primarily due to concerns about safety or losing the hearing aids. There were also situations that were easier for achieving consistent hearing aid use, including mealtimes, one-on-one playing time with parents, and especially book sharing opportunities (essentially, all times when the mothers were able to monitor their children closely). Walker et al. (2013) used a similar questionnaire with a wider age range (6 months to 6 years). As children grew older, situations such as riding in the car became less of an issue, while child-specific factors such as degree of hearing loss were more significant. For both going out in public and school, parents of children with milder hearing losses reported less consistent hearing aid use than children with more severe hearing losses.

The take-home message from both of these studies is that hearing aid use consistency varies among children. Consistent use differs across families and across developmental periods. The process of achieving consistent hearing aid use is multifaceted and is affected by child-specific issues, parent-child issues, situational issues, and parental adjustment issues (Moeller et al., 2009). By working with the AV practitioner and using a rating scale for determining consistency of use in different contexts (Table 5–2), parents can formulate plans for creating positive listening environments, and monitoring progress related to hearing aid use over time. Parents who make an informed choice of AVT usually *buy into* the notion of consistent hearing aid use during all waking hours from the beginning.

Strategies for Enhancing Hearing Aid Use

Once parents have begun to identify challenging situations, there are direct and indirect strategies that can be implemented to overcome barriers and integrate hearing aid use. Given the fact that many challenging situations seem to be related to parental safety concerns, hearing aid retention devices may be a feasible option for reducing the risk of losing the hearing aids. Retention devices include bonnets, Oto or Critter Clips, toupee tape, EarGear, and Hearing Aid Headbands, to name a few options (Figure 5–7).

Infants, toddlers, and preschoolers are persistent, however, and will likely find many innovative ways to remove their hearing aids even while wearing retention devices. For example, some

Table 5–2. Example of Parent Rating Questionnaire for Situational Hearing Aid Use

Situation	Never (0)	Rare (1)	Sometimes (2)	Often (3)	Always (4)	N/A
10. Car						
11. Preschool/ school						
12. Day care						
13. Mealtime						
14. Playing alone						
15. Book sharing						
16. Playground						
17. Public (store, zoo, restaurant)						

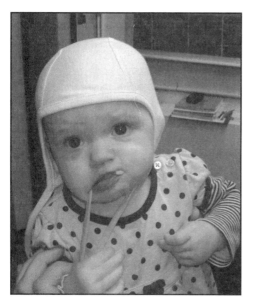

Figure 5–7. Caps and bonnets are one option for keeping hearing aids secure on infants and toddlers.

young children will remove the hearing aids to get attention or during tantrums. Parents need to learn to respond neutrally to behaviors such as throwing hearing aids, and reinsert the hearing aids after a few minutes when the child has had time to regulate himself (Moeller et al., 2009). In difficult situations such as the car or going to the park or zoo, using a remote microphone system, such as personal FM, may address some of the challenges because it will improve communication issues related to distance and background noise between the parent and an active child (Thibodeau & Schafer, 2002) (see Chapter 7). The website Supporting Success for Children with Hearing Loss (http://successforkidswithhearingloss .com/hearing-aids-on) lists additional recommendations for supporting full-time hearing aid use, including survey results describing the options parents and audiologists preferred.

Data logging may also be useful in trying to enhance hearing aid use (McCreery, 2013). The term *data logging* may make parents feel slightly apprehensive about privacy, because it is not clear what data are being collected. Parents need to be assured that the information collected via hearing aid data logging is related to the number of hours that the battery is activated, and no conversations are being recorded. Data logging needs to be considered as a strategy to monitor the function of the hearing aids, in collaboration with the audiologist and AV practitioner. Occasionally, parents' estimations of hours of daily hearing aid use do not correspond with the reported average number of hours obtained through data logging. Parents, AV practitioners, and audiologists can view this as an opportunity to discuss the situations that pose challenges to hearing aid use and prompt conversations about effective strategies for addressing these challenges.

AVT purports that parents become the primary facilitators of their child's listening and spoken language development. Research shows that parents who feel more engaged and involved in the early intervention tend to have children who wear amplification more often (Desjardin, 2003, 2005). This is particularly true for mothers who are confident in their abilities to troubleshoot and maintain their child's sensory device (hearing aids and/or cochlear implants). Desjardin proposed that this relationship is the result of personal beliefs of self-efficacy, and that these

beliefs lead to more persistence in the challenge of achieving consistent hearing aid use. Parents who perceive that they have the knowledge and competence to manage their child's amplification are more likely to persist with meeting specific goals related to AVT. Although this is not a direct strategy for keeping hearing aids on a child, parents who take an active role in hearing aid management, including performing daily listening checks and troubleshooting the equipment, feel more empowered (Desjardin, 2005). Families also can embrace the hearing aids as something that makes their child unique (Figure 5–8). For younger children, this can include customizing their devices by choosing colorful earmolds. Older children can add removable tube decorations such as TubeRiders, which can be selected to fit children's personalities and hobbies.

SPECIAL CASES: MILD HEARING LOSS

Children with mild hearing loss have significant amounts of residual hearing and often appear to be able to *get by* without hearing aids during conversation. At the same time, there are a number of studies that indicate that this population of children is at risk of experiencing difficulties in language, academic, and psychosocial outcomes (Bess, Dodd-Murphy, & Parker, 1998; Đoković et al., 2014; Porter, Sladen, Ampah, Rothpletz, & Bess, 2013). There is also evidence that children with mild hearing loss are less likely to wear their hearing aids on a consistent basis

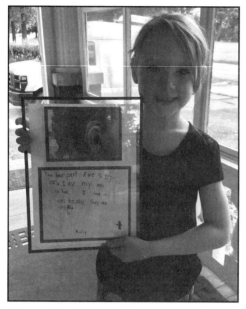

A

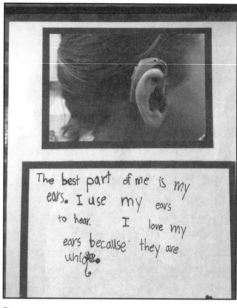

B

Figure 5–8. We encourage families and children to talk to classmates about hearing aids and how they work. Children who are comfortable with talking about their hearing aids are more likely to wear them on a regular basis.

(Fitzpatrick, Durieux-Smith, & Whittingham, 2010; Walker et al., 2013). Is there evidence to support that these children need to wear hearing aids during all waking hours? The Outcomes of Children with Hearing Loss (OCHL) project is a longitudinal, multicenter study that followed a large group of children with bilateral mild to severe hearing loss. The OCHL team looked specifically at the question of hearing aid use and language outcomes in a subset of 38 children with mild hearing loss (Walker et al., 2015b). The children were divided into three groups based on their amount of daily hearing aid use. The researchers determined amount of daily hearing aid use by a combination of parent-report measures and hearing aid data logging. Group 1 consisted of children with mild hearing loss who had never worn hearing aids, Group 2 consisted of children who wore hearing aids part time (on average, 5.5 hr per day), and Group 3 consisted of children who wore their hearing aids full time (on average, 11 hr per day). Results showed that the full-time users had significantly higher scores on grammar and vocabulary measures, compared to children who did not wear hearing aids. Children who wore hearing aids part time had average language scores between the nonusers and the full-time users. These findings are a powerful example of how consistent hearing aid use can benefit language development, even for children who have some access to speech sounds. These findings also have implications for AVT practitioners and audiologists. Cumulative auditory experience influences outcomes even in cases of children with very mild hearing loss. AVT practitioners can facilitate consistent device use and help optimize language development potential for children with all degrees of hearing loss.

When working with children with mild hearing loss who do receive hearing aids, it is critical for audiologists to follow best-practice guidelines when fitting and verifying hearing aids. Earlier, we described the real-ear-to-coupler difference (RECD) as a tool for measuring a child's individual ear canal acoustics during hearing aid verification. Children's ear canals change rapidly in size over time, and this change affects the loudness of sounds as they are presented through the hearing aid. The size of the child's ear canal can also affect the loudness of sounds used to test hearing. The equipment used to test hearing is calibrated on a coupler that is designed to mimic the volume of an adult ear canal. As in the case with hearing aids, the level of the sound in the child's ear canal during the hearing test may be higher than the level indicated on the equipment. This is particularly the case for foam insert earphones that are placed in the child's ear canal. Another potential application of the RECD is to estimate the child's hearing thresholds, while taking into account the effect of their ear canal acoustics on the level of sound in the ear. In many cases, hearing loss that appears to be in the mild range for infants and young children can be more significant because the actual sound level used during the hearing test is much higher in the ear canal.

When ear canal acoustics are taken into account using the RECD, the impact of the child's hearing loss and ear canal acoustics on audibility for speech can be more accurately determined. As with any degree of hearing loss, obtaining regular audiograms and individually measured RECDs ensures that the audiologist is providing adequate gain at soft and average conversational speech levels, as the child gets older and the acoustic properties of the ear canals change (Bagatto & Tharpe, 2013).

SPECIAL CASES: AUDITORY NEUROPATHY SPECTRUM DISORDER (ANSD)

ANSD is a relatively rare subtype of sensory/neural hearing loss in which the auditory nerve or auditory brainstem is functioning abnormally, but the outer hair cells in the cochlea are working appropriately. For infants with ANSD, it is critical to identify this type of hearing loss as early as possible, because our methods for clinical management are less straightforward than other types of sensorineural hearing loss. The reason for this lies in the measures that we use to diagnose and determine severity of the hearing loss in infants who cannot participate in behavioral audiometry. In children with ANSD, ABR responses are absent or abnormal and may not correspond with auditory thresholds that are documented on an audiogram, making it more of a challenge to accurately determine how much residual hearing the child has.

Clinical management for ANSD is further complicated by the fact that individuals who have ANSD with similar amounts of residual hearing can have very different abilities in terms of how they understand speech. Speech recognition abilities in ANSD may be better or poorer than what we expect based on their audibility levels (Rance, 2005). This feature of ANSD is different from having a sensorineural hearing loss, in which level of audibility corresponds with the ability to understand speech (in other words, people with better audibility with sensorineural hearing loss tend to have higher speech recognition scores; people with poorer audibility tend to have lower speech recognition scores). In addition, understanding speech in noise is particularly difficult for people with ANSD, even more so than for people with sensorineural or conductive hearing losses (Kraus et al., 2000; Rance & Barker, 2008). It is not entirely clear why speech recognition skills vary so much in individuals with ANSD. Researchers suspect that it may be related to the degree to which ANSD affects the ability of the auditory system to process timing differences in speech (Rance, McKay, & Grayden, 2004). Currently, an important area of research involves developing appropriate evidence-based clinical interventions for this population, given the challenges in diagnosing and providing clinical management with ANSD (Roush, Frymark, Venediktov, & Wang, 2011).

Children with ANSD may be candidates for three different types of hearing technology: cochlear implants, hearing aids, or remote microphone technology. Chapter 6 by Wolfe and Neumann describes the use of cochlear implants as an intervention for ANSD. Regardless of whether or not children with ANSD eventually receive a cochlear implant, however, the American Academy of Audiology (AAA) recommends that they receive hearing aids as soon as it is determined that their hearing loss limits their ability to understand speech. In general, children with ANSD who have thresholds in the severe-to-profound range show only minimal benefit from hearing aids, and therefore are better candidates for cochlear implants (Rance, Cone-Wesson, Wunderlich, & Dowell, 2002). Evidence for appropriate intervention for children with significant residual hearing is mixed. Some children with ANSD may have the potential to greatly benefit from the audibility provided by hearing aids (Ching et al., 2013; Rance, Barker, Sarant, & Ching, 2007). At the same time, some children with ANSD who have residual hearing have difficulty understanding speech, even when wearing hearing aids (Rance et al., 2002). The AV practitioner has an important role in carefully monitoring children with ANSD, to establish if they are receiving benefit from hearing aids, or if cochlear implantation is warranted.

Earlier, we described how audiologists may use electrophysiological measures of hearing to determine how much amplification should be provided via hearing aids. Unfortunately, electrophysiological measures such as ABR cannot provide valid estimates of behavioral thresholds for children with ANSD, in contrast to children with sensorineural hearing loss. The AAA Pediatric Amplification guidelines suggest that hearing aids may initially be fit based on careful behavioral observations to sound, by the clinician and/or the parent until a reliable behavioral audiogram can be obtained. Because of the difficulty in obtaining reliable behavioral audiometry, children with ANSD who wear hearing aids may need to see their audiologist a minimum of every 3 months until the child is 6 years old.

Once the audiologist is able to obtain behavioral responses to sound, the child should be fitted with behind-the-ear hearing aids using prescriptive targets that will optimize audibility of speech (Bagatto et al., 2005). Similar to children with sensorineural hearing loss, the output of the hearing aids should be verified using probe microphone measures, at soft, average, and loud conversational levels of speech. These measures may be obtained in the child's ear canal or via simulated measurements of the hearing aid output in a coupler with a real-ear-to-coupler-difference measure (AAA, 2013; Bagatto, Scollie, Hyde, & Seewald, 2010; King, 2010).

Since ANSD was first identified in children and adults with hearing loss, researchers and clinicians have debated about what is the best approach for providing hearing aids to children with ANSD. Some have argued for using a conservative approach of providing low-gain hearing aids, similar to how a hearing aid would be fit for someone with mild hearing loss. There is no empirical evidence to support this conservative approach for children who have ANSD with mild-severe behavioral thresholds, however. Using this approach could limit the ability to acquire listening and spoken language, because it underamplifies sounds and reduces the child's access to the speech spectrum and environment sounds. The major differences in hearing aid fitting and verification for children with ANSD, compared to children with sensorineural hearing loss, are that audiologists

will not be able to use ABR results to help estimate auditory thresholds and fitting amplification, and children with ANSD will need to be monitored more closely, both before and after the hearing aid fitting. This close monitoring will allow the audiologist to determine that behavioral thresholds are stable and that appropriate progress is being made.

One of the hallmark features of ANSD is poor performance in background noise (Rance, 2005; Starr et al., 1998). Therefore, another important recommendation for this population is the use of remote microphone systems to improve the ability to listen in noise (Kraus et al., 2000; Rance, 2005). This is particularly important for children with ANSD who have significant residual hearing. Just like children with normal hearing and children with sensorineural hearing loss, children with ANSD are expected to learn academic material while listening in noisy, reverberant acoustics conditions in mainstream classroom settings (Crandell & Smaldino, 2000). Remote microphone technology will help with understanding speech in these adverse listening conditions.

Guidance for the AV Practitioner

AV practitioners should be aware that children with ANSD may or may not show improvements in speech understanding once they have been fit with hearing aids. Questionnaires such as the LittlEARS (Coninx et al., 2009) or the Parents' Evaluation of Aural/Oral Performance of Children (PEACH; Ching & Hill, 2007) may help with the counseling process, in that they will provide information about functional auditory skills and developmental progress. *The AV practitioner may ask the child's audiologist:* Is the child is showing any improvement with or without the hearing aids using speech perception measures? What type of remote microphone technology should be used in combination with the hearing aids?

CONCLUSION

This chapter provided an overview of the importance of hearing aids in the AVT for children with hearing loss. Hearing aids are an essential component to providing auditory access for listening and the development of spoken language. Hearing aids maximize residual hearing and make speech and other environmental sounds audible to give each child the greatest opportunity to develop the skills needed for listening and spoken language. A wide range of advanced signal processing features in hearing aids can benefit children and increase auditory access, if appropriately prescribed. Consistent audibility and use of hearing aids can provide children with an essential foundation for development. By providing an overview of the hearing aid fitting process, we hope that parents, AV practitioners, and other professionals may have a greater understanding of how hearing aids work and what questions to ask audiologists who provide these services for children.

REFERENCES

Akhtar, N. (2005). The robustness of learning through overhearing. *Developmental Science, 8*(2), 199–209.

American Academy of Audiology. (2013). *Clinical practice guidelines: Pediatric amplification*. Reston, VA: Author.

American National Standards Institute. (1997). *American National Standard: Methods for calculation of the Speech Intelligibility Index*. Melville, NY: Acoustical Society of America.

Bagatto, M., Moodie, S., Scollie, S., Seewald, R., Moodie, S., Pumford, J., & Liu, K. R. (2005). Clinical protocols for hearing instrument fitting in the Desired Sensation Level method. *Trends in Amplification, 9*(4), 199–226.

Bagatto, M., Scollie, S. D., Hyde, M., & Seewald, R. (2010). Protocol for the provision of amplification within the Ontario infant hearing program. *International Journal of Audiology, 49*(Suppl. 1), S70–S79.

Bagatto, M. P., & Tharpe, A. M. (2013). Decision support guide for hearing aid use in infants and children with minimal/mild bilateral hearing loss. *Proceedings from a Sound Foundation in Amplification*. Chicago, IL: Phonak

Bess, F. H., Dodd-Murphy, J., & Parker, R. A. (1998). Children with minimal sensorineural hearing loss: Prevalence, educational performance, and functional status. *Ear and Hearing, 19*(5), 339–354.

Ching, T. Y., Day, J., Dillon, H., Gardner-Berry, K., Hou, S., Seeto, M., . . . Zhang, V. (2013). Impact of the presence of auditory neuropathy spectrum disorder (ANSD) on outcomes of children at three years of age. *International Journal of Audiology, 52*(S2), S55–S64.

Ching, T. Y., & Hill, M. (2007). The parents' evaluation of aural/oral performance of children (PEACH) scale: Normative data. *Journal of the American Academy of Audiology, 18*(3), 220–235.

Ching, T. Y., O'Brien, A., Dillon, H., Chalupper, J., Hartley, L., Hartley, D., . . . Hain, J. (2009). Directional effects on infants and young children in real life: Implications for amplification. *Journal of Speech, Language, and Hearing Research, 52*(5), 1241–1254.

Coninx, F., Weichbold, V., Tsiakpini, L., Autrique, E., Bescond, G., Tamas, L., . . . Le Maner-Idrissi, G. (2009). Validation of the LittlEARS® Auditory Questionnaire in children with normal hearing. *International Journal of Pediatric Otorhinolaryngology, 73*(12), 1761–1768.

Crandell, C. C., & Smaldino, J. J. (2000). Classroom acoustics for children with normal hearing and with hearing impairment. *Language, Speech, and Hearing Services in Schools, 31*(4), 362–370.

Desjardin, J. L. (2003). Assessing parental perceptions of self-efficacy and involvement in families of young children with hearing loss. *Volta Review, 103*(4).

Desjardin, J. L. (2005). Maternal perceptions of self-efficacy and involvement in the auditory development of young children with prelingual deafness. *Journal of Early Intervention, 27*(3), 193–209.

Đoković, S., Gligorović, M., Ostojić, S., Dimić, N., Radić-Šestić, M., & Slavnić, S. (2014). Can mild bilateral sensorineural hearing loss affect developmental abilities in younger school-age children? *Journal of Deaf Studies and Deaf Education, 19*, 484–495.

Fitzpatrick, E. M., Durieux-Smith, A., & Whittingham, J. (2010). Clinical practice for children with mild bilateral and unilateral hearing loss. *Ear and Hearing, 31*(3), 392–400.

Glista, D., Scollie, S., Bagatto, M., Seewald, R., Parsa, V., & Johnson, A. (2009). Evaluation of nonlinear frequency compression: Clinical outcomes. *International Journal of Audiology, 48*(9), 632–644.

Holte, L., Walker, E., Oleson, J., Spratford, M., Moeller, M. P., Roush, P., . . . Tomblin, J. B. (2012). Factors influencing follow-up to newborn hearing screening for infants who are hard of hearing. *American Journal of Audiology, 21*(2), 163–174.

Jones, C. & Feilner, M. (2013). What do we know about the fitting and daily life usage of hearing instruments in pediatrics? In *A Sound Foundation through Early Amplification: Proceedings of the 2013 international conference* (pp. 97–103). Chicago, IL: Phonak AG.

Kimlinger, C., McCreery, R., & Lewis, D. (2015). High-frequency audibility: The effects of audiometric configuration, stimulus type, and device. *Journal of the American Academy of Audiology, 26*(2), 128–137.

King, A. M. (2010). The national protocol for paediatric amplification in Australia. *International Journal of Audiology, 49*(Suppl. 1), S64–S69.

Koehlinger, K., Van Horne, A. O., Oleson, J., McCreery, R., & Moeller, M. P. (2015). The role of sentence position, allomorph, and morpheme type on accurate use of s-related morphemes by children who are hard of hearing. *Journal of Speech, Language, and Hearing Research, 58*(2), 396–409.

Kraus, N., Bradlow, A., Cheatham, M., Cunningham, J., King, C., Koch, D., . . . Wright, B. (2000). Consequences of neural asynchrony: A case of auditory neuropathy. *Journal of the Association for Research in Otolaryngology, 1*(1), 33–45.

Kuhl, P. K., Conboy, B. T., Padden, D., Nelson, T., & Pruitt, J. (2005). Early speech perception and later language development: Implications for the "Critical Period." *Language Learning and Development, 1*(3–4), 237–264.

Ling, D. (1978). Speech development in hearing-impaired children. *Journal of Communication Disorders, 11*(2), 119–124.

McCreery, R. (2013). Data logging and hearing aid use: Focus on the forest, not the trees. *Hearing Journal, 66*(12), 18–19.

McCreery, R. W., Alexander, J., Brennan, M. A., Hoover, B., Kopun, J., & Stelmachowicz, P. G. (2014). The influence of audibility on speech recognition with nonlinear frequency compression for children and adults with hearing loss. *Ear and Hearing, 35*(4), 440–447.

McCreery, R. W., Venediktov, R. A., Coleman, J. J., & Leech, H. M. (2012a). An evidence-based systematic review of amplitude compression in hearing aids for school-age children with hearing loss. *American Journal of Audiology, 21*(2), 269–294.

McCreery, R. W., Venediktov, R. A., Coleman, J. J., & Leech, H. M. (2012b). An evidence-based systematic review of directional microphones and digital noise reduction hearing aids in school-age children with hearing loss. *American Journal of Audiology, 21*(2), 295–312.

McCreery, R. W., Venediktov, R. A., Coleman, J. J., & Leech, H. M. (2012c). An evidence-based systematic review of frequency lowering in hearing aids for school-age children with hearing loss. *American Journal of Audiology, 21*(2), 313–328.

McCreery, R. W., Walker, E. A., Spratford, M., Oleson, J., Bentler, R., Holte, L., & Roush, P. (2015). Speech recognition and parent ratings from auditory development questionnaires in children who are hard of hearing. *Ear and Hearing, 36*, 60S–75S.

Moeller, M. P. (2000). Early intervention and language development in children who are deaf and hard of hearing. *Pediatrics, 106*(3), e43.

Moeller, M. P., Hoover, B., Peterson, B., & Stelmachowicz, P. (2009). Consistency of hearing aid use in infants with early-identified hearing loss. *American Journal of Audiology, 18*(1), 14–23.

Moeller, M. P., Hoover, B., Putman, C., Arbataitis, K., Bohnenkamp, G., Peterson, B., . . . Stelmachowicz, P. (2007). Vocalizations of infants with hearing loss compared with infants with normal hearing: Part I —phonetic development. *Ear and Hearing, 28*(5), 605–627.

Mueller, H. G. (2007). Data logging: It's popular, but how can this feature be used to help patients? *Hearing Journal, 60*(10), 19–26.

Pisoni, D. B. (2000). Cognitive factors and cochlear implants: Some thoughts on perception, learning, and memory in speech perception. *Ear and Hearing, 21*(1), 70–78.

Porter, H., Sladen, D. P., Ampah, S. B., Rothpletz, A., & Bess, F. H. (2013). Developmental outcomes in early school-age children with minimal hearing loss. *American Journal of Audiology, 22*(2), 263–270.

Rance, G. (2005). Auditory neuropathy/dys-synchrony and its perceptual consequences. *Trends in Amplification, 9*(1), 1–43.

Rance, G., & Barker, E. J. (2008). Speech perception in children with auditory neuropathy/dyssynchrony managed with either hearing aids or cochlear implants. *Otology and Neurotology, 29*(2), 179–182.

Rance, G., Barker, E. J., Sarant, J. Z., & Ching, T. Y. (2007). Receptive language and speech production in children with auditory neuropathy/dyssynchrony type hearing loss. *Ear and Hearing, 28*(5), 694–702.

Rance, G., Cone-Wesson, B., Wunderlich, J., & Dowell, R. (2002). Speech perception and cortical event related potentials in children with auditory neuropathy. *Ear and Hearing, 23*(3), 239–253.

Rance, G., McKay, C., & Grayden, D. (2004). Perceptual characterization of children with auditory neuropathy. *Ear and Hearing, 25*(1), 34–46.

Roush, P., Frymark, T., Venediktov, R., & Wang, B. (2011). Audiologic management of auditory neuropathy spectrum disorder in children: A systematic review of the literature. *American Journal of Audiology, 20*(2), 159–170.

Sharma, A., Dorman, M. F., & Kral, A. (2005). The influence of a sensitive period on central auditory development in children with unilateral and bilateral cochlear implants. *Hearing Research, 203*(1), 134–143.

Sharma, A., Dorman, M. F., & Spahr, A. J. (2002). A sensitive period for the development of the central auditory system in children with cochlear implants: Implications for age of implantation. *Ear and Hearing, 23*(6), 532–539.

Starr, A., Sininger, Y., Winter, M., Derebery, M., Oba, S., & Michalewski, H. (1998).

Transient deafness due to temperature-sensitive auditory neuropathy. *Ear and Hearing, 19*(3), 169–179.

Stelmachowicz, P., Lewis, D., Hoover, B., Nishi, K., McCreery, R., & Woods, W. (2010). Effects of digital noise reduction on speech perception for children with hearing loss. *Ear and Hearing, 31*(3), 345.

Thibodeau, L. M., & Schafer, E. (2002). Issues to consider regarding use of FM systems with infants with hearing loss. *SIG 9 Perspectives on Hearing and Hearing Disorders in Childhood, 12*(1), 18–21.

Tomblin, J. B., Harrison, M., Ambrose, S. E., Walker, E. A., & Moeller, M. P. (2015). Language outcomes in young children with mild to severe hearing loss. *Ear and Hearing, 36*, 76S–91S.

Tsao, F.-M., Liu, H.-M., & Kuhl, P. K. (2004). Speech perception in infancy predicts language development in the second year of life: A longitudinal study. *Child Development*, 1067–1084.

Walker, E. A., Holte, L., McCreery, R. W., Spratford, M., Page, T., & Moeller, M.P. (2015b). The effects of hearing aid use on outcomes of children with mild hearing loss. *Journal of Speech, Language, and Hearing Research, 58*, 1611–1625.

Walker, E. A., Holte, L., Spratford, M., Oleson, J., Welhaven, A., & Harrison, M. (2014). Timeliness of service delivery for children with later-identified mild-to-severe hearing loss. *American Journal of Audiology, 23*(1), 116–128.

Walker, E. A., McCreery, R. W., Spratford, M., Oleson, J. J., Van Buren, J., Bentler, R. A., . . . Moeller, M. P. (2015a). Trends and predictors of longitudinal hearing aid use for children who are hard of hearing. *Ear and Hearing, 36*, 38S–47S.

Walker, E. A., Spratford, M., Moeller, M. P., Oleson, J., Ou, H., Roush, P., & Jacobs, S. (2013). Predictors of hearing aid use time in children with mild-to-severe hearing loss. *Language, Speech, and Hearing Services in Schools, 44*(1), 73–88.

Wolfe, J., John, A., Schafer, E., Nyffeler, M., Boretzki, M., Caraway, T., & Hudson, M. (2011). Long-term effects of non-linear frequency compression for children with moderate hearing loss. *International Journal of Audiology, 50*(6), 396–404.

6

IMPLANTABLE HEARING TECHNOLOGIES AND AUDITORY-VERBAL THERAPY

Jace Wolfe and Sara Neumann

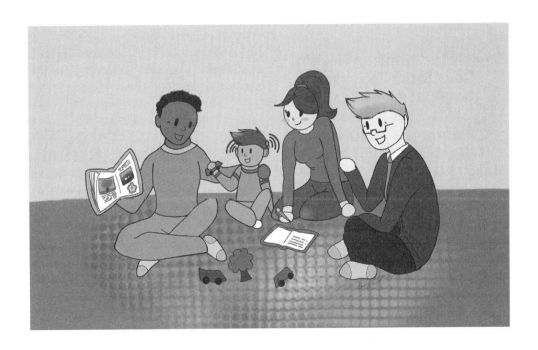

INTRODUCTION

Implantable hearing technologies encompass a wide range of cochlear implants, auditory brainstem implants, bone conduction devices, and middle ear devices. Recent developments in implantable hearing technology have created opportunities for children with all degrees, types, and configurations of hearing loss to develop age-appropriate auditory skills and spoken language that are commensurate with their peers with typical hearing. The majority of this chapter, therefore, focuses on cochlear implants and bone conduction hearing devices, the implantable hearing technologies most commonly used by children with hearing loss, and the implications of such technologies for Auditory-Verbal Therapy (AVT).

Pediatric Hearing Health Care Team Providing Services to Children With Implantable Hearing Technology

Children who are being considered for implantable hearing technology or who are current users of implantable hearing technology need to be managed by a team of professionals who are highly experienced in the use and provision of services involved with these technologies. At a minimum, this team needs to include the child's caregivers (e.g., parents, grandparents, legal guardians), a pediatric audiologist, an AV practitioner, a pediatric otologist, and the child's pediatrician. A social worker may also provide a valuable contribution to the team, particularly for families with limited resources and/or special needs. It is important that the basic needs of families (e.g., food, shelter, safety, transportation, etc.) are met so that the family is well equipped to devote the time, attention, energy, and resources required to optimize the potential listening and spoken language abilities of the child with hearing loss.

The team providing services for children with additional challenges or special needs may also include other medical specialists, a neurodevelopmental specialist, and an early intervention coordinator. It is imperative that these team members consistently and effectively communicate in an interdisciplinary approach to ensure that the child's needs are being met, that the child is making satisfactory auditory and spoken language progress, and that the child is appropriately equipped with hearing technology that will facilitate optimal development and hopefully realize the outcomes that everyone desires.

COCHLEAR IMPLANTS

Cochlear implants are sensory prosthetic devices that deliver electrical stimulation to the cochlear nerve in an effort to restore access to a wide range of acoustic input levels throughout the speech frequency range. Cochlear implantation is generally considered to be the standard of care for children and adults with severe to profound sensory hearing loss. Many children with auditory neuropathy spectrum disorder also receive substantial benefit from cochlear implantation.

Assessment of Cochlear Implant Candidacy for Children

Pediatric cochlear implant guidelines vary by manufacturer and global region. Differences in indication of use of cochlear implants in children vary by age of implantation, degree of hearing loss, aided auditory performance, and so on. For instance, in some countries, indications for cochlear implant use state that children should be 12 months old, while other countries have approved cochlear implantation for children under one year of age.

Although industry guidelines do offer a framework for suggesting children who should be considered for cochlear implantation, there are many important factors that influence the evaluation process and outcomes that are not explicitly discussed in the indications for use. The following describes a number of instrumental components of the pediatric cochlear implant candidacy assessment.

Hearing Aid Verification

Verification of a child's performance with hearing technology involves the use of a variety of measures and assessments that evaluate the user's ability to overcome the hearing loss. Suggested by Bagatto (2012), this is to be completed as part of the clinical process.

Electroacoustic probe microphone measures need to be completed with every child undergoing cochlear implant candidacy assessment. Often referred to as in situ assessment, in situ probe microphone measures provide the most accurate representation of the output of the hearing aid worn by the child, but the child must be capable of sitting still and facing the loudspeaker of the hearing aid analyzer for several minutes while in situ assessment is being completed (Figure 6–1). The goal of electroacoustic hearing aid verification is to ensure that the output of the child's hearing aids matches the target output level defined by a generic, evidenced-based prescriptive method, such as Desired Sensation Level 5.0 (DSL 5.0)

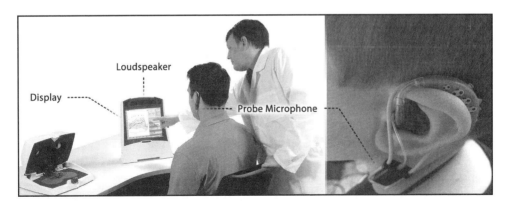

Figure 6-1. An example of a real-ear hearing aid analyzer (right side) and an in situ real-ear probe microphone assessment used to fit hearing aid output to the Desired Sensation Level v5.0 prescriptive targets for a young child (left side).

(Scollie et al., 2005) or the National Acoustic Laboratories Non-linear 2 (NAL-NL2) (Dillon & Keidser, 2013).

If the child is incapable of remaining still for several minutes, then it is perfectly acceptable for the clinician to complete simulated probe microphone measures with the hearing aid connected to a 2cc hearing aid measurement coupler (Figure 6–2). For both in situ and simulated measures, the clinician needs to measure the real-ear-to-coupler difference (RECD) prior to the probe microphone measurement (Moodie, Seewald, & Sinclair, 1994).

Aided Thresholds

Although electroacoustic probe microphone measures are the primary staple of the battery a clinician uses to evaluate the appropriateness of pediatric amplification, they do not inform the clinician of a very important piece of information. Probe microphone measures do not indicate the lowest-level (softest) sound a hearing aid wearer can detect. For that reason, the clinician needs to consider obtaining aided thresholds in an effort to determine the lowest-level sound a child can detect across the speech frequency range. The audiogram in Figure 6–3 shows that the softest sounds of average conversational level speech reside between 20 and 25 dB HL. As a result, children using hearing technology ideally should have aided thresholds between 20 and 25 dB HL in order to allow for consistent access to the lowest-level phonemes of speech. In short, the audiologist needs to consider measuring aided thresholds in conjunction with probe microphone measures in order to obtain a comprehensive understanding of the benefit a child is likely to receive from hearing aids.

Hearing Technology Validation Measures

The aforementioned measures of aided function are all verification measures. In contrast, validation measures evaluate the efficacy of the hearing technology when used in functional situations; in another words, it measures the user's ability to perceive speech in quiet and in noise, the effect of various hearing aid settings/adjustments on speech perception, and the effect the hearing technology has on the user's social or emotional well-being (Weinstein, 1997). Bagatto (2012) has suggested that validation measures should be completed to evaluate the functional outcomes of children using hearing technology. These measures may be administered by asking the family to complete norm-referenced, standardized questionnaires that are designed to evaluate auditory and spoken language development and performance in the child's day-to-day life. An AV practitioner's formal and informal assessments of a child's auditory and spoken language development are also an example of a validation measure of aided benefit and performance.

In many ways, validation measures are the most important component of the cochlear implant candidacy assessment battery. For instance, an audiologist may be satisfied with the results of probe microphone assessment of hearing aid performance, but cochlear implantation may be strongly considered if the responses provided to standardized questionnaires or the findings of a child's AV practitioner suggest the

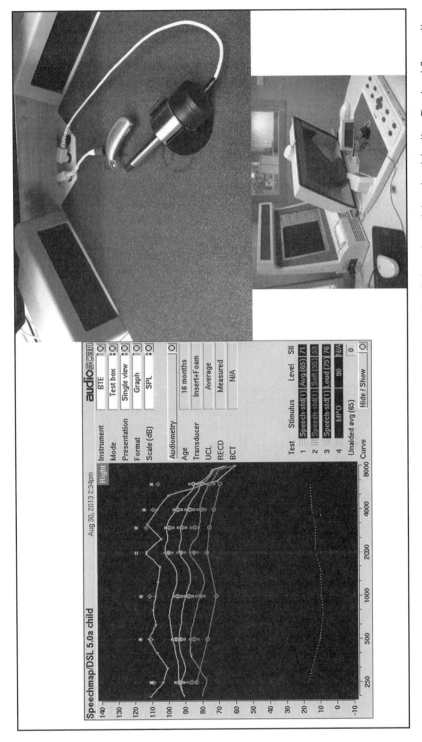

Figure 6–2. Simulated real ear probe microphone assessment used to fit hearing aid output to the Desired Sensation Level v5.0 prescriptive targets for a young child.

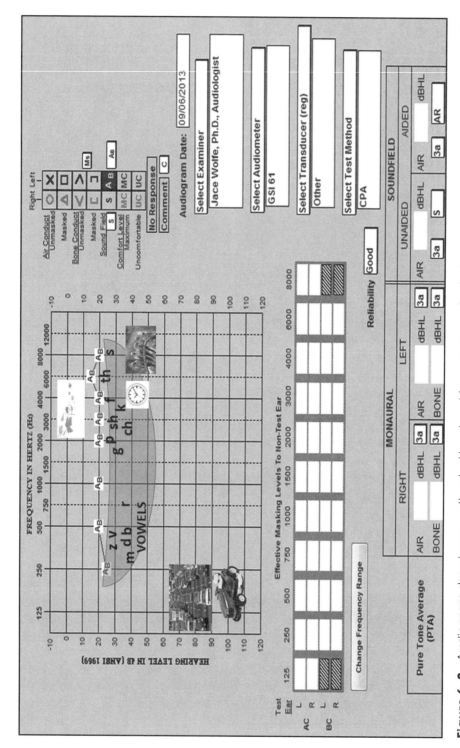

Figure 6-3. Audiogram showing an estimated level and frequency content of speech and everyday sounds along with binaurally aided sound-field detection thresholds indicating satisfactory audibility for low-level sounds (aided thresholds in the 20–25 dB HL range).

child is making poor progress in auditory and spoken language development. The quality of a pediatric hearing aid fitting or cochlear implant program cannot be determined until the child's family and AV practitioner report that the child is making excellent progress with use of the hearing technology. As a result, all professionals involved in the child's hearing and spoken language intervention need to be equipped with the proper resources to evaluate a child's functional progress with hearing technology.

Questionnaires to Evaluate Auditory Aptitude

A number of questionnaires exist that evaluate functional auditory development and performance. The use of questionnaires to evaluate functional auditory development is particularly important for younger children who are unable to participate in traditional audiological tests such as speech recognition assessments. Examples of this type of questionnaire include the LittlEARS Auditory Questionnaire (Tsiakpini et al., 2004) and the Parents' Evaluation of Aural/Oral Performance of Children (PEACH) (Ching & Hill, 2005) The reader is referred to the work of Bagatto and colleagues (2011) for more information on the use of standardized, norm-referenced questionnaires to evaluate auditory skill development in children with hearing loss.

Speech Recognition Assessments

Aided speech recognition capacity is another important component of the cochlear implant assessment battery.

Pediatric cochlear implant guidelines often indicate an aided speech recognition criterion a child should meet in order to be considered for cochlear implantation (e.g., 30% correct or less on an age- and linguistically appropriate measure of open-set word recognition with use of binaural hearing aids). The following section will address a number of factors that are relevant to the assessment of speech recognition for the purposes of determining cochlear implant candidacy in children.

Speech Material

The speech recognition measure selected to evaluate aided performance is an important factor in the process of determining implant candidacy in children. The most important objective is to select a speech recognition material that is cognitively and linguistically appropriate for the child's developmental age. The selection of a particular speech recognition test to use for candidacy determination is an important decision, because the degree of difficulty can vary considerably across test measures. For instance, research has shown the HINT (Nilsson, Soli, & Sullivan, 1994) sentence test to be a relatively easy measure of open-set speech recognition for cochlear implant users and hearing aid wearers being considered for cochlear implant candidacy, particularly when compared to monosyllabic word recognition tests (Gifford, Shallop, & Peterson, 2008). The HINT measure is composed of linguistically simple words with a high level of predictability and presented by one male speaker at a relatively slow rate. In contrast, monosyllabic (single-syllable) words possess no contextual cues, so the listener is forced to resolve the phonetic elements in order to identify a word correctly. Use of HINT sentences for CI candidacy may not be representative of the difficulties a child with hearing loss may have in real-world settings. Of course, sentence recognition assessments, such as the HINT, may be inappropriate for use with young children because the difficulty of the task exceeds the linguistic capabilities expected for the child's age.

Many of the current pediatric cochlear implant guidelines mention the Lexical Neighborhood Test (LNT) or Multisyllabic Lexical Neighborhood Test (MLNT) (Kirk, 1998) as a measure for assessing aided speech recognition in the implant candidacy evaluation. The LNT and MLNT were designed for the purpose of evaluating performance of implant candidates and recipients. Although suitable measures for these purposes, they do have one drawback. The LNT and MLNT each possess two "easy" lists (e.g., words with few lexical neighbors) and two "hard" lists (e.g., words with several lexical neighbors). Therefore, it is not possible to evaluate performance in the right, left, and binaurally aided conditions with lists of equivalent difficulty. Consequently, many clinicians tend to use PBK-50 words with younger children (4–6 years old) and CNC words with older children (7 years and up).

Presentation Level for Speech Recognition Assessment

It is widely appreciated that one of the many benefits of cochlear implantation is the fact that unlike hearing aids, cochlear implants are not limited by the audibility that can be provided for low-level (20–30 dB SPL) inputs. Firszt and colleagues (2004) recommended that speech recognition assessments for the purpose of cochlear implant candidacy evaluation or postimplant outcome evaluation be conducted at 60 dB SPL rather than 70 dB SPL. They also note that average conversational level speech typically occurs at around 60 dB SPL. Although a presentation level of 70 dB SPL is more akin to loudly spoken speech, evaluating speech recognition at levels lower than 70 dB SPL likely provides a better indication of the difficulty a prospective candidate would experience in daily situations. In addition, softly spoken and distant speech often reaches a listener at a level of 40 to 50 dB SPL. As a result, the audiologist needs to consider evaluating speech recognition at a presentation level of 60 and 50 dB SPL in order to gain an understanding of the child's ability to understand low-level speech, a skill that is crucial considering the fact that some estimates suggest that 90% of a child's language development is acquired through incidental listening (Cole & Flexer, 2007).

Recorded Versus Live Voice

Recorded presentations of speech recognition materials need to be conducted, if at all possible, when evaluating a candidate for cochlear implantation. Use of recorded materials eliminates the variability in talker characteristics that exists among clinicians, and it allows for a valid comparison of scores obtained across time (Roeser & Clark, 2008). A recent study (Uhler, Biever, & Gifford, 2016) revealed that use of recorded material resulted in a 13% decrease in performance on compared to results with monitored live voice (MLV).

Quiet Versus Noise

Audiologists need to consider evaluating speech recognition in noise for cochlear implant candidacy assessments and also for post-activation outcomes assessment. Crukley, Scollie, and Parsa (2011) reported that over 70% of the day in a day care setting and 90% of the day in an elementary school is composed of listening to speech in the presence of competing noise. Therefore, it is imperative that the audiologist determine how well a child with hearing loss is able to understand speech in noise. The signal-to-noise ratio (SNR) in typical listening situations ranges from −5 to +10 dB SNR, so any child with a double-digit SNR required for 50% speech recognition needs to be considered at considerable risk for experiencing substantial difficulty understanding speech in daily conditions. When speech recognition in noise is evaluated at a fixed SNR, it is reasonable to assess performance at a SNR routinely encountered in realistic settings. The authors of this chapter recommend a +5 dB SNR when evaluating performance at a fixed SNR.

Right, Left, and Binaurally Aided

Aided performance (aided warble tone threshold assessment and aided speech recognition) needs to be evaluated in each monaural condition (e.g., right and left aided) as well as in the binaurally aided condition. The audiologist needs to determine whether the speech recognition of one ear is considerably

poorer than the other and to determine whether performance in the binaural condition is better or poorer than performance in the better monaural condition. Additionally, speech recognition in noise in the binaural condition needs to be compared to performance in each monaural condition to ensure that binaural benefit is observed in noise. If performance in noise in the binaural condition is not significantly better than performance in the better ear, monaural condition, then the poor ear is not adequately supporting binaural hearing processes and cochlear implantation may be considered.

Factors Influencing Candidacy

The decision to pursue cochlear implantation for a child needs to be based on two questions. First, will the provision of a cochlear implant (or cochlear implants) most likely improve a child's quality of life? Second, will the provision of a cochlear implant (or cochlear implants) most likely optimize a child's auditory and spoken language abilities? If the answer to one or both of those questions is yes, then cochlear implantation needs to be considered.

A number of recent studies indicate that the benefits typically obtained from cochlear implantation suggest that current pediatric guidelines for cochlear implantation are too conservative (Carlson et al., 2015; Ching & Dillon, 2013; Geers, Strube, Tobey, & Moog, 2011; Niparko et al., 2010). Specifically, Ching and Dillon (2013) reported on outcomes for a large group of children with hearing loss who were receiving intervention through the Australian Hearing Services. It was demonstrated that spoken language outcomes of children with cochlear implants were as good as the outcomes of children who used hearing aids and had a four-frequency pure tone average (500, 1000, 2000, and 4000 Hz) of 66 dB HL. Likewise, Carlson and colleagues (2015) reported on cochlear implant outcomes for a group of 51 children who underwent off-label cochlear implantation (e.g., users who receive a cochlear implant even though they did not meet the criteria specified in the manufacturer's indications for use). A mean improvement of 63 percentage points was found for speech recognition of the implanted ear and of 40 percentage points in the bimodal condition. Furthermore, all 51 subjects experienced significant improvement in speech recognition after cochlear implantation, and there was significant improvement in speech and language development.

In summary, the decision to move forward with cochlear implantation for any child needs to be made by a team of professionals who are experienced in the evaluation of auditory, speech, and language development of children with hearing loss. A cochlear implant needs to be considered for a child when it is likely that implantation will improve the child's quality of life and the child's auditory, speech, and language abilities. The cochlear implant team needs to consider a cochlear implant for young children with severe to profound hearing loss when standard, norm-referenced measures (e.g., LittlEARS, PEACH) indicate that the child is not making satisfactory progress. Additionally, cochlear implantation can be considered when speech and language progress does not meet age-appropriate norms or when the child does not achieve 1 year of

development in speech and language over the time of 1 year. Finally, limited speech understanding on a linguistically appropriate measure of speech recognition is an indicator for cochlear implantation. Children need to score at least 80% correct in the best-aided condition. Otherwise, they will be inclined to experience considerable difficulty in real-world situations. Certainly cochlear implantation should be strongly considered for children who cannot achieve this criterion with the use of well-fitted current hearing aid technology.

Factors That Complicate the Cochlear Implant Candidacy Process

A number of factors can complicate the decision to move forward with cochlear implantation. First, 40% of children with hearing loss have additional disabilities, many of which affect cognitive/neurological status (Gallaudet Research Institute, 2008). Cognitive challenges obviously present the potential to delay speech and language progress. In the case of children who have *cognitive disabilities* and profound hearing loss, cochlear implantation will likely optimize the child's potential to communicate by using spoken language. For children who have cognitive challenges and moderately severe to severe hearing loss (e.g., pure-tone average of 70–80 dB HL), the decision to pursue cochlear implantation is more complicated. It is possible that the speech and language of these children is hindered by cognitive challenge as much, or more so than the hearing loss. In these cases, it may be worthwhile to evaluate the child's nonverbal IQ. If speech and language aptitude is poorer than expected from the nonverbal IQ assessment, then cochlear implantation needs to be considered.

Poor progress with hearing aids may also occur when a child does not receive adequate support in the home. This can be manifested in the form of poor hearing aid usage as indicated by data logging (e.g., user information, such as number of hours used per day, types of acoustic environments encountered by the child, etc., collected by a child's hearing aid and displayed within the audiologist's fitting software at hearing aid checkups), infrequent attendance to audiology appointments, and a lack of commitment to AVT. Data logging can indicate that a child is using hearing technology during all waking hours. If this is not the case, the cochlear implant team must strive to assist the family in achieving full-time hearing aid use prior to cochlear implantation. Otherwise, the child may be implanted with a device that is rarely used. Likewise, the cochlear implant team needs to seek solutions to facilitate full-time participation in audiology and AVT sessions. It is necessary to develop these habits, because the cochlear implant will not provide a successful outcome if the family does not attend audiology appointments to ensure the device is programmed properly or attend AVT appointments to ensure the child learns to listen to the signal provided by the cochlear implant. Again, in these cases, the cochlear implant team needs to include a social worker who can assist the family in locating the resources required in order to meet the needs of the child. Failing to offer the supports necessary to develop language in a child with hearing loss constitutes neglect. It is the cochlear implant team's responsibility to make certain the family is aware of the consequences of a lack of action and to provide the support required to optimize the child's potential be successful in mainstream society.

Audiologic Management of Children With Cochlear Implants

In order to facilitate optimal responses from a child to a cochlear implant, the prudent practitioner lays a solid foundation for success well before the sound processor is activated.

The family is provided with information about the child's cochlear implant external equipment, user manuals, and video tutorials. With these, the family has an opportunity to become acquainted with the equipment prior to the activation appointment, which is helpful considering that cochlear implant activations are often emotional experiences making it difficult to absorb information about device use provided toward the end of the appointment.

Underpromise and Overdeliver/Three Categories of Initial Responses

It may seem trivial on the surface, but it is important to establish realistic expectations that the family associates with cochlear implantation. Audiologists and AV practitioners strive to underpromise and overdeliver. In other words, we attempt to manage expectations prior to the cochlear implant activation process and then do everything in our power to exceed these expectations once implant use commences.

Practitioners prepare the family so their child may respond to cochlear implant activation in one of three ways. First, some children smile, vocalize, and become quite happy when they first receive sound from their new cochlear implant. Although this is the most desirable outcome, it does not always occur.

Second, some children are fairly ambivalent to the sound they receive and show little to no emotion or reaction to stimulation from the implant, even when the audiologist can be absolutely certain the signal is audible because of its relationship to stimulation levels required to elicit neural responses. This response can be unsettling to parents, because they may assume that the child will be unable to hear with the implant. However, the family will be more comfortable with an inconclusive response if they have been adequately prepared for the possibility prior to activation.

Third, the child may become upset when he or she hears for the first time. Specifically, the child may cry, vocalize displeasure, remove the implant, and/ or seek out reassurance and comfort from a caregiver, and so on. Although this response is certainly undesirable, it is understandable given it is possibly the first time the child has experienced auditory stimulation. Once again, parents will be less concerned with this type of response if they have been adequately informed of the possibility ahead of time.

It is perfectly acceptable for a child to become upset to stimulation that is new and different as long as it is not uncomfortable for the child. The experienced audiologist will proceed conservatively with increases in stimulation in an effort to avoid overstimulating the child and eliciting an adverse response to the implant. A primary objective of the cochlear implant activation process is to promote a bond between the child and the new implant. Early overstimulation (e.g., stimulation that is too loud or uncomfortable) may cause the child to refuse the implant. In such cases, it can be a challenge to reacquire the child's trust in order for him or her to willingly wear the cochlear implant. The AV practitioner plays a key role in providing feedback to the audiologist regarding child's level of acceptance to the cochlear implant.

Eyes Open, Ears On

It is also imperative to establish the adage, "eyes open, ears on!" In other words, when a child's eyes are open, his or her hearing technology must be on to allow full-time access to all auditory stimuli. If a child does not have consistent access to intelligible speech throughout the first few years of life, the auditory centers of the brain will not develop fully and spoken language and auditory skill development will suffer (Buckley & Tobey, 2011; Ching & Dillon, 2013; Sharma, Dorman, & Spahr, 2002). Practitioners and families must work together to strive for an eyes open, ears on lifestyle. This requires the child's cochlear implant to be programmed appropriately, the family to understand the importance of full-time hearing technology use, and the family to be equipped with resources that facilitate full-time use (e.g., sound processor retention strategies/accessories, alarms/indicators that inform the caregiver when the device is not functioning properly, etc.).

Cochlear Implant Activation

Physical and Audiologic Examination

The audiologist needs to begin the appointment by examining the child's implant site. Otoscopy and tympanometry are likely also conducted. The audiologist selects the appropriate magnet strength for the child's transmitting coil that is strong enough to allow for consistent adherence of the coil to the head but not so strong that it compromises blood flow to the implant site. The coil site will be monitored at each implant checkup to ensure satisfactory health of the soft tissue at the implant site.

For children who have a considerable amount of low-frequency acoustic hearing prior to implantation (70 dB HL or better from 125–750 Hz), it is prudent to complete an audiometric assessment prior to cochlear implant activation to determine whether it may be preferable to provide acoustic stimulation in the low-frequency range rather than electrical stimulation. Low-frequency acoustic stimulation needs to be considered for all frequencies (125–1000 Hz) at which the air conduction threshold is 75 dB HL or better.

Cochlear Implant Programming

Setting Stimulation Levels

In order to optimize a child's auditory performance with a cochlear implant, it is imperative that stimulation levels are set appropriately. There are a number of different techniques used to set stimulation levels. Methods used to determine stimulation levels, however, vary considerably as a function of the age of a child. The following section highlights a number of ways that stimulation levels may be determined for pediatric cochlear implant recipients.

Optimizing T Levels to Ensure Consistent Audibility

T Levels represent the minimum amount of electrical stimulation a child can detect. T Level settings determine the stimulation a child will receive for low-level sound inputs. The clinician needs to set T levels according to the manufacturer's recommended definition in order to promote consistent audibility of desirable, low-level sounds while avoiding persistent exposure to constant electrical noise or overstimulation of low-level ambient noise (Holden et al., 2011). The techniques used to measure the electrical thresholds (e.g., T levels) of pediatric implant users are similar to techniques used to measure behavioral audiometric thresholds. Visual reinforcement audiometry (VRA) is often the procedure of choice to measure T levels in children between the ages of 8 and 24 months. All clinicians who use VRA with children need to be familiar with excellent resources that address this topic (Gravel, 2000; Gravel & Hood, 1999; Widen, 1993).

Conditioned play audiometry (CPA) is another excellent technique for measuring T levels. CPA involves setting up a game in which the child performs an action every time he or she hears a sound. A conditioned play response needs be developed as early as possible, because young children often become uninterested in the VRA tasks after multiple programming sessions.

The child's AV practitioner may strive to establish a CPA response in weekly therapy sessions. With focused practice, it is possible for children with hearing loss to develop a CPA as young as 18 months of age, although expected to perform these consistently at 24 months. As with VRA, an assistant is often necessary for CPA to be successful in the programming session.

T Level responses obtained from young children are probably best described as minimal response levels (MRL). In other words, the T levels do not represent the child's true detection threshold for electrical stimuli but rather the lowest suprathreshold (e.g., stimulation that exceeds the listener's true threshold of audibility) level at which the child will respond to electrical stimulation. In fact, it has been suggested that audiologists need to globally decrease measured T levels for small children in order to account for the possibility that the child's responses to programming stimuli are suprathreshold in nature (Zwolan & Griffin, 2005). Ultimately ideal sound-field detection thresholds are obtained between 20 and 25 dB HL. If sound-field detection thresholds are elevated, the audiologist needs to re-measure T levels and increase them as necessary to achieve acceptable sound-field detection thresholds.

Optimizing Upper Stimulation Levels to Ensure Comfort, Sound Quality, and Speech Recognition

Upper stimulation levels determine the amount of electrical stimulation a child will receive for high-level sound inputs. For older children and adults, upper stimulation levels may be set by psychophysical loudness scaling. The recipient's task is to point to a psychophysical loudness scaling chart to indicate the loudness associated with the signal that is presented. Figure 6–4 provides an illustration of a loudness scaling chart. The measure is completed on a given channel when the loudness reaches upper stimulation level as defined by the manufacturer.

Infants and young children do not possess sufficient expressive language to allow for their participation in loudness scaling and balancing tasks. Determining sufficient upper stimulation levels in infants and young children can be challenging. Audiologists must rely on their knowledge of typical electrical dynamic range and upper stimulation levels for particular cochlear implant systems as well as their observations of the child's behavior and responsiveness to sound as upper stimulation levels are increased. As the upper stimulation levels are slowly increased, the audiologist and assistant observe the child's behavior for signs that the stimulation from the implant is too loud. It may be helpful to use noisemakers, such as a xylophone, a drum, a tambourine, electronic toys, and so on, that produce moderate to high-level noise while upper stimulation levels are being increased in live speech mode. The child's caregiver may also speak to the child while upper stimulation levels are being increased.

The child's responses to increasing upper stimulation levels may be subtle and may occur in many forms. If the child is playing with the noisemakers, then he or she may stop playing with the toy, push it away, and/or decrease the intensity with which he or she is playing with it (e.g., banging on a drum

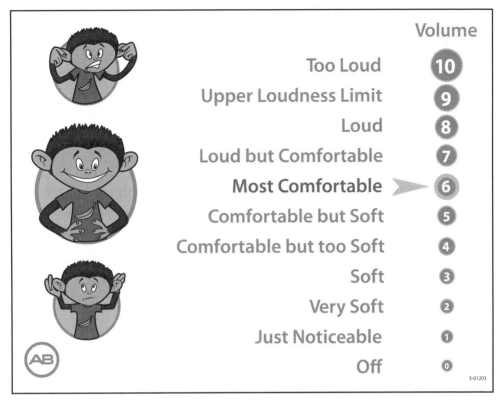

Figure 6–4. An example of a conventional loudness scaling chart (right side), and a loudness rating chart for young children (left side).

may change to tapping). Also, as upper stimulation levels are increased to a point that may be too loud, the child may change facial expression and/or his or her breathing pattern (e.g., stop smiling, hold breath, etc.), reach for a caregiver for affirmation, throw a toy from the highchair tray, attempt to remove the sound processor, and so on. The practitioners observe these behaviors closely in an effort to avoid increasing upper stimulation levels that are too loud. If they feel the child is exhibiting behaviors suggesting that the stimulation may be approaching the child's upper loudness limits, then upper stimulation levels will be decreased slightly, until they may confirm that the stimula-

tion is comfortable. If the child appears to be fine, then upper stimulation levels may be increased in small steps again, while the practitioners continue to observe the child's responses. These steps continue until the desired upper stimulation levels are reached or until the child exhibits behavior suggesting the stimulation is approaching a level that may be too loud.

Some children may show signs of discomfort prior to reaching the aforementioned upper stimulation levels, particularly during the early stages of implant use. In these cases, the practitioners refrain from aggressively pursuing the typical upper stimulation levels previously mentioned. Instead, upper stimulation levels are set at a level that will provide audibility and avoid any discomfort. Subsequently, the audiologist may seek to increase upper stimulation levels at future appointments.

Getting Objective: The Use of Objective Measures to Estimate Upper Stimulation Levels

Objective measures of auditory responsiveness to electrical stimulation may also be used as a guide to create programs for children with cochlear implants. A number of different objective measures have been used to evaluate a child's response to a cochlear implant including the electrically evoked compound action potential (eCAP) (e.g., Neural Response Telemetry [NRT]), the electrically evoked auditory brainstem response (eABR), the electrically evoked cortical auditory-evoked potential (eCAEP), and the electrically evoked stapedial reflex threshold (eSRT). The eABR and eCAEP have largely been used for research purposes only and will not be discussed in detail in this chapter. However, the eCAP and eSRT are routinely used in clinical settings and will be addressed here. A comprehensive discussion of the eCAP and eSRT are beyond the scope of this chapter. However, the eCAP can be used to determine a level of stimulation that is audible to the recipient, but it is not a satisfactory predictor of T levels or upper stimulation levels. The eCAP may be used in conjunction with behavioral measures to aid in the determination of stimulation levels for children who cannot provide verbal feedback about the auditory stimulation they receive from their cochlear implant. In contrast, the eSRT has been shown to be an excellent predictor of upper stimulation level

and needs to be used routinely as a guide to determine upper stimulation levels in children (Hodges, Balkany, Ruth, et al., 1997; Spivak, Chute, Popp, & Parisier, 1994; Wolfe & Kasulis, 2008). Wolfe and Schafer (2015) provide more information regarding the use of the eCAP and eSRT for cochlear implant programming in children.

Follow-Up: Touching Base to Ensure Optimal Performance for the Long Run

Children with cochlear implants need to be scheduled for frequent audiology appointments to evaluate postactivation outcomes, ensure the cochlear implant system is functioning appropriately, and ensure the cochlear implant program/MAP is set to optimize recipient performance. Table 6–1 provides a recommended audiologic management schedule for pediatric cochlear implant recipients. The family needs to be encouraged to contact the audiologist to report any concerns that arise regarding the child's performance and/or progress with the cochlear implant. Also, the child's AV practitioner and audiologist need to maintain a continual dialogue, and an unscheduled appointment may be set if the AV practitioner believes the child's progress is being impeded by his or her inability to hear optimally with the cochlear implant. At follow-up audiology appointments, attempts are made to measure aided sound-field thresholds to ensure the child has good access to low-level sounds (as indicated by sound-field thresholds between 20 and 25 dB HL). Also, speech recognition in quiet (at a presentation level consistent with average and soft-level speech) and in noise need to be evaluated. Finally, standard-

Table 6-1. Overview of Audiologic Appointment Schedule for Pediatric CI Recipients

Appointment	Duration	Basic Overview of Typical Procedures
Activation	2–3 hours	• Visual examination of incision site and otoscopy • Device programming/activation • Objective measures (ECAP) • Counseling regarding care, use, maintenance
One-day checkup	1–2 hours	• Same as activation procedures • Objective measures (ESRT* and ECAP) • Adjust and fine-tune per recipient report
One-week checkup	1–2 hours	• Assessment of aided performance in sound-field • Evaluation of cochlear implant/hearing aid hardware • Repeat procedures from one-day appointment
One-month checkup	1–2 hours	Repeat previous procedures
Quarterly checkups	1–2 hours	Repeat previous procedures

Note. * = if recipient will tolerate procedure; ECAP = electrically evoked compound action potential; ESRT = electrically evoked stapedius reflex threshold.

ized questionnaires are recommended to assess the child's functional auditory development.

Etiologies of Deafness and Cochlear Implant Outcomes

As previously mentioned, cochlear implants are the standard of care for children with severe to profound hearing loss. Although children with cochlear implants share this common trait, divergent etiologies of severe to profound hearing loss result in considerable variability in the underlying cause as well as the anatomic and physiologic bases responsible for the hearing loss. As a result, children with cochlear implants make up a fairly heteroge-

neous group. Variability in cochlear implant outcomes depends on many factors including the underlying etiology of the auditory disorder. As such, practitioners strongly consider referring children with hearing loss for a comprehensive genetic evaluation. Programs such as the University of Iowa's OtoSCOPE, which is a platform that relies on the newest DNA sequencing methods to screen all genes known to cause sensorineural hearing loss, are now available to provide a thorough evaluation of over 100 genes known to cause hearing loss. Additionally, otologists will commonly recommend magnetic resonance imaging (MRI) and/or computed tomography (CT) scans prior to cochlear implantation to evaluate the anatomical structures of the cochlear and vestibular organs. (Ellul, Shelton, Davidson, & Harnsberger, 2000, Parry, Booth, & Roland, 2005).

The following section addresses many common causes of hearing loss along with information pertaining to cochlear implantation.

Connexin 26

Connexin 26 mutations account for about 50% of autosomal recessive nonsyndromic congenital hearing loss (McGuirt & Smith, 1999). Connexin 26 mutations interfere with the metabolic state of the cochlea and often result in severe to profound hearing loss. Children with connexin 26 mutations typically have no other comorbidities and usually receive little to no benefit from hearing aid use when the hearing loss is severe to profound in degree. However, they typically excel with cochlear implants (Bauer, Geers, Brenner, Moog, & Smith, 2003; Wu, Lui, Wang, Hsu, & Wu, 2011), which bypass the site of lesion and stimulate the intact cochlear nerve directly.

Enlarged Vestibular Aqueduct

A diagnosis of enlarged vestibular aqueduct is usually accompanied by a significant high-frequency hearing loss that is frequently, but not always, progressive. Mild head trauma may result in progression of the hearing loss, so families need to be cautioned of the potential of further hearing loss from contact sports. Also, many children with enlarged vestibular aqueduct possess some low-frequency hearing loss with an air-bone gap in the absence of middle ear dysfunction. The air-bone gap is likely attributed to the force that the abnormally high pressure of

cochlear fluid places on the footplate of the stapes. It is also not uncommon for these children to have other associated inner ear abnormalities (Valvassori & Clemis, 1978).

Children who have enlarged vestibular aqueduct and mild to moderate hearing loss usually do quite well with hearing aids. However, these children may encounter frustration and difficulty with communication when hearing sensitivity fluctuates with changes in the ionic composition of endolymph and/or the pressure of cochlear fluids secondary to the abnormal function of the vestibular duct and endolymphatic sac. When hearing loss progresses to the severe to profound range, children with enlarged vestibular aqueducts are often better served with a cochlear implant, at least for one ear. Fortunately, because the site of lesion resides in the inner ear, children who have enlarged vestibular aqueducts and undergo cochlear implantation typically achieve favorable outcomes (Miyamoto, Bichey, Wynne, & Kirk, 2002).

Cochlear Abnormalities

Approximately 20% of children with hearing loss possess an anatomic abnormality of the temporal bone (Jackler, Luxford, & House, 1987; Papsin, 2005), and many of these children have severe to profound hearing loss and receive limited benefit from hearing aids (Park et al., 2000). Although many professionals may assume that abnormal cochlear anatomy might preclude a child from cochlear implantation, a number of studies suggest that children with a wide range of temporal bone abnormalities frequently receive considerable benefit from cochlear implantation (Buchman et al., 2004; Papsin, 2005). The potential benefit obtained from cochlear implantation is inversely related to the extent of the cochlear malformation.

Cochlear implant programming may be more challenging for these children. Specifically, the audiologist needs to communicate with the implant surgeon to determine whether all electrodes are in the cochlea and whether complications, such as facial nerve stimulation, might be expected. Also, children with significant cochlear anatomy abnormalities need to undergo more frequent checkups including audiologic assessment and implant programming, as these children are more likely to have performance that fluctuates over time requiring fine-tuning to the program/MAP.

Cochlear Nerve Deficiency

In contrast to the favorable outcomes observed in children with cochlear abnormalities, children diagnosed with cochlear nerve deficiency generally achieve limited benefit from cochlear implantation (Govaerts et al., 2003; Wu et al., 2015; Young, Kim, Ryan, Tournis, & Yaras, 2012). Clinically, cochlear nerve deficiency presents as an absent or abnormally small cochlear nerve on a magnetic resonance imaging (MRI) scan. High resolution computed tomography can also be beneficial for further evaluation of the anatomy involving the cochlear nerve (Adunka, Jewells, & Buchman, 2007). For the most part, children diagnosed with cochlear nerve deficiency struggle to develop spoken language with the use of a cochlear implant. When outcomes are poor after cochlear implantation, children with cochlear nerve deficiency may be considered for an auditory brainstem implant.

Cytomegalovirus

Cytomegalovirus (CMV) is likely responsible for 15% to 20% of moderate to profound congenital sensorineural hearing loss (Fowler & Boppanna, 2006; Grosse, Ross, & Dollard, 2008). Of all infants who contract congenital CMV, about 15% develop some degree of hearing loss, and 3% to 5% develop moderate to profound bilateral hearing loss (Grosse et al., 2008). Hearing loss associated with congenital CMV is not always present at birth, and it is may be progressive throughout the first few years of life. Children who have congenital CMV need to undergo audiometric evaluations every 6 months and every 3 months if hearing loss is identified. CMV is a well-known cause of neurological disorders. As a result, spoken language outcomes and, for that matter, general developmental outcomes, may be limited. Cochlear implantation is most certainly a viable (and likely beneficial) alternative for children who have congenital CMV-induced severe to profound hearing loss, but parents need to be cautiously counseled about the potential comorbidities associated with CMV and the impact those deficits may have on the child's overall development.

Auditory Neuropathy Spectrum Disorder

A finding of ANSD can be associated with dysfunction at a variety of different sites of lesion. If an inner hair cell disorder is the primary factor responsible for an absent ABR, then a cochlear implant can be expected to provide significant benefit. Indeed, research has suggested that a history of neonatal anoxia may be tied to a loss of inner hair cells. Furthermore, if a disorder of the auditory synapse is responsible for ANSD, then cochlear implantation can likely produce a successful outcome because the site of lesion would be bypassed when the cochlear nerve receives direct stimulation from the implant. An identified genetic disorder known as OTOF affects how a protein called *otoferlin* is coded (Rodriguez-Ballesteros et al., 2003). Otoferlin is present at the synapse between the cochlea and cochlear nerve. Research suggests that children with OTOF mutations do not spontaneously develop spoken language with the use of hearing aids (Berlin et al., 2010), but they do achieve favorable outcomes with cochlear implants (Rouillon et al., 2006; Wu et al., 2011).

Cochlear implant outcomes may be poorer for children for whom the site of lesion responsible for ANSD resides in the cochlear nerve or auditory brainstem. Pathologies of the cochlear nerve and brainstem can theoretically be quite variable in nature. Cochlear nerve pathologies may range from demyelination of the auditory axonal nerve fibers to complete absence of the spiral ganglion cell bodies of the cochlear nerve. The former case may show some benefit from cochlear implantation, while the latter can most likely be associated with a poor outcome from implantation. Likewise, a site of lesion at the auditory portion of the brainstem may be attributed to demyelination, a vascular disorder, or compression from a space-occupying lesion, such as a vestibular schwannoma, and so on. Further information can be obtained through a recommended review of Rapin and Gravel (2003, 2006) and Rance (2005) pertaining to the use of audiologic

diagnostic assessment to determine the site of lesion of ANSD.

A hearing aid trial needs to be completed on children with ANSD prior to pursuing cochlear implantation. Mixed results have been reported in studies examining the benefit children with ANSD receive from cochlear implantation. Berlin and colleagues (2010) reported that 85% of children who had ANSD and received a cochlear implant showed significant improvement in speech recognition and language comprehension. The methods used to evaluate speech recognition and language development were not clearly defined and the criteria that constituted significant benefit were not elucidated in the manuscript. Furthermore, Zeng and Liu (2006) reported that participants with ANSD and cochlear implants performed better than those with ANSD and hearing aids.

Teagle and colleagues (2010) reported on the speech recognition of 140 children with ANSD. Fifty-two of these children received cochlear implants after demonstrating limited benefit with hearing aids. Almost 30% achieved a word recognition score of 30% correct or less with use of their cochlear implant. Mean word recognition of the children who had been diagnosed with ANSD and had received a cochlear implant was 54% correct. Several children did perform quite well with their cochlear implant. Of particular importance, Teagle et al. reported that all of the children with open-set word recognition scores exceeding 30% correct also had present and robust eCAP responses (e.g., ART, NRI, NRT). In contrast, children with absent eCAP responses typically had poor word recognition.

Ching and Dillon (2013) reported on speech, language, and auditory skill outcomes for 47 children who had ANSD and were part of a larger cohort of 451 children with hearing loss who are being evaluated as part of a longitudinal population study. Ching and Dillon found that outcomes of the children with ANSD were similar to children with cochlear hearing loss when evaluated at 3 years of age. Also, the speech, language, and auditory skill development at 3 years of age was similar between the children with ANSD and hearing aids compared to children with ANSD and cochlear implants.

The variability reported across studies of outcomes of children with ANSD and cochlear implants is likely attributed to whether a child has additional challenges that may influence performance and also to the site of lesion causing ANSD. As previously mentioned, if the site of lesion occurs within the cochlea (e.g., inner hair cells) or at the synapse between the inner hair cells and cochlear nerve, cochlear implantation will most likely produce benefit and a successful outcome. However, benefit and outcomes may be more likely to be limited if the site of lesion occurs at the cochlear nerve or auditory brainstem.

Additional Considerations Pertaining to Pediatric Cochlear Implantation

Bilateral Cochlear Implantation

A wealth of research suggests that children with bilateral severe to profound hearing loss are typically best served through the use of bilateral cochlear implantation (Litovsky, Johnstone, & Godar, 2006; Schafer, Amlani, Paiva, Nozari, & Verret, 2011). Namely, speech recognition in quiet and in noise as well as localization are typically better with use of two cochlear implants relative to the unilateral condition (Litovsky et al., Murphy, Summerfield, O'Donoghue, & Moore, 2011). 2006). It has also been suggested that better language outcomes are prevalent among children who use bilateral cochlear implants. But, in order to obtain maximum benefit from bilateral cochlear implantation, research has suggested that implantation needs to occur at an early age with a relatively short delay in implantation between ears (Gordon, Jiwani, & Papsin, 2011, 2013; Peters, Litovsky, Parkinson, & Lake, 2007; Wolfe et al., 2007).

Bimodal

The bimodal condition (use of a cochlear implant on one ear and a hearing aid on the other ear) generally provides better hearing performance than that obtained with use of a cochlear implant alone (Ching et al., 2014; Ching, van Wanrooy, & Dillon, 2007; Litovsky et al., 2006). Specifically, children understand speech better in noise with bimodal use compared to performance with the implant alone (Ching et al., 2007, 2014; Litovsky et al., 2006). Bimodal use typically provides a limited improvement in localization, because electrical stimulation does not adequately preserve low-frequency timing cues necessary for localization via interaural time differences, while the hearing aid typically provides poor audibility of high-frequency sounds necessary for localization via interaural level differences. Bimodal use can be considered essential for children with bilateral hearing loss who are not deemed to be good candidates for bilateral cochlear implantations. Additional research is needed to determine whether bimodal or bilateral cochlear implant use needs to be recommended for children with bilateral, severe to profound hearing loss. In the absence of evidence-based guidelines, the authors of this chapter suggest the following criteria for selection of technology for children with bilateral hearing loss:

- When better ear thresholds are flat and better than 75 dB HL, try bimodal.
- When low-frequency thresholds are better than 70 dB HL with severe to profound high-frequency hearing loss, consider hybrid cochlear implantation.
- When hearing loss is flat and in the 75 to 85 dB HL range, lean toward bimodal until evidence of bilateral disruption or poor progress exists.
- When hearing loss exceeds 85 dB HL for both ears, consider bilateral implantation.

(*Note.* Low-frequency = 125–750 Hz; high-frequency = 1500 Hz and up)

Single-Sided Deafness

An emerging trend in pediatric cochlear implantation is the consideration of a cochlear implant for children with single-sided deafness (e.g., severe to profound hearing loss in one ear and normal hearing sensitivity in the poorer ear). Historically, children with single-sided deafness (SSD) have been considered as candidates for contralateral-routing-of-signal (CROS) hearing aids, implantable bone conduction hearing devices, and/or remote microphone technology. However, none of these technologies are able to effectively stimulate the impaired ear, and as a result, binaural processing cannot be restored. Also, the continuation of auditory deprivation for the impaired ear may result in irreversible changes in the auditory cortex opposite the impaired ear (Bilecen et al., 2000; Gordon, Henkin, & Kral, 2015; Kral, Heid, Hubka, & Tillein, 2013; Kral, Hubka, Heid, & Tillein, 2013; Schmithorst et al., 2005, Schmithorst, Plante, & Holland, 2014; Vasama, Mäkelä, Parkkonen, & Hari, 1994). Consequently, pediatric hearing health care professionals have begun to consider cochlear implantation for children with SSD. Indeed, if an MRI indicates that the child has an intact cochlear nerve for the impaired ear, then cochlear implantation is the only hearing technology that allows for auditory stimulation to the poorer ear. Early cochlear implantation may prevent negative effects associated with auditory deprivation and may serve to partially restore interaural auditory cues, and subsequently may improve localization and speech recognition in noise. Additional research is needed to further clarify the advantages and limitations of cochlear implantation for children with SSD.

Noise Management Technologies for Children With Cochlear Implants

It is well known that speech recognition in noise of persons with cochlear implants is typically 30 to 60 percentage points worse than speech recognition in quiet (Schafer & Thibodeau, 2004; Wolfe, Morais, Neumann, et al., 2013; Wolfe, Morais, Schafer, et al., 2013).

Cochlear implant manufacturers have introduced several technologies that aim to improve performance in noise. Signal processing strategies that reduce stimulation in channels dominated by noise and enhance stimulation in channels containing speech need to be considered for use in children of all ages (e.g., autosensitivity control [ASC; Gifford & Revitt, 2010; Wolfe, Schafer, Heldner, et al., 2009; Wolfe, Schafer, John, et al., 2011], ClearVoice [Wolfe, Morais, et al., 2015], and SNR-NR (Wolfe, Neumann, et al., 2015; Wolfe, Morais, et al., 2015).

Directional microphone technology has been introduced to modern cochlear implant sound processors. Modern directional devices automatically switch from omnidirectional to directional mode when the recipient moves from a quiet to a noisy environment and change the microphone's sensitivity in an attempt to provide maximum attenuation for the direction from where the most intense noise arrives. These devices are sometimes referred to as fully adaptive systems. Directional microphone technology has certainly been shown to improve speech recognition in noise of cochlear implant users (Wolfe et al., 2012; Wolfe, Neumann, Marsh, et al., 2015). However, a potential drawback of directional microphone use is that it may result in a reduction in audibility for desirable sounds that arrive from behind a child (e.g., a parent speaking behind the child). Consequently, there is not unanimous agreement among professionals.

The authors suggest the following recommendations for directional technology for infants and children. Infants and toddlers are less likely to orient toward a caregiver who may be speaking to them. As a result, fully adaptive directional technology may not be the best choice for this age group. However, preschool-age (3–5 years old) children are fully able to orient toward the signal of interest (Ricketts & Galster, 2008), so fully adaptive directional technology may at least be considered for this group. Audiologists need to counsel families about the intent of fully adaptive directional systems and note the importance of making frequent observations of the child's behavior in noisy situations to determine the benefit of directional technology. School-age children (6 years old and up) are capable in most cases of providing verbal feedback about their listening experiences. Fully adaptive directional systems can definitely be considered for use with this group. If a child reports difficulty associated with the introduction of the technology, then the feature may be removed.

Electric-Acoustic Stimulation

An emerging trend in cochlear implantation is the use of atraumatic electrode arrays and surgical techniques in an attempt to preserve low-frequency acoustic hearing. Recipients who do possess residual, low-frequency acoustic hearing after surgery may be fitted with an electric-acoustic stimulation (EAS) processor that provides acoustic stimulation in the low frequencies and electrical stimulation in the high frequencies. Research has shown that EAS provides better speech recognition in quiet and noise, localization, music appreciation and performance, and sound quality when compared to electric-only stimulation (Adunka, Pillsbury, Adunka, & Buchman, 2010; Cochlear Nucleus Hybrid L24 Implant System P130016, 2014; Incerti, Ching,

& Cowan, 2013). As a result, EAS can be considered a viable option for children who have mild to moderate low-frequency hearing loss and severe to profound high-frequency hearing loss. There is no consensus as to whether short, hybrid electrode arrays need to be considered for use with children. A shorter array likely improves the chances for preservation of low-frequency hearing, but it may not provide sufficient stimulation across the frequency range for children who lose their low-frequency hearing during surgery or progressively across time. More research is needed to determine potential benefits and limitations of EAS, and in particular hybrid electrode arrays, for children.

AUDITORY BRAINSTEM IMPLANTS

The overwhelming majority of those who have severe to profound hearing loss and are candidates for an implantable hearing device will receive and benefit from a cochlear implant. However, a small number will be unresponsive to or unsuitable for a cochlear implant. Some may be candidates, therefore, for an *auditory brainstem implant* (Kaplan, Kozin, Puram, et al., 2015).

An auditory brainstem implant is similar to a cochlear implant, but the electrode array is typically inserted on the cochlear nucleus at the inferior, dorsolateral area of the pons. Figure 6–5 provides an example of an auditory brainstem implant system.

Auditory brainstem implants function in a similar manner to cochlear implants, but instead of providing stimulation to the auditory nerve, the cochlea is bypassed and electrical stimulation is delivered via a paddle electrode array to the auditory brainstem. A neurotologist places the paddle electrode in the lateral recess of the fourth ventricle over the cochlear nucleus.

Typical Outcomes With Auditory Brainstem Implants

Auditory brainstem implants were originally developed for persons with neurofibromatosis type 2 (NF2), a condition that causes tumors to proliferate along the central nervous system. In some

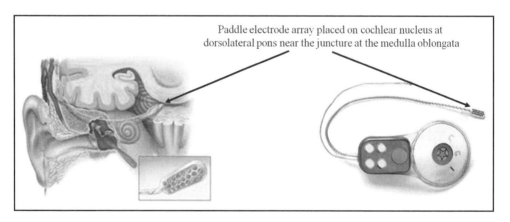

Paddle electrode array placed on cochlear nucleus at dorsolateral pons near the juncture at the medulla oblongata

Figure 6–5. An example of an auditory brainstem implant.

patients with NF2, the cochlear nerve is severed during the process of tumor removal, and as a result, a cochlear implant is unsuccessful. The auditory brainstem implant bypasses the damaged cochlear nerve and stimulates the auditory areas of the lower brainstem directly. Unfortunately, many persons with NF2 experience a substantial amount of degeneration of the neurons in the cochlear nerve as well as in the auditory centers of the brainstem. As such, the auditory brainstem may not produce a favorable outcome for many persons with NF2 (Behr et al., 2014; Colletti & Shannon, 2005; Colletti, Shannon, Carner, Veronese, & Colletti, 2009).

Outcomes appear to be more favorable in studies examining performance of persons with auditory brainstem implants and etiologies other than NF2 (Colletti et el., 2009; Colletti & Shannon, 2005; Noij et al., 2015). For example, Colletti et al. (2009) reported on the open-set speech recognition of 48 auditory brainstem implant users who did not have NF2. These participants achieved a mean score of 59% correct with performance ranging from 10% to 100% correct. Of note, participants with cochlear nerve deficiency and cochlear nerve injury typically performed quite well with their auditory brainstem implants. In short, auditory brainstem implants are a worthy consideration for children who have cochlear nerve deficiency or cochlear ossification.

IMPLANTABLE BONE CONDUCTION HEARING DEVICES (IBCHD)

Implantable bone conduction hearing devices (IBCHDs), also commonly re-ferred to as bone-anchored hearing aids (BAHAs), and were created as an option to treat conductive or mixed types of hearing losses as well as SSD. IBCHDs aim to transmit acoustic information to the cochlea via vibratory transmission through the skull. IBCHDs essentially operate on the same physiologic bases as what is found in bone conduction hearing assessment. All IBCHD devices possess an external sound processor and a titanium-implanted component. In short, sound is received at the microphone of the external sound processor and converted from acoustic to mechanical energy. Then, the mechanical, vibratory signal is transmitted to the implanted component either across the skin or via direct connection. The vibratory oscillations are then delivered from the implanted component through the bones of the skull to vibrate the structures of the cochlea.

Bone conduction hearing devices have been available for over 60 years (Mudry & Tjellstrom, 2011). The original bone conduction hearing devices featured a vibratory device that was worn on an uncomfortable metal headband or built into bulky glasses frames. The bone conduction oscillator was typically worn on the skin at or near the mastoid process, and the vibratory signal was delivered across the skin to the skull. There was no implantable component in these early devices. As a result, the signal of interest was attenuated by approximately 15 dB as it traveled across the skin (Tjellstrom, Hakansson, & Granstrom, 2001). Also, these devices often obtained inferior technology (e.g., no digital signal processing, limited bandwidth, limited output, high distortion).

To overcome the loss of energy that occurs when vibratory signals are delivered across the skin, Tjellstrom introduced the concept of implanting a titanium fixture into the skull allowing the vibratory transducer to be coupled directly to the skull via the fixture (Mudry & Tjellstrom, 2011). Since the advent of implantable, direct bone conduction technology and bone conduction hearing devices have steadily evolved over the past several decades. Additionally, usage has increased, and the performance of and benefit from IBCHD has improved (Hakansson, Tjellstrom, & Rosenhall, 1984; Mudry& Tjellstrom, 2011).

IBCHDs are typically classified into two broad categories, *percutaneous* and *transcutaneous* systems. Percutaneous devices contain an implantable fixture that is surgically inserted into the mastoid bone of the skull. An abutment, which is connected to the fixture, protrudes through the skin so that the surface resides just over the skin. The IBCHD external sound processor is connected to the abutment so that the mechanical oscillations of the sound processor may be delivered directly to the skull via the implanted fixture/abutment. Figure 6–6 provides examples of percutaneous IBCHDs.

Transcutaneous IBCHDs feature an implantable titanium component that is surgically fixed to the mastoid bone of the skull by biocompatible titanium screws. The implanted component also possesses a magnet or magnets. The external sound processor is connected to a magnetic plate that adheres to the magnet(s) of the implanted component residing under the skin. As such, the external sound processor sits on the skin above the mastoid bone by way of magnetic attraction to the implanted component. The vibratory oscillations of the external sound processor are delivered across the skin to the implanted component and then to the cochlea via bone conduction through the skull. Figure 6–7 provides examples of transcutaneous IBCHDs.

A recently introduced IBCHD does not necessarily fall into either of the aforementioned broad categories of

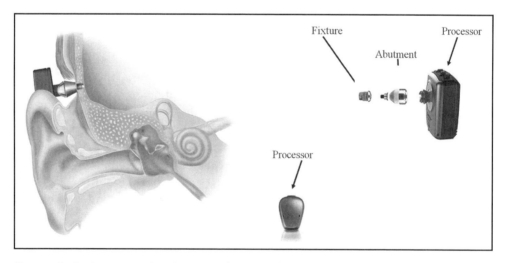

Figure 6-6. An example of a percutaneous implantable bone conduction hearing system.

IBCHDs. Figure 6–8 provides an example of an IBCHD that possesses a titanium implant that is surgically fixed to the mastoid bone with titanium screws. This IBCHD also contains an electromagnetic receiving coil that is used to receive an electromagnetic radio frequency signal from the external sound processor. A magnet resides in the center of the internal receiving coil and the external sound processor to allow for adherence of the external sound processor to the internal device. Acoustic inputs are captured by the microphone of the external sound processor, processed by the digital signal processor within the external sound processors, and delivered to the internal receiving

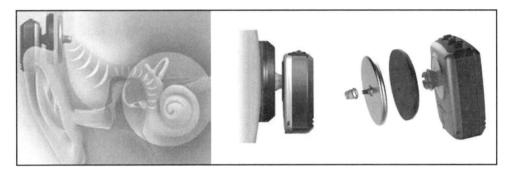

Figure 6-7. An example of a transcutaneous implantable bone conduction hearing system.

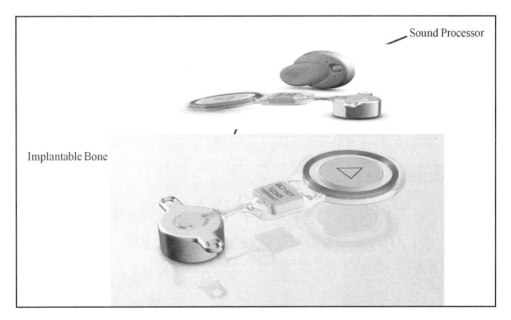

Sound Processor

Implantable Bone

Figure 6-8. An example of an implantable bone conduction hearing device in which the signal of interest is delivered from a sound processor to a titanium-implanted device via electromagnetic induction.

coil by way of a short-range electro-magnetic induction link. Then, the signal is sent to a mechanical oscillator that creates vibratory oscillations that are delivered to the skull. The external sound processor of an IBCHD may also be connected to a "softband" so that the processor resides on the head similar to a conventional nonimplantable bone conduction device (Figure 6–9). IBCHDs are typically not surgically inserted until 5 years of age or older. This is necessary in order to allow for maturation of the skull so that it is thick enough to accommodate the implantable component. The technology of IBCHDs is more sophisticated than early model bone conduction hearing aids, and substantial benefit may be obtained from the use of a contemporary external sound processor coupled to a softband. However, the signal is attenuated in a frequency-specific manner as it crosses the skin to be delivered to the skull.

Assessment of IBCHD Candidacy With Various Indications for Use

IBCHDs are considered to be the standard of care for treating children with permanent conductive hearing loss (CHL) or mixed hearing loss (MHL) that may not be ameliorated through surgical intervention. Children diagnosed with congenital aural atresia and/or microtia or other outer and middle ear hearing losses are the most common candidates for an IBCHD. These hearing losses can occur in one or both ears, but more commonly occur unilaterally. Other common causes of CHL and MHL include chronic otitis media and chronic otitis externa (middle and outer ear infections) with resulting hearing loss, cholesteatoma, and ossicular chain abnormalities such as congenital stapes fixation. Specific examples of children who commonly benefit from an IBCHD include those who have congenital syndromes such as Goldenhar, Treacher-Collins, and Down syndrome. Individuals with single-sided deafness (severe to profound hearing loss in one ear) are also common candidates for an IBCHD.

Bone conduction hearing devices are recommended over conventional air conduction hearing aids for those with CHL or MHL with an air-bone gap exceeding 30 dB and normal to near-normal bone conduction hearing sensitivity (Hol, Bosman, Snik, Mylanus, &

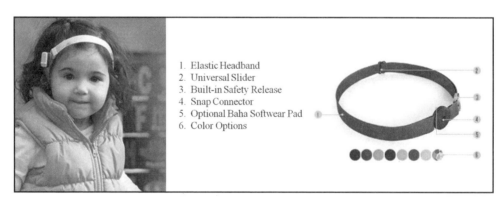

1. Elastic Headband
2. Universal Slider
3. Built-in Safety Release
4. Snap Connector
5. Optional Baha Softwear Pad
6. Color Options

Figure 6-9. An example of how a bone conduction sound processor may be worn on the head with a soft headband connector.

Cremers, 2005; Hol, Snik, Mylanus, & Cremers, 2005b; Mylanus, van der Pouw, Snik, & Cremers, 1998; Snik et al., 2005). IBCHDs can bypass the affected middle ear and directly stimulate the intact inner ear(s). As a result, a higher-fidelity signal with lower distortion can be provided.

IBCHDs may also be considered for children with SSD. In such cases, an IBCHD may be used to send the signal captured at the side of the poorer ear to the better ear via bone conduction. In essence, the IBCHD works like a CROS hearing instrument by delivering the signal of interest from the poor ear to the better ear by way of bone conduction, which assists in overcoming the head shadow effect. However, the impaired ear is not being stimulated in this situation. Also, use of an IBCHD for children with SSD will not improve localization, and speech recognition in quiet and in noise will not improve unless the signal of interest arrives on the side of the impaired ear.

Audiologic Criteria for Candidacy

From an audiologic perspective, children must have a conductive or mixed hearing loss with an average air-bone gap (average bone conduction thresholds at 500, 1000, and 2000 Hz) of at least 30 dB, to benefit from an IBCHD. The U.S. Food and Drug Administration (FDA) guidelines state that the bone conduction pure tone average (an average of bone conduction thresholds at 500, 1000, and 2000 Hz) has to be less than or equal to 55 to 65 dB HL. Ideally, however, bone conduction thresholds should be in the normal to near-normal rage. IBCHD sound processor selection is an important consideration when

the sensorineural component is more severe (e.g., bone conduction 25 dB HL or poorer), because those individuals may do best with a more powerful external sound processor. The manufacturers of IBCHD have delineated the selection of external sound processors on the basis of bone conduction pure-tone average criteria. For example, "standard" sound processors are recommended for persons with bone conduction pure tone averages of 45 dB HL or better, while "power" processors are suggested for persons with poorer bone conduction hearing thresholds (45–65 dB HL).

Of course, the stimulation an IBCHD user receives from a device is also substantially influenced by the coupling mechanism. Less output is achieved with conventional transcutaneous use (e.g., sound processor placed on the mastoid with no implantable component). Greater output will be obtained with use of transcutaneous system that contains an implanted component fixed to the skull. The highest output is achieved with the use of a percutaneous system, which allows for direct delivery of the vibratory signal to the skull. As a result, percutaneous systems are the ideal choice for those with bone conduction thresholds falling outside of the normal range.

Additional Candidacy Assessments

Additional testing to determine candidacy needs to involve a trial with a modern IBCHD sound processor that is deemed appropriate for the candidate's audiologic profile. The candidate can be given the opportunity to listen with the sound processor coupled to a softband or a metal headband. Additionally, the sound processor may be attached to an oral post on which the candidate may bite down to receive the bone conducted signal directly by way vibration from the teeth to the skull. If adequate output is achieved with use of the softband, then a transcutaneous system will likely provide satisfactory performance. If the listening experience with the softband is unsatisfactory, then the candidate most likely needs to be considered for a percutaneous implant.

Aided thresholds can be measured with the trial device (with the better ear plugged or masked as needed) to ensure that adequate audibility is provided for soft sounds. Ideally, aided thresholds should be no poorer than 30 dB HL. Furthermore, aided speech recognition needs to be assessed when possible to determine whether adequate speech recognition can be obtained at presentation levels consistent with average and soft-level speech (Snapp, Fabry, Telischi, Arheart, & Angeli, 2010). This information is especially important to establish a baseline to compare with future performance and also to ensure that the most appropriate type of coupling and sound processor is prescribed.

The Trade-Off Associated With Use of Percutaneous and Transcutaneous Devices

There are advantages and disadvantages to selecting either a transcutaneous or percutaneous device. Use of a percutaneous device provides better sound transfer with less energy loss, which would likely translate, to better sound quality. Additionally, the lower gain requirements result in a reduced chance of acoustic feedback. The primary drawback associated with a percutaneous device is the protruding screw, which can be problematic from a psychosocial (e.g., cosmetic concerns, peer pressure, etc.) and medical perspective (e.g., soft tissue complications, fixture extraction, healing time, time required for osseointegration, etc.). For example, in order to allow for osseointegration to occur, children have to wait up to 6 months before coupling their external sound processor to the abutment.

For the transcutaneous devices, soft tissue complications are less likely, and the recipient is not burdened with the responsibility of maintaining hygiene around the abutment as is the case with percutaneous devices. Also, recipients may consider transcutaneous devices to be more aesthetically pleasing. However, transcutaneous devices must overcome the attenuation that occurs when the vibratory signal is sent across the skin. It is reasonable to expect that the transcutaneous coupling will result in attenuation of 5 dB around 1000 Hz ranging up to 20 to 25 dB at 6000 Hz compared to that of the percutaneous coupling (Kurz, Flynn, Caversaccio, & Kompis, 2014). As a result, transcutaneous devices generally cannot provide as much stimulation as percutaneous systems, and they may not be appropriate for persons with elevated bone conduction thresholds. Additionally, a higher-powered (and larger) sound processor may be required to generate sufficient stimulation. Finally, recipients of transcutaneous systems may begin using their sound processor within 1 month compared to the 3 to 6 month delay required for osseointegration with most percutaneous systems (Briggs et al., 2015).

Single-Sided Deafness and IBCHDs

Candidacy guidelines also exist for children with SSD. Specifically, labeling indicates that hearing sensitivity in the contralateral ear must be within normal limits. Normal limits for this population is defined as the air conduction pure tone average at 500, 1000, 2000, and 3000 Hz that is equal to or better than 20 dB HL. The hearing loss in the poorer ear must fall within the severe to profound hearing loss range.

In the case of SSD candidacy, it is important to have a discussion with the family about outcomes with an IBCHD versus a cochlear implant. As new research continues to emerge suggesting that a cochlear implant is the more effective option for treating SSD, IBCHDs may not be recommended as regularly. However, there is still a place for IBCHDs in SSD in the case that imaging shows a child has cochlear malformations or an absent or small auditory nerve or for other reasons that a cochlear implant may be contraindicated. A study has shown that in a group of 69 pediatric (0–15 years) patients, almost 67% had inner ear and/or auditory canal malformations (Masuda, Usi, & Matsunaga, 2013).

Bilateral IBCHD Use

Those with bilateral CHL or MHL may be considered for bilateral IBCHD use. Research suggests that bilateral IBCHD use may improve sound localization (Priwin, Stenfelt, Granstrom, Tjellstrom, & Hakansson, 2004; Priwin, Jonsson, Hultcranz, & Granstrom, 2007; van der

Pouw et al., 1998), speech reception thresholds (SRTs) in quiet and in noise (Priwin et al., 2004) and speech perception in quiet and in noise (Dutt et al., 2002b; Priwin et al., 2007; van der Pouw, Snik, & Cremers, 1998). In adult patients, bilateral IBCHDs were also associated with improved quality of life and perceived well-being (Dutt et al., 2002a). This was affirmed with children who reported an improvement in sound quality and global benefit in a majority of patients (Dun et al., 2010).

Assessment of Auditory Outcomes of Children With IBCHD/Expectations

Beyond the provision of an IBCHD, verification and validation are necessary to ensure ongoing benefit. For children using IBCHDs, the expectations and outcomes need to be similar to children who wear traditional hearing aids or cochlear implants. Aided sound-field warble tone thresholds need to be ideally no less than 30 dB HL. Most real-ear verification systems do not have the ability to allow for the completion of real-ear measures on those with an IBCHD. The exception is the Interacoustics SKS skull stimulator that works with the Interacoustics Affinity real-ear hearing aid analyzer system (Interacoustics, n.d.) to verify output in the test box.

Speech recognition assessments need to be completed at normal (60 dBA/45 dB HL) and soft (50 dBA/35 dB HL) conversational levels in quiet and in noise. Given the normal to near-normal cochlear status for children with IBCHD, substantial open-set speech recognition capacity can be expected with device use.

The youngest children fit with IBCHDs may be at a disadvantage because practitioners are not always able to assess benefit objectively through audiologic measures, at least not at first. Instead, subjective measures can be administered. Questionnaires can be an effective way to validate the IBCHD fitting. Also, the child's AV practitioner can provide valuable information regarding auditory and spoken language development. At least 1 year of growth in auditory and spoken language development needs to occur for each chronological year.

IMPLICATIONS OF IMPLANTABLE HEARING TECHNOLOGIES FOR THE AV PRACTITIONER

Many children with severe to profound hearing loss, auditory neuropathy spectrum disorder, or significant, permanent conductive hearing loss may receive limited benefit from hearing aids. In such cases, the AV practitioner needs to consult with the child's hearing health care team (e.g., audiologist, otologist, etc.) to determine whether the child's needs may be met more effectively with implantable hearing technology. Implantable hearing technologies are continuously evolving, and AV practitioners who coach and guide parents, need to have current knowledge of the changes in these technologies in order to optimize the child's listening and spoken language development.

Determination of a child's candidacy for implantable hearing technology is a multifaceted process that involves audiological, otological, and speech and language assessments. The AV practitioner plays a critical role in the cochlear implant candidacy process. The status of a child's auditory skills and spoken language development is one of the primary and most instrumental factors governing the cochlear implant candidacy decision-making process. With modern hearing technology and AVT, many children with hearing loss can achieve age-appropriate auditory and spoken language abilities and make at least 1 year of progress in spoken language development for every chronological year. Thus, sessions with the AV practitioner are critical both pre- and postcochlear implantation.

The AV practitioner is required to have a thorough understanding of a child's unaided and aided auditory function including the degree, type, and configuration of the hearing loss, aided thresholds, and aided speech recognition in quiet (at an average and soft conversational level) as well as in noise. With this knowledge and ongoing diagnostic sessions in AVT, the practitioner can move forward or consider modifying the child's services (e.g., hearing technology) when aided performance is inadequate.

Audiologists and AV practitioners work together in order to effectively optimize the progress and performance of the child. This partnership (see Chapter 16) takes place throughout the assessment and management processes. Management of implantable hearing technologies (e.g., device programming, troubleshooting, evaluation of aided performance, etc.) is a complex process that is best navigated when the audiologist and AV practitioner work in tandem. Ideally, the AV practitioner needs to be an intimate part of managing the child's implantable hearing technology, including the provision of assistance in device programming, assessment, and troubleshooting. The audiologist and AV practitioner can work collaboratively to improve hearing performance when aided assessment of auditory function, or the AV practitioner's assessment of auditory and spoken language development, indicate insufficient performance and/or progress.

SUMMARY

Implantable hearing technology makes age-appropriate spoken language a possibility for the vast majority of children with hearing loss, regardless of their degree, configuration, or type of hearing loss. Pediatric hearing health care providers need to be vigilant about the advances in implantable hearing technology to ensure that children with hearing loss are able to reach their full potential in the development of listening and spoken language abilities. Audiologists, AV practitioners, otologists, and families work together in order to optimize the benefit children receive from implantable hearing devices.

REFERENCES

Adunka, O. F., Jewells, V., & Buchman, C. A. (2007). Value of computed tomography in the evaluation of children with cochlear nerve deficiency. *Otology and Neurotology*, *28*(5), 597–604.

Adunka, O. F., Pillsbury, H. C., Adunka, M. C., & Buchman, C. A. (2010). Is electric acoustic stimulation better than conventional cochlear implantation for speech perception in quiet? *Otology and Neurotology*, *31*(7), 1049–1054.

AG Bell Academy of Listening and Spoken Language. (2007). *Principles of LSLS Auditory-Verbal Therapy (LSLS Cert. AVT™)*. Retrieved August 25, 2015, from http://www.listeningandspoken language.org/AcademyDocument.aspx?id=563

Bagatto, M. (2012). 20Q: Baby steps following verification—outcome evaluation in pediatric hearing aid fitting. *Audiology Online*. Retrieved August 28, 2015, from http://www.audiologyonline.com/articles/20q-baby-steps-following-verification-783

Bagatto, M. P., Moodie, S. T., Malandrino, A. C., Richert, F. M., Clench, D. A., & Scollie, S. D. (2011). The University of Western Ontario audiological monitoring protocol (UWO PedAMP). *Trends in Amplification*, *15*(1), 57–76.

Bauer, P. W., Geers, A. E., Brenner, C. Moog, J. S., & Smith, R. J. (2003). The effect of GJB2 allele variants on performance after cochlear implantation. *Laryngoscope*, *113*(12), 2135–2140.

Behr, R., Colletti, V., Matthies, C., Morita, A., Nakatomi, H., Dominique, L., . . . Skarzynski, H. (2014). New outcomes with auditory brainstem implants in NF2 patients. *Otology and Neurotology*, *35*(10), 1844–1851.

Berlin, C. I., Hood, L. J., Morlet, T., Wilensky, D., Li, L., Mattingly, K. R., & Frisch, S. A. (2010). Multi-site diagnosis and management of 260 patients with auditory neuropathy/dys-synchrony (Auditory Neuropathy Spectrum Disorder*). *International Journal of Audiology*, *49*(1), 30–43.

Berninger, E., & Westling, B. (2011). Outcome of a universal newborn hearing-screening programme based on multiple transient-evoked otoacoustic emissions and clinical brainstem response audiometry. *Acta Oto-laryngologica, 131*(7), 728–739.

Bess, F. H., Dodd-Murphy, J., & Parker, R. A. (1998). Children with minimal sensorineural hearing loss: Prevalence, educational performance, and functional status. *Ear and Hearing, 19*(5), 339–354.

Bilecen, D., Seifritz, E., Radü, E. W., Schmid, N., Wetzel, S., Probst, R., & Scheffler, K. (2000). Cortical reorganization after acute unilateral hearing loss traced by fMRI. *Neurology, 54*(3), 765–767.

Briaire, J. J., & Frijns, J. H. (2005). Unraveling the electrically evoked compound action potential. *Hearing Research, 205*(1–2), 143–156.

Briggs, R., Van Hasselt, A., Luntz, M., Goycoolea, M., Wigren, S., Weber, P., & Cowan, R. (2015). Clinical performance of a new magnetic bone conduction hearing implant system: Results from a prospective, multicenter, clinical investigation. *Otology and Neurotology, 36*(5), 834–841.

Brown, C. J., Abbas, P. J., Fryauf-Bertschy, H., Kelsey, D., & Gantz, B. J. (1994). Intraoperative and postoperative electrically evoked auditory brainstem responses in nucleus cochlear implant users: Implications for the fitting process. *Ear and Hearing, 15*(2), 168–176.

Brown, C. J., Abbas, P. J., & Gantz, B. J. (1998). Preliminary experience with neural response telemetry in the nucleus CI24M cochlear implant. *American Journal of Otology, 19*(3), 320–327.

Buchman, C. A., Copeland, B. J., Yu, K. K., Brown, C. J., Carrasco, V. N., & Pillsbury, H. C. (2004). Cochlear implantation in children with congenital inner ear malformations. *Laryngoscope, 114*(2), 309–316.

Buckley, K. A., & Tobey, E. A. (2011). Crossmodal plasticity and speech perception in pre- and postlingually deaf cochlear implant users. *Ear and Hearing, 32*(1), 2–15.

Carlson, M. L., Sladen, D. P., Haynes, D. S., Driscoll, C. L., DeJong, M. D., Erickson, H. C., & Gifford, R. H. (2015). Evidence for the expansion of pediatric cochlear implant candidacy. *Otology and Neurotology, 36*(1), 43–50.

Centers for Disease Control and Prevention (CDC). (2007). *Risk of bacterial meningitis in children with cochlear implants.* Retrieved August 29, 2015, from http://www.fda.gov/MedicalDevices/Safety/AlertsandNotices/PatientAlerts/ucm064671.htm

Chen, J., Gittleman, A., Barnes, P., & Chang, K. W. (2008). Utility of temporal bone computed tomographic measurements in the evaluation of inner ear malformations. *Archives in Otolaryngology—Head and Neck Surgery, 134*(1), 50–56.

Ching, T.Y.C. & Dillon, H. (2013). Major findings of the LOCHI study on children at three years of age and implications for audiological management. *International Journal of Audiology, 52*(Suppl. 2) S65-S68.

Ching, T. Y., & Hill, M. (2005). *The parents' evaluation of Aural/Oral Performance of Children (PEACH) rating scale.* Chatswood, New South Wales, Australia: Australian Hearing. Retrieved from http://www.outcomes.nal.gov.au/LOCHI%20assessments.html

Ching, T. Y., & Hill, M. (2007). The parents' evaluation of aural/oral performance of children (PEACH) scale: Normative data. *Journal of American Academy of Audiology 18*(3), 220–235. Retrieved from http://www.audiology.org/resources/journal/Pages/default.aspx

Ching, T. Y. C., Day, J., Van Buynder, P., Hou, S., Zhang, V., Seeto, M., . . . Flynn, C. (2014). Language and speech perception of young children with bimodal fitting or bilateral cochlear implants. *Cochlear Implants International, 15*(Suppl. 1), S43–S46.

Ching, T. Y. C., van Wanrooy, E., & Dillon, H. (2007). Binaural-bimodal fitting or bilateral l implantation for managing severe to profound deafness: A review. *Trends in Hearing, 11*(3), 161–192.

Cochlear Nucleus Hybrid L24 Implant System P130016. (2014). Retrieved on May 19, 2015, at http://www.fda.gov/Advisory Committees/CommitteesMeetingMate rials/MedicalDevices/MedicalDevices AdvisoryCommittee/EarNoseandThroat DevicesPanel/ucm373789.htm

Cole, E. B., & Flexer, C. (2007). *Children with hearing loss: Developing listening and talking: Birth to six* (2nd ed.). San Diego, CA: Plural.

Colletti, V., & Shannon, R. V. (2005). Open set speech perception with auditory brainstem implant? *Laryngoscope, 115*(11), 1974–1978.

Colletti, V., Shannon, R., Carner, M., Veronese, S., & Colletti, L. (2009). Outcomes in nontumor adults fitted with the auditory brainstem implant: 10 years' experience. *Otology and Neurotology, 30*(5), 614–618.

Crukley, J., Scollie, S., & Parsa, V. (2011). An exploration of non-quiet listening at school. *Journal of Educational Audiology, 17*, 23–35.

Dillon, H., & Keidser, G. (2013). Siemens Expert Series: NAL-NL2—Principles, background data, and comparison to other procedures. *Audiology Online.* Retrieved from http://www.audiology online.com/articles/siemens-expert-series-nal-nl2-11355

Dun, C. A., de Wolf, M. J., Mylanus, E. A., Snik, A. F., Hoi, M. K. & Cremers, C. W. (2010). Bilateral bone-anchored hearing aid application in children. The Nijmegen experience from 1996 to 2008. *Otology and Neurotology, 31*(4), 615–623.

Dutt, S. N., McDermott, A. L., Burrell, S. P., Cooper, H. R., Reid, A. P., & Proops, D. W. (2002a). Patient satisfaction with bilateral bone-anchored hearing aids: The Birmingham experience. *Journal of Laryngology and Otology, 116*(S28), 37–46.

Dutt, S. N., McDermott, A. L., Burrell, S. P., Cooper, H. R., Reid, A. P., & Proops, D. W. (2002b). Speech intelligibility with bilateral bone-anchored hearing aids: The Birmingham experience. *Journal of Laryngology and Otology, 116*(S28), 47–51.

Ellul, S., Shelton, C., Davidson, H. C., & Harnsberger, H. R. (2000). Preoperative cochlear implant imaging: Is magnetic resonance imaging enough? *American Journal of Otology, 21*(4), 528–533.

Firszt, J. B., Holden, L. K., Skinner, M. W., Tobey, E. A., Peterson, A., Gaggl, W., . . . Wackym, P. A. (2004). Recognition of speech presented at soft to loud levels by adult cochlear implant recipients of three cochlear implant systems. *Ear and Hearing, 25*(4), 375–387.

Fowler, K. B., & Boppanna, S. B. (2006). Congenital cytomegalovirus (CMV) and hearing deficit. *Journal of Clinical Virology, 35*(6), 226–231.

Gallaudet Research Institute. (2008). *Regional and national summary report of data from the 2007–08 annual survey of deaf and hard of hearing children and youth.* Retrieved August 28, 2015, from http://research.gallaudet.edu/Demographics/2008_National_Summary.pdf

Geers, A. E., Strube, M. J., Tobey, E. A., & Moog, J. S. (2011). Epilogue: Factors contributing to long-term outcomes of cochlear implantation in early childhood. *Ear and Hearing, 32*(1 Suppl.), 84S–92S.

Gifford, R. H., & Revit, L. R. (2010). Speech perception for adult cochlear implant recipients a realistic background noise: Effectiveness of preprocessing strategies and external options for improving speech recognition in noise. *Journal of the American Academy of Audiology, 21*(7), 441–451.

Gifford, R. H., Shallop, J. K., & Peterson, A. M. (2008). Speech recognition materials and ceiling effects: Considerations for cochlear implant programs. *Audiology and Neurotology, 13*(3), 193–205.

Gordon, K., Henkin, Y., & Kral, A. (2015). Asymmetric hearing during development: The aural preference syndrome and treatment options. *Pediatrics, 136*(1), 141–153.

Gordon, K. A., Jiwani, S., & Papsin, B. C. (2011). What is the optimal timing for bilateral cochlear implantation in children? *Cochlear Implants International, 12*(2), 8–14.

Gordon, K. A., Jiwani, S., & Papsin, B. C. (2013). Benefits and detriments of unilateral cochlear implant use on bilateral auditory development in children who are deaf. *Frontiers in Psychology, 4*(719), 1–14.

Gordon, K. A., Papsin, B. C., & Harrison, R. V. (2004). Toward a battery of behavioral and objective measures to achieve optimal cochlear implant stimulation levels in children. *Ear and Hearing, 25*(5), 447–463.

Govaerts, P. J., Casselman, J., Daemers, K., De Beukelaer, C., Yperman, M., & De Ceulaer, G. (2003). Cochlear implants in aplasia and hypoplasia of the cochleovestibular nerve. *Otology and Neurotology, 24*(6), 887–891.

Gravel, J. S. (2000). Audiologic assessment for the fitting of hearing instruments: Big challenges from tiny ears. In R. C. Seewald (Ed.), *A Sound Foundation Through Early Amplification: Proceedings of an International Conference* (pp. 33–46). Stafa, Switzerland: Phonak AG.

Gravel, J. S., & Hood, L. J. (1999). Pediatric audiologic assessment. In F. E. Musiek & W. F. Rintelmann (Eds.), *Contemporary perspectives in hearing assessment* (pp. 305–326). Needham Heights, MA: Allyn & Bacon.

Grosse, S. D., Ross, D. S., & Dollard, S. C. (2008). Congenital cytomegalovirus (CMV) infection as a cause of permanent bilateral hearing loss: A quantitative assessment. *Journal of Clinical Virology, 41*(2), 57–62.

Hakansson, B., Tjellstrom, A., & Rosenhall, U. (1984). Hearing thresholds with direct bone conduction versus conventional bone conduction. *Scandinavian Audiology, 13*(1), 3–13.

Hodges, A. V., Balkany, T. J., Ruth, R. A., Lambert, P. R., Dolan-Ash, S., & Schloffman, J. J. (1997). Electrical middle ear muscle reflex: Use in cochlear implant programming. *Otolaryngology-Head and Neck Surgery, 117*(3), 255–261.

Hol, M. K. S., Bosman, A. J., Snik, A. F., Mylanus, E. A. M., & Cremers, C. W. R. J. (2005).Bone-anchored hearing aids in unilateral inner ear deafness: An evaluation of audiometric and patient outcome measurements. *Otology and Neurotology, 26*(5), 999–1006.

Hol, M. K. S., Nelissen, R. C., Agterberg, M. J. H., Cremers, C. W. R. J., & Snik, A. F. M. (2013). Comparison between a new implantable transcutaneous bone conductor and percutaneous bone-conduction hearing implant. *Otology and Neurotology, 34*(6), 1071–1075.

Hol, M. K. S., Snik, A. F., Mylanus, E. A., & Cremers, C. W. (2005). Long-term results of bone-anchored hearing aid recipients who had previously used air-conduction hearing aids. *Archives of Otolaryngology-Head and Neck Surgery, 131*(4), 321–325.

Holden, L. K., Reeder, R. M., Firszt, J. B., & Finley, C. C. (2011). Optimizing the perception of soft speech and speech in noise with the Advanced Bionics cochlear implant system. *International Journal of Audiology, 50*(4), 255–269.

Incerti, P. V., Ching, T. Y. C., & Cowan, R. (2013). A systematic review of electric-acoustic stimulation: Device fitting ranges, outcomes, and clinical fitting practices. *Trends in Hearing, 17*(1), 3–26.

Interacoustics, Inc. (n.d.). *The SKS10 skull stimulator.* Retrieved August 29, 2015, from http://www.interacoustics.com/affinity/sks10

Jackler, R. K., Luxford, W. M., & House, W. F. (1987). Congenital malformations of the inner ear: A classification based on embryogenesis. *Laryngoscope, 97*(3 Pt. 2 Suppl. 40), 2–14.

Kaplan, A. B., Kozin, E. D., Puram, S. V., Owoc, M. S., Shah, P. V., Hight, A. E., & Lee, D. J. (2015). Auditory brainstem implant candidacy in the United States in children 0–17 years old. *International Jour-*

nal of Pediatric Otorhinolaryngology, 79(3), 310–315.

Kirk, K. I. (1998). Assessing speech perception in listeners with cochlear implants; The development of the lexical neighborhood tests. *Volta Review, 100* (2), 63–85.

Kral, A., Heid, S., Hubka, P., & Tillein, J. (2013). Unilateral hearing during development: Hemispheric specificity in plastic reorganizations. *Frontiers in Systems Neuroscience, 7*, 93.

Kral, A., Hubka, P., Heid, S., Tillein, J.(2013) Single-sided deafness leads to unilateral aural preference within an early sensitive period. *Brain, a Journal of Neurology, 136*(Pt. 1), 80–193.

Kurz, A., Flynn, M., Caversaccio, M., & Kompis, M. (2014). Speech understanding with a new implant technology: A comparative study with a new nonskin penetrating baha system. *Biomed Research International, 2014,* Article ID 416205, 9 pages.

Lieu, J. E. (2013). Unilateral hearing loss in children: speech-language and school performance. *B-ENT,* (Suppl. 21) 107–115.

Litovsky, R. Y., Johnstone, P. M., & Godar, S. P. (2006). Benefits of bilateral cochlear implants and/or hearing aids in children. *International Journal of Audiology, 45*(Suppl. 1), S78–S91.

Masuda, S., Usi, S., & Matsunaga, T. (2013). High prevalence of inner-ear and/or internal auditory canal malformations in children with unilateral sensorineural hearing loss. *International Journal of Pediatric Otorhinolaryngology, 77*(2), 228–232.

McDermott, A-L., Williams, J., Kuo, M., Reid, A., & Proops, D. (2009b). Quality of life in children fitted with a bone-anchored hearing aid. *Otology and Neurotology, 30*(3), 344–349.

McGuirt, W. T., & Smith, R. J. H. (1999). Connexin 26 as a cause of hereditary hearing loss. *American Journal of Audiology, 8*(2), 93–100.

Miyamoto, R. T., Bichey, B. G., Wynne, M. K., & Kirk, K. I. (2002). Cochlear implantation with large vestibular aqueduct syndrome. *Laryngoscope, 112*(7 Pt. 1), 1178–1182.

Moodie, K. S., Seewald, R. C., & Sinclair, S. T. (1994). Procedure for predicting real-ear hearing aid performance in young children. *American Journal of Audiology, 3*, 23–31.

Mudry, A., & Tjellstrom, A. (2011). Historical background of bone conduction hearing devices and bone conduction hearing aids. *Advances in Otorhinolaryngology, 71*, 1–9.

Murphy, J., Summerfield, A. Q., O'Donoghue, G. M., & Moore, D. R. (2011). Spatial hearing of normally hearing and cochlear implanted children. *International Journal of Pediatric Otorhinolaryngology, 75*(4), 489–494.

Mylanus, E. A., van der Pouw, K. C., Snik, A. F., & Cremers, C. W. (1998). Intraindividual comparison of the bone-anchored hearing aid and air-conduction hearing aids. *Archives of Otolaryngology-Head and Neck Surgery, 124*(3), 271–276.

Nilsson, M., Soli, S. D., & Sullivan, J. A. (1994). Development of the Hearing in Noise Test for the measurement of speech reception thresholds in quiet and in noise. *Journal of the Acoustical Society of America, 95*(2), 1085–1099.

Niparko, J. K., Tobey, E. A., Thal, D. J., Eisenberg, L. S., Wang, N. Y., Quittner, A. L., & Fink, N. E. (2010). Spoken language development in children following cochlear implantation. *Journal of the American Medical Association, 303*(15), 1498–1506.

Noij, K. S., Kozin, E. D., Sethi, R., Shah, P. V., Kaplan, A. B., Herrmann, B., & Lee, D. J. (2015). Systematic review of nontumor pediatric auditory brainstem implant outcomes. *Otolaryngology-Head and Neck Surgery, 153*(5), 739–750.

Papsin, B. C. (2005). Cochlear implantation in children with anomalous cochleovestibular anatomy. *Laryngoscope, 115* (Suppl. 1), S1–S25.

Park, A. H., Kau, B., Hotaling, A., Azar-Kia, B., Leonetti, J., & Papsin, B. (2000). Clinical course of pediatric inner ear malformation. *Laryngoscope, 110*(10 Pt. 1), 1715–1719.

Parry, D. A., Booth, T., & Roland, P. S. (2005). Advantages of magnetic imaging over computed tomography in preoperative evaluation of pediatric cochlear implant candidates. *Otology and Neurotology, 26*(5), 976–982.

Peters, B., Litovsky, R., Parkinson, A., & Lake, J. (2007). Importance of age and post-implantation experience on speech perception measures in children with sequential bilateral cochlear implants. *Otology and Neurotology, 28*(5), 649–657.

Priwin, C., Jonsson, R., Hultcranz, M., & Granstrom, G. (2007). BAHA in children and adolescents with unilateral or bilateral conductive hearing loss: A study outcome. *International Journal of Pediatric Otorhinolaryngology, 71*(1), 135–145.

Rance, G. (2005). Auditory neuropathy/dys-synchrony and its perceptual consequences. *Trends in Amplification, 9*(1), 1–43.

Rapin, I., & Gravel, J. (2003). "Auditory neuropathy": Physiologic and pathologic evidence calls for more diagnostic specificity. *International Journal of Pediatric Otorhinolaryngology, 67*(7), 707–728.

Rapin, I., & Gravel, J. (2006). Auditory neuropathy: A biologically inappropriate label unless acoustic nerve involvement is documented. *Journal of American Academy of Audiology, 17*(2), 147–150.

Ricketts, T. A., & Galster, J. (2008) Head angle and elevation in classroom environments: Implications for amplification. *Journal of Speech, Language, and Hearing Research, 51*, 516–525.

Rodrıguez-Ballesteros, M., del Castillo, F. J., Yolanda Martın, Y., Moreno-Pelayo, M. A., & Morera, C. (2003). Auditory neuropathy in patients carrying mutations in the otoferlin gene (OTOF). *Human Mutations, 22*(6), 451–456.

Roeser, R. J., & Clark, J. L. (2008). Live voice speech recognition audiometry—Stop the madness. *Audiology Today, 20*(1), 32–33.

Rouillon, I., Marcolla, A., Roux, I., Marlin, S., Feldmann, D., Couderc, R., . . . Loundon, N. (2006). Results of cochlear implantation in two children with mutations on the OTOF gene. *International Journal of Pediatric Otorhinolaryngology, 70*(4), 689–696.

Schafer, E. C., Amlani, A. M., Paiva, D., Nozari, L., & Verret, S. (2011). A meta-analysis to compare speech recognition in noise with bilateral cochlear implants and bimodal stimulation. *International Journal of Audiology, 50*(12), 871–880.

Schafer, E. C., & Thibodeau, L. M. (2004). Speech recognition abilities of adults using cochlear implants interfaced with FM systems. *Journal of the American Academy of Audiology, 15*(10), 678–691.

Schafer, E. C., Wolfe, J., Algier, K., Morais, M., Price, S., Monzingo, J., . . .Ramos, H. (2012b). Spatial hearing in noise of young children with cochlear implants and hearing aids. *Journal of Educational Audiology, 18*, 38–51.

Schmithorst, V. J., Holland, S. K., Ret, J., Duggins, A., Arjmand, E., & Greinwald, J. (2005). Cortical reorganization in children with unilateral sensorineural hearing loss. *Neuroreport, 16*(5), 463–467.

Schmithorst, V. J., Plante, E., & Holland, S. (2014). Unilateral deafness in children affects development of multi-modal modulation and default mode networks. *Frontiers in Human Neuroscience, 8*, 164.

Scollie, S., Seewald, R., Cornelisse, L., Moodie, S., Bagatto, M., Laurnagaray, D., . . . Pumford, J. (2005). The Desired Sensation Level Multistage Input/Output Algorithm. *Trends in Amplification, 9*(4), 159–197.

Sharma, A., Dorman, M. F., & Spahr, A. J. (2002). A sensitive period for the development of the central auditory system in children with cochlear implants: Implications for age of implantation. *Ear and Hearing, 23*(6), 532–539.

Siegert, R., & Kanderske, J. (2013). A new semi-implantable transcutaneous bone conduction device: Clinical, surgical, and audiologic outcomes in patients with congenital ear canal atresia. *Otology and Neurotology, 34*(5), 927–934.

Snapp, H. A., Fabry, D. A., Telischi, F. F., Arheart, K. L., & Angeli, S. I. (2010). A clinical protocol for predicting outcomes with an implantable prosthetic device (Baha) in patients with single-sided deafness. *Journal of the American Academy of Audiology, 21*(10), 654–662.

Snik, A. F., Mylannus, E. A., Proops, D. W., Woolfaardt, J. F., Hodgetts, W. E., Somers, T., . . . Tjellström, A. (2005). Consensus statements on BAHA system: Where do we stand at present? *Annals of Otology, Rhinology, and Laryngology, 195*, 2S–12S.

Spivak, L. G., Chute, P. M., Popp, A. L., & Parisier, S. C. (1994). Programming the cochlear implant based on electrical acoustic reflex thresholds: Patient performance. *Laryngoscope, 104*(10), 1225–1230.

Teagle, H. F. B., Roush, P. A., Woodard, J. S., Hatch, D. R., Buss, E., Zdanski, C. J., & Buchman, C. A. (2010). Cochlear implantation in children with auditory neuropathy spectrum disorder. *Ear and Hearing, 31*(3), 325–335.

Tjellstrom, A., Hakansson, B., & Granstrom, G. (2001). Bone-anchored hearing aids: Current status in adults and children. *Otolaryngologic Clinics of North America, 34*(2), 337–364.

Tsiakpini, L., Weichbold, V., Kuehn-Inacker, H., Coninx, F., D'Haese, P., & Almadin, S. (2004). *LittlEARS Auditory Questionnaire.* Innsbruck, Austria: MED-EL.

Uhler, K., Biever, A., & Gifford, R. (2016). Method of speech stimulus presentation impacts pediatric speech recognition: Monitored live voice versus recorded speech. *Otology and Neurotology, 37*(2), e70–e74.

Valvassori, G., & Clemis, J. (1978). The large vestibular aqueduct syndrome. *Laryngoscope, 88*(5), 723–728.

van der Pouw, K., Snik, F. M., & Cremers, C. W. R. J. (1998). Audiometric results of bilateral bone-anchored hearing aid application in patients with bilateral congenital aural atresia. *Laryngoscope, 108*(4), 548–553.

Vasama, J. P., Mäkelä, J. P., Parkkonen, L., & Hari, R. (1994). Auditory cortical responses in humans with congenital unilateral conductive hearing loss. *Hearing Research, 78*(1), 1–97.

Weinstein, B. E. (1997). Outcomes measures in the hearing aid fitting process/selection process. *Trends in Amplication, 2*(4), 117–137.

Whitton, J. P., & Polley, D. B. (2011). Evaluating the perceptual and pathophysiological consequences of auditory deprivation in early postnatal life: A comparison of basic and clinical studies. *Journal of the Association for Research in Otolaryngology, 12*(5), 535–546.

Widen, J. E. (1993). Adding objectivity to infant behavioral audiometry. *Ear and Hearing, 14*(1), 49–57.

Wolfe, J., Baker, S., Caraway, T., Kasulis, H., Mears, A., Smith, J., & Wood, M. (2007). 1-year postactivation results for sequentially implanted bilateral cochlear implant users. *Otology and Neurotology, 28*(5), 589–596.

Wolfe, J., Gilbert, M., Schafer, E. C., Litvak, L., Spahr, T., & Saoji, A. (in preparation). *Optimization of the electrically-evoked stapedial reflex threshold measurement in cochlear implant recipients.*

Wolfe, J., & Kasulis, H. (2008). Relationships among objective measures and speech perception in adult users of the HiResolution Bionic Ear. *Cochlear Implants International, 9*(2), 70–81.

Wolfe, J., Morais, M., Neumann, S., Schafer, E., Mulder, H., Wells, N., & Hudson, M. (2013). Evaluation of speech recognition with personal FM and classroom audio distribution systems. *Journal of Educational Audiology Association, 19*, 65–79.

Wolfe, J., Morais, M., Schafer, E. C., Agrawal, S., & Koch, D. (2015). Evaluation of speech recognition of cochlear implant recipients using adaptive, digital remote microphone technology and a speech enhancement sound processing algorithm. *Journal of the Academy of Audiology, 26*(5), 502–508.

Wolfe, J., Morais, M., Schafer, E. C., Mills, E., Mülder, H. E., Goldbeck, F., . . . Lianos, L. (2013). Evaluation of speech recognition of cochlear implant recipients using a personal digital adaptive radio frequency system. *Journal of the American Academy of Audiology, 24*(8), 714–724.

Wolfe, J., Parkinson, A., Schafer, E. C., Gilden, J., Rehwinkel, K., Mansanares, J., & Gannaway, S. (2012). Benefit of a commercially available cochlear implant processor with dual-microphone beamforming: A multi-center study. *Otology and Neurotology, 33*(4), 553–560.

Wolfe, J., & Schafer, E. C. (2015). *Programming cochlear implants* (2nd ed.). San Diego, CA: Plural.

Wolfe, J., Schafer, E. C., Heldner, B., Mulder, H., Ward, E., & Vincent, B. (2009). Evaluation of speech recognition in noise with cochlear implants and dynamic FM. *Journal of the American Academy of Audiology, 20*(7), 409–421.

Wolfe, J., Schafer, E. C., John, A., & Hudson, M. (2011). The effect of front-end processing on cochlear implant performance of children. *Otology and Neurotology, 32*(4), 533–538.

Wu, C. C., Lee, Y. C., Chen, P. J., & Hsu, C. J. (2008). Predominance of genetic diagnosis and imaging results as predictors in determining the speech performance outcome after cochlear implantation in children. *Archives in Pediatric and Adolescent Medicine, 162*(3), 269–276.

Wu, C. C., Liu, T. C., Wang, S. H., Hsu, C. J., & Wu, C. M. (2011). Genetic characteristics in children with cochlear implants and the corresponding auditory performance. *Laryngoscope, 121*(6), 1287–1293.

Wu, C. M., Lee, L. A., Chen, C. K., Chan, K. C., Tsou, Y. T., & Ng, S. H. (2015). Impact of cochlear nerve deficiency determined using 3-dimensional magnetic resonance imaging on hearing outcome in children with cochlear implants. *Otology and Neurotology, 36*(1), 14-21.

Young, N. M., Kim, F. M., Ryan, M. E., Tournis, E., & Yaras, S. (2012). Pediatric cochlear implantation of children with eighth nerve deficiency. *International Journal of Pediatric Otorhinolaryngology, 76*(10), 1442–1448.

Zeng, F. G., & Liu, S. (2006). Speech perception in individuals with auditory neuropathy. *Journal of Speech, Language, and Hearing Research, 49*(2), 367–380.

Zwolan, T. A., & Griffin, B. L. (2005). How we do it: Tips for programming the speech processor of an 18-month-old. *Cochlear Implants International, 6*(4), 169–177.

7

ASSISTIVE HEARING AND ACCESS TECHNOLOGIES AND AUDITORY-VERBAL THERAPY

Samuel R. Atcherson, Tina Childress, and Sarah Warren Kennett

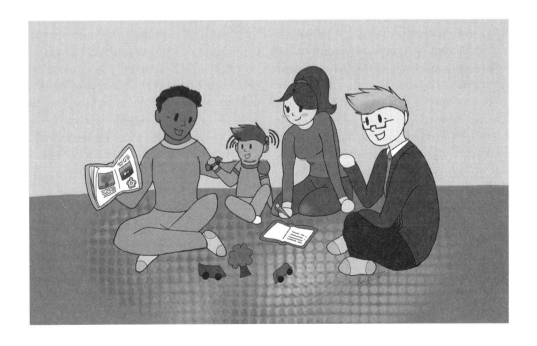

INTRODUCTION

Hearing assistive and access technologies can be used by individuals with hearing loss across the life span, but the focus here is primarily on children ages 0 to 6 years of age with some application to school-aged children. Two principles of Auditory-Verbal Therapy (AVT) are addressed here. Principle 2 is for AV practitioners to "recommend immediate assessment and use of state-of-the-art hearing technology to maximize benefits of auditory stimulation." Immediately, technology such as hearing aids and cochlear implants come to mind. However, hearing technology limited to placement on a child's ear (i.e., ear-level technology) is only a first step toward truly maximizing the benefits of acoustic stimulation. Although hearing aids and implantable devices provide individuals with benefit in ideal listening environments, they are often not sufficient where background noise is present and the person who is talking may be far away from the listener (e.g., classroom setting). Technologies are available to maximize auditory stimulation in environments that are noisy and when access to a speaker's face is not always possible or necessary. Technologies are also available that may be useful when hearing aids and implantable devices are not worn, such as alerting and warning devices that use flashing lights and vibrations. The key, after all, is ensuring access to sound (e.g., the speech signal) while minimizing obstacles to sound (e.g., noise or other physical barriers). Related to the second principle of AVT is Principle 5, which calls for the AV practitioner to "guide and coach parents to create

environments that support listening for the acquisition of spoken language throughout the child's daily activities."

As a first step, we subscribe to the term *hearing assistive technology* (HAT) as any device or system that helps to overcome hearing loss by way of delivering or enhancing sound to improve audibility while counteracting poor signal-to-noise ratios and the effect of distance (Atcherson, Franklin, & Smith-Olinde, 2015). Other terms used, often interchangeably, include *hearing assistive technology system* (HATS), *assistive listening device* or *assistive listening system* (ALD or ALS), and *remote microphone technology*. Hearing aids and implantable devices are personal ear-level technologies that can be coupled with hearing assistive technologies. We also subscribe to the term *access technology* as any device, system, or even a technical service that may provide equal access for an individual with hearing loss, but will not necessarily provide equal opportunity (Atcherson et al., 2015). Ultimately, the goal is to use both hearing assistive *and* access technologies to "maximize" success in an auditory world. Used appropriately, these technologies may be especially important in the intervention of listening and spoken language success of children with hearing loss.

To understand how hearing assistive technology is beneficial to children with hearing loss, first one must understand some basic information about acoustics and speech. All children, hearing loss or not, need sounds to be louder (more audible) to understand what is being said. Making sounds more audible also helps to reduce overall listening effort and fatigue. Although hearing aids and implantable devices indeed provide access to sound, they do not have the natural ability of the brain to "filter" or "squelch" background noise that most people with normal hearing sensitivity have. Individuals with typical hearing (as well as typical auditory processing) are able to maximize speech in noisy listening situations by taking advantage of subtle sound cues using the shape of their ears, the powerful filtering characteristics of the inner ear, and the precision of neural firing patterns in the brainstem and midbrain to detect subtle differences between the ears. These anatomical and physiological parts of the auditory system help to cause speech to become much more accessible. However, children with hearing loss must rely much more greatly on their ear-level hearing technology to make these subtle sound distinctions, and even then, access to sound is not truly maximized. As advanced as these devices may be, they cannot completely separate speech from noise. Instead, any manipulations made by hearing aids or implantable devices to enhance or remove portions of sound will undoubtedly affect both speech and noise. The degree to which speech is enhanced (or noise is minimized) varies across hearing aids and implantable devices. Some are quite good, but no ear-level hearing technology will be sufficient for all listening situations.

What makes environmental noise complex? In general, *noise* is anything a listener does not (or should not) want to hear. Noise that interferes with the speech signal can result in poor understanding. In some circumstances, the amount of noise can be controlled and reduced, and other times it cannot. *Reverberation* is commonly thought of as the "echoing" of sound in a room, and

can add unintended noise when sounds bounce off hard surfaces such as tile floors and bare walls. The echoes produced by reverberation are extra copies of the same sound that linger around for a long time. Reverberation can be physically measured as the amount of time (in seconds) to determine how long it takes a loud sound to decrease by 60 dB (or *RT60*). Rooms with long RT60s will be more reverberant. As an example, a small, carpeted therapy room will have less reverberation compared to a noncarpeted therapy room (e.g., short RT60 of 0.20 s compared to long RT60 of 0.55 s). Reverberation can be reduced by adding materials that can absorb sound such as carpet, curtains, and acoustic tiles. The reverberation of cafeterias and gymnasiums often cannot be altered without significant cost. Another factor that contributes to a difficult listening environment is the distance a listener is from the sound source. At short distances from the sound source, this "direct" sound is generally unaffected by reverberant characteristics of the room as it gradually loses intensity. The traveling sound is no longer "direct" when it begins to mix with the reverberant characteristics of the room, a point beyond which is considered the *critical distance*. Maximum sound access is best achieved when the listener is within a critical distance. The combination of noise, reverberation, and not being within the critical distance can result in a confusing sound received by the listener. This can be overcome by increasing the *signal-to-noise-ratio* (SNR or S/N ratio). The signal is the sound of interest (e.g., speech), and the noise is any interfering sound, including reverberation. For the signal to be clearly perceived by individuals with hearing loss, it has to have a "positive" signal-to-noise ratio. This simply means that the intensity of the signal of interest must be louder than the noise. When the signal-to-noise ratio is poor ("negative"), individuals with hearing loss will have greater difficulty understanding speech compared to individuals who have normal hearing. Optimal listening occurs when sound is +20 to +25 dB. As an example, adults with normal hearing do best with a signal-to-noise ratio of +6 dB (Kramer, 2004). Young children with brains that are still developing require a higher signal-to-noise ratio (Chermak, Bellis, & Musiek, 2014), and children with hearing loss need even more.

HEARING ASSISTIVE TECHNOLOGY

The primary role of hearing assistive technology is to provide direct access to sound, which may involve the need to improve the signal-to-noise ratio. In this section, we address five broad areas of hearing assistive technology: frequency-modulation/digital-modulation (FM/DM), induction, infrared (IR), Bluetooth, and direct audio input. For each broadly defined hearing assistive technology, there may be one or more ways to gain acoustic access and "listen" to sounds at home, in therapy, in school, and out in public. As this section is approached, refer to Table 7–1, which offers a condensed view of some of the many listening and connectivity options for hearing aids and implantable devices using a remote microphone, phone, media player, television, and sound boards. The audiologist and/or

the AV practitioner will be the first step toward determining which of these hearing assistive technologies are appropriate. Although several different hearing assistive technologies exist, they share some common terminology:

- *Microphone Transmitter:* Many hearing assistive technology systems allow for the person who is talking to wear a small device that contains a microphone, and what is picked up by the microphone is transmitted to another device called a *receiver.* Oftentimes, the microphone transmitter is simply referred to as a "microphone" or "mic." The microphone is either clipped to a shirt ("lapel" style), worn on the head ("boom mic" style), worn around the neck ("lavalier" style), or handheld (sometimes known as a "pass-around" style). For the strongest signal, the microphone is best used within 1 to 6 inches from the mouth. Any further away, the overall intensity is less effective and the signal-to-noise is not ideal.
- *Receiver:* The receiver is an ear-level or body-worn device that picks up the transmitted signal from a microphone transmitter and delivers it to the listener via a hearing aid or an implantable device. In some cases, the receiver may be built directly into the hearing aid or implantable device.
- *Coupling:* Coupling refers to how the technology connects the receiver and the device used for hearing, whether a hearing aid or an implantable device.

Table 7–1. Hearing Assistive Technology Listening and Connectivity Options

	Remote Microphone	Phone	Media Player[a]	Television	Sound Board[b]
Acoustic					
Headphones (wired or Bluetooth)		•	•	•	
External speaker	•	•	•	•	•
Induction					
T-coil setting on HA/CI		•			
Amplified neckloop					
Wired		•	•		
Bluetooth		•	•	•	
Induction earhooks/HATIS					
Wired		•	•		
Bluetooth		•	•	•	
Room loop (large area)	•		•	•	•
Personal loop (small area)			•	•	
Neckloop receiver					
FM/DM[c]	•		•	•	•
Infrared	•			•	•
Near-field/streamer					
FM/DM[c]	•			•	•
Bluetooth	•	•	•	•	
Direct audio input					
Auxiliary cable		•	•	•	
FM/DM[c]	•	•	•	•	•

[a]e.g., MP3/MP4, tablet, game console, laptop, etc. [b]e.g., music, worship center, movie, or live theater sound system. [c]Transmitter for FM/DM system is connected to the input.

Options might be *wired* or *wireless*. Technology that is wired together may be described as "hard-wired" or "direct audio input." Wireless technology can encompass "frequency or digital modulation," "electromagnetic induction," "infrared light," and "Bluetooth®" to name a few of the most common. For the devices to be coupled, they sometimes need to be specially programmed or "fit" by an audiologist.

- *Compatibility:* Compatibility is the notion that different devices or technologies may or may not work well with one another. Some hearing assistive technologies are designed to be universally compatible, whereas others are not.

Frequency/Digital Modulation (FM/DM)

Frequency modulation (FM) and *digital modulation* (DM) are forms of wireless connectivity that are used in systems to transmit an audio signal to a receiver. FM/DM systems are used with children with hearing loss to overcome the detrimental effects of background noise, reverberation, and distance as well as provide a more robust audio signal. These systems consist of two parts: a microphone transmitter ("mic") worn by the person who is speaking and a receiver worn by the listener.

With FM technology, the analog signal is broadcast on a specific channel or frequency, similar to how a radio signal that is sent to a station on your car stereo. You need to synchronize the channels on the transmitter and the receiver

in order for these two parts to work with each other. This can be as simple as pressing a button on the transmitter to connect the two devices. Multiple children with receivers can listen from a single microphone transmitter time as long as they are all on the same channel. A disadvantage to FM technology is that a child's receiver might pick up an unintended transmitter signal (e.g., hear another teacher's voice) or get interference if the channels are too close. If the child is in a school setting and uses FM technology, the audiologist who provided the equipment needs to determine which channel is appropriate for the child—this is only a concern if there are multiple children using FM systems within the same school.

With the newer DM technology, the signal uses digital frequency hopping technology to provide a digital signal and also overcome the effects of channel interaction (since the DM signal is constantly changing). With a DM system, the transmitter and receiver merely need to be in the same "network" in order to communicate with each other. As with FM technology, multiple children can listen with a single microphone transmitter if they are on the same network.

Children can use FM/DM systems in a variety of settings. Families of toddlers might use a system when they are working on any AVT materials to maximize their hearing input. Children in school often use FM/DM systems to hear their teachers and peers better. Outside of school, a child might use a system to have conversations with parents in the car, or to hear their sports coach while on the field.

Transmitters come in various forms and sizes and can also be referred to as microphones. Some microphones are *omnidirectional* (picks up signals all around it) and some are *directional* (focuses on a narrower, specific location). Microphones can be worn on the lapel of your clothing, worn around your neck like a necklace ("lavalier" style), worn next to your mouth like what you see many singers use ("boom mic" style), or can be handheld. Lapel, lavalier, and boom microphones work best in the directional mode because they focus on the mouth of whoever is talking and provide a very clear signal. In the case of handheld microphones, these can be used as *auxiliary* microphones in addition to the teacher's microphone and passed around from child to child ("pass around microphone"). There is also a new style of handheld microphone in the shape of a wand or pen that the child controls. Be merely pointing the device at the sound source, the directional microphone can pick up the signal. This newer technology has gained wide acceptance by teenagers who want to be in control and not stand out by having to give the teacher a microphone, as well as in group settings where there are several talkers. Transmitters can also be plugged into audio sources. An example would be a child listening to a signal from his or her computer. Instead of using headphones, the child merely has to connect an audio cable from his or her transmitter to the headphone jack of the audio source, and then the signal is wirelessly transmitted via FM/DM to the receiver(s) that the child is already wearing.

Receivers come in various styles. There are receivers that can directly plug into a child's hearing aid, implant, or streamer/near-field device, and neckloop receivers that are accessed via the telecoil setting. Classroom and toteable/desktop speakers are even considered receivers since they can pick up a transmitter signal.

Selecting an appropriate receiver style involves several factors. Receivers that directly plug into the hearing aid or implantable device can provide a cleaner signal because of the direct connection, but this is only appropriate for children who are already good users and reporters of their device. If the FM/DM system is not working, the child may or may not be able to provide this information because it is not obvious. Some companies have receivers that have an LED indicator on them to indicate function. These receivers are quite small and can be easily lost if they become dislodged. One receiver may only connect to one hearing aid or implantable device, so if a child is listening in binaural/bimodal condition, two receivers may be necessary. *Neck-loop* receivers are larger, have an indicator light, and can transmit to both ears, but they are more prone to interference because they use the telecoil setting. Sound-field speaker systems work well for amplifying a whole classroom or even a smaller area in the case of a toteable/desktop system, and it is obvious when it is working, but speaker systems can still be susceptible to the effects of background noise and distance because the signal needs to travel across a distance to reach the listener.

Obtaining an FM/DM system involves a process that includes evaluation, verification, and validation. If the child (subjectively or objectively) appears to be having problems hearing in background noise, hearing at a distance, or receives limited benefit from his or her hearing aids or implantable devices, the child might be a candidate for such a system. After this has been established, there are specific algorithms and protocols that an audiologist follows to make sure that the FM/DM system is adequately and appropriately providing amplification. The default setting for using an FM/DM system is that the child is able to hear through the system *and* is able to hear as received through the environmental microphone. AV practitioners, parents, and audiologists know that there are many opportunities for *incidental learning* throughout the day, and no child should miss out on hearing classmates talking. Finally, it is important that the whole team monitors the child to make sure that the FM/DM system is working as intended. Sometimes children are distracted by this extra equipment. Sometimes teachers need to relearn how to appropriately use the equipment and will require guidance as to when and where it should be used (e.g., recess versus lunchtime versus one-on-one teaching with another student). Different listening situations may even require a different configuration for transmitters or receivers, so it is important to discuss these options with the audiologist. More recently, advances in DM technology using a *dynamic/adaptive* strategy show great advantages over fixed FM technology when environmental noise changes from soft to loud (Thibodeau, 2014; Wolfe et al., 2009, 2013, 2015). As environmental noise increases, a dynamic/adaptive DM system will adjust to keep the signal-to-noise ratio as high as possible. Although increasing noise levels cause poorer speech understanding, the dynamic/adaptive DM system will consistently outperform a fixed FM system.

Induction

Induction is a method of coupling where sound input is converted into an electromagnetic signal and then picked up by the *telecoil* (also known as *T-coil*) on a hearing aid or implantable device. The electromagnetic signal may be transmitted *directly* as in the case of holding a phone up to the hearing aid or implantable device. It can also be transmitted *indirectly* via a device worn around the neck (*neckloop*), via hooks that sit on the ear next to the hearing aid or cochlear implant (*induction earhook*), or a physical loop of wire installed under carpeting or in a ceiling (*induction or hearing loop*) that picks up the electromagnetic signal. Another way to look at it is this: any time you use the telecoil setting, you are using induction to pick up the signal.

For younger children, the default telecoil setting allows the child to hear a combination of the signal coming through the telecoil as well as through their environmental microphone ("T+EM"). This means that they should be able to hear any incidental sounds or conversations happening around them even when they are in the telecoil setting. The AV practitioner and the parent(s) can monitor children's ability to understand speech through this setting during the AVT session or home environment. Older children and adults may select a "telecoil only" setting so that their device(s) only picks up the electromagnetic signal and blocks out any environmental sounds. Because most hearing aids and implantable devices come with multiple program slots, it is possible to have both of these telecoil settings on their device. It is important that the AV practitioner assess the child's performance in both settings as the child gains greater listening experience and linguistic competence. The goal is to ensure the child gains independence and the ability to articulate which listening condition is preferred.

In the *direct* induction scenario, a child holds a telephone up to his or her ear, and the electromagnetic signal from the phone transmits the voice signal directly to the child's hearing aid or implantable device that is in the telecoil setting. The advantage of using a phone in this matter is that there is less likelihood of feedback from hearing aids. If the child is set in "telecoil only," he or she will only hear the phone signal on one ear and can monitor the loudness of his or her voice with the other ear. Currently, all landline wired and wireless phones and a percentage of cellular phones are required by the Federal Communications Commission (FCC) in the United States to be *hearing aid compatible* (HAC). This means that HAC phones need to have a strong telecoil signal and not have interference in the form of static. An adult can help the child by selecting phones with known compatibility of M3 or M4 (when the microphone is used) and T3 or T4 (when the telecoil is used) to be used with hearing aids or implantable devices (Atcherson & Highley, 2013). The overall sound quality may differ from phone to phone depending on the hearing technology used. When shopping for new phones, parents are encouraged to consider listening to the sound quality of HAC phones through their child's hearing technology to judge which phone has the best sound quality.

Considering *indirect* induction, a discussion of neckloop devices is important. A neckloop device is a single loop of wire worn around the neck like a necklace. The neckloop emits a wireless signal to the telecoil of a hearing aid or implantable device. One advantage here is that there are no additional devices worn on or near the ear. Rather, the neckloop can be worn conspicuously around the neck and under a person's shirt. A person can use a neckloop to transmit audio information to both ears, whether the person is in the bilateral or bimodal condition. There are neckloop receivers that can pick up an FM/DM signal. For example, a teacher wears an FM/DM transmitter, the sounds travels via the FM/DM signal to the neckloop receiver, and the neckloop receiver sends the sound *via* an electromagnetic signal to the child's hearing aid or implantable device in the telecoil setting. These work well for younger children because the neckloop receivers are larger and less likely to get lost, and they have a light indicator that is easily visible for parents and teachers to see if the device is operational and connected. *Personal amplified neckloops* can be used to connect with cell phones, personal media devices, and computers. If they are set in "telecoil only," the person will only hear the input from whatever he or she is listening to. This can be problematic in the case of telephone use because the person will not be able to hear or monitor the loudness of his or her own voice. One solution is to have "telecoil only" on one ear and "T+EM" on the other ear. If a person is only using one ear to listen, he or she can choose the "T+EM" setting for phone use and "telecoil only" for listening to a media device. There are neckloops that have an audio cable where one end plugs into the neckloop and the other end plugs into the headphone jack of the phone or media device. There are also amplified neckloops that connect via Bluetooth to any Bluetooth-compatible device. To emphasize this point, induction loops with cell phones were found to be better than using a landline phone or cell phone with the hearing aid microphone alone (Sorri et al., 2003). *Induction earhooks* work in the same way that an amplified neckloop does except that there is a hook that sits on the ear next to the hearing aid or implantable device. There are systems that have one and some that have two earhooks. As with neckloops, there are wired configurations as well as Bluetooth connections to phones and media players (see "Bluetooth Technology" below). The reason to use an earhook as opposed to a neckloop is that an earhook is the only way to get a true stereo signal (e.g., left channel presents instrumentals and right channel presents vocals) to each ear individually. With a neckloop, if the audio input is in true stereo, the neckloop combines both channels (i.e., mono signal) and sends the signal to both ears—essentially a binaural mono signal.

An *induction* or *hearing (room) loop system* can be found in larger areas such as theaters, public meeting spaces, or places of worship. They can also be installed in small areas like a family room or even in a favorite chair (which might be hooked up to the television) or in a car (where one person wears a microphone). The system picks up the sound input, sends it through a series of looped wires strategically installed under the carpet or above in the ceiling in the case of a hearing (room) loop system or individual area to be looped, and converts the sound into an electromagnetic signal that is then picked up by the child via the telecoil setting. The child needs to be situated within this loop in order to access the signal; however, no additional receiver or attachment is needed—just the telecoil setting. In a looped meeting space, the presenter speaks into a microphone (which is often connected to a speaker system as well as to the hearing loop system), and the child sits within the looped area to pick up the signal directly to his or her device(s). In theaters and cinemas, the audio input is connected to the overall sound system that connects to the hearing device(s). Again, there is no problem with reverberation and distance. Letowski, Donahue, and Nábělek (1986) demonstrated in listeners with hearing loss that using a classroom induction loop system was better for speech understanding than with no system at all. One disadvantage, seen in poorly installed loop systems, is the possibility of induction "bleed over" when there are two or more loop systems in the same building. When "bleed over" happens, the individual with telecoil may hear sounds from two or more rooms. Hearing loop systems are becoming more prevalent around the world due to a concerted effort by various hearing loss advocacy groups.

Sometimes a child may need to move around within a looped room, or reposition the phone or neckloop, in order to find the best signal (often called the "sweet spot"). The reason for this is that the orientation of the telecoil within a hearing aid or implantable device is not universal and, thus, may need to search for the right orientation. Individuals who have telecoils situated in the horizontal orientation are better able to hear input. Such is the case with phones held directly to the ear, and when using an induction earhook. For those who have telecoils situated in the vertical position, they are better able to hear in larger hearing loop areas and when using a personal neckloop. Consulting the audiologist or manufacturer can help to determine the telecoil orientation for a particular device. This information is helpful in terms of knowing what to expect for different listening situations through induction. One needs to also be aware that buzzing or interference may occur if a child is an area with excessive electromagnetic fields. Examples include under fluorescent lighting or near lots of electronics like a computer room. Perhaps most importantly, the telecoil strength of hearing aids can (and should) be assessed and adjusted by the audiologist using a hearing aid test box to meet ANSI S3.22-2003 standards (American National Standards Institute, 2003; Atcherson et al., 2015). The AV practitioner can guide parents and teachers in how to listen through some devices directly with a listening stethoset (scope) or headphones and try to seek the best location in a room, or the best position for a neckloop or phone.

Infrared System

An *infrared system* (or *IR system*) picks up sounds from a microphone transmitter and converts the sound from an electric signal to invisible light waves. The light waves are sent from a transmitter (sometimes called an emitter) to a receiver that converts the signal back into acoustic sound and is presented to the listener. The energy conversion is the same technology used in a television's remote control, and just like the remote control, the receiver must be in the line of sight of the transmitter because the signal moves by light waves. By using light rays, the infrared system has an advantage over FM technology because the signal is contained within one room and will not interfere with nearby systems, nor is it sensitive to electrical noise or other transmitting systems. Because the receiver has to be in line of sight with the transmitter, the transmitter will not send signals to a receiver that is in another room. This is an attractive feature because the person wearing the infrared transmitter (e.g., teacher, AV practitioner, or parent) does not have to be concerned with "bleedover" from room to room, and the user also does not have to turn the transmitter off when leaving the room such as with an FM transmitter. This also means the system is ideal in situations where it is important that the signal stay confidential, such as a courtroom or private meeting. One disadvantage to that feature is that infrared systems work better in rectangular rooms, and they do not work well around corners or when the pathway between the transmitter and receiver may be blocked. In addition, these systems cannot be used outside because sunlight interferes with the signal transmission.

Infrared systems are not built into any hearing aid and implantable devices; therefore, an additional receiver is needed. These systems are often used with neckloops or headphones, or with speakers often mounted to the walls or ceilings. Disadvantages of infrared systems include that they can be more difficult to install and maintain, and in general they are more expensive than other available options. Maintenance also requires either external or rechargeable batteries for the system. Because the technology relies on direct sight between the transmitter and receiver, often clothing and other items can impede the pathway and briefly interrupt the signal. The elegance of an infrared system is clear as a hearing assistive technology, but research is generally scarce. Infrared systems are better than a public address system (Nábělek, Donahue, & Letowshi, 1986); however, the location of the infrared transmitter (e.g., ceiling) may not provide the benefit as imagined (Anderson & Goldstein, 2004). Certainly, the design of infrared systems is important, and the sound quality must be evaluated.

Bluetooth Technology

Bluetooth is a specific standard used for short-range, wireless connectivity that can be used by a variety of devices (up to 10 meters in open space). Some examples that can apply to children with hearing loss include remote microphones, headphones/headsets, external speakers, phones, media devices like MP3 players, tablets, game consoles, and computers. There are several other short-range, wireless connectivity options (e.g., near-field communication, 900 MHz, and 2.4 GHz), but here the focus is on Bluetooth as it is fairly well recognized.

Currently, direct Bluetooth technology is not available in hearing aids and implantable devices. Although Bluetooth technology uses relatively little power (current) consumption, it still requires more power than what today's hearing technology can offer. In addition, there is not enough space available in the body of hearing aids/implantable devices to accommodate a Bluetooth receiver. As technology and miniaturization continue to evolve and miniaturization, perhaps future devices can have Bluetooth technology built-in. Therefore, at this time, an *intermediary device* is needed to utilize today's Bluetooth technology. For example, an intermediary device such as a neckloop has the electronic requirements to function as a "bridge" or wireless connection between the hearing aid and/or cochlear implant to a Bluetooth transmitter such as a cell phone.

Examples of *intermediary devices* that pick up the audio signal include streamers or near-field communication devices, amplified neckloops, headphones, and speakers. These intermediary devices communicate via the Bluetooth wireless protocol to *audio sources* such as remote microphones, phones, and media players. One needs to know how the *intermediary device* can connect with a hearing aid or implantable device. There are several options. An auditory signal provided by Bluetooth headphones and speakers can simply be received by the environmental microphone (EM) on a child's device. Bluetooth-amplified neckloops communicate with hearing aids and implantable devices via the telecoil setting. Streamers and near-field communication devices use a proprietary signal to communicate with hearing aids and implantable devices. An advantage to Bluetooth connectivity is that it can be secure and only accessible to one person. Another advantage is that a person does not have to worry about interference or picking up the signal of other audio sources at the same time because audio sources and intermediary devices are specifically "paired."

Directions on "pairing" audio sources with intermediary devices can vary so one needs to consult the user manual for more information. It is most important to determine if the user needs a special access code (typically "0000" or "1234") to pair devices. Many devices do not require such a code, but if required, the code needs to be kept in a safe place for easy access should it later be needed if the user changes devices. In general, permission needs to be "granted" to connect devices. This ensures that outside devices cannot connect to the user's cell phone or tablet, for example. Pairing of devices needs to occur only one time, and thereafter, connections should be automatic.

Because Bluetooth technology is wireless, the child can connect without the hassle of wires. Children can get a more robust signal using Bluetooth headphones with their tablet when using apps that work on auditory skill development. Older children can use a Bluetooth-amplified neckloop to hear their cell phone better. One of the newer applications of Bluetooth are remote microphones that connect with streamers that help with listening in background noise and across distances. The possibilities are endless.

Direct Audio Input

Direct audio input (DAI) involves using an auxiliary cable to directly connect a hearing aid or implantable device with an audio source. An advantage to DAI, unless there is a short in the wire, is that there is almost no possibility for interference. One disadvantage is that it is completely wired, and thus, you are tethered to that device. For hearing aids, a special battery door or adapter is necessary to accept one end of the auxiliary cable. This male end is usually three-pronged, so you also need a three-pronged female part to accept this connection. The other male end plugs into the headphone jack of the audio source. Each implant company has proprietary cables that are used with their device. One end of these proprietary cables plugs into a port or receptacle accessory on the implant and the other end plugs into the headphone jack of the audio source.

A message of caution is necessary with cochlear implants and DAI connections because of the electrical pathway across the scalp from the external implant device to the internal receiver stimulator inside the child's head. Cochlear implants should never be "electrically connected" (i.e., DAI) to any device that is still plugged into the wall. In the event of a power surge, the extra current could enter the building, travel through the electrical circuitry, travel through the DAI cable, and damage a child's cochlear implant and perhaps cause a serious injury. It is highly recommended that an auxiliary cable with surge protection be obtained if the cochlear implant is going to be plugged directly into a device such as a desktop computer that also plugs into a wall outlet. As a safety precaution, electronic devices should never be plugged in for charging during DAI use. Similarly, DAI should not be used with portable music devices (e.g., iPod, tablet, or laptop) while they are still plugged into the wall.

Considerations for Bilateral/Bimodal Users

Not only can hearing assistive technology be used with both hearing aids and cochlear implants, they can be used whether the child wears similar (bilateral; such as two hearing aids or two cochlear implants) or different (bimodal; one hearing aid and one cochlear implant) ear-level technology. Although the level of integration for bimodal technologies is not as seamless as bilateral technologies, audiologists can work with children to incorporate a setup that takes advantage of bimodal arrangements. Universal FM/DM receivers do exist so that one system can be used for both devices. Induction loop systems and direct audio input can also be used with hearing aids and implantable devices simultaneously. Because signal delivery is fundamentally different through CIs and HAs, audiologists have to fit the system independently for the two devices. As with ALD fitting with the devices separately, the goal of the fitting is to establish an output where speech is perceived of appropriate loudness and clarity, and that the outputs are balanced between ears.

ALERTING AND WARNING DEVICES

There are times when hearing aids or implantable devices are being repaired or when they are not being worn (e.g., sleeping or taking a shower). With or without amplification or implantation, it is vitally important to know if there is an alarm going off. As young children with hearing loss grow and mature, this promotes environmental awareness and independence. Some devices can be simple, single-function devices such as an alarm clock with a very loud audible signal. Other devices may have multiple functions with very loud alarms (for those that still have residual hearing) and built-in flashing lights. Some devices will accept bed-shaker attachments or can be used to cause an external lamp to flash. Some systems have remote receivers so one can keep the main system at the bedside with the bed shaker and have a remote system in the living room connected to a lamp that flashes. Older children may be able to take advantage of specific alarm apps using a "Smart Device" such as a cell phone, tablet, or even a watch (see below). There are also stand-alone fire/smoke or carbon monoxide detector systems that have a strobe light or a bed shaker attached, or a special low-pitched and very loud tone. Some local fire departments may distribute these free of charge. Otherwise, there are online vendors that have these specialized products.

A family emergency plan is mandatory, especially if there is someone in the family with a hearing loss. In an emergency, there may not be time to grab the hearing aids or implantable devices. The child will have great difficulty without his or her hearing technologies, especially at night. A serious discussion of the emergency plan is imperative ahead of time so that everyone knows what to do. The AV practitioner can help families develop emergency plans and perhaps help determine appropriate alert devices that are truly accessible to all members of the family, regardless of hearing abilities.

SMART DEVICE APPLICATIONS

Greater opportunities for access, independence, and more learning have come with the advent of technology available on cell phones and tablets ("smart devices") and their accompanying apps. Their portability and easy manipulations with swipes, taps, and pinches make them very appealing due to their multimodal capabilities. In addition, using smart devices can be instantly stimulating with many apps from which to choose. Couple these advantages with the fact that they are widely adopted in childhood education; they are powerful tools.

There are concerns about using smart devices with children, especially infants and toddlers. These devices should not become electronic parents, babysitters, or teachers and used by the child in isolation. Parents need to limit the time that children use these, instead providing children with opportunities for interactive dialogue, engaging in calorie-burning activities, playing with and manipulating physical toys, and unplugging their brains from technology.

There are several features to smart devices that make them accessible to those with hearing loss: Front-facing

cameras can provide more opportunities for lipreading for those children who need it when communicating with relatives and friends. Although the sound quality of a smart device may be questionable at times, the AV practitioner and parent can certainly use their own voices to repeat what was misheard or to provide the linguistic input that goes with the images. If the AV practitioner or anyone else uses the smart device, a powered or battery-operated external loudspeaker can be plugged into the headphone jack to provide a more audible signal to the child.

For young, emerging readers, most of the television and movie streaming apps now have the ability to display text options (e.g., closed captions or subtitles). For the hours a child might be in front of a screen, they can have many opportunities to connect print (captions) with auditory information and improve their literacy skills.

As mentioned earlier, there are plenty of ways to connect hearing aids and implantable devices to smart devices. One can use headphones or speakers, wired or Bluetooth-amplified neckloops and induction loops, DAI, personal streamers, or near-field devices. These options need consideration for times like riding in a car, listening in a place with excessive background noise, or even just to bring a more robust signal to the child's ear(s).

When determining whether an app is appropriate for a child, the AV practitioner and parent consider many questions. Does it fulfill a therapy goal such as expanding vocabulary, a higher-level auditory task, or self-advocacy? Does it have features that are accessible for the child, like being able to turn text on/off for working on reading? Does it have record keeping options so that one can track progress and data?

Buying apps can become expensive, but there are opportunities to get apps free or at reduced prices. Popular times for sales are April/May and September/October/November. Social media and developer websites also provide information about sales, and parents can sign up for developer magazines. Social media can also be used to preview apps in action, and some tutorials are available. There are sites that categorize apps by IEP goal and video channels that demonstrate the app.

At http://bit.ly/Apps4HL, you will find the list entitled "Apps for Kids (and Adults) With Hearing Loss." This is a list compiled and maintained by Tina Childress since 2011 when apps first started becoming popular. The apps are grouped into categories including Accessibility, Advocacy, Audiology, Classroom Tools, Hearing Test, Listening Therapy, Media Player, Personal Amplifier, Sound Level Meter, Speech/Language, and Telecommunication. By and large, the most popular and most populated category is Listening Therapy. Here, parents and kids can find engaging apps for working on specific auditory skills. Smart devices and apps are tools to put in the toolbox of the parent and AV practitioner.

AGE APPROPRIATENESS

Determining if and when to use hearing assistive and access technology with a child needs to be done on an individual and situational basis. The child's age and developmental skills, the technology and connectivity options available on his or her device, the child's wants and needs for using this technology, the setting where access is needed, and even the adult's technological savviness all need to be considered when settling on a device. Technology is of no use if it sits on a shelf or in a box. One tool that can help narrow the focus for technology needs can be found at http://www.wati.org/content/supports/free/pdf/Ch13-Hearing.pdf. The Assessing Students' Needs for Assistive Technology (ASNAT) document is also helpful in guiding one through the process of deciding on whether technology is necessary or available.

Before purchasing any kind of equipment, one should see if there are opportunities to *try it before you buy it*. The local clinic or hospital, a local audiology program, vendors with demonstration rooms, Centers for Independent Living, and consumer event exhibit halls are all places where one could touch and play with a piece of technology before purchasing it. One needs to check the return policy. With the evolution of technology, this goal of independence is more achievable, especially if one can *think outside the (tool)box*.

SUMMARY

A great deal of information on hearing assistive and access technology needs to be known by the AV practitioner and parents, and a concerted effort needs to be made to learn about and stay current with existing, new, and developing technology. It can be overwhelming at times, but the underlying motivation is to anticipate all the ways to help maximize access to the auditory world given the available technologies. For very young children and school-aged children with hearing loss, it is incumbent upon a collaborative team, including the AV practitioner and the parents, to facilitate listening and maximize access to spoken language by acquiring as much knowledge and expertise as possible about hearing assistive and access technologies. This knowledge and expertise can help parents in their quest to not only help their children maximize their listening and spoken language potential, but help their children develop the tools and independence to gain and maintain consistent auditory access to all the sounds of the world.

REFERENCES

American National Standards Institute. (2003). *Specification of hearing aid characteristics*. (ANSI S3.22-2003). Melville, NY: Acoustical Society of America.

Anderson, K. L. & Goldstein, H. (2004). Speech perception benefits of FM and infrared devices to children with hearing aids in a typical classroom. *Language, Speech, and Hearing Services in Schools, 35*(2), 169–184.

Atcherson, S. R., Franklin, C. A., & Smith-Olinde, L. (2015). *Hearing assistive and access technology*. San Diego, CA: Plural.

Atcherson, S. R., & Highley, P. (2013, Spring). Cell phones decoded. *Hearing Health, 29*(2), 22–27.

Chermak, G. D., Bellis, T. J., & Musiek, F. E. (2014). Neurobiology, cognitive science, and intervention. In G. D. Chermak & F. E. Musiek (Eds.), *Handbook of central auditory processing disorder: Comprehensive intervention* (Vol. 2, 2nd ed., pp. 3–38). San Diego, CA: Plural.

Kramer, S. (2014). *Audiology: Science to practice* (2nd ed.). San Diego, CA: Plural.

Letowski, T., Donahue, A. M., & Nábělek, A. K. (1986). Induction loop listening system designed for a classroom. *Journal of Rehabilitation Research and Development, 23*(1), 63–69.

Nábělek, A. K., Donahue, A. M., & Letowski, T. R. (1986). Comparison of amplification systems in a classroom. *Journal of Rehabilitation Research and Development, 23*(1), 41–52.

Sorri, M., Piiparinen, P., Huttunen, K., Haho, M., Tobey, E., Thibodeau, L., & Buckley, K. (2003). Hearing aid users benefit from induction loop when using digital cellular phones. *Ear and Hearing, 24*(2), 119–132.

Thibodeau, L. (2014). Comparison of speech recognition with adaptive digital and FM remote microphone hearing assistance technology by listeners who use hearing aids. *American Journal of Audiology, 23*(2), 201–210.

Wolfe, J., Morais, M., Schafer, E., Agrawal, S., & Koch, D. (2015). Evaluation of speech recognition of cochlear implant recipients using adaptive, digital remote microphone technology and speech enhancement sound processing algorithm. *Journal of the American Academy of Audiology, 26*(5), 502–508.

Wolfe, J., Morais, M., Schafer, E., Mills, E., Mülder, H. E., Goldbeck, F., . . . Lianos, L. (2013). Evaluation speech recognition of cochlear implant recipients using personal digital adaptive radio frequency system. *Journal of the American Academy of Audiology, 24*(8), 714–724.

Wolfe, J., Shafer, E. C., Heldner, B., Mülder, H., Ward, E., & Vincent, B. (2009). Evaluation of speech recognition in noise with cochlear implants and dynamic FM. *Journal of the American Academy of Audiology, 20*(7), 409–421.

SELECTED RESOURCES

http://www.listeningandspokenlanguage
.org/AcademyDocument.aspx?id=563

http://www.asha.org/public/hearing/
Induction-Loop-Systems/

https://www.fcc.gov/guides/hearing-
aid-compatibility-wireline-and-wireless-
telephones http://bit.ly/Apps4HL

http://www.wati.org/content/supports/
free/pdf/Ch13-Hearing.pdf

8

MILESTONES IN AUDITORY-VERBAL DEVELOPMENT

Auditory Processing, Speech, Language, Emergent Literacy, Play, and Theory of Mind

Karen MacIver-Lux, Stacey R. Lim,
Ellen A. Rhoades, Lyn Robertson,
Rosie Quayle, and Louise Hönck

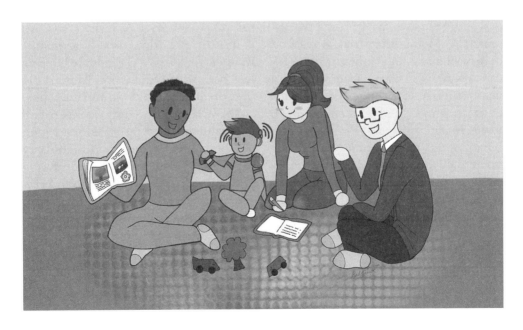

INTRODUCTION

Age-specific milestones are guidelines for skill acquisition in children with typical hearing who are considered *average*. Some children reach these milestones earlier and some reach them later than others, and they are not predictable across the domains represented. In Auditory-Verbal Therapy (AVT), these milestones become benchmarks by which the AV practitioner and the parent measure the development and progress of the child, as we work in tandem to close the listening and linguistic gap created by the child's hearing loss.

AUDITORY PROCESSING SKILLS

From infancy through adolescence, the peripheral auditory system (outer, middle, inner ear, and auditory nerve) and the central auditory nervous system (CANS) (auditory pathways and cortex of the brain) undergo significant changes that reflect growth and maturation. As a result, listening skills become refined, and spoken language emerges and evolves.

Many factors contribute to the development of the CANS, and the development of discrete auditory processing skills that contribute to listening (Sanes & Woolley, 2011). Along with growth and maturation of the outer ear canals and middle ear structures, the quantity and quality of auditory experiences, the integrity and maturation of the auditory neural networks and the auditory cortex of the brain (Eggermont & Moore, 2012), attention, self-regulation, and cognitive skills (Werner, 2012) contribute to the strength and effectiveness of the child's auditory processing skills. When conditions are ideal, children become proficient at processing various types of auditory input (e.g., accents, degraded speech signals, soft speech) across all types of listening conditions (e.g. noisy environments, reverberation). This proficiency has a significant impact on the development of skills in spoken language, literacy, and learning.

Prolonged periods of auditory deprivation and/or poor auditory access to linguistic structures and sounds of the environment cause the auditory system to undergo cross modal reorganization resulting in diminished connections within the auditory nerve and the auditory centers of the brain (Teoh, Pisoni, & Miyamoto, 2004). As the period of auditory deprivation increases, auditory performance regresses (Teoh et al., 2004). When the brain receives a diminished amount of auditory input, the neural networks reorganize themselves for other senses (e.g., vision) (Coez et al., 2011; Sharma, Gilley, Dorman & Baldwin, 2007). A child with hearing loss needs immediate provision of the best-quality auditory stimulation possible with appropriately selected and programmed hearing technology, and an abundance of meaningful auditory experiences that stimulate maturation of the CANS and the auditory and language association areas of the brain. AV practitioners guide and coach parents to create conditions in the daily environment that hopefully help the child develop exquisite auditory processing skills despite the presence of hearing loss.

Discrete Auditory Processing Skills

Although there are many neurophysiological and cognitive components and different auditory processes that contribute to the understanding of verbal and nonverbal sounds, presented here are five auditory processing skills that are commonly monitored in the AV session and their corresponding stages of development in children with typical hearing. These include *frequency resolution and discrimination, intensity, localization, temporal resolution, auditory attention,* and *speech discrimination in the presence of background noise.*

The better the auditory processing skills, the better the child is able to listen, especially in nonideal acoustic environments. Early auditory access to the sounds of speech and the environment plays a critical role in strengthening the auditory neural pathways (Werner, 2007) and, ultimately, the child's listening skills. When AV practitioners know the stages of development of these auditory processing skills, they are to help parents know (a) *which* strategies and conditions facilitate development of the select auditory processing skills (see Chapter 11), (b) *when* these strategies can be used to facilitate this development quickly, (c) how much listening time it takes to refine those auditory processing skills within all listening conditions, and (d) the auditory processes that are affected by certain auditory disorders (see Chapter 20). Knowledge of the stages of development of discrete auditory processing skills helps the AV practitioner to determine the level of the child's progress based on his or her hearing age.

Ages and Stages of Development

Frequency Discrimination and Resolution

Frequency resolution and discrimination abilities in the newborn are underdeveloped. They have poorer speech discrimination abilities in the higher frequencies (e.g., 4000 Hz) than in the low frequencies (e.g., 500 Hz) (Tharpe & Ashmead, 2001; Werner, 2011), that is most likely due to the immaturity of the auditory system (i.e., smaller ear canals and smaller middle ear space). Early exposure to high-frequency information such as high-frequency consonants (/s/, /f/) is essential for developing the auditory pathways associated with those frequencies (Werner, 2007). Newborns have sufficient discrimination skills, however, to support the perception of musical pitch. Thus, incorporating music, singing, and melodic speech has benefits because they activate cortical areas associated with sensorimotor skills (Grahn & Brett, 2007), memory and cognition (Janata, 2009; Koelsch & Siebel, 2005), and socioemotional skills (Blood & Zatorre, 2001).

From *3 months* onward, infants can discriminate different melodies (Plantinga & Trainor, 2009); can discriminate commonly used words better than uncommonly used words; and can attend to sentences that contain more familiar words than those that contain novel, or unfamiliar, words (Seidl & Johnson, 2006). Starting at approximately *4 months* of age, infants begin to prefer maternal and paternal infant-directed speech (IDS) to maternal and paternal adult-directed speech (ADS) (van Heugten & Johnson, 2012). Infant-directed speech is characterized by a slightly slower rate of speaking, more prosody (melodic intonation), and simpler sentence structures (McMurray, Kovack-Lech, Goodwin, & McEchron, 2013). Furthermore, infants show much more interest in IDS than in synthetic sounds (Shultz & Vouloumanos, 2010; Vouloumanos & Werker, 2007), such as those created by a noisemaker. Thus, the AV practitioner coaches the parent(s) to prioritize using melodic speech and singing over the use of noisemakers. At *6 months* of age, frequency discrimination becomes better at 4000 Hz (and adult-like) than at 500 Hz and 1000 Hz (Olsho et al., 1988; Werner, 2007; Werner et al., 2011). Speech discrimination skills continue to mature from toddlerhood well into childhood, reaching adult-like skills by 10 years of age. It is thought that the improvement of pitch discrimination is likely because of improvement in auditory memory (Keller & Cowan, 1994). During this preteen age, the child's ability to discriminate speech in the presence of background noise and with speakers who have accents has been refined and continues to grow into late adolescence.

Intensity

Between *1 and 6 months*, infants begin to have improved ability to detect differences in intensity (loudness) thresholds, but intensity processing is not fully mature until *10 years of age* (Werner, 2002). One reason for the slower maturation of intensity processing is the underdeveloped outer and middle ear structures. Unlike the cochlea, the outer and middle ear continue to grow throughout childhood (Werner, 2002, 2007). AV practitioners encourage parents to get *up close and personal* (when the speaker is close to the microphone of the hearing technology, the intensity of speech increases) so that children have an easier time hearing the quieter and higher-frequency sounds of speech.

Localization

Localization (ability to determine the origin of a sound within a physical space) is one of the skills that develop in the *early months of life*. Newborns exhibit localization abilities by turning their heads, or orienting, to the left or right in response to the presentation of a sound (Werner, 2007). Although not precise, the baby can orient to the general region from where the sound comes. By *7 months of age*, the infant can determine the distance to the sound (Gomes, Molholm, Christodoulou, Ritter, & Cowan, 2000). As a result, they are able to more accurately judge where to reach for an object that is making a sound. By *24 months of age*, he or she is able to localize speakers in many different directions. Because infants are highly interested in their parents' voices, the AV practitioner coaches them to use their voices for localization tasks, rather than using noisemakers or other toys. Localization skills continue to improve through late childhood.

Temporal Resolution

Temporal resolution is an essential skill for understanding speech and has been shown to affect children with auditory neuropathy spectrum disorder (ANSD;

Rance, Cone-Wesson, Wunderlich, & Dowell, 2002). Briefly stated, as sound is produced, there are rapid changes in frequency and intensity, and these changes carry information about voicing and prosody (Werner, 2002). Temporal resolution skills are developed *early*, and by *3 months of age*, are adult-like (Stuart, .2005;Werner, 2002). AV practitioners, therefore, coach parents to use nursery rhymes and infant-directed speech to refine this skill.

Auditory Attention

Auditory attention is a higher-level skill, one of the last to reach maturation in children (Werner, 2002). Throughout the child's early auditory development, there are different components of attention: *arousal*, the ability to detect and respond to a sound (Gomes et al., 2000), appears to develop rapidly in the *first two months* of life (Leibold, 2012); and *orienting*, an automatic behavioral response where the listener turns toward the sound (Gomes et al., 2000). There are two types of auditory attention: *attentiveness* (or *sustained attention*) and *selective attention*. Attentiveness is the listener's ability to maintain interest or listen while the sound is being presented, and to remain "on task" (Leibold, 2012). *Selective attention* occurs when a child focuses on a desired speech signal, ignoring other sounds that may be present (Werner, Fay, & Popper, 2011). AV practitioners coach parents to engage in frequent infant-parent exchanges as a way to extend the child's auditory attention, and these exchanges contribute significantly to listening and spoken language development.

Speech Understanding in the Presence of Competing Noise

Infants and young children have difficulty separating speech from noise (Werner, 2007). This, of course, has implications for spoken language learning. These stages of increasingly complex listening skills in less than ideal listening situations are due in part to brain maturation and myelination of various neural structures (Eggermont & Moore, 2012). This skill matures throughout childhood, with better processing of masked and degraded speech developing between the ages of *5 and 12 years* (Eggermont & Moore, 2012). Some children may exhibit adult-like skills around the age of *8 or 9 years*. However, they may rely more on slightly different cues (e.g., contextual cues, temporal cues, or frequency resolution cues) than adults when separating speech from noise (Werner, 2007). Adults have had more listening experience, so they are able to use these cues to a greater extent. Speech understanding capabilities in the presence of competing noise are more like adults' after *11 years of age* (Stuart, 2005). After *the age of 12*, children are better able to understand reverberant (echoey) speech and speech in noise. During the preteen and adolescent ages, the child's ability to discriminate speech in the presence of background and that of speakers who have accents has been refined and continues to grow into *late adolescence*. AV practitioners realize that early listeners need a quiet environment for AV sessions, and they coach parent(s) in ways to create quieter and more acoustic friendly environments in the home. As the child develops more advanced listening skills, the AV practitioner and parent(s) can incrementally add competing noise (such as opening the window in the therapy room or playing soft music at home).

Auditory Processing Skills: Conclusion

The discrete auditory processing skills form the foundation for listening skills (see Chapter 4) that the AV practitioner and parents work to develop in children with hearing loss. For example, if a child has poor temporal resolution skills or poor frequency discrimination skills, he or she will have more difficulty discriminating between similar phonemes or understanding speech in background noise. Being aware of the cognitive and developmental stages of auditory skills is critical for the AV practitioner. This way, the AV practitioner can ensure that the child is able to maximize his or her listening potential by using developmentally appropriate activities that promote the strengthening of discrete auditory processing skills. See Table 8–1 for the stages of auditory processing discussed in this section.

SPEECH

Speech is defined as the verbal means of communication and refers to the way speech sounds are made (articulation), the use of vocal folds and breathing that makes a sound (voice), and the rhythm of speech (fluency) (ASHA, 2015). Speech involves the coordination of many neurological and motor acts;

the brain plans which sounds need to be produced and communicates to the muscles that control breathing, voicing, articulation, and resonance. These all enable production of the planned sounds that need to happen quickly, fluently, and consistently in a controlled manner (Bennett, 2012). When there is a disconnect or disruption in the brain's ability to pass the motor-planning messages to the muscles that are responsible for speech production, it is referred to as apraxia; if there is impaired movement of the muscles responsible for speech production, it is referred to as dysarthria (ASHA, 2015). The following is a brief description of speech milestones beginning at birth and continuing throughout early childhood, and are typically refined by the time the child is 7 years old.

Stages of Speech Development

During the first two months of life, newborns make automatic and reflexive noises and vocalizations; they cry, cough, grunt, burp, and sneeze. Many researchers agree that these vocalizations seem to follow the melody of their surrounding language models (Mampe, Friederici, Chriostopher, & Wernke, 2009; Oller, 2000). Newborns also make quasi-vowel sounds that mimic the quality of speech but involve only the vocal cords that vibrate while the rest of the vocal tract (throat, oral cavity, nasal passage ways) and articulators (lips, tongue) remain at rest (Bennett, 2012). At this time, young infants are gaining early experience with turning on their voices and coordinating phonation and respiration (Oller, 2000).

Table 8–1. Ages and Stages of Auditory Processing

0–1 month	Demonstrates poorer discrimination at 4 kHz compared to 500 Hz (Olso et al., 1987; Tharpe & Ashmead, 2001).
	Prefers their mother's voices compared to unfamiliar voices (De Casper & Fifer, 1980).
	Prefers consonant-vowel sounds compared to synthetic sounds (Vouloumanos & Werker, 2007).
	Higher-frequency nonverbal and speech sounds are not clearly represented (Werner, 2008).
	Demonstrates perception of musical pitch and singing (Werner, 2012).
	No preference between maternal ADS and maternal IDS (Panneton-Cooper et. al., 1997).
	Discriminates two unknown languages of different rhythmic classes (Nazzi et. al., 1998).
1–2 months	Turns head to left or right in response to presentation of a sound (Werner, 2008).
	Infants have behavioral alerting thresholds higher than adults (Werner, 2007).
	Difficulty separating speech from noise (Werner, 2007).
2–3 months	Discriminates different melodies (Plantinga & Trainor, 2009).
	Discriminates commonly used words more accurately than uncommonly used words (Seidl & Johnson, 2006).
	Attends to sentences with highly used words than those with novel words (Seidl & Johnson, 2006).
	Temporal resolution skills adult-like by 3 months of age (Werner, 2007).
3–4 months	Aroused from sleep by sound of 90 dB in noisy environments and 50–70 in quiet (McConnell & Ward, 1967).
	Show preference for maternal IDS to maternal ADS (Panneton-Cooper et al., 1997).
	Makes rudimentary head turn toward a sound signal 50–60 dB.
	Begins paying attention to emotional tone of voice (Nygaard & Lunders, 2002.
4–5 months	Detects differences in intensity (Werner, 2007).
	Infants prefer maternal IDS over maternal ADS; is more important in early infancy rather than later infancy (Panneton-Cooper et al., 1997).
	Processing of lexically ambiguous words enhanced by emotional tone (Nygaard & Lunders, 2002).
5–6 months	Turns head to the side of the signal 40–50 dB SPL but cannot find it above or below (McConnell & Ward, 1967).
	Demonstrates a "listening attitude" (McConnell & Ward, 1967).
	Fine-tunes localization skills to direct localization of sounds to side and indirectly below (McConnell & Ward, 1967).

continues

Table 8-1. *continued*

6–7 months	Demonstrates better and more adult-like discrimination at 4 kHz than at 500 Hz and 1 kHz (Olsho et al., 1987).
7–8 months	Exaggerated pitch contours facilitate vowel discrimination in 6- to 7-month-old infants and serves to enhance segmental properties of fluent speech (Trainor & DesJardins, 2002). Becomes more precise in determining the location and distance of the sound (Werner, 2008). Directly locates sound source 30–40 dB to the side and directly below (McConnell & Ward, 1967).
8–9 months	Locates quieter sound sources (30–40 dB) directly to the side and below (McConnell & Ward, 1967). Attends more to sentences that have frequently occurring words (Seidl & Johnson, 2006). Treats high-probability sequences as potential word (Graf Estes et al., 2007). Fine-tunes ability to segment utterances with key words in initial and final position rather than in medial position of utterances (Seidle & Johnson, 2006).
9–10 months	Reaction time to detection tasks drops to adult-like levels (McConnell & Ward, 1967) Directly locates sound source of 25–35 dB to the side and below indirectly (McConnell & Ward, 1967).
10–12 months	Directly locates sounds to side, directly below ear level and indirectly above ear level to sounds that are 25–35 dB SPL (McConnell & Ward, 1967). (9–13 months).
12 months and up	Speech discrimination skills continue to develop and mature during toddlerhood well into childhood, reaching adult-like skills by 10 years of age. The improvement of pitch discrimination is likely because of improvement in auditory memory (Keller & Cowan, 1994). Children tend to judge sounds as being louder than adults would judge them to be (Leibold & Werner, 2002). Toddlers have difficulty recognizing words across gender, accents, although with practice, they learn (Ross & McMurray, 2010). During this time, the child's ability to discriminate speech in the presence of the background and with speakers who have accents has been refined and continues to grow into late adolescence. As with frequency resolution, intensity processing is not fully mature until 10 years of age (Werner, 2002). By the time the child is 24 months of age, he or she is able to localize speakers from many different directions. Localization skills are continually refined throughout late childhood (Werner, 2008). Direct localization of sounds on side, above, and below to 25 dB SPL (McConnell & Ward, 1967).

This stage of speech development is referred to as the Phonation Stage. During the second and third months of life, babies enter the Gooing/Cooing and Laughing Stage of speech development. They begin to move their mouths as they phonate, and vowel and consonant-like sounds emerge. These vocalizations often occur in interactions with caregivers as they make eye contact with them and take turns making sounds with them, a behavior that is fundamental to the development of social and language skills. At 4 to 5 months of age they enter the Expansion Stage, when many new sounds begin to occur as the baby engages in playful exploration of the vocal tract. At this stage babies are also starting to make movements that produce a sequence of sounds that resemble consonant-vowel combinations (e.g., "ba," "da"). At 6 to 7 months of age, babies enter the Canonical Babbling Stage and combine consonant (C) and vowel (V) sounds with rapid, speech-like transitions between the sounds. They are developing greater coordination of the articulators (jaw, lips), resonators (throat, oral cavity), and larynx that results in sounds recognized as real syllables (Bennett, 2012). When parents are responsive and provide feedback to their babies' babbling, phonological learning is facilitated (Goldstein & Schwade, 2008). The last stage of early speech development is the Integrative/Jargoning Stage at age 10 to 15 months. Now, babies produce long strings of syllables with a variety of sounds, varied stress, and varied intonation patterns. Real words may be included in these productions. By this time, the young child has spent a significant amount of time playing with sounds and begins to attach meaning to the form. A child's first words typically emerge around 12 months and often resemble the sound sequences produced in babbling (e.g., wawa for water, a da for all done, ba for ball). Children need to hear their own voices and the voices of others so that they are able to perceive the sounds necessary for speech development. They also require meaningful social interactions with their caregivers to gain practice developing motor control of the speech mechanism as they progress through the stages from infant vegetative sounds to jargon and first words. Therefore, speech development is strongly influenced by babies' auditory access to all sounds of speech and their environment, their social interactions, experiences making sounds, and maturation. See Table 8–2 for a summary of the ages and stages of speech development in young children.

Phonological Processes/Errors

As the child learns to pronounce new sounds and words, he or she may make errors that follow developmental patterns. The frequency of use varies from child to child and reduces with age and/or increased speaking (McIntosh & Dodd, 2008; Newton & Wells, 2002). For example, a common error of 2-year-olds is final consonant deletion (the final consonant in the word is dropped (e.g., ha for hat or coe for comb) due to difficulties perceiving it (e.g., otitis media with effusion), lack of attention, or reduced speech motor control. This typically is resolved about the age of 3. The AV practitioner needs to be knowledgeable about typical speech development in order to distinguish between

Table 8-2. Ages and Stages of Speech Development in Young Children

0–2 months	• Phonation Stage (e.g., cry, grunt, burp, cough, sneeze) (McIntosh & Dodd, 2008; Newton & Wells, 2002).
2–3 months	• Gooing/Cooing/Laughter Stage (e.g., being able to hear consonant sounds) (McIntosh & Dodd, 2008; Newton & Wells, 2002).
4–5 months	• Expansion Stage (e.g., many new sounds arise, resonant vowel sounds, pitch, and intensity) (McIntosh & Dodd, 2008; Newton & Wells, 2002).
6–7 months	• Canonical Babbling (e.g., sounds recognized as syllables) (McIntosh & Dodd, 2008; Newton & Wells, 2002). • From 6–12 months, their vocalization patterns reflect the dominant prosodic contours (e.g., falling versus rising pitch; Whalen, Levitt, & Wang, 1991) of the baby's native language. • Stress patterns parallel to the dominant stress patterns of native language in late babbling and early words (e.g., predominantly trochaic stress-first patterns in English; iambic stress-last patterns in French; Vihman, DePaolis, & Davis, 1998).
7–18 months	• Integrative/Jargoning Stage (10–15 months of age) (e.g., child produces long strings of syllables with a variety of sounds and varied stress and intonation patterns) (McIntosh & Dodd, 2008). • Jaw control is developed by 15 months, before control is established for the upper and lower lips (Green, Moore, Higashikawa, & Steeve, 2000; Green, Moore, & Reilly, 2002). • Motor development is slower for structures, such as the lips, that have more degrees of freedom of movement (Green et al., 2002). • Tongue development continues, with extrinsic tongue movements used for swallowing and sucking developed first followed by intrinsic tongue movements used for fine motor control to produce syllables (Fletcher, 1973; Kahane, 1988). • First words typically appear (McIntosh & Dodd, 2008).
18–24 months	• Jargoning Stage (e.g., nonsense gibberish combines with real words paired with gestures, body language, and eye contact) (McIntosh & Dodd, 2008; Newton & Wells, 2002). • Babbling decreases and word production increases. • Slight differences in frequencies of sounds and word shapes are reported cross-linguistically (Boysson-Bardies & Vihman, 1991; Maneva & Genesee, 2002), the considerable cross-linguistic similarities observed in babbling also exist in first words.
24–36 months 2–3 years	• /b/, /d/, /h/, /m/, /n/, /p/ in initial position of words is achieved. • /b/, /m/, /n/ in medial position of words is achieved. • /m/, /p/ in final position of words is achieved. (Goldman-Fristoe Test of Articulation 2, 2000).

Table 8-2. *continued*

36–48 months 3–4 years	• /t/, /g/, /k/, /t/, /w/ in initial position of words is achieved. • /t/, /g/, /k/, /ng/, /p/, /t/ in medial position of words is achieved. • /b/, /d/, /g/, /k/, /n/, /t/ in final position of words is achieved. (Goldman-Fristoe Test of Articulation 2, 2000). • Prevocalic voicing resolved (e.g., big for pig) (Bowen, 1998). • Word-final devoicing resolved (e.g., pick for pig) (Grunwell, 1997). • Stopping /f/ resolved (e.g., tish for fish) (Bowen, 1998) • Stopping /s/ resolved (e.g., dope for soap) (Bowen, 1998). **At 3.3 years** • Final consonant deletion resolved (e.g., ha for hat) (Bowen, 1998). **At 3.6 years** • Fronting is resolved (e.g., tar for car, sip for ship) (Grunwell, 1997). • Stopping /v/ is resolved (e.g., berry for very) (Bowen, 1998). • Stopping /z/ is resolved (e.g., doo for zoo) (Grunwell, 1997). **At 3.9 years** • Consonant harmony is resolved (e.g., mime for mine; titty tat for kitty cat) (Bowen, 1998).
48–60 months 4–5 years	• /kw/ in initial position of words is achieved. • /d/ in medial position of words is achieved. • /f/ in final position of words is achieved (Goldman-Fristoe Test of Articulation 2, 2000). • Weak syllable deletion resolved (e.g., efant for elephant, tato for potato) (Bowen, 1998). • Cluster reduction (e.g., poon for spoon, chain for train, keen for clean) (Bowen, 1998). **At 4.6 years** • Stopping "sh" resolved (e.g., dop for shop) (Bowen, 1998). • Stopping /dz/ "j as in jump" resolved (e.g., dump for jump) (Bowen, 1998). • Stopping "ch" resolved (e.g., tare for chair) (Bowen, 1998).
60–72 months 5–6 years	• ch, /dz/ (j as in judge), /l/, /s/, "sh", /j/ ("y" as in yellow), /bl/ in initial position of words is achieved. • "ch", /dz/ (j as in judge), /l/,/s/, "sh," /z/ in medial position of words is achieved. • /l/, /ng/ (ing as in cooking), "ch," /dz/ (j as in judge), /s/, "sh," /r/, /v/, /z/ in final position of words is achieved (Goldman-Fristoe Test of Articulation 2, 2000).

continues

Table 8–2. *continued*

60–72 months	• Gliding of liquids is resolved (e.g., one for run, weg for leg, yeg for leg) (Bowen, 1998).
5–6 years	• Stopping voiceless "th" is resolved (e.g., ting for thing) (Bowen, 1998).
	• Stopping voiced "th" is resolved (e.g. dem for them) (Bowen, 1998).
	• The primary period for the development of prosody occurs from approximately 5 to 8 years of age (Local, 1980; Wells, Peppe, & Goulandris, 2004).
	6–7 years
	• /r/, /v/, /br/, /dr/, /fl/, /fr/, /gl/, /gr/, /kl/, /kr/, /pl/, /st/, /tr/ in initial position of words is achieved.
	• /r/, /v/ in medial position of words is achieved (Goldman-Fristoe Test of Articulation 2, 2000).
	7 years
	• /z/, /sl/, /sp/, /sw/, "th" is achieved in initial position of words.
	• "th" in medial position of words is achieved.
	• "th" in final position of words is achieved (Goldman-Fristoe Test of Articulation 2, 2000).

speech errors that are developmental because of a young hearing age (e.g., phonological processes/errors), motor speech issues (e.g., dysarthria or childhood apraxia) and those that result due to compromised auditory access.

Speech Errors Related to Inadequate Auditory Access

Children typically say what they hear. It is possible, therefore, for a child with hearing loss to have speech errors that are caused by changes in hearing levels/hearing technology, insufficient gain or overamplification by the hearing aids, or a problem with the cochlear implant. Whenever the child's speech production does not follow typical developmental patterns, it is critical that the audiologist examine the child's hearing status and hearing technology immediately. When necessary, adjustments to the hearing technology need to be made immediately, before the speech errors become habitual (Ling, 1989). The following speech errors may occur when there is insufficient auditory access at the stated specific frequencies.

Low Frequencies 250 to 500 Hz

■ Voice is weak, breathy, high in pitch
■ Nasalization or denasalization
■ Voiced consonant deletions (b, m, n, ing, d)

- Vowel confusions (oo, ee)
- Nasal/plosive confusions (b/m, d/n)
- Voiced/voiceless consonant confusions (p/b, k/g)

Mid Frequencies 500 to 2000 Hz

- Voice may be too quiet or too loud
- Poor pitch control
- Omission of unstressed vowels in words
- Omission of unstressed words in sentences
- Neutralization of vowels

High Frequencies 2000 to 5000 Hz

- Voiceless consonant confusions (p, t, and k)
- Production of high-frequency consonants poor (s, f, th)
- Vowel confusions (oo, ee)
- Omission of final consonants in words
- Omission of markers for plurals, past tense (Estabrooks, 2006; Ling, 1990; Pollack et al., 1997)

SPOKEN LANGUAGE

During the first year of life, the infant transitions from being *an examiner* to *an experimenting scientist* determined on discovering the patterns of what is seen and heard (Gopnik, Meltzoff, & Kuhl, 1999). During the second year of life, the toddler is *an explorer* whose "communicative universe" is continually expanding (Boysson-Bardies, 1999).

Then, across the preschool years, the child becomes *an exhibitor* demonstrating the linguistic skills that have been learned (Yang, 2006). These learning stages enable the child to become language proficient and ready for academic learning (Pinker, 2007).

Hearing and listening, and understanding and speaking a language are influenced by *all* the developmental areas including the cognitive and socioemotional domains (Tomasello, 2003). The depth and range of the child's spoken language are built upon the scaffolding of many concepts (Ferguson & Waxman, 2014). For example, when a child has learned to vocalize a combination of several words in appropriate order, his or her spoken language is dependent on what was previously heard and understood as well as on short-term, long-term, and working memory and other social and cognitive skills (Galinsky, 2010). Because skills from different developmental domains lead up to the production of spoken language, the language scales below reflect some skills from auditory, cognitive, speech, and social domains.

A milestone indicates a developmental change from one age to the next; it serves as a benchmark or guideline for skill acquisition. Milestones tend to be age-specific markers that the "average" child demonstrates. Not every child, however, follows the same timetable. Some children reach age-appropriate milestones in one developmental domain at an earlier age than they might in another area of growth. The fact that some children attain milestones a bit later is not as disconcerting as those who do not progress from one skill to another in sequential order (Owens, 2005).

There are many reasons why children demonstrate great heterogeneity in learning a spoken language. Of course, the quantity and quality of parental input as well as access to sound are enormous factors, particularly for children with hearing loss (e.g., Ambrose, Walker, Unflat-Berry, Oleson, & Moeller, 2015). But other influential factors must also be considered: cultural differences; psychosocial contexts; the child's learning capacities; and environmental stressors, such as poverty and low birth weight (e.g., Madigan, Wade, Plamondon, Browne, & Jenkins, 2015).

Therefore, the "average" child usually reflects the "mean"—the midway point between two extremes. There is a wide range in the attainment of any skill; half of all children reach the milestone earlier and the other half reach that same milestone at later points in time (Owens, 2005). This normal distribution of skill acquisition is associated with the "bell curve." For parents and AV practitioners involved in the planning of objectives, goals, and AVT activities, developmental milestones are of importance because they are *hierarchical* in nature, representing *attainable* skills for children with hearing loss.

Developmental milestones are sometimes culture specific (e.g., Taverna, Waxman, Medin, Moscoloni, & Peralta, 2014). Some milestones that apply to young children in westernized nations may not apply to children from other nations such as those in Asia, the Arab Gulf, or Eastern Europe (Glennen & Masters, 2002). However, across all cultures, the first three years of life is the most intensive period for acquiring speech and language skills. The second three years of life, while not as linguistically intensive, are also important for developing the morphological, syntactical, and lexical aspects of language (Owens, 2005). Ultimately, by the time children with typical hearing reach grade school, their knowledge and use of spoken language is essentially equivalent to that of adults whose grammar is both correct and complete (Pinker, 2007). And once the young child learns the native language, it will never be lost (Pierce, Klein, Chen, Dekenserie, & Genesee, 2014). This is the benchmark by which AV practitioners measure progress in our children with hearing loss. See Table 8–3 for a breakdown of the stages of spoken language.

Table 8–3. Ages and Stages of Spoken Language

Birth	
Knowledge/Receptive Language	**Expressive Language**
• Exhibits startle reflex in response to sudden loud noises; will stiffen, quiver, blink, screw eyes up, fan out fingers and toes, or cry as a response. • Sensitive to a wide range of sounds, including prosodic and rhythmic cues. • Recognizes and prefers mother's voice; quiets if crying. • Sounds of different frequencies have different effects on the infant. • Low-frequency sounds and rhythmic sounds have a calming effect. • Higher-frequency sounds result in a more violent reaction. • Increases or decreases sucking sound in response to sound.	• Cries. • Begins to coo when content.
Three Months	
Knowledge/Receptive Language	**Expressive Language**
• Awareness of human speech; attends to voice. • Shows excitement at sound of approaching footsteps, running bath water, etc. • Awakens or quiets to sound of mother's voice. • Searches for human voice. • Begins to localize sound by turning eyes toward the general sound source. • Begins to enjoy sound-making toys; listens to a bell near him. • Listens to music.	• Cries are meaningful, e.g., different cries for hunger, discomfort, pain. • Coos and gurgles when happy, playful, or content. • Imitates own noises as he hears them, e.g., ooh, baba. • Vocally responds to mother's voice. • Begins to babble.
Six Months	
Knowledge/Receptive Language	**Expressive Language**
• Distinguishes between friendly and angry voices; reacts appropriately • Discriminates between sounds of strangers and familiar people.	• Vocal play occurs when playing. • Responds to human speech by vocalizing.

continues

Table 8-3. *continued*

Six Months *continued*	
Knowledge/Receptive Language	**Expressive Language**
• Specifically locates sound anywhere such as the bell that is rung out of sight (downward localization develops before upward localization).	• Chuckles and laughs; vocalizes excitement and displeasure.
• Responds to human speech by smiling.	• Emerging repetition of select sounds.
• Turns immediately to mother's voice across the room.	• Makes speech-like babbling sounds, especially using /p/, /b/, /m/ sounds.
• Responds differentially to emotional tones of mother's voice.	• Begins to communicate by using sounds with gestures to indicate wants and needs.
• Responds to baby hearing tests at one and a half feet from each ear by correct visual localization, but may show slightly delayed response.	
• Associates hearing with sound production, in that select sounds are repeated.	
• Attends to own name, to music, and to toys that make sounds.	
• Knows names associated with primary caregivers, e.g., mommy, daddy.	
• Understands the meaning of no.	
Nine Months	
Knowledge/Receptive Language	**Expressive Language**
• Turns head and shoulders toward familiar sounds, even when cannot see what is happening.	• Babbling is frequent, including consonants and vowels.
• Begins to understand some words in context.	• Says one- or two-syllable sounds that indicate items is wanted, e.g., baba (for bottle)
• Recognizes familiar sounds, e.g., dog bark, door knock, doorbell.	• Babbles to get caregiver's attention as well as to indicate needs and wants.
• Responds to a telephone ringing, a human voice, his own name, e.g., no-no, bye-bye.	
• Enjoys simple games, e.g., pat-a-cake, peek-a-boo.	
• Looks at daddy and other family members when named.	
• Raises arms when mother says, Come up and reaches toward child.	

Table 8-3. *continued*

Nine Months *continued*	
Knowledge/Receptive Language • Responds more discriminatingly to adult verbalizations. • Listens with selective interest; increases "listening attitude" for conversation. • Understands a few words for common items, e.g., juice, milk, shoe. • Responds when called to or when gestured to, e.g., Come here, Want more? • Begins following through on a simple direction, e.g., Give it to mommy.	

Twelve Months (1 year)	
Knowledge/Receptive Language	**Expressive Language**
• Understands approximately 50+ words. • Has precise localization of sound. • Turns head when hears own name. • May cry when there is thunder or frown when scolded. • Enjoys listening to sounds, words, simple stories. • Recognizes and differentiates appropriately between vocalizations, e.g., ow, uh-oh, no, shhh, all gone. • Responds to simple commands (at first, responds only when command is accompanied by gesture), e.g., giving a toy on request or going someplace as directed. • Understands an assortment of action words (verbs), e.g., drink, go, come, give. • Understands some simple directions, e.g., wave bye-bye. • No real understanding of questions is shown. • Interested in environmental noises beyond his immediate surroundings.	• Jabbers in response to human voice, with intonational contours of native language. • When babbling, sometimes uses gestures such as pointing. • Begins to use jargon, i.e., babbling mixed up with made-up and real words. • Sound imitations indicate that child hears the sounds and matches them with his own sound productions. • Imitates novel sounds. • Imitates a few words inexactly. • Says approximately 1–5 different words.

continues

Table 8–3. *continued*

Twelve Months (1 year) *continued*	
Knowledge/Receptive Language • Likes jingles and rhymes; moves to music. • Begins to recognize 12 or more objects when he hears the names of them. • Comprehension of spoken words begins to increase by at least one new word a week. • Points to pictures when they are named.	

Eighteen Months (one-and-a-half years)	
Knowledge/Receptive Language • Understands about 150–250 words. • Words are understood outside of routine games. • Understands simple sentences. • Understands simple questions, e.g., What's this? Where's daddy? • Consistently responds to own name. • Overhears familiar words not directed to child. • Recognizes sounds out of context. • Understands the pronouns: you, me. • Begins to understand prepositional phrases, but only within the total unit, e.g., putting something in or on something. • Begins to follow one-step directions and short series of simple commands, e.g., Wipe the doll's nose. • Points to real and pictured objects as well as body parts on request. • Comprehension of spoken words begins to increase by at least several new words per day.	**Expressive Language** • Echoes prominent or last word addressed to him. • Says new words every month. • Uses many different consonant sounds at the beginning of words. • May begin using two words together, e.g., Where ball? No doggie. More push. • Most words are not yet intelligible to strangers. • Says approximately 25–100 different words.

Table 8-3. *continued*

Twenty-Four Months (2 years)	
Knowledge/Receptive Language	**Expressive Language**
• Understands approximately 200–500 words. • Shows interest in the sounds of radio or TV commercials. • Listens to the reason (logic) of language. • Enjoys listening to simple stories. • Responds to command, e.g., Show me the —. • Understands simple wh- questions, e.g., Where is your —? • Waits in response to: just a minute. • Identifies five body parts. • Understands family names by selecting appropriate pictures. • Understands many phrases, e.g., have candy after lunch • Carries out four separate directions with a ball, e.g., Give it to me. Put the ball down. Go get the block. • Follows a direction with two critical elements, e.g., Get your socks and put them in the basket. • Responds appropriately to directions involving simple prepositions: in, on, under • Understands some action verbs by selecting appropriate pictures. • Recognizes the syntactic order of words when context, semantics, and prosody are coherent.	• Repeats two numbers, letters, or words. • Begins using two-word utterances in correct word order. • Makes appropriate differentiations between talking loudly, talking softly, and whispering; can modify own loudness level of talking. • Uses "telegraphic speech" with articles/conjunctions missing. • Says own name on request. • Names own body parts, favorite toys, familiar objects. • Emerging use of verbs and adjectives. • Emerging use of oral narrative skills. • Says: What's that? • Begins having a word for everything. • Approximately 25% of what child says is intelligible to strangers. • Says approximately 100–300 different words.
Thirty Months (two-and-a-half years)	
Knowledge/Receptive Language	**Expressive Language**
• Understands approximately 250–700 words. • Listens to stories read from a picture book for longer periods of time.	• Has a word for just about anything. • Says two- to three-word sentences. • Recalls and repeats only first, second, or third item of a series.

continues

Table 8-3. *continued*

Thirty Months (two-and-a-half years) *continued*	
Knowledge/Receptive Language	**Expressive Language**
• Differentiates between nearly all sounds in the mother tongue.	• Answers simple wh- questions, e.g., Where is your —?
• When child hears pleasurable sounds, he reacts to them by running to look or by telling someone what he hears.	• Tells a very simple story that usually revolves around one event.
• Responds to descriptive or locative information about things from pictures, e.g., Show me the one that is up in the sky.	• Tries to get a reaction from others by repeating phrases that earn a big laugh.
• Enjoys listening to songs.	• Uses pronouns like me and you but may get them mixed up.
• Understands the concept of more, e.g., more cats.	• Says some phrases, e.g., no want cookie, my turn.
• Differentiated understanding of: one, many, all	• Production of vocabulary explodes; rapid expansion in use of new words.
• Understands gross size differences and polar opposites, e.g., hot/cold, stop/go, nice/yucky, in front of/behind, big/little, up/down, fast/slow, push/pull.	• Approximately 50% of what child says is intelligible to strangers.
• Identifies object by use: brush is for hair; spoon is for mouth	• Says approximately 150–400 different words.
• Follows simple two-step directions, e.g., Get the book and then sit here.	
• Understands more who/what/where questions, e.g., What do you hear with?	
• Understands prepositions: in, on, under, in front of, in back of, around, behind.	
• Understands and responds appropriately: give me just one block	
• Understands differences between sentences varying in syntax: Show me the car pushing the truck versus The truck is pushing the car.	
• Understands conjunction: and	
• Comprehends nearly all sentence structures.	
• Understands /s/ (plural) and /-ing/ (present progressive verb tense).	

Table 8–3. *continued*

Three Years	
Knowledge/Receptive Language	**Expressive Language**
• Understands approximately 500–1,500 words.	• Imitates a 5- to 7-syllable sentence, based on short-term memory.
• Carries out commands using two different prepositions.	• Remembers and repeats three items of a story.
• Responds to two unrelated commands, e.g., Put your cup on the table and turn off the TV.	• Recalls and repeats three numbers, letters, or words.
• Listens eagerly to stories and demands his favorite ones over and over again.	• Recalls and repeats a nonsense syllable after 15 s.
• Identifies the use of things in pictures, e.g., Show me the one you wear.	• Produces sentences that are longer, combining four words.
• Understands and responds to simple questions: who, what, where?	• Uses regular past tense of regular verbs, tending to overgeneralize the past tense with irregular verbs, e.g., swimmed.
• Understands the why question.	• Uses present progressive tense -ing of regular verbs, e.g., swimming.
• Begins to match simple sound tones.	• Uses negation between subject and verb: no, not, can't, don't, e.g., I don't want it.
• Recognizes several melodies.	• Uses contracted form of is, e.g., he's.
• Knows third-person pronouns, e.g., he/she.	• Uses 's for possession, e.g., Juan's.
• Understands regular past tense forms of verbs.	• Uses adverbs of location, e.g., here, there.
• Understands articles: a, the.	• Uses prepositions, e.g., in, on.
• Expanded understanding of common opposites, e.g., empty/full, give/take, heavy/light, long/short, loud/soft.	• Uses present tense of auxiliary verbs, e.g., I can help.
• Follows a direction with three critical elements.	• Uses be verbs, e.g., I am happy.
• Understands taking turns.	• Uses articles, e.g., a, the, that.
• Understands most common adjectives, including sizes, colors, shapes.	• Emerging use of semi-auxiliary verbs, e.g., wanna, gotta, hafta.
• Shows an interest in explanations of why and how.	• Answers simple wh- questions, e.g., What do you have? Which one is broken?
	• Can sing a familiar song, e.g., Twinkle, twinkle little star.
	• Talks about things that happened away from home, e.g., preschool, outings.
	• Spoken language is fluent and most sentences are complete.
	• Talks about absent objects and make-believe things.

continues

Table 8-3. *continued*

Three Years *continued*	
	Expressive Language • Lies and teases. • Approximately 75% of what child says is intelligible to strangers. • Says approximately 900–1,000 different words.

Four Years	
Knowledge/Receptive Language	**Expressive Language**
• Understands approximately 4,000–6,000 words.	• Imitates a 9- to 11-syllable sentence, based on short-term memory.
• Listens to and understands most preschool children's stories.	• Remembers and repeats four items of a story.
• Listens to electronic media at the same loudness level as other family members.	• Recalls and repeats two numbers backward.
• Carries out a sequential command of three action parts, e.g., Pick up the ball, put it on the table, and bring me the book.	• Recalls four numbers, letters, or words.
• Carries out four separate commands using different prepositions, e.g., in back of, beside, beneath.	• Tells longer tales with multiple sentences that may include several events.
• Understanding of prepositions expands to include: between/above/below/top/bottom.	• Answers simple questions about children's stories.
• Emerging ability to follow a four-step command, i.e., a direction with four critical elements.	• Constructs detailed sentences, e.g., We went to the zoo but had to come home early.
• Understands and replies appropriately with a word or gesture to questions, e.g., What do you do when you are sleepy? Which one is bigger? Why is it broken?	• Can tell long and involved imaginative stories using adult-like grammar.
• Comprehends time phrases: all the time, all day, for 2 weeks.	• Completes opposite analogies, e.g., Daddy is a boy, mommy is a __.
• Understands regular plurals, e.g., hat/hats, box/boxes.	• Uses pronouns appropriately: I, me, you, your, they, us, we, they, our.
• Understands possessives. e.g., dog's	• Enjoys reciting rhyming words, e.g., hat, fat, cat.
• Understands the number three, e.g., Give me three.	• Uses possessives, e.g., Juan's.
	• Uses variations of to be, e.g., I <u>am</u> happy. It <u>was</u> gone.
	• Uses articles, e.g., a, the, that, this, these, those.
	• Uses present tense of auxiliary and semi-auxiliary verbs, e.g., can, help, gonna, wanna, gotta, hafta.

Table 8–3. *continued*

Four Years *continued*	
Knowledge/Receptive Language	**Expressive Language**
• Emerging understanding of more advanced polar opposites, e.g., alike/unlike, same/different. • Identifies four colors. • Understands dependent clause: if, because, when, why. • Hears and understands most of what is said at home and school.	• Appropriately uses regular plurals, e.g., birds, buses. • Communicates easily with adults and other children. • Asks open-ended questions, e.g., when, how, why. • Can easily engage people in conversations. • Approximately 90% of what child says is intelligible to strangers. • Says approximately 1,500–1,600 different words.
Five Years	
Knowledge/Receptive Language	**Expressive Language**
• Understands 3,000–6,000 words • Loves stories; emerging appreciation for humor and surprise elements. • Comprehends more complex time phrases, e.g., for a long time, for years, a whole week, in the meantime, two things at once. • Understands comparatives and superlatives: tall/taller/tallest, same/more/less, most/least, several/few, some/many, before/after, now/later. • Follows classroom paper-and-pencil directions, e.g., On your paper, draw a circle around something that you eat. • Understands most, if not all, pronouns and contractions, e.g., she's. • Knows function of body parts. • Knows the meaning of some words signifying time, e.g., now, later, yesterday, today, tomorrow, before, after; What happens after lunch? • Understands: the opposite of – is –. • Identifies some indefinite pronouns, e.g., any, every, both, few, many, each.	• Imitates a 14-syllable sentence, based on short-term memory. • Recalls and repeats five items of a story. • Recalls and repeats five numbers, letters, or words. • Borrows characters from TV and stories for own narratives. • Tells stories of past and present events, in which several events are logically connected. • Uses an average of 6 words per sentence. • Says complete sentences. • Uses conjunctions that introduce conditional clauses in sentences: if, so. • Can keep a conversation going. • States simple similarities and differences of items when presented with pictures. • Answers what-if questions, e.g., What happens if it breaks? • Emerging use of auxiliary verb have, e.g., I have the car. • Asks for permission to others' items, e.g., Can I borrow_? May I use _?

continues

Table 8–3. *continued*

Five Years *continued*	
Knowledge/Receptive Language	**Expressive Language**
• Knows the difference between real life and fantasy stories.	• Uses present, past, future tense of verbs.
• Understands that zero represents nothing.	• Use conjunctions to string words together, e.g., A bear <u>and</u> a wolf. A book <u>or</u> a toy.
• Knows the meaning of words signifying order, e.g., first, next, last	• Uses polite expressions, e.g., Thank you. I'm sorry. Please.
• Points to correct coins when named.	• Uses superlatives -est, e.g., biggest, smartest.
• Responds correctly to complicated sentences, but may still be confused by long complex sentences, particularly those contains compound clauses.	• Uses -er to form nouns from verbs, e.g., teach/teacher.
	• Responds to: What did you say?
• Comprehends just about everything said in school and at home.	• Can define objects by use and composition, e.g., Napkins are made of paper; you wipe your mouth with them.
	• Adapts talking style according to listener and place, e.g., uses shorter and simpler sentences with very young children, or talks louder outside than inside.
	• Uses different strategies for recounting events.
	• Recites letters and numbers.
	• Emerging use in naming the positions of items: first, second, third, last.
	• Emerging use of adverbial word endings, e.g., -ly -> sadly, quickly.
	• Uses possessives and negatives more consistently.
	• Uses irregular plurals, e.g., children, mice, teeth.
	• Uses irregular past tense verbs, e.g., was, said, found, ate, thought.
	• Tells some very involved adult-like tall tales.
	• Sentences are complex and include clauses, e.g., I want to get a horse but daddy says that won't happen until he wins the lottery, and then, just maybe, then he will buy one for me.
	• Says approximately 2,500+ different words.

Table 8–3. *continued*

Six Years	
Knowledge/Receptive Language	**Expressive Language**
• Understands approximately 20,000–25,000 words.	• Imitates a 16-syllable sentence, based on short-term memory.
• Differentiates right and left of own body but not in others.	• Remembers and repeats six items of a story.
• Knows irregular comparatives, e.g., good, better, best	• Recalls and repeats three numbers backward.
• Responds appropriately to numbers, e.g., Give me four pennies.	• Provides a word that rhymes with a given word.
• Understands seasons of the year, and knows what we do in each season.	• Use complex, compound sentences.
	• Learns letter-sound associations.
• Understands riddles and idioms, e.g., hold your horses.	• Tells own address and phone number.
• Becoming aware of mistakes in other people's speech.	• Emerging use of irregular comparatives/superlatives, e.g., good, better, best, worst, worse.
	• Uses past perfect tense, e.g., She had been shopping.
	• Continues to improve correct use of irregular part tense and plurals.
	• Asks 'have' questions with present perfect, e.g., Have you been there before?
	• Can use the passive voice.
	• Emerging use of derivational morphemes in which verbs are changed into nouns, e.g., catch becomes catcher.
	• Begins to produce gerunds (a nun form produced by adding -ing to a verb infinitive, e.g., fish → fishing: Fishing with my dad is fun.
	• Uses most morphological markers fairly consistently, e.g., Both boys walked to the store.
	• Learning to name days of the week in order and months of the year.
	• Learning to count up to 100, and to tell time.
	• Tells jokes and well-formed narratives.
	• May start to use slang, e.g., That's cool. Awesome!
	• Says approximately 3,000+ different words.

EMERGENT LITERACY

Emergent literacy (Chapter 9) as discussed by most scholars is a stage that begins at birth and lasts until around age 6. During this period, children learn to listen and talk, gradually building a repertoire of experiences, sounds, vocabulary, language structures, and ways to use language for different purposes. Children move through this rather long stage of becoming aware of reading and writing in various ways and at individual paces. As children encounter language in all forms—listening, speaking, reading, and writing—they create the background knowledge necessary to begin to learn to read and write, literacy processes whose foundations are listening and speaking.

Full-fledged literacy, the ultimate goal for children with and without hearing loss, is becoming more complex. The National Council of Teachers of English (2013) definition asserts that 21st century demands include multiple literacies that include proficiency with technology, working across cultures to solve problems, collaborating with global communities, working at complex levels with "multiple streams of simultaneous information" and multimedia texts, and employing ethical responsibilities in complex settings.

Historically, few individuals with hearing loss have learned to read at adult levels, creating low expectations for this population. With the advent of Auditory-Verbal Therapy (AVT), reading levels have increased in individuals who followed AVT, and while no approach guarantees high levels of literacy in children with or without hearing loss, AVT and other auditory-based learning

provide the most likely route to literacy development (Robertson, 2014).

During the emergent period, the main task for the child is that of spoken language acquisition. During the first years, beginning as early as possible, parents and caregivers need to talk extensively with the child, play with sounds and language, engage in imaginative play, and read many books with their little one. As this continues, it is common to see older babies and toddlers choose favorite books and begin to retell the stories and recite the rhymes and words read from the books. People who read to the children make the books meaningful for them, and they can add the language of books to his or her repertoire. Repeated experiences with books help children learn book-sharing routines and book-handling skills, and guided access to writing materials leads to scribbling, drawing, and an emerging concept that symbols stand for meanings (McGee & Richgels, 2012). Along the way, children pick up on "Concepts About Print," a list of what children need to learn and an assessment system with for gauging readiness for formal reading instruction (Clay, 2000). These concepts include reading from left to right and from top to bottom; moving from one line to the next with a return sweep; letters and words represent a message that one can turn into spoken words; pictures are related to the print; and a book has a front, a back, and an author. Writing begins with scribbling and moves through creating lines and shapes, and onward to attempting to copy letters and write one's name.

Stimulating development through the emergent literacy stage involves the practitioner, teacher, and parent(s) introducing reading and writing materials with which to advance language acquisition and understanding. Reading with a child, talking about the book, and writing and reading Language Experience Books (see Chapter 9) provide valuable opportunities for children to listen, talk, and "write"; these can be used in AV sessions, and parents can learn how to do these literacy activities with their children themselves. Without any direct teaching, many children will pick up knowledge of literacy and its purposes, and they will use this when formal reading and writing instruction begin in first kindergarten or first grade. The practitioner can document children's responses during reading and writing times, as well as spontaneous instances of prereading and prewriting behaviors and reflect upon whether and how these connect to the language development the child is demonstrating.

Table 8–4 demonstrates ages and stages of emergent literacy. The goal at the end this stage is that the child be linguistically and experientially prepared to enter school where formal literacy instruction begins.

PLAY

Play is often defined as "engaging in an activity for enjoyment rather than a practical purpose," (Oxford English Dictionary, 2015). However, it has long been accepted that "play is a child's work (Piaget, 1977)" and can be used in the transition from the living room into a world of possibilities—the chair can become a bus, a boat, or a fantasy castle. *"Play is a transition from the purely situational constraints of early childhood, to the adult capability for abstract thought"* (Vygotsky, 1978). The important links in all the areas of child development, including the development of language, motor skills, social skills, literacy, mathematical ability, and self-concept have been well documented in literature (Brown, 1999; Singer et al., 2006). Play gives children time to practice and hone their skills and develop interactions in ways that are engaging, fun, and "easy." Play teaches children to be creative, solve problems, make choices, negotiate, use ideas, experiment, set goals, and explore emotions. Consequently, play stimulates and coaxes children into new learning. As the child becomes immersed in various auditory, visual, and social environments, play provides a platform for the development of vocabulary, language structures, attention span, and motor skills.

Developmental Sequence of Play Behaviors

The desire to connect with another human being through playful interaction starts *from birth* when an infant imitates an adult's facial expressions. Although this imitation is reflexive at first, the continuing positive reinforcement from parents leads the child to intent gazing and preference for human faces *before 6 months* of age. Next, babies explore their world through cause and effect, mouthing, and hiding and finding games between *6 and 9 months of age*. Play becomes a bit more schematic just before *12 months of age* when babies delight in books demonstrating early pretend play. Pretending

Table 8–4. Ages and Stages of Emergent Literacy

Prereading/ emerging Literacy Birth–6 years	Age-appropriate behavior: evidence-based expectations and norms
	Birth–2 years • Learns to listen and begins to speak • Enjoys word play and being read with by an adult
	2–4 years • Continues to learn to listen and speak • Enjoys word play and being read with by an adult • Names some items in books • Enjoys and responds to Language Experience Books • Enjoys rhyming games • Exhibits book handling skills • Identifies some logos and symbols encountered in daily life • Enjoys scribbling

	4–6 years
	 • Continues to learn to listen and speak
	 • Demonstrates knowledge of basic concepts about print
	 • Enjoys word play and being read with by an adult
	 • Enjoys and responds to Language Experience Books
	 • Enjoys retelling simple stories
	 • Draws lines and shapes
	 • By the end of this stage, the child
	    ◦ knows and uses the structures of his/her spoken language;
	    ◦ converses in complete sentences;
	    ◦ comprehends, remembers, and formulates stories;
	    ◦ interacts with some printed words;
	    ◦ pretends to read and write;
	    ◦ understands thousands of spoken words, but can read only a few of them
	    ◦ has established a beginning level of phonemic awareness

Note. The goal at the end of this stage is that the child is prepared linguistically and experientially to enter school where formal literacy instruction will begin.

to feed dollies and other people in sequenced steps and taking turns with adults, come at about *18 months*. At just about 2 years of age, play develops rapidly to include more complex actions. Although still playing parallel, children start to transition from playing with large objects to small world–play figures and props at that time. Role-play with themes is established by *36 months,* and role-play that includes peers, imaginary friends, and negotiation is seen at about *42 months of age.* Fantasy play and using voices in play to reflect the drama of life develops around *42 to 48 months,* and by *54 months of age,* play typically takes the form of creative narrative and story structures with peers. Table 8–5 summarizes the ages and stages of play.

Play and the Child With Hearing Loss

Research on children with hearing loss and the effects of play are limited to studies in the 20th century, where findings were relatively consistent (Blum, Fields, Scharfman, & Silber, 1994; Higgingbotham & Baker, 1981; Kretschemer, 1972; Schirmer, 1989). Specifically, there were documented delays of several months at various stages (pretend play, problem-solving activities, cooperative play, dramatic play, imaginary play, symbolic play) in children with hearing loss as compared to children with typical hearing. By the time the latter enjoyed a range of dramatic play schemas and played in cooperation with peers, children with hearing loss still preferred solitary, constructive activities.

Links were found between degrees of hearing loss, age at amplification, and the associated level of social play (Gross, 1982). Spencer and Deyo (1993), however, concluded that it is not hearing loss that is associated with delays in pretend play, but rather the accompanying language delay. Children may be stuck in a repetitive play loop that does not move to a higher level of play because those children lack the language to incorporate more pretend ideas into their play (Gross, 1982). *Children with hearing loss may not*

know the sequence or potential of a toy, because they lack world knowledge; they have not overheard the social conversations of children who are playing around them (Brown, 1999). The challenges in social interaction due to auditory deprivation (auditory information not reaching their brain) may cause children with hearing loss to disengage from cooperative and dramatic play, and consequently make significantly fewer verbal initiations than those with typical hearing (Weisel, Most, & Efron, 2004).

Strategies for Facilitating Play Development

Parents often report that it is difficult to know how to play with their child when there is a mismatch between his or her language and play abilities. For example, if a child's language is only at a single-word level, it is tempting to work with single-object naming. However, reducing linguistic complexity does not cognitively stimulate a 2-year-old the way it might a 1-year-old. A 2-year-old child typically lives in the world of pretend play, and the parent needs skills in creating opportunities for the child to think and play at a level that matches the child's cognitive abilities, and even slightly beyond (Vygotsky, 1978). In AVT, the AV practitioner knows when he or she is *in the child's zone* because the child wants to play.

The AV practitioner coaches parents to "push in," to enhance their child's play within the zone of proximal development, even in the face of delayed play (Vygotsky, 1978). The play must be purposeful, and the reward for play needs to be intrinsic so that the child thinks and remains motivated and

Table 8-5. Ages and Stages of Play

0–6 months	• Reflexively imitate adult facial expressions (e.g., sticks out tongue) from birth (Meltzoff, 2007; Nadel et al., 1999) • Gaze intently at mother's face (Trevarthan, 1979) • Prefer to look at human faces over other stimuli at 3 months (Rosser, 1994) • Reach out for toys and grasp them by 4–6 months (Sheridan, 2006)
6–9 months	• Development of cause and effect—shake a rattle deliberately make a sound (Sheridan, 2006) • Explore objects by touching, stroking, and patting them (Meggit, 2012) • Search for a partially hidden object (Sheridan, 2006) • Explore toys through mouthing (Sheridan, 2006)
9–12 months	• Object permanence has developed—loves peekaboo games (Adamson et al., 1996; Sheridan, 2006) • Development of early play schemas—takes objects in and out of containers, opens and closes doors (Sheridan, 2006) • Early pretend play when acting on a book to pretend to feed/wipe the baby in the photographs from 10 months • Relates objects to one another—puts a spoon in a bowl, keys in the door (Sheridan, 2006) • Does actions in simple play routines, e.g., waving bye bye, pat a cake (Sheridan, 2006)
12–18 months	• Real objects are used according to their function, e.g., Sweeping the floor. (Brown, 1999; Sheridan, 2006) • Acts on self (e.g., pretending to drink) (Adamson, 1996; Watson et al., 1977) • De-centred (15 months); begin to pretend on others (Sheridan, 2006). • Early pretend play on objects (once they already pretend on people), e.g., feeding dolly, putting teddy to sleep (Adamson 1996) • Begin to take turns with adults in (Brown, 1999) • Play becomes more sequenced with three steps around 12–15 months (Lowe & Costello, 1976)
18–24 months	• Object transformation—Substitute objects in pretend play—instead of needing a toy car, a brick can be used to represent a gas station, etc. (Belsky et al., 1981; Casby, 2003) • Actions on dolls and other people become increasingly sequenced—pours water into a cup, gives baby a drink, wipes its mouth (Casby, 2003) • Sequences become less linear—the same doll has a number of actions before moving to the next (Brown, 1999) • Transition from larger objects to small-world play figures • Play in parallel alongside other children but not with them (Sheridan, 2006)

Table 8–5. *continued*

24–30 months	• Pretend to be another agent, e.g., doll or teddy—speaking and acting for them (Casby, 2003; Sheridan, 2006) • Act out short sequences of familiar everyday activities, e.g., shops (Sheridan, 2006) • Ask for multiple repetitions of favorite stories (Trelease, 2013)
30–36 months	• Role-play less familiar themes, e.g., going to the doctor (Sheridan, 2006) • Use words to describe pretend worlds or scenarios, e.g., "The monster in the corner is eating all the food!" (Saarni, 1999) • Talk through toys—toys have increasing personalities or characters (Brown, 1999) • Play sequence follows a logical order (Brown, 1999)
36–42 months	• Take on themes beyond own personal experience, e.g., being a fireman (Sheridan, 2006) • Play cooperatively with other children (Ginsburg, 2007) • Negotiates roles—"you be . . . I'll be . . . " (Garvey, 1984) • May have an imaginary friend who could persist until age 7 (Taylor et al., 2004)
42–48 months	• Fantasy role-play—pretend to be knights, pirates, or fairy tale characters (Sheridan, 2006) • Dresses up in imaginative play (Sheridan, 2006) • Use voices for the characters to reflect age, gender, or characteristics (Garvey, 1984) • Plan cooperatively with other children, using language (Ginsburg, 2007)
48–54 months	• Create miniature worlds with their toys, rich in narrative and story structure (Sheridan, 2006) • Share miniature worlds cooperatively with other children (Sheridan, 2006) • Spontaneously take turns and share with peers (Rivera, Girolametto, Greenberg & Weitzman, 2005) • Negotiate to resolve arguments (Saarni, 1999)
54–60 months	• Increased use of emotion-based language and schemas in play (Saarni, 1999) • Reliably judge "fact" versus "fiction" (Woolley & Cox, 2006) • Plays complex board games needing literacy/number skills (Ramani et al., 2008)

attentive, while still achieving short-term objectives.

Active engagement of the parents is essential because *"children should be taught to play as intentionality and systematically as you would teach literacy or math"* (Leong & Bodrova, 2012). Research has found that active and intentional parental behaviors such as turn taking, modeling, verbal suggestions, contingent commentary (Brown, 1999), and explicit teaching (Leong & Bodrova, 2012) rather than passive observation, have a significant positive effect on play development.

In AVT, children often learn through parental modeling about the specific schemas for play scenarios (e.g., going shopping, going to the library, going on holiday). When the child becomes a *more experienced player*, he or she eventually generates his or her own schemas and scenarios, and subsequently develops higher levels of listening, language, and learning.

THEORY OF MIND

The term *Theory of Mind* (ToM) first coined by Premack and Woodruff in 1978 is defined as "the ability to attribute mental states—beliefs, intents, desires, pretending, knowledge, etc.—to oneself and others and to understand that others have beliefs, desires and intentions that are different from one's own." ToM allows us to perceive and interpret the thoughts and feelings of others (Peterson & Wellman, 2009). Language is fundamental to the development of ToM (Astington & Jenkins, 1999). As children's language abilities develop, they are able to take part in increas-

ingly long conversations, giving them further insight into the mental states of others and allowing them to acquire a wider range of mental state verbs such as "imagine," "dream," "hope," and "pretend," and also to understand more about how others think and feel (Remmel & Peters, 2008).

Ages and Stages of ToM Development

The development of ToM begins in infancy. By *4 months of age,* infants can not only smile to evoke a response from an adult, but can also indicate needs and emotions by their facial expressions. Joint attention develops between *6 and 9 months*, with a declarative point established around a child's first birthday. Children develop a need for autonomy, and can express emotions such as frustration and anxiety between *12 and 18 months* when they start to attribute mental states to others based on what they observe around them. The expression of emotion to do with self-consciousness happens shortly before a child's second birthday, and he or she starts using the word "want" to describe his or her own desires between *18 and 24 months.* Early mental state words to do with feelings and likes and dislikes develop between *24 and 30 months,* and a wide range of these terms are understood and used by the time a child is *36 months* old. Mental state words enable the child to understand behavior and consequences because about this time, he or she can discriminate between more complex terms such as "know" and "think." This leads the child to explain his or her reasoning using the word "because" by the time they are *42 months.* By 48 months, the child uses mental state verbs to explain the actions and emotions of themselves and others. At this time, they also understand and pass the *false belief testing* that underpins ToM knowledge. Table 8–6 summarizes the ages and stages of ToM development.

False Belief

False belief is defined as recognizing that others can have beliefs about the world that are wrong. To do this, a child needs to understand how knowledge is formed, and that one's beliefs are based on knowledge—what one knows. The milestone false belief tasks have led to well-established evidence that ToM cannot be fully attributed until *4 to 5 years of age* in children with typical hearing (Astington & Gopnik, 1991; Gopnik & Wellman, 1994).

ToM and Children With Hearing Loss

Children with a hearing loss have been found to have significantly delayed ToM compared to children with typical hearing (Hoffmeister, De Villiers, De Villiers, & Schick, 2007; Peterson & Siegal, 1999; Russell et al., 1998), even when the linguistic demands of the false belief tests are adjusted, indicating that the reduced access to language, rather than demands of the task are correlated to reduced ToM development (Figueras-Costa & Harris, 2001). There is a paucity of research on the ToM of children with a hearing loss with reference to their language outcomes, although more recent studies suggest that increased auditory

brain access may mean children with cochlear implants can achieve the same levels of ToM understanding as their hearing peers (Remmel et al., 2009).

ToM develops along an orderly, developmental sequence in children with typical hearing (Wellman & Liu, 2004). Executive functioning, language competence, learning through social-interactive experiences, and increased exposure to mental state vocabulary are all important underpinnings for the developing sequence of ToM. These ToM attributes underlie a child's ability to make and keep friends (De Villiers, 2005; Peters, Remmel, & Richard, 2009; Peterson & Siegal, 2009; Scholl & Leslie, 2001). Poor acoustic input of auditory information to the brain of a child with a hearing loss causes a language delay that has been attributed to the late onset of ToM (Milligan, Astington, & Dack, 2007). That is, a child with a hearing loss has reduced opportunities to overhear the conversation and social-interactive experiences of others in their environment (Moeller & Schick, 2006), and so misses out on many opportunities to learn how others are expressing their feelings.

Strategies for Developing ToM Skills

As AV practitioners, we know that standardized assessments only provide a snapshot of a child's overall language ability. Age-appropriate language scores do not necessarily mean the child has all the social-cognitive and verbal reasoning skills necessary to make friends and cope in the classroom (Peters et al., 2009). Specific attention to and work on ToM skills is essential to ensure that

Table 8-6. Ages and Stages of ToM Development

0–6 months	• Imitates facial expressions (Meltzoff, 2005) • Indicates interest (sustained attention) versus disgust (facial expressions), sadness and anger by 4 months (Carr, 2006) • Smiles to evoke smile response at 4 weeks (Meltzoff, 2005) • Develops skills for regulating attention so caregivers can soothe them (Melzoff, 2005)
6–9 months	• Follows an adult's gaze to an object (Senju & Csibra, 2008) • Looks longer at face looking at him (Farroni, Massaccesi, Menon, & Johnson, 2007) • Develops joint attention (Gray, Hoise, Russell, & Ormel, 2001)
9–12 months	• Attends to the emotional expressions of caretakers and begin to replicate to express emotion (Feinman, 1992) • Develops declarative pointing—point with index finger to direct attention to shared object • Indicates fear when separated from an adult (Meltzoff, 2005)
12–18 months	• Develops sustained imperative point—point with index finger to ask for something (Callaghan et al., 2011) • Attributes mental states to others based on visual information (Senju, Southgate, Snape, Leonard, & Csibra, 2011) • Recognizes mother is leaving and reacts sharply with separation anxiety (Diessel & Tomasello, 2001) • Becomes increasingly frustrated when parents place limits on need for autonomy (Saarni, 1999)
18–24 months	• Uses "want" to describe own desires (Lahey, 1988) • Understands what others intend to do (Meltzoff, 1999) • Expresses emotions involving self-consciousness—shame, pride, or coyness (Senju et al., 2011)
24–30 months	• Talks about likes and dislikes (Babu, 2009) • Talks about early feelings using mental state vocabulary, e.g., happy, scared, sad (Meltzoff, 1999) • Begins to use language to regulate their emotions through internal speech and conversations with others (Senju et al., 2011)
30–36 months	• Uses wider range of mental state terms (Shatz, Wellman, & Silber, 1983) • Refers to past events that were personally experienced with increasing length (Miller & Sperry, 1988) • Has increasing emotions involving self-consciousness, e.g., embarrassment (Meltzoff, 2005) • Discriminates between certainty "know" and uncertainty "think" (Diessel & Tomasello, 2001)

Table 8-6. *continued*

36–42 months	• Takes on roles beyond own experience in play (Sheridan, 2006) • Uses "because" to explain reasoning (Lahey, 1988) • Explains why others may experience an emotion (Saarni et al., 2007)
42–48 months	• Imitates a wide variety of roles and perspectives • Uses mental state verbs such as "think," "know," "remember" (to explain the emotions and actions of others) (Babu, 2009) • Passes "false belief" tasks at age 4 years (Baron-Cohen, 1999; Peterson, Wellman, & Liu, 2005)
48–54 months	• Develops sense of humor—understands irony (Recchia, How, Ross, & Alexander, 2010) • Uses some modal auxiliaries, e.g., "Shouldn't," "can't" (Papafragou, 1998) • Tailors the amount of information they give to their perception of the listener's knowledge (Saylor, Baird, & Gallerani, 2006)
54–60 months	• Imitates the social behavior of others considered "cool" (Meltzoff et al., 2007) • Presents "cool" emotional front to peers (Senju et al., 2011) • Becomes increasingly concerned with equality and fairness (Meltzoff, 2005)

the child whose family has chosen AVT will thrive in school. This work can help the child access the emotion-based language and conceptual thoughts that will help develop a good ToM, and make and keep friends.

We see from the literature that social interaction with familiar peers and siblings, social play, and exposure to mental state language are key factors in the development of ToM (Moore, Bosacki, & Macgillivray, 2011; Taumoepeau & Ruffman, 2006, 2008; Taylor & Carlson, 1997). By using play throughout AV sessions, practitioners can help parents understand ToM by coaching them to scaffold the play (see Chapter 11) between them and the child, and between the child and his familiar peers or siblings. Showing the child how to take part in sociodramatic play helps him or her learn how to appreciate how other people feel, how to share in pretend ideas, how to guess, how to make predictions, and how to negotiate roles to include everyone (see Table 8–6) (Brendsen, 2005; Schwebel, Rosen, & Singer, 1999). Through play, the child also learns how to discuss and respond to other's emotions by congratulating, encouraging, comforting, and commiserating in a way that will help make and keep friends. Pretend play with others also increases use of mental state language.

AV practitioners can demonstrate how to be explicit (Brendsen, 2005) in the use of emotion and mental state language when giving children reasons for actions of others. The practitioner can coach parents to read books to provide explanation of a character's thoughts and feelings (Slaughter, Peterson, & Mackintosh, 2007), and use the child as a referent when talking about thoughts and feelings (Gola-Howard, 2012) (e.g., "You feel upset when you have to come in and tidy up. Maybe you can tell me, I feel upset when you say come in!").

In more recent studies, there appears to be a relationship between ToM development and the timing and use of mental state language, even when talking with a baby (Moore et al., 2011; Taumoepeau & Ruffman, 2006, 2008). Examples are:

- reading the baby's *thought bubble* and attaching emotional intent to it at 6 months of age: "You're excited to see Daddy!";
- talking about desires (not thoughts and feelings) around the age of 15 months, "I can see you really want that biscuit!"; and
- talking about people's thoughts and feelings by the time their child is around 2 years of age, "Harry's cross because you took his toy!"

Therefore, there is a need for ToM intervention, through parent coaching, right from the start. The practitioner is encouraged to scaffold ToM development in AV sessions by providing parents with a systematic framework of how to introduce and use mental state vocabulary in their everyday conversations and play with their baby/child.

REFERENCES

Adamson, L. B. (1996). *Communication development during infancy.* Madison, WI: Brown & Benchmark.

Ambrose, S. E., Walker, E. A., Unflat-Berry, L. M., Oleson, J. J., & Moeller, M. P. (2015). Quantity and quality of caregivers' linguistic input to 18-month and 3-year-old children who are hard of hearing. *Ear and Hearing, 36*(Suppl. 1), S48–S59.

American Speech-Language-Hearing Association (ASHA). (n.d). *Childhood apraxia of speech.* Retrieved from http://www.asha.org/public/speech/disorders/ChildhoodApraxia/

American Speech-Language-Hearing Association (ASHA). (n.d). *Dysarthria.* Retrieved from http://www.asha.org/public/speech/disorders/dysarthria/

American Speech-Language-Hearing Association (ASHA). (n.d). *What is language? What is speech?* Retrieved from http://www.asha.org/public/speech/development/language_speech/

Astington, J. W., & Gopnik, A. (1991). Theoretical explanations of children's understanding of the mind. In G. E. Butterworth, P. L. Harris, A. M. Leslie, & H. M. Wellman (Eds.), *Perspectives on the child's theory of mind* (pp. 7–31). New York, NY: Oxford University Press.

Astington, J. W., & Jenkins, J. M. (1999). A longitudinal study of the relation between language and theory-of-mind development. *Developmental Psychology, 35,* 1311–1320.

Babu, N. (2009). *Development of theory of mind and mental state language in children.* New Delhi, India: Concept.

Baron-Cohen, S. (1999). Evolution of a theory of mind. In M. Corballis, & S. Lea (Eds.), *The descent of mind: Psychological perspectives on hominid evolution.* New York, NY: Oxford University Press.

Bennett, D. L. (2012). *Understanding the stages of baby babble.* Retrieved November 2, 2015, from http://www.sentinel source.com/parent_express/pregnancy_ babies/understanding-the-stages-of-baby-babble/article_611d18f4-a11d-11 e1-8120-0019bb2963f4.html

Blood, A. J., & Zatorre, R. J. (2001). Intensely pleasurable responses to music correlate with activity in brain regions implicated in reward and emotion. *Proceedings of the National Academy of Sciences, 98*(20), 11818–11823.

Blum, Fields, Scharfman, & Silber. (1994). Development of symbolic play in deaf children aged 1 to 3. In *Children at play.* New York, NY: Oxford University Press.

Bowen, C. (1998). *Developmental phonological disorders. A practical guide for families and teachers.* Melbourne, Australia: ACER Press.

Boysson-Bardies, B. (1999). *How language comes to children: From birth to two years.* Boston, MA: MIT.

Boysson-Bardies, B. D., & Vihman, M. M. (1991). Adaptation to language: Evidence from babbling and first words in four languages. *Language, 67,* 297–319.

Brendsen, M. (2005). Theory of mind: Implication for intervention. Retrieved September 15, 2007, from http://www .speechpathology.com/articles/article_ detail.asp?article_id=249 cited in Peters, K., Remmel, E., & Richard, D. (2009). Language, mental state vocabulary and false belief understanding in children with cochlear implants. *Language, Speech and Hearing Services in School, 40,* 245–255.

Brown, M. (1999). Early development in deaf and hard of hearing children: The state of play. *Australian Journal of Education of the Deaf, 5,* 27–36.

Callaghan, T., Moll, H., Rakoczy, H., Behne, T., Liszkowski, U., & Tomasello, M. (2011). Early social cognition in three cultural contexts. *Monographs of the Society for Research in Child Development, 76*(2), 1–142.

Carr, A. (2006). *The handbook of child and adolescent clinical psychology. A contex-*
tual approach (2nd ed.). London, UK: Routledge.

Casby, M. (2003). Developmental assessment of play: A model for early intervention. *Communication Disorders Quarterly, 24,* 175.

Clay, M. (2000). *Concepts about print: What have children learned about the way we print language?* Portsmouth, NH: Heinemann.

Coez, A., Zilbovicius, M., Ferrary, E., Bouccara, D., Mosnier, I., Bozorg-Grayeli, A., . . . Sterkers, O. (2011). A neuro-imaging approach to evidencing bilateral cochlear implant advantages in auditory perception. *Cochlear Implants International, 12*(Suppl. 1), S124–126.

De Villiers, J. G. (2005). Can language acquisition give children a point of view? In J. W. Astinton & J. Baird (Eds.), *Why language matters for theory of mind* (pp. 186–219). New York, NY: Oxford University Press.

Diessel, J., & Tomasello, M. (2001). The acquisition of finite complement clauses in English: A corpus based analysis. *Cognitive Linguistics, 12,* 97–141.

Eggermont, J. J., & Moore, J. K. (2012). Morphological and functional development of the auditory nervous system. In *Human auditory development* (pp. 61–105). New York, NY: Springer.

Estabrooks, W. (Ed.). (2006). *Auditory-verbal therapy and practice.* Washington, DC: A.G. Bell

Farroni, T., Massaccesi, S., Menon, E., & Johnson, M. H. (2007). Direct gaze modulates face recognition in young infants. *Cognition, 102*(3), 396–404.

Feinman, S. (1992). *Social referencing and the social construction of reality in infancy.* New York, NY: Plenum.

Ferguson, B., & Waxman, S. R. (2014). Communication and categorization: New insights into the relation between speech, labels, and concepts for infants. In M. Knauff, M. Pauen, N. Sebanz, & I. Wachsmuth (Eds.), *Proceedings of the 35th*

Annual Conference of the Cognitive Science Society (pp. 2267–2272). Austin, TX: Cognitive Science Society.

Figueras-Costa, B., & Harris, P. (2001). Theory of mind development in deaf children: A nonverbal test of false-belief understanding. *Journal of Deaf Studies and Deaf Education, 6,* 92–102.

Fletcher, S. G. (1973). Maturation of the speech mechanism. *Folia Phoniatrica, 25,* 161–172.

Galinsky, E. (2010). *Mind in the making: The seven essential life skills every child needs.* New York, NY: HarperCollins.

Glennen, S., & Masters, M. G. (2002). Typical and atypical language development in infants and toddlers adopted from Eastern Europe. *American Journal of Speech-Language Pathology, 11,* 417–433.

Gola-Howard, A. A. (2012). Mental verb input for promoting children's Theory of Mind: A training study. *Cognitive Development, 27*(1), P64–76.

Goldman, R. *GFTA-2: Goldman-Fristoe 2 Test of Articulation* (2nd ed.). Circle Pines, MN: American Guidance Service.

Goldstein, M. H., & Schwade, J. A. (2008). Social feedback to infants' babbling facilitates rapid phonological learning. *Psychological Science, 19*(5), 515–523.

Gomes, H., Molholm, S., Christodoulou, C., Ritter, W., & Cowan, N. (2000). The development of auditory attention in children. *Frontiers in Bioscience, 5,* 108–120.

Gopnik, A., Meltzoff, A., & Kuhl. P. (1999). *The scientist in the crib: Minds, brains, and how children learn.* New York, NY: William Morrow.

Gopnik, A., & Wellman, H. M. (1994). The theory theory. In L. A. Hirschfeld & S. A. Gelman (Eds.), *Mapping of the mind* (pp. 257–293). Cambridge, UK: Cambridge University Press.

Grahn, J. A., & Brett, M. (2007). Rhythm and beat perception in motor areas of the brain. *Journal of Cognitive Neuroscience, 19*(5), 893–906.

Gray, C. D., Hoise, J. A., Russell, P. A., & Ormel, E. A. (2001). Emotional development in deaf children: Facial expressions, display rules, and theory of mind. In M. D. Clark, M. Marshack, & M. Karchmer (Eds.), *Context, cognition, and deafness* (pp. 135–160). Washington, DC: Gallaudet University Press

Green, J. R., Moore, C. A., Higashikawa, M., & Steeve, R. W. (2000). The physiologic development of speech motor control: Lip and jaw coordination. *Journal of Speech, Language, and Hearing Research, 43,* 239–255.

Green, J. R., Moore, C. A., & Reilly, K. J. (2002). The sequential development of jaw and lip control for speech. *Journal of Speech, Language, and Hearing Research, 45,* 66–79.

Greenberg, J., & Weitzman, E. (2005). *Fostering peer interaction in early childhood settings.* Ontario, Canada: Hanen Early Language Programme.

Gross, H. (1982). *Language and play in the deaf nursery school.* Paper presented at the British Psychological Society Developmental Conference, 17–20 September. Cited in Brown, M. (1999). Early development in deaf and hard of hearing children: The state of play. *Australian Journal of Education of the Deaf, 5,* 27–36.

Grunwell, P. (1997). Natural phonology. In M. Ball & R. Kent (Eds.), *The new phonologies: developments in clinical linguistics.* San Diego, CA: Singular.

Heugten, M. V., & Johnson, E. K. (2012). Infants exposed to fluent natural speech succeed at cross-gender word recognition. *Journal of Speech Language and Hearing Research, 55*(2), 554.

Higgingbothham, D. J., & Baker, B. M. (1981). Social participation and cognitive play differences in hearing impaired and normally hearing pre-schoolers. *The Volta Review, 83,* 135–149. Cited in Brown, M. (1999). Early development in deaf and hard of hearing children: The state of play. *Australian Journal of Education of the Deaf, 5,* 27–36.

Hoffmeister, R., De Villiers, J., De Villiers, P., & Schick, B. (2007). Language and theory of mind: A study of deaf children, *Child Development, 78,* 376–396.

Janata, P. (2009). The neural architecture of music-evoked autobiographical memories. *Cerebral Cortex, 19*(11), 2579–2594.

Kahane, J. C. (1988). Anatomy and physiology of the organism of the peripheral speech mechanism. In M. H. Lass, L. V. McReynolds, J. L. Northern, & D. E. Yoder (Eds.), *Handbook of speech-language pathology and audiology* (pp. 2–51). Philadelphia, PA: B.C. Decker.

Keller, T. A., & Cowan, N. (1994). Developmental increase in the duration of memory for tone pitch. *Developmental Psychology, 30*(6), 855.

Koelsch, S., & Siebel, W. A. (2005). Towards a neural basis of music perception. *Trends in Cognitive Sciences, 9*(12), 578–584.

Kretschemer, R. R. (1972). A study to assess the play activities and gesture output of hearing handicapped preschool children. Bureau of Education for the Handicapped. Washington, DC. Cited in Brown, M. (1999). Early development in deaf and hard of hearing children: The state of play. *Australian Journal of Education of the Deaf, 5,* 27–36.

Lahey, M. (1988). *Language disorders and language development* (pp. 186–187). New York, NY: Macmillan.

Leibold, L. J. (2012). Development of auditory scene analysis and auditory attention. In *Human auditory development* (pp. 137 161). New York, NY: Springer.

Leong, D. J., & Bodrova, E. (2012). Assessing and scaffolding: Make believe play. In Spotlight on young children—exploring play. *NAEYC.*

Ling, D. (1989). *Foundations of spoken language for hearing-impaired children.* Washington, DC: A.G. Bell

Local, J. (1980). Modeling intonational variability in children's speech. In S. Romaine (Ed.), *Sociolinguistic variation in speech communication* (pp. 85–103). London, UK: Edward Arnold.

Lowe, M., & Costello, A. (1976). Symbolic Play Test *(SPT).* NFER Nelson.

Madigan, S., Wade, M., Plamondon, A., Browne, D., & Jenkins, J. M. (2015). Birth weight variability and language development: Risk, resilience, and responsive parenting. *Journal of Pediatric Psychology, 40,* 869–877.

Maneva, B., & Genesee, F. (2002). Bilingual babbling: Evidence for language differentiation in dual language acquisition. *Proceedings of the Annual Boston University Conference on Language Development, 26,* 383–392.

Mampe, B., Friederici, A. D., Christophe, A., & Wermke, K. (2009). Newborns' cry melody is shaped by their native language. *Current Biology, 19*(23), 1994-1997.

McGee, L. & Richgels, D. (2012). *Literacy's beginnings: Supporting young readers and writers* (6th ed.). Boston, MA: Pearson Education.

McIntosh, B., & Dodd, B. J. (2008). Two-year-olds' phonological acquisition: Normative data. *International Journal of Speech-Language Pathology, 10*(6), 460–469.

McMurray, B., Kovack-Lesh, K. A., Goodwin, D., & Mcechron, W. (2013). Infant directed speech and the development of speech perception: Enhancing development or an unintended consequence? *Cognition, 129*(2), 362–378.

Meggit, C. (2012). *Children's development, an illustrated guide, birth to 19 years.* London, UK: Pearson.

Meltzoff, A. N. (1999). Origins of theory of mind, cognition, and communication. *Journal of Communication Disorders, 32,* 251–269.

Meltzoff, A. N. (2005). Imitation and other minds: The "Like Me" hypothesis. In S. Hurley & N. Chater (Eds.), *Perspective on imitation: From neuroscience to social science* (Vol. 2, pp. 55–77). Cambridge, MA: MIT Press.

Meltzoff, A. N. (2007). 'Like me': A foundation for social cognition. *Developmental Science, 10*(1), 126–134.

Miller, P. J., & Sperry, L. (1988). Early talk about the past: The origins of conversational stories of personal experience. *Journal of Child Language, 15,* 293–315.

Milligan, K., Astington, J. W., & Dack, L. A. (2007). Language and theory of mind. Meta-analysis of the relation between language ability and false-belief understanding. *Child Development, 78,* 622–646.

Moore, C., Bosacki, S. L., & Macgillivray, S. (2011). Theory of mind and social interest in zero-acquaintance play situations. *Child Development, 82*(4), 1163–1172.

Nadel, J., Guérini, C., Pezé, A., & Rivet, C., (1999). The evolving nature of imitation as a format for communication. In J. Nadel & G. Butterworth (Eds.), *Imitation in infancy. Cambridge studies in cognitive perceptual development* (pp. 209–234). New York, NY: Cambridge University Press.

National Council of Teachers of English. (2013). *The NCTE Definition of 21st Century Literacies.* Retrieved from http://www.ncte.org/positions/statements/21stcentdefinition

Newton, C., & Wells, B. (2002). Between-word junctures in early multi-word speech. *Journal of Child Language, 29*(2), 275–299.

Oller, D. K. (2000). *The emergence of the speech capacity.* Mahwah, NJ: Lawrence Erlbaum.

Olsho, L. W., Koch, E. G., & Carter, E. A. (1988). Nonsensory factors in infant frequency discrimination. *Infant Behavior and Development. 11,* 205–222.

Owens, R. E. (2005). *Language development: An introduction* (6th ed.). New York, NY: Pearson.

Papafragou, A. (1998). The acquisition of modality: Implications for theories of semantic representation. *Mind and Language, 13,* 370–399.

Peters, K., Remmel, E., & Richard, D. (2009). Language, mental state vocabulary and false belief understanding in children with cochlear implants. *Language, Speech, and Hearing Services in School, 40,* 245–255.

Peterson, C. C., & Siegal, M. (2006). Deafness, conservation and theory of mind. *Journal of Child Psychology and Psychiatry, 36,* 459–474.

Peterson, C. C., & Wellman, H. M. (2009). From fancy to reason: Scaling deaf and hearing children's understanding of theory of mind and pretence. *British Journal of Developmental Psychology, 27,* 297–310.

Peterson, C. C., Wellman, H. M., & Liu, D. (2005). Steps in theory-of-mind development for children with deafness or autism. *Child Development, 76,* 502–517.

Piaget, J. (1977). *Insights and illusions of philosophy.* New York, NY: Routledge.

Pierce, L. J., Klein, D., Chen, J-K., Dekenserie, A., & Genesee, F. (2014). Mapping the unconscious maintenance of a lost first language. *Proceedings of the National Academy of Sciences, 111*(48), 17314–17319.

Pinker, S. (2007). *The stuff of thought: Language as a window into human nature.* New York, NY: Viking.

Plantinga, J., & Trainor, L. J. (2009). Melody recognition by two-month-old infants. *Journal of the Acoustical Society of America., 125*(2).

Premack, D. G., & Woodruff, G. (1978). Does the chimpanzee have a theory of mind? *Behavioral and Brain Sciences, 1,* 515–526.

Rance, G., Cone-Wesson, B., Wunderlich, J., & Dowell, R. (2002). Speech perception and cortical event related potentials in children with auditory neuropathy. *Ear and Hearing, 23*(3), 239–253.

Reading is fundamental. (n.d.). *Literacy milestones from birth to age six.* Retrieved from http://www.rif.org/us/literacy-resources/articles/literacy-milestones-from-birth-to-age-six.htm

Reading rockets. (n.d.). *The stages of reading development.* Retrieved from http://www.readingrockets.org/article/stages-reading-development

Recchia, H. E., How, N., Ross, H. S., & Alexander, S. (2010). Children's understanding and production of verbal irony in family conversations. *British Journal of Developmental Psychology, 28*(2), 255–274.

Remmel, E., & Peters, K. (2008). Theory of mind and language in children with cochlear implants. *Journal of Deaf Studies and Deaf Education, 14*(2), 218–236.

Remmel, E., & Peters, K. (2009). Theory of mind and language in children with cochlear implants. *Journal of Deaf Studies. Deaf Education, 14*(2), 218–236.

Rivera, C. D., Girolametto, L., Greenberg, J., & Weitzman, E. (2005). Children's responses to educators' questions in day care play groups. *American Journal of Speech-Language Pathology, 14*(1), 14.

Robertson, L. (2014). *Literacy and deafness: Listening and spoken language* (2nd ed.). San Diego, CA: Plural.

Rosser, R. (1994). *Cognitive development: Psychological and biological perspectives.* Boston, MA: Allyn & Bacon.

Russell, P. A., Hosie, J. A., Gray, C. D., Scott, C., Hunter, N., Banks, J. S., & Macaulay, M. C. (1998). The development of theory of mind in deaf children. *Journal of Child Psychology and Psychiatry and Allied Disciplines, 39*, 903–910.

Saarni, C. (1999). *Developing emotional competence.* New York, NY: Guilford.

Saarni, C., Campos, J. J., Camras, L. A., & Witherington, D. (2007). Emotional development: Action, communication, and understanding. *Handbook of Child Psychology, III*, 5.

Sanes, D. H., & Woolley, S. M. (2011). A behavioral framework to guide research on central auditory development and plasticity. *Neuron, 72*(6), 912–929.

Saylor, M. M., Baird, J. A., & Gallerani, C. (2006). Telling others what's new: Preschoolers adherence to the given-new contract. *Journal of Cognition and Development, 7*(3), 341–379.

Schirmer, B. R. (1989). Relationship between imaginative play and language development in hearing impaired children. *American Annals of the Deaf, 134*(3), 219–222. Cited in Brown, M. (1999). Early development in deaf and hard of hearing children: The state of play. *Australian Journal of Education of the Deaf, 5*, 27–36.

Scholl, B. J., & Leslie, A. M. (2001). Minds, modules and meta-analysis. *Child Development, 72*, 696–701. Cited in Peterson, C. C., & Wellman, H. M. (2009). From fancy to reason: Scaling deaf and hearing children's understanding of theory of mind and pretence. *British Journal of Developmental Psychology, 27*, 297–310.

Schwebel, D., Rosen, C., & Singer, J. (1999). Pre-schooler's pretend play and theory of mind, *British Journal of Developmental Psychology, 17*, 734–751.

Seidl, A., & Johnson, E. K. (2006). Infant word segmentation revisited: Edge alignment facilitates target extraction. *Developmental Science, 9*(6), 565–573.

Senju, A., & Csibra, G. (2008). Gaze following in human infants depends on communicative signals. *Current Biology, 18*(9), 668–671.

Senju, A., Southgate, V., Snape, C., Leonard, M., & Csibra, G. (2011). Do 18 month olds really attribute mental states to others? A critical test. *Psychological Science, 22*(7), 878–880.

Sharma, A., Gilley, P. A., Dorman, M. F., & Baldwin, R. (2007). Deprivation-induced cortical reorganization in children with cochlear implants. *International Journal of Audiology, 46*, 494–499.

Shatz, M., Wellman, H. M., & Silber, S. (1983). The acquisition of mental verbs: A systematic investigation of the first reference to mental state. *Cognition, 14*(3), 301–321.

Sheridan, M. (2006). *From birth to five years: Children's developmental progress.* Oxon, UK: Routledge.

Shultz, S., & Vouloumanos, A. (2010). Three-month-olds prefer speech to other naturally occurring signals. *Language Learning and Development, 6*, 241–257.

Singer, D. G., Golinkoff, R. M., & Hirsch-Pasek, K., (2006). *Play = learning. How play motivates and enhances children's cognitive and social-emotional growth.* New York, NY: Oxford University Press.

Slaughter, V., Peterson, C. C., & Mackintosh, E. (2007). Mind what mother says:

Narrative input and theory of mind in typical children and those on the autism spectrum. *Child Development, 78*(3), 839–858.

Spencer, P. E., & Deyo, D. (1993). Cognitive and social aspects of deaf children's play. In M. Marschark & M. D. Clark (Eds.), *Psychological perspectives on deafness* (pp. 65–92). Hillsdale, NJ: Lawrence Erlbaum. Cited in Brown, M. (1999). Early development in deaf and hard of hearing children: The state of play. *Australian Journal of Education of the Deaf, 5,* 27–36.

Stuart, A. (2005). Development of auditory temporal resolution in school-age children revealed by word recognition in continuous and interrupted noise. *Ear and Hearing, 26*(1), 78–88.

Taumoepeau, M., & Ruffman, T. (2006). Mother and infant talk about mental states relates to desire language and emotion understanding. *Child Development, 77,* 465–481.

Taumoepeau, M., & Ruffman, T. (2008). Stepping stones to others' minds: Maternal talk relates to child mental state language and emotion understanding at 15, 24 and 33 months. *Child Development, 79,* 284–302.

Taverna, A. S., Waxman, S. R., Medin, D. L., Moscoloni, N., & Peralta, O. A. (2014). Naming the living things: Linguistic, experiential and cultural factors in Wichí and Spanish speaking children. *Journal of Cognition and Culture, 14,* 213–233.

Taylor, M., Carlson, S. M., Maring, B. L., & Charlye, C. M. (2004). The characteristics and correlates of fantasy in school-age children: Imaginary companions, impersonation, and social understanding. *Developmental Psychology, 40*(6), 1173–1187.

Teoh, S. W., Pisoni, D. B., & Miyamoto, R. T. (2004). Cochlear implantation in adults with prelingual deafness. Part II. Underlying constraints that affect audiological outcomes. *Laryngoscope, 114*(10), 1714–1719.

Tharpe, A. M., & Ashmead, D. H. (2001). A longitudinal investigation of infant auditory sensitivity. *American Journal of Audiology, 10*(2), 104.

Tomasello. M. (2003). *Constructing a language.* Cambridge, MA: Harvard University Press.

Tomblin, J. B., Harrison, M., Ambrose, S. E., Walker, E. A., Oleson, J. J., & Moeller, M. P., (2015). Language outcomes in young children with mild to severe hearing loss. *Ear and Hearing, 36*(Suppl. 1), S76–S91.

Trelease, J. (2013). *The read-aloud handbook* (7th ed.). New York, NY: Penguin.

Trevarthan, C. (1979). Communication and cooperation in early infancy: A description of primary intersubjectivity. Cited in M. Bullowa (Ed.), *Before speech: The beginning of interpersonal communication* (pp. 321–347). New York, NY: Cambridge University Press.

Vihman, M. M., Depaolis, R. A., & Davis, B. L. (1998). Is there a "trochaic bias" in early word learning? Evidence from infant production in English and French. *Child Development, 69*(4), 935.

Vouloumanos, A., & Werker, J. F. (2007). Listening to language at birth: Evidence for a bias for speech in neonates. *Developmental Science, 10*(2), 159–164.

Vygotsky, L. (1978). *Mind in society. Development of higher psychological processes.* Cambridge, MA: Harvard University Press.

Whalen, D. H., Levitt, A. G., & Wang, Q. (1991). Intonational differences between the reduplicative babbling of French- and English-learning infants. *Journal of Child Language 18*(3), 501.

Weisel, A., Most, T., & Efron, C. (2004). Initiations of social interactions by young hearing impaired pre-schoolers. *Journal of Deaf Studies and Deaf Education, 10*(2), 161–170.

Wellman, H. M. (2009). From fancy to reason: Scaling deaf and hearing children's understanding of theory of mind and pretence. *British Journal of Developmental Psychology, 27,* 297–310.

Wells, B., Peppe, S., & Goulandris, N. (2004). Intonation development from five to thirteen. *Journal of Child Language, 31,* 749–778.

Werner, L. A. (2002). Infant auditory capabilities. *Current Opinion in Otolaryngology and Head and Neck Surgery, 10*(5), 398–402.

Werner, L. A. (2007). Issues in human auditory development. *Journal of Communication Disorders, 40*(4), 275–283.

Werner, L., Fay, R. R., & Popper, A. (Eds.). (2011). *Human auditory development* (Vol. 42). New York, NY: Springer Science and Business Media.

Woolley, J. D., & Cox, V. (2007). Development of beliefs about storybook reality. *Developmental Science, 10*(5), 681–693.

Yang, C. (2006). *The infinite gift: How children learn and unlearn the languages of the world.* New York, NY: Scribner.

9

EMERGENT LITERACY IN CHILDREN WITH HEARING LOSS AND AUDITORY-VERBAL THERAPY

Lyn Robertson and Denise Wray

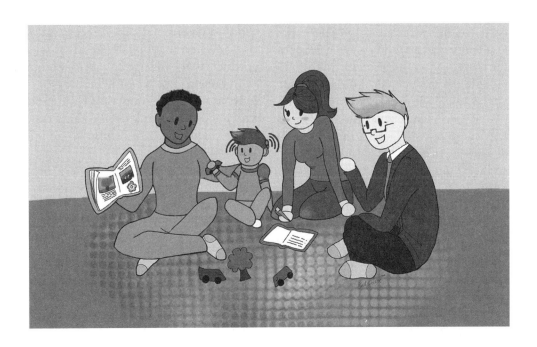

INTRODUCTION

All the goals of Auditory-Verbal Therapy (AVT) are foundational to the development of solid literacy achievement. Had the AV pioneers sought to create a plan that fosters emergent reading and writing skills and the valuing of them, they would not have needed to do anything different. Indeed, if all children, including those with typical hearing, were presented with AV environments, practitioners and teachers would encounter fewer reading and writing problems, as all children thrive in such language-rich settings. The overarching purpose of AVT is to immerse children in so much meaningful listening and conversation that they develop a complete mastery of the language(s) spoken around them as they interact with people in their daily lives. Here at the beginning, though, a caveat is in order: although such spoken language capability is necessary for the development of literacy in an individual, it is not always sufficient; some individuals, with and without hearing loss, experience processing differences that interfere with literacy development despite the presence of a well-developed spoken language base. Likewise, some individuals, with and without hearing loss, have difficulties learning spoken language for reasons unrelated to hearing and listening. These situations are beyond the scope of this book.

COMPREHENSION: THE GOAL OF LITERACY PROCESSES

The most important place to begin when thinking about literacy, hearing, and hearing loss is to specify comprehension as the goal of reading and writing. In general, comprehension takes place because the reader uses his or her array of prior knowledge to construct a logical sense about a passage of text and is able to store that understanding in memory for later use. The flip side of reading for comprehension is the production of writing that makes sense to the writer and to others. To create a spoken utterance or a passage of writing meaningful to another, the child needs to learn to think about what she or he knows and wants to express and what the recipient of the message will recognize and connect with.

Reading and writing, the receptive and expressive processes we cluster under *literacy*, depend on the individual making use of letter, word, and sentence structure knowledge, as well as content knowledge drawn from firsthand and symbolic experiences in the world. Taken together, these processes produce that *click of recognition* one feels during a successful reading episode and that feeling of satisfaction when one has completed a writing task and receives validation from someone who reads it.

Because comprehension is a lifelong task, so is the mastery of literacy (see Chapter 8). Learning to read and write involves far more than learning to look at the print on the page and pronounce it or learning to spell and put words to paper. In the words of the National Council of Teachers of English:

> Becoming a reader is a gradual process that begins with our first interactions with print. As children, there is no fixed point at which we suddenly become readers. Instead, all of us bring our understanding

of spoken language, our knowledge of the world, and our experiences in it to make sense of what we read. We grow in our ability to comprehend and interpret a wide range of reading materials by making appropriate choices from among the extensive repertoire of skills and strategies that develop over time. These strategies include predicting, comprehension monitoring, phonemic awareness, critical thinking, decoding, using context, and making connections to what we already know. (National Council of Teachers of English Statement on Reading, 1999, http://www.ncte.org/positions/statements/position onreading)

Because of this complexity, preparing children with hearing loss to become literate, active adults who are capable of functioning in every part of society has been a daunting task. Over many decades, AVT has enabled many children to become ready for literacy; now, though, we are in a new era of technological advances that make the learning necessary for literacy to emerge more easily available to children with hearing loss.

Brief History of Reading Achievement Among Individuals With Hearing Loss

Studies that have attempted to gauge the academic and literacy levels of children with hearing loss are available from as far back as the beginning of the 20th century (see, for example, Pintner & Paterson, 1916). Having the requisite spoken language maturity figures prominently in the progression of studies of literacy development in students with hearing loss. Individuals who could hear better, individuals who had had spoken language exposure due either to post-lingual hearing loss or to intensive therapy that made use of their residual hearing, and individuals who made use of well-fitted hearing technologies began to emerge in the studies as more successful with reading as measured by standardized tests. As these outcomes were mounting, theorizing about reading pointed increasingly to the relationship between spoken language capability and reading achievement. As well, parents and AV practitioners began reporting that the dire predictions about low levels of reading and academic achievement they had received at the time of their child's diagnosis were not being borne out (Robertson, 2014).

PREREQUISITE KNOWLEDGE NECESSARY FOR LITERACY DEVELOPMENT

Literacy involves complex interactions among the components of spoken language: vocabulary (semantics), phonology (sounds), structure (syntax), word functions (grammar), intonation, conventional ways of speaking and writing (pragmatics and discourse), and sound-to-symbol relationships (graphophonemic knowledge). When a child learns to listen and talk, she or he is also learning to shift attention between short-term (working) memory and long-term memory stores, to recognize sequencing and cause and effect, to make predictions and confirm or disconfirm them, to identify affirmation and negation, to make comparisons and contrasts, and to draw inferences. The growing ability to use all of these aspects of language in listening and talking is critical for literacy acquisition; the reader must be able to do in listening and speaking what is demanded in reading and writing.

Phonological Awareness and Knowledge

During the past two decades, research has revealed a direct connection between insufficient phonological skill, specifically phonemic awareness, and an increased risk of reading difficulties in children with typical hearing (Catts, Fey, Zhang, & Tomblin, 2001; Schuele & Boudreu, 2008; Yopp, 1997). In the United States, the *National Reading Panel* (2000) identified phonemic awareness as a key building block in reading acquisition. Children with phonological awareness sensitivity understand the sound structure of a spoken language and can manipulate this sound structure of spoken words at the syllable, onset-rime, and phoneme levels (Gillon, 2004). Phonological awareness sensitivity enables the child to make the connection between graphemic symbol (letter) and the phonemic (letter sound), thus supporting word decoding skills that help the child connect written symbols with spoken language stored in memory. An awareness of the phoneme as it relates to the spoken sound structure supports reading acquisition and is necessary to discovering the logic of the written system (Yopp, 1999).

> ### Phonological Awareness is Possible for Children with Hearing Loss
>
> Phonological awareness and its finer-grained form, phonemic awareness, require full auditory access to the entire speech spectrum. In the past, this requisite skill underlying literacy development posed major obstacles for children with hearing loss due to the obvious difficulty of accessing adequate speech sound perception. Today, however, the combination of early identification, state-of-the-art hearing technologies, and early AVT intervention has ameliorated the debilitating factors that hearing loss poses, thereby opening the door to age-appropriate listening, talking, reading, writing, and thinking skills that define literacy achievement.

For the child with hearing loss, the absence or instability of phonological knowledge is highly problematic, because so much is conveyed by the sounds in phonemes (the smallest unit of speech), syllables, words, phrases, sentences, and longer utterances represented as paragraphs and chapters. For the beginning reader, a growing ability to listen and then segment a phrase into words, a word into syllables, and a syllable into phonemes is needed in order to begin to make sense of how words are put together. As the child hears and uses more of the spoken language, she or he becomes better prepared to identify words and word parts in print. Such phonological discovery takes place in the presence of spoken language, and we have known for some time that most children with typical hearing have learned to recognize and produce the sounds spoken around them by the time they are six or seven (Fry, 1966), making first grade a reasonable time for most children to begin receiving formal instruction in reading. Formal instruction that includes word identification strategies (*sounding out* and *whole word*) is comprehensible at this time, because it depends upon the auditory and semantic language base of the child. Learning to read, in the presence of both formal instruction at school and experience and informal instruction at home, helps children fill in whatever sounds they have not already mastered (Adams, 2000; Goswami, 2000). This is particularly advantageous to the child with hearing loss who still has a few gaps. Attempting to teach letter sounds to children who cannot already listen and talk with the goal of their learning to identify written words, has met with less success.

Geers and Hayes (2011) report results of a longitudinal study that followed the performance of language-related skills in 184 students who had severe-to-profound hearing loss and who received cochlear implants prior to age 5. They had followed these students throughout elementary school and were able to reassess the reading, writing and phonological processing skills of 112 of those original subjects in high school. They found that, depending upon the test, between 47% and 66% performed within or above the average range for reading in comparison to hearing peers, an encouraging outcome in view of previous research findings. However, two areas continued to pose serious challenges for the subjects, that of written expression and phonological processing. Processing skills in particular have been found to be critical predictors of high school literacy skills.

Background Knowledge: Content and Process Schemas

First-hand knowledge of the world is built from experiences, and the wider the world of the individual, the more background knowledge the person has in terms of both content and processes. The experiences children have with language and its connections to what they see, hear, touch, taste, and feel, as well as to their emotions create their knowledge base. Experiences in society provide access to commonly held knowledge about objects, actions, descriptors, relationships, and interpretations, as well as the referential, culturally appropriate language used to talk about them. Interacting in meaningful ways with as many people as possible about the full range of such experiences is essential to the processes foundational to comprehension.

Virtual knowledge constructed through indirect experience such as photos, images in books and electronic devices, stories and descriptions, and pretend play (imaginative play) is vital, as well. Other important kinds of knowledge include how to carry out particular processes and how to interpret feelings. First-hand, virtual, and procedural knowledge combine and come to represent a child's knowledge base, and this base becomes foundational to all future learning. In cognitive psychology, each such memory structure is called a schema (Anderson, 2004, provides an interesting account of this robust theory). Schemas (the alternate plural is schemata) overlap and connect what the person stores away in memory; the ability to tap into one's memory network in the presence of new experiences is what enables us to learn.

Comprehension, whether through listening, reading, or using one's senses, and expression, whether through speaking or writing, *depends upon connecting this base of background knowledge to the language that represents its many parts.* AVT serves children well in that it encourages many experiences and meaningful conversations about them thereby enabling them to apply spoken words to their schemas.

Spoken Vocabulary Knowledge

For a child with hearing loss, any decrease in the number of spoken words heard completely and in connected, meaningful contexts, jeopardizes the development of many aspects of spoken language needed for reading.

For over 20 years, the devastating effects of spoken language deprivation on children with typical hearing have been known in a specific, quantifiable way (Hart & Risley, 1995; Hart & Risley, 1999). While Hart and Risley focused on children with typical hearing, their findings carry salient implications for thinking about children with hearing loss. Their interest was in quantifying the amount of spoken language in the home environments of children, hypothesizing that at least one cause of the differences in school progress among children from homes where the parents were professionals, working-class homes, or homes where

the family was on welfare, might be the sheer number of words the children encountered during their earliest, language-acquisition years. On a monthly basis, they tape recorded the language used in these homes and extrapolated estimates of the number of words, repetitions included, each group of children had heard by age 4. The differences were substantial: the children of the professionals had had access to 45 million words, the children of parents in the working class had had 26 million words, and the children of parents on welfare had had 13 million. Hart and Risley observe, "parents who talked a lot . . . or only a little ended up with 3-year-olds who talked a lot, or only a little" (1999, p. xii). This phenomenon associated with parental style in talking with their children has been termed the *30 Million Word Gap,* and this knowledge is being used as the basis for programs aimed at enriching the language abilities of children unfortunate enough to be born into the chaos that poverty often creates (Suskind, Thirty Million Words Initiative, http://thirtymillionwords.org/). We hasten to note that Hart and Risley's work dealt with vocabulary development and was not about identifying socioeconomic strengths and weaknesses; indeed, in some families with few resources, talk was rich and productive. The point of their findings highlights the importance of entering school with an extensive vocabulary. Such knowledge is connected directly to the progress a child can make with reading; it has been established that a child's spoken language ability at preschool age has a relationship to the child's reading ability in second grade (Scarborough, 1989) and beyond. The more spoken words the child recognizes and understands, the better chance the child has of excelling in reading and writing.

The implications of these findings for children with hearing loss must be stressed emphatically. During the early years when the brain is most receptive for language development, the child with hearing loss whose hearing is not augmented via amplification is in a similar and damaging situation to that of the child who hears typically but has little opportunity to listen and speak. Constant and consistent access to increasingly complex interactions using spoken language is imperative for creating the conditions for emerging reading.

Practical Approaches for Building a Foundation for Literacy

Moving from theory into practice is the exciting task of the AV practitioner and the parent. Table 9–1 links LSLS Domain 9 and literacy theory with auditory-verbal practice, and demonstrates how AVT is intentional in fostering emerging literacy.

The underlying reason for the practical approaches offered in this section is the fostering of auditory memory in order to facilitate auditory-based thinking, the goal of AVT. A critical element in auditory processing involves phonological memory. The combination of phonological awareness, phonological memory, and phonological retrieval comprises a cluster of requisite skills for learning to read and read fluently (Justice & Cabell, 2010); these skills underlie the ability to become aware of, store, and retrieve phonologically

encoded information in words and sentences, including that found in extended discourse (Catts & Kamhi, 2005).

The following sections offer practical strategies that can be employed as one coaches the parent to work with their child. The use of each strategy begins with a simple application and can be made increasingly complex as the child's abilities mature.

Intentional Development of Phonological Awareness in Children

Research has demonstrated that intervention can positively influence phonologic awareness skills and has documented improvement in word identification and decoding skills (Schuele & Boudreu, 2008). Substantial support in the literature suggests that phonological instruction needs to be initiated in preschool and no later than kindergarten (Schuele & Boudreu, 2008); AVT begins such instruction even earlier. It is important that the AV practitioner and the parents of young children with hearing loss recognize a hierarchy of phonological awareness knowledge that moves from the global to the specific so that appropriate intervention can take place (Adams, 1990); particular emphasis needs to shift focus progressively toward the level of the phoneme, as intervention that leads the child from phonological to phonemic awareness promotes the child's use of strategies for effective decoding and spelling (Price & Ruscher, 2006). Because children with hearing loss in AVT have early access to hearing the full speech spectrum, formal attention to phonological awareness can realistically begin in preschool.

Table 9-1. Linking LSLS Domain 9 and Literacy Theory With Auditory-Verbal Therapy

Domain 9	National Reading Panel Category	Auditory-Verbal Therapy
a. Reciting finger plays and nursery rhymes	Phonemic awareness Phonics Fluency Vocabulary Comprehension	Targeted listening practice • Example: Discriminating between one- and two-syllable words whose phonemes differ by one (e.g., mat-bat, bat-bam, batter-matter, batter-badger) • Exposing child to melody, expression, rhythm, rhyme, intonation • Using repetition
b. Telling and/or retelling stories	Vocabulary Comprehension	Targeted listening practice • Responding with spoken language • Waiting for and requiring child to use spoken language Daily read-alouds with the child • Positioning close to the microphone • Using acoustic highlighting • Pausing, waiting (providing thinking time for the child) • Changing voices for characters • Asking and answering questions in a conversational manner • Using classic literature, songs, nursery rhymes
c. Activity and story sequencing	Vocabulary Comprehension	Targeted listening practice • Responding with spoken language • Waiting for and requiring child to use spoken language
d. Singing songs and engaging in musical activities	Phonemic awareness Phonics Fluency Vocabulary Comprehension	Targeted listening practice • Exposing child to melody, pitch, expression, rhythm, rhyme, intonation • Using repetition

Table 9–1. *continued*

Domain 9	National Reading Panel Category	Auditory-Verbal Therapy
e. Creating experience stories/ experience books	Vocabulary Comprehension	Targeted listening practice • Developing conversations using natural interactions • Highlighting vocabulary • Paying attention to word order • Changing words by adding • prefixes and suffixes
f. Organization of books (e.g., cover; back; title; author page)	Vocabulary Comprehension	Incorporating book-reading vocabulary during read-alouds
g. Directionality and orientation of print	Vocabulary Comprehension	Incorporating book-reading vocabulary during read-alouds

h. Distinguishing letters, words, sentences, spaces, and punctuation	Phonemic awareness Phonics	Targeted listening practice
		• Acoustic highlighting
		  ○ Suprasegmental
		  ○ Segmental
		• Asking, "What did you hear?"
		• Pointing out and talking about letters, words, sentences, spaces, and punctuation

i. Phonics (e.g., sound-symbol correspondences and letter-sound correspondences)	Phonemic awareness Phonics	Targeted listening practice • Preparing a child who listens for formal instruction that leads to understanding the alphabetic principle
j. Phonemic awareness (e.g., sound matching; isolating; substituting; adding; blending; segmenting; deleting)	Phonemic awareness Phonics	Targeted listening practice • To one's own speech • Six-Sound Test • Nursery rhymes • Music and singing
k. Sight word recognition	Fluency	Allowing sight word identification to develop naturally during read-alouds without focusing directly on this aspect of reading during the emergent reading period

continues

Table 9–1. *continued*

Domain 9	National Reading Panel Category	Auditory-Verbal Therapy

l. Strategies for the development of listening, speaking, vocabulary, reading and writing	Phonemic awareness
	Phonics
	Fluency
	Vocabulary
	Comprehension
		Targeted listening practice
		• Focus on building:
		  ○ auditory memory
		  ○ receptive and expressive spoken language
		• Providing the child with mature models of spoken and written language structure and function
		• Playtime alone, with parent, and with other children

m. Contextual clues to decode meaning	Vocabulary Comprehension	Having frequent conversations with the child in the course of daily activities fosters meaning making
n. Oral reading fluency development	Fluency	Having frequent conversations with the child in the course of daily activities fosters fluency in spoken language and reading
o. Text comprehension strategies (e.g., direct explanation; modeling; guided practice; and application)	Vocabulary Comprehension	Narrating life as it happens Bringing sounds to life through meaningful experiences Having frequent conversations Learning through exposure: • Semantics • Morphology • Syntax Learning to: • Turn statements into questions, exclamations, etc. • Apply words to objects, actions, relationships modifiers, and ideas • Use pragmatic aspects of language • Apply memories of experiences to text
p. Abstract and figurative language (e.g., similes; metaphors)	Vocabulary Comprehension	Focusing on abstract and figurative language with the child during: • Frequent conversations • Daily read-alouds

Table 9–1. *continued*

Domain 9	National Reading Panel Category	Auditory-Verbal Therapy
q. Divergent question comprehension (e.g., inferential questions; predictions)	Vocabulary Comprehension	Asking divergent questions of the child during: • Frequent conversations • Daily read-alouds

Note. *The focus of Domain 9 is the development of the auditory and language skills that underlie and support the acquisition and advancement of literacy.

In fact, Johnson and Goswami (2010) conclude that early cochlear implantation is associated with improved phonological awareness skills as well as improved spoken language and auditory memory. Studies have demonstrated that the sequential acquisition of these skills is similar for children with and without typical hearing and instruction can be conducted in small group or one-on-one settings.

The following hierarchy of phonemic awareness levels is recommended:

1. Rhythm and Rhyme: the ability to recognize, complete, and produce word patterns and detect spoken syllables
2. Parts of a Word: the ability to blend, segment, and delete syllables
3. Sequencing of Sounds: the ability to recognize initial and final sounds
4. Separation of Sounds: the ability to segment sounds in words and blend sounds
5. Manipulation of Sounds: the ability to add, delete, and/or substitute sounds
   (Fitzpatrick, 1997; Yopp & Yopp, 2000)

Price and Ruscher (2006) suggest a naturalistic approach that provides phonological awareness instruction within the context of children's picture books and literature; this instruction is consistent with the principles first described by Justice and Kaderavek (2004). Such instruction promotes explicit and hierarchical phonological awareness training while providing socially meaningful encounters with literacy experiences throughout the day complemented by structured lessons that target specific emergent literacy goals. Price and Ruscher's *Embedded-Explicit Approach* suggests the following sequence of instruction for phonologic awareness skills:

1. Instruction progresses in the following order at these sound unit levels:
   a. Syllables
   b. Rhyming with onset-rime
   c. Sound-symbol associations and alliteration
   d. Phonemes
2. Within these sound unit levels, instruction about tasks and operations progresses in the following order:

a. Blending
b. Segmenting
c. Counting
d. Deleting
(Price & Ruscher, 2006, pp. 23–77)

Important intervention tenets supported by evidence-based research include the following:

- Explicit instruction is systematic.
- Intervention occurs within authentic reading and writing contexts and class curriculum.
- Phonemic awareness skills are causally related to word decoding and spelling.
- Instruction is done in small groups.
- Focus is on a small set of skills (e.g., blending or segmenting) rather than a large number of operations at once.
- Total instruction should occupy approximately 20 hr spread across a 10-week period (Carson, Gillon, & Boustead, 2013).
- The strongest effects will occur during the preschool and/or kindergarten years.
- Close collaboration is necessary between the speech-language pathologist and the teacher.
- Students at risk must be identified early, with identification followed by instruction tailored for each student.
- Instruction needs to be organized in a logical order from easier to more difficult skills (e.g., blending, segmenting, counting, and deleting) within each of the sound unit levels of syllable awareness, rhyming with onset-rime, sound-symbol

identification/alliteration, and finally, phoneme awareness (Justice, 2006).

Over two decades of research suggests that children with and without hearing loss can benefit from intense phonological awareness instruction, that such instruction matters in reading acquisition, and that it must occur early and intensively with attention given to the challenges facing the individual child. Tailored to meet the needs of the child, an explicit and systematic plan can be implemented with positive impact on word identification, decoding, spelling, and comprehension (Carson, Gillon, & Boustead, 2013; Price & Ruscher, 2006; Schuele & Boudreu, 2008; Yopp & Yopp, 2006). The child who is receiving AVT is positioned well to be receptive of and benefit from such intervention.

Story Retelling

Story retelling strategies (Robertson, Dow, & Hainzinger, 2006) involve the child interacting with the reader of the story while engaged in read-alouds. As the child gains more competence in listening, remembering, and talking, he or she begins to repeat words and sentences that are presented verbally, and verbatim utterances become possible. Comprehension builds as the child learns how to make sense of what he or she hears in a story, and spoken language develops accordingly. This tactic can easily be implemented at home between the parent and child and any significant others using children's literature. Using toy figures to relate narratives is highly motivating, and the resulting speaker-listener dialogue involves auditory memory recall. For example, in the story, Kellie says, *"The trip to the zoo will be the first time I see tigers!"* This might prompt the adult to ask, *"What does Kellie say?"* and the child to progress over time and repeated reading from saying, *"See tigers!"* to *"First time see tigers!"* to *"This will be the first time I see tigers!"*

Lengthening Auditory Attention Span

Engaging the child in interactive book reading also expands auditory memory span (Trelease, 2007). Exposing children to literature carries many benefits in that it is motivating and emotionally bonding, in addition to being intellectually stimulating. For the child with hearing loss, there cannot be a better signal-to-noise ratio than that achieved with a child sitting on the caregiver's lap. While listening and discussing the details shared in children's books, the adult and child can explore lands never traveled and discuss narratives with intriguing story lines. The conversation that ensues between the reader and the listener strengthens conversational competency and encourages the child's inferential and critical thinking skills. The child's personal Language Experience Book (LEB) as described by Robertson (2014) makes a narrative and its language more memorable. The LEB is about the child's own experience and makes it easy for the parent to pose questions that initiate interactions involving the story, fact recall, feelings, and predictions. Repetitive reading of the LEB stories also contributes to developing fluency in oral reading (Rasinski, 2010).

Reading and auditory recall can also be promoted by creating and introducing a *Poetry Notebook* containing various kinds of poetry and rhymes, song lyrics, famous speeches, jump rope chants, cheers, jokes, and movie scripts. Each passage in the notebook can be accompanied by an object or a picture that represents the main feature (e.g., a poem about apples has a pointer with an apple sticker at the end of it to use while reading the poem). This demonstrates to the child the connection between spoken and written language and plants the seeds of fluency and phonemic awareness, two of the building blocks for reading. Reading with significant others is encouraged daily, and the child is asked to obtain *signatures* from the listeners of their *Poetry Notebook*. Initially, the task involves auditory memory, and then it is used to encourage children to actually see and read the words in the text as they develop fluency in guided reading practice (Rasinski, 2010).

Guided Reading

Byrd and Westfall (2002) outline several strategies for use in guided reading; these appear in their *Guided Reading Coaching Tool*. Their use involves listening, speaking, and learning about books and stories.

To Teach Directionality to the Child

Ask the child:

- Show me the front of the book.
- Point to the title.
- Open the book.
- Which page do we read first?

- Point to the first word we will read.
- In which direction should we turn the page?
- Where do our eyes go next after we get to the end of the line?

To Teach the Child How to Gain Information from the Illustrations

Ask the child:

- Who do you see in the picture?
- Tell me all of the names that a character could be called. (e.g., girl, daughter, princess, sister, classmate).
- How is the character feeling?
- What details do you see in the background?
- Where is the story taking place?
- Can you make any predictions from this picture?
- Does it look like there may be any problems in this story?

To Teach the Child to Use Background Knowledge to Make Sense of the Text/To Draw the Child's Attention to Visual Cues, Words, and Sentence Structure

Say to the child:

- Does ____ make sense in that sentence?
- Try a new word that may make more sense.
- When you said ____ did it make more sense?
- Let's use our common sense to determine what this means.
- Does that new word look right and sound right?

- Does the sentence make sense when you hear it?

The reader is encouraged to explore Byrd and Westfall's text, as it offers additional guided reading suggestions involving decoding unfamiliar and frequently occurring words that enhance every child's ability to recall and comprehend many genres of text. These practical suggestions can lead children in AVT on their journey toward literacy in a motivating and engaging manner.

Shared Reading

Reading aloud to children has been identified as one of the most important activities for promoting the skills that lead to the eventual success in reading for children (Trelease, 2006). Initially, it is not so important to teach the child *how* to read, but rather to *want* to read. The parent needs to entice the child to want to *break the code* of squiggles (*letters*) on the page. Consequently, reading becomes a *labor of love*, not a symbol of labor and struggle.

Research suggests that guided and shared reading experiences with a child struggling with reading can have a significantly positive impact on the child's early language development and subsequent ability to read. Whitehurst and his research team (1988) suggest that adults create a highly interactive reading experience, similar to a *dialogue* in which the adult invites and maintains the child's active participation while reading both *to* and *with* the child. Specific strategies that define *dialogic reading* include the following:

- Labeling objects and events
- Presenting simple *wh* questions

- Posing more complex *what* questions about function and attributes
- Repeating the child's verbal attempts
- Requesting that the child imitate verbally
- Offering praise
- Providing verbal expansions
- Posing open-ended questions

Williams (2006) suggests an integrated approach, *Enhanced Dialogic Reading* (EDR) that integrates instruction in phonological sensitivity (associated with decoding skills) and spoken language (associated with comprehension skills) while engaging with the child. The goal of EDR is to make the two precursors of reading become interactive, so that phonological sensitivity and spoken language will create fluent, accurate readers.

Similarly, Marsha Spears (2004) published a *Shared Reading Coaching Tool* that promotes print conventions such as directionality, text conventions, picture cues, letter activities, and phonemic awareness while simultaneously focusing on spoken language skills such as asking the child to predict, self-monitor, guess vocabulary meaning, re-tell and repeat story elements, and note repetitive patterns in the language of the text. Spears' step-by-step process to teach shared reading uses an intense 3-day protocol.

In yet another shared reading approach, Moore, Perez-Mendez, and Boerger (2006) suggest what they refer to as a *4-Squares Technique* in which parents read favorite stories to their child. The experience is videotaped while the parent follows a discussion framework with a facilitator afterwards.

The observation instrument includes strengths of the caregiver and the child as well as the next steps to be taken by both the parent and the child. A parent's strengths might include pointing to familiar letters, using emotion while reading, and waiting for the child to respond. These techniques are all familiar to the AV practitioner. Strengths of the child might include turning the pages and watching intently, asking various questions, and pointing to pictures. Next steps for the parent might include asking the child to predict the rest of the plot and re-tell the story, while relating the story to the child's everyday life. The child's subsequent steps may include filling-in words that appear in the story, something that encourages the child to continue talking about the story or re-telling the plot.

These shared reading paradigms reflect the philosophy that there is no one way to teach children to read. Rather, an integrated approach that prepares a child for the demands of decoding (phonological sensitivity) and spoken language (comprehension) increases the probability that a child with hearing loss will develop the requisite skills for a successful reading acquisition experience and will go on to become a lifetime reader.

Shared Writing

Calkins (1994) and Graves (2003) explain that children often engage in writing prior to or along with experiences with reading, and it is the writing experience that incites a desire to learn to read. Graves suggests reading and writing are "synergistic," with each feeding off the other's characteristics.

A Framework for the Writing Process

Newman (2001) identifies four concepts in the writing process that provide a framework when analyzing children's writing: intention, organization, experimentation, and orchestration. In *intention,* the child writes with purpose or meaning. The child is intent on conveying a meaningful message. A child learns to communicate verbally to express desires, needs, requests, denials, or refusals, and likewise learns that the written word manipulates the environment as well. In *organization,* the child displays awareness that writing has various formats to which it must adhere. In English, there are three directional principles to be learned: we read and write top to bottom, left to right and return quickly from the right to left and begin again (Clay, 1987, 2010). In *experimentation,* the child explores punctuation conventions she or he may see but not yet fully understand. Risk-taking is an integral part of experimentation, and the child is attempting to learn what she or he can control in the writing process. Last, the child learns that writing is a matter of *orchestration.* The child learns the necessity of juggling many aspects of writing at once, such as spelling, grammar, printing, and meaning, while simultaneously making decisions about prioritizing those aspects. When they receive responses to their writing from others, children learn that writing is a powerful, and complex, process.

The Language Experience Book (LEB)

As an approach to helping the child understand the relationship between reading and writing, the LEB offers an excellent opportunity for a child with hearing loss in AVT to experience the process of writing and its power to function as another form of communication. Because children are developmentally egocentric, participating in the writing of the LEB can fascinate the child and help him or her to recall actions, narratives, concepts, and feelings, along with the words that represent them. As a way of chronicling daily activities, the LEB compiles and illustrates step-by-step details of the child's experiences. Working on understanding of sequence provides one example of how the LEB can be extended; one might number or transfer events in a sequence to index cards for shuffling and sequencing at a later time. Such sequenced events can first be described by the AV practitioner and/or parent and then be reviewed and enumerated repeatedly for others with whom the child shares the LEB. Documenting daily events in a notebook provides purpose for the child and parent to interact using shared writing as they record events and ideas important to the child. The parent fosters the child's desire to share with others using a form that goes beyond speaking—writing words down on paper.

Thoughts on Fostering Writing

The following incentives are used routinely with eager young authors:

- Weekly surprises are always literacy based such as pens, markers, crayons, notepads, diaries, books, printable books, or props such as popsicle stick pointers to follow words of songs, finger plays, or nursery rhymes; all can be found at home, at flea markets, or as freebies from family and friends.

- Writing is a social experience, so the graduate student models the writing process for the child by writing alongside the child on the floor, at the table, or wherever it is comfortable. It is not surprising when children imitate, as imitation is the way children learn from experienced writers.

- Adults create their own Language Experience Books as well as expecting the children to do so. They love to hear the adults share their weekly challenges and dramas. They love to listen and laugh at life experiences chronicled in the LEBs.

- Parents need to be involved throughout the sharing of the LEB to demonstrate the importance of making reading and writing a part of everyday living. Once they observe the motivation of the LEB, they recognize the contribution that writing makes in creating a lifetime reader and writer in their child.

A Few Words Concerning Digital Literacy

The question of whether and how to use digital, electronic devices with children is becoming increasingly frequent, as we are experiencing a profound change in the ways we record, store, and retrieve information. Digital technology is powerful and useful. Some embrace using it with children, thinking it will work wonders, and others will not let their children near it, fearing it will damage them. Its potential benefits for children need to be pursued and researched. Currently, the American Academy of Pediatrics and the White House Task Force on Childhood Obesity recommend strongly that children under age 2 not be exposed to screen media and that a limit of 1 to 2 hr of screen time per day be enforced for children older than 2 (National Association for the Education of Young Children [NAEYC], 2002).

The concerns associated with exposing children with typical hearing to digital media range from sleep and behavior problems to diminished academic achievement to a lesser development of language and social skills. Of particular concern is noninteractive technology, as it hampers both physical and linguistic activity. From a listening and spoken language point of view, the major worry concerning using digital media with children with hearing loss is that it could interfere with language acquisition and the learning of social skills. If a caregiver believes that use of such media can substitute for the presence and interaction with an adult, then precious time with the child who needs more spoken language input than children with typical hearing is lost, never to be regained. Anything that gets in the way of spoken language learning likely limits the acquisition of literacy, so if *screen time* replaces listening and speaking or gets in the way of vocabulary growth, the child will not make the same progress she or he would if someone were conversing with or creating interesting experiences with him or her.

Used in ways that stimulate interaction and connection making, digital media can bring the outside world to a child in enriching ways; photographs, videos, and interactive programs can offer much to a child, and the best use of them is in the presence of an adult who uses well-formed language to talk about what is appearing on the screen. Such use is similar to using traditional materials for reading or writing with a child. For example, there are several phone and tablet apps on which one can create language experience books with a child, so that a parent can have an LEB ready for daily use and even while waiting for an appointment.

In reporting on a study done in British classrooms with children ages 3 to 4, 4 to 5, and 7 to 13, Flewitt, Messer, and Kucirkova (2004) distinguish between closed and open content in apps being used with children. Closed content apps assume a transmission model of learning that attempts to fill the learner with particular knowledge. Such knowledge often includes phonics and vocabulary, and the approach of such apps is one of drilling and rewarding correct responses. Children often tire of this quickly, whether it is presented on paper or by electronic means. Open content apps assume that children learn through extensive interaction; they invite children's creative engagement in activities such as composing stories, and they support children as they learn how to develop ideas and the words for them. Children learn how to use a particular electronic device by using it, regardless of the open or closed character of instruction. Flewitt's exploratory study observed older children exhibiting enthusiasm for complex planning while using iPads to collaborate in writing a play, acting out their writing, and then using a camera to preserve their work. Flewitt, Messer, and Kucirkova

conclude that such use of electronic devices can provide "a rich platform for language and communication, collaborative problem-solving, negotiating meanings and sharing experiences" (p. 302), but they caution that "unless 'new' digital devices are woven innovatively into the fabric of classroom practice, then their potential could all too easily be reduced to being no more than a device for delivering repetitive curriculum content, albeit with added interactive multimedia appeal" (p. 303). Flewitt, Messer, and Kucirkova challenge practitioners to explore and develop interactive ways to use the technology offered by phones, tablets, and computers so that children's language and vocabulary grow in ways that support literacy.

Critical to a child's learning and particularly in AVT, are interactions with an adult who provides high-quality narration to the joint experience the child has with that person, regardless of the medium used. Rather than focusing on the technology, parents, teachers, and AV practitioners need to focus on the content that children can learn and use multiple ways to present and interact with it. This content can come in the form of real-life experiences or in virtual (digital) experiences, but, it is the spoken and written language provided by the adults that makes the difference; "the most logical conclusion to be drawn from the existing scholarly literature is that it is the educational content that matters—not the format in which it is presented" (NAEYC, 2002).

In sum, the position of the NAEYC and the Fred Rogers Center offers suitable guidance for those who work with and care about young children with hearing loss:

Technology and interactive media are tools that can promote effective learning and development when they are used intentionally by early childhood educators, within the framework of developmentally appropriate practice (NAEYC, 2009a), to support learning goals established for individual children. (http://www.naeyc.org/files/naeyc/file/positions/PS_technology_WEB2.pdf)

Concluding Where we Began: Becoming Literate is a Lifelong Process

We conclude this chapter where we began. Drawing on the immense literature concerning literacy processes, we remind ourselves that becoming literate begins with listening and that such listening must begin as early in a child's life as possible. The ability to read and write at proficient levels carries with it access to human knowledge, the world of work, creativity, personal growth, and enjoyment. Reading and writing are important means to thinking, and children with hearing loss have the need, indeed the right, to become part of the literate world. We turn again to the National Council of English for their helpful statements:

Reading is the complex act of constructing meaning from print. We read in order to better understand ourselves, others, and the world around us; we use the knowledge we gain from reading to change the world in which we live. (National Council of Teachers of English position statement on reading, http://

www.ncte.org/positions/statements/positiononreading)

Writing for real purposes is rewarding, and the daily activities of families present many opportunities for purposeful writing. Involving your child may take some coaxing, but it will be worth your patient effort. (National Council of Teachers of English position statement on writing, http://www.ncte.org/positions/statements/howtohelpenglish)

We close with these important points:

- ■ Reading and writing are thought processes associated with and dependent on listening and speaking.
- ■ The active construction and communication of meaning are the purposes of literacy.
- ■ Knowledge of the spoken language is the prerequisite for becoming literate in that language.
- ■ Literacy involves mastery of complex interactions among the components of spoken language.
- ■ Auditory-verbal approaches provide excellent preparation for literacy acquisition.

Where it was once exceedingly rare, it is now commonplace to find highly literate young adults who have used hearing technology all their lives. These individuals have few communication difficulties working as professionals alongside of and in sustained communication with people with typical hearing. These young adults are doctors, lawyers, psychologists, information technology experts, teachers, and so on; indeed, they can be found throughout the world of work (Robertson, 2014). The primary difference between mature and diminished literacy development is learning the spoken language to be read by listening to it and using it to interact in speech with others from an early age. This is a common practice in AVT. AVT sets children with hearing loss on their way toward emerging literacy by helping them establish a solid foundational knowledge of spoken language on which to build a lifetime of discovery and learning of language and content.

REFERENCES

Adams, M. (1990). *Beginning to read*. Cambridge, MA: MIT Press.

Alexander Graham Bell Association for the Deaf and Hard of Hearing, the Academy for Listening and Spoken Language. Retrieved September 21, 2015, from http://www.listeningandspokenlanguage.org/AcademyDocument.aspx?id=563

Anderson, R. (2004). Role of the reader's schema in comprehension, learning, and memory. In R. Ruddell & N. Unrau (Eds.), *Theoretical models and processes of reading* (5th ed., pp. 594–606). Newark, DE: International Reading Association.

Byrd, D., & Westfall, P. (2002). *Guided reading teaching tool*. Peterborough, NH: Crystal Springs Books.

Calkins, L. (1994). *The art of teaching writing* (2nd ed.). Portsmouth, NH: Heinemann.

Carson, K. L., Gillon, G. T., & Boustead, T. M. (2013). Classroom phonological awareness instruction and literacy outcomes in the first year of school. *Language, Speech, and Hearing Services in Schools, 44*, 147–160.

Catts, H. W., Fey, M. E., Zhang, X., & Tomblin, J. B. (2001). Estimating the risk of future reading difficulties in kindergarten children: A research-based model and its clinical implementation. *Language, Speech, and Hearing Services in Schools, 32*, 38–50.

Catts, H. W., & Kamhi, A. G. (Eds.). (2005). *Language and reading disabilities* (2nd ed.). Boston, MA: Allyn & Bacon.

Clay, M. (1987). *Writing begins at home: Preparing children for writing before they go to school*. Hong Kong: Heinemann.

Clay, M. (2010). *How very young children explore writing*. Hong Kong: Heinemann.

Fitzpatrick, J. (1997). *Phonemic awareness: Playing with sounds to strengthen beginning reading skills*. Cypress, CA: Creative Teaching Press.

Flewitt, R., Messer, D., & Kucirkova, N. (2014). New directions for early literacy in a digital age: The iPad. *Journal of Early Childhood Literacy, 15*(3), 289–310.

Fry, D. (1966). The development of the phonological system in the normal and the deaf child. In F. Smith & G. Miller (Eds.), *The genesis of language: A psycholinguistic approach* (pp. 187–206). Cambridge, MA: MIT Press.

Geers, A., & Hayes, H. (2011). Reading, writing, and phonological processing skills of adolescents with 10 or more years of cochlear implant experience. *Ear and Hearing, 32*, 49S–59S.

Gillon, G. T. (2004). *Phonological awareness: From research to practice*. New York: NY: Guilford Press.

Goswami, U. (2000). Phonological and lexical processes. In M. Kamil, P. Mosenthal, P. D. Pearson, & R. Barr (Eds.), *Handbook of reading research, Volume III* (pp. 251–267). Mahwah, NJ: Lawrence Erlbaum.

Graves, D. (2003). *Writing: Teachers and children at work* (2nd ed.). Portsmouth, NH: Heinemann.

Hart, B., & Risley, T. (1995). *Meaningful differences in the everyday experience of young American children*. Baltimore, MD: Brookes.

Hart, B., & Risley, T. R. (1999). *The social world of children learning to talk*. Baltimore, MD: Brookes.

Johnson, C., & Goswami, U. (2010). Phonological awareness, vocabulary, and reading in deaf children with cochlear implants. *Journal of Speech, Language, and Hearing Research*, *53*, 237–261.

Justice, L. M. (Ed.). (2006). *Clinical approaches to emergent literacy intervention*. San Diego, CA: Plural.

Justice, L. M., & Cabell, S. (2010). Reading disabilities. In Justice (Ed.), *Communication sciences and disorders: A contemporary perspective* (pp. 248–279). Boston, MA: Allyn & Bacon.

Justice, L. M., & Kaderavek, J. N. (2004). An embedded-explicit model of emergent literacy intervention for young at-risk children: Part I. *Language, Speech, and Hearing Services in Schools*, *35*, 201–211.

Moore, S. M., Perez-Mendez, C., & Boerger, K. (2006), Meeting the needs of culturally and linguistically diverse families in early language and literacy intervention (pp. 29–70). In L. M. Justice, *Clinical approaches to emergent literacy intervention*. San Diego, CA: Plural.

National Association for the Education of Young Children. (2002). *Technology and interactive media as tools in early childhood programs serving children from birth through age 8: A joint position statement of the National Association for the Education of Young Children and the Fred Rogers Center for Early Learning and Children's Media at Saint Vincent College*. Retrieved from http://www.naeyc.org/files/naeyc/file/positions/PS_technology_WEB2.pdf

National Council of Teachers of English. (1999). *NCTE position statement on reading*. Retrieved from http://www.ncte.org/positions/statements/positiononreading

National Council of Teachers of English. (2004). *A call to action: What we know about adolescent literacy and ways to support teachers in meeting students' needs*. Retrieved from http://www.ncte.org/positions/statements/adolescentliteracy

National Council of Teachers of English. *How to help your child become a better writer (English version)*. Retrieved from http://www.ncte.org/positions/statements/howtohelpenglish

National Institute of Child Health and Human Development (NICHD). (2000). *Report of the National Reading Panel. Teaching children to read: An evidence-based assessment of the scientific research literature on reading and its implications for reading instruction: Reports of the subgroups* (NIH Publication No. 00-4754). Washington, DC: U.S. Government Printing Office.

Newman, J. (2001). *The craft of children's writing* (2nd ed.). Spring, TX: Absey & Company.

Pintner, R., & Paterson, D. (1916). Learning tests with deaf children. *Psychology Monographs*, 20.

Price, L. H., & Ruscher, K. Y. (2006). Fostering phonological awareness using shared book reading and an embedded-explicit approach. In A. van Kleeck, *Sharing books and stories to promote language and literacy* (pp.15–77). San Diego, CA: Plural.

Rasinski, T. V. (2010). *The fluent reader: Oral and silent reading strategies for building fluency, word recognition and comprehension*. New York, NY: Scholastic.

Robertson, L. (2014). *Literacy and deafness: Listening and spoken language* (2nd ed.). San Diego, CA: Plural.

Robertson, L., Dow, G., & Hainzinger, S. (2006). Story retelling patterns among children with and without hearing loss: Effects of repeated practice and parent-child attunement. *Volta Review*, *106*(2), 147–170.

Scarborough, H. (1989). Prediction of reading disability from familial and individual differences. *Journal of Educational Psychology*, *81*(1), 101–108.

Schuele, C. M., & Boudreau, D. (2008). Phonological awareness intervention: Beyond the basics. *Language, Speech, and Hearing Services in Schools, 39*, 3–20.

Spears, M. (2004). *Shared reading coaching tool.* Peterborough, NH: Crystal Springs Books.

Suskind, D. (n.d.). *Thirty Million Words Initiative.* Retrieved from http://thirtymillion words.org/

Trelease, J. (2007). *The read-aloud handbook* (7th ed.). New York, NY: Penguin Books.

Whitehurst, G., Falco, F. L., Lonigan, C. J., Fischel, J. E., DeBaryshe, B. D., Valdez-Menchaca, M. C., & Caulfield, M. (1988). Accelerating language development through picture book reading. *Developmental Psychology, 24*(4), 552–559.

Williams, A. L. (2006). Integrating phonological sensitivity and oral language instruction into enhanced dialogic reading. In L. M. Justice, *Clinical approaches to emergent literacy intervention* (pp. 261–294). San Diego, CA: Plural.

Yopp, H. K. (1997, November). *Research developments in phonemic awareness and implications for classroom practice.* Presentation at the Research Institute at the annual meeting of the California Reading Association, San Diego, CA.

Yopp, H. K. (1999). Phonemic awareness: Frequently asked questions. *The California Reader, 32*, 21–27.

Yopp, H. K, & Yopp, R. H. (2000). Supporting phonemic awareness development in the classroom, *The Reading Teacher, 54*, 130–143.

Yopp, H. K, & Yopp, R. H. (2006). *Literature-based reading activities* (4th ed.). Boston, MA: Pearson Education.

10

STRATEGIES FOR LISTENING, TALKING, AND THINKING IN AUDITORY-VERBAL THERAPY

Ellen A. Rhoades, Warren Estabrooks,
Stacey R. Lim, and Karen MacIver-Lux

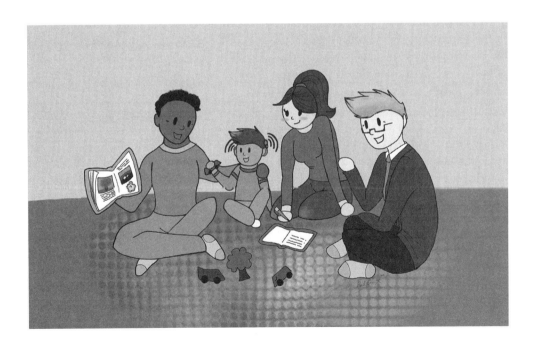

INTRODUCTION

Many language facilitative strategies have been studied specifically for outcome effectiveness with children who have typical hearing and language delays/disorders. Consequently, there are considerable evidence-based strategies targeting that large pediatric population. Yet, for children with hearing loss, evidence-based strategies to facilitate listening and spoken language skills remain relatively scarce. Nevertheless, there are many *evidence-informed* strategies that the auditory-verbal (AV) practitioner can use to facilitate listening and spoken language (Nevo & Slonim-Nevo, 2011). The purpose of this chapter, therefore, is to present these *evidence-informed strategies* in detail.

Evidence-informed practice is guided by research that the practitioner finds in peer-review journals. AV practitioners use the best available knowledge and research to guide strategy selection and implementation, and they try to familiarize themselves with outcome studies across related disciplines such as psychology, general education, child development, neurobiology, reading, and so forth. Research findings concerning all issues in communication disorders, therefore, need to be appropriately incorporated into AVT (Nevo & Slonim-Nevo, 2011). Throughout this chapter, we refer to the AV practitioner although we also expect that *the parents of children with hearing loss* (as a result of ongoing coaching) will learn, practice, and apply the strategies in daily life.

Parents and children with typical hearing usually interact *in tandem* from birth, meaning that their biological rhythms, gaze, affect, and vocal behaviors are coordinated (Feldman, Magori-Cohen, Galili, Singer, & Louzon, 2011). This *natural* parent-child "interaction synchrony," however, may be disrupted when the child does not respond appropriately because of a hearing loss. It is imperative, therefore, that parent-child interaction synchrony be restored.

In general, the best evidence-informed practice is considered to be *naturalistic intervention.* Many characteristics of this are embraced by AV practitioners as it is child-directed, play, based on the child's interests, and involves incidental and responsive teaching. *Naturalistic intervention* includes *strategies* that encourage joint attention, turn-taking, and other reciprocal adult-child interactions (Dunst, Raab, & Trivette, 2011; Snyder et al., 2015). Thus, with the use of strategies that facilitate listening, speech, and language, AV practitioners coach and guide parents to develop the same skills.

STRATEGIES

A *strategy* generally refers to a plan of action or method designed to achieve a goal; it tends to be behavioral or mental in nature. Effective and appropriate strategies are based on good knowledge of the situation/problem with reasonable expectations of outcomes. A *technique* is a way of doing something by using a particular skill or special knowledge. There are sometimes many techniques or ways in which a strategy can be executed. AV practitioners and parents may differ in their techniques when implementing a strategy, and the techniques may vary from child to child. Nevertheless, everyone needs to work in harmony to achieve the outcomes they want for the child. Sometimes it is difficult to agree on the correct term, so for the purpose of clarity throughout this chapter, the word *strategies* includes both.

One *historical strategy* that has been associated with AVT is the *hand cue* (the adult's "hand over mouth" to eliminate speech reading). For many compelling reasons, however, this is no longer considered an effective strategy. Evidence for this indicates that

- Covering the mouth disrupts sensorimotor input during infancy and may have negative implications for the development of speech motor control (Yeung & Werker, 2013).
- Covering up visual cues (lip movements) in an obvious way can instigate stress in young children which, in turn, negatively affects speech perception (Wang, Lee, Sigman, & Dapretto, 2006).
- Placing one's "hand over mouth" is considered negative body language among adults (Fast, 2002).
- Covering the mouth can alter the child's visual learning and visual memory (Brockmole, Davoli, Abrams, & Witt, 2013).
- Seeing the mouth purposefully hidden from view can detract from full auditory attention, thus slightly delaying speech perception (Musacchia, Sams, Nicol, & Kraus, 2006).
- Obstructing the mouth provides an acoustic barrier for the child with hearing loss. For example, high-frequency sounds tend to distort or diminish in

clarity when passing through a barrier or an acoustic filter. High-frequency audibility for children with hearing loss is critical (Stelmachowicz, Pittman, Hoover, Lewis, & Moeller, 2004). Speech directed to young children with hearing loss must not involve degraded spectral content (Zangl, Klarman, Thal, Fernald, & Bates, 2005).

Some practitioners use "speech hoops" (acoustic screens) to cover their faces. Their reason for using these to replace the "hand cue" is to avoid compromising the sound quality. However, preventing adult-child eye contact can negatively affect the child's overall development. The speaker's eyes give children important cues about the direction of visual attention as well as an emotional and/or mental state gaze necessary for joint attention, spoken language, and social skills (Frischen, Bayliss, & Tipper, 2007; Nappa, Wessel, McEldoon, Gleitman, & Trueswell, 2009; Rigato, Menon, Johnson, Faraguna, & Farroni, 2011). *Consequently, the use of the* hand cue *(or any substitute for it) is no longer recommended in AVT.*

A precept underlying *all* strategies presented in this chapter is that sound must be meaningful. The child with hearing loss will learn to "tune out" sound if it is has no meaning since the brain learns to ignore nonmeaningful sounds (Kotz, Opitz, & Friedrici, 2007). A young child wearing hearing aids with ear molds that inadequately fit, for example, may hear a high-pitched squeal and will eventually ignore the acoustic feedback if it persists.

Another example is when, after activation and programming of the child's cochlear implant, an adult calls the child's name while he or she is happily playing. The child hears his or her name and turns in the direction of the adult. Subsequently, the adult becomes excited, gleefully remarking to the AV practitioner, "See, he heard me! He knows his name!" In fact, there was no *payoff* for the child, and consequently had no real value, except to indicate detection of a sound.

The AV practitioner coaches the parent to call the child's name and make it meaningful by saying something such as: "Yes, you heard me call you. Great! Come here and help me" or "Come here! I want to show you this" *Sound must be meaningful* if it is to be processed and retained by the brain.

Learning how to become an effective communicator is a dynamic process that also involves cumulative *practice*. Listening, in part, involves a set of *skills* that can be taught, developed, and enhanced through the use of various strategies (Graham, Santos, & Vanderplank, 2011). This chapter, therefore, identifies SIX GOALS of the AV practitioner and discusses many effective strategies used by the AV practitioner to foster the growth of listening and spoken language across the years 0 to 6.

Table 10–1 provides an outline of these SIX GOALS and strategies recommended for each of them.

SIX GOALS OF THE AUDITORY-VERBAL PRACTITIONER (FOR EVERY AVT SESSION)

There are essentially *SIX GOALS* that the AV practitioner typically addresses in the planning and delivery of every AVT session. Parents usually learn these goals quickly as the practitioner creatively coaches them on using various strategies to accomplish them. Some strategies may be specific to AVT while some are used to help children with a variety of communication disorders. These strategies encourage children to listen and talk in AVT sessions and are not to be confused with general parent guidance and coaching practices found in Chapter 12.

Table 10–1. Six Goals and Selected **Strategies** of the AV Practitioner

GOAL 1: CREATE A LISTENING ENVIRONMENT
Strategies   • Controlling the environment; setting the stage   • Speaking within earshot; leaning to the child's better hearing side
GOAL 2: FACILITATE AUDITORY ATTENTION
Strategies   • Presenting a look of concentration with a verbal prompt   • Pointing to the ear and saying, "I heard something!"   • Using auditory hooks   • Using visual distractors   • Preparing the child to "listen first and last"

Table 10-1. *continued*

GOAL 3: ENHANCE AUDITORY PERCEPTION OF SPEECH

Strategies
- Speaking parentese
- Engaging in vocal play
- Associating sounds with objects and words
- Whispering
- Singing
- Stressing selected syllables, words, and phrases

GOAL 4: PROMOTE KNOWLEDGE OF LANGUAGE

Strategies
- Focusing on the "knowing" rather than the "using"
- Taking turns
- Imitating the child's early vocalizations
- Verbalizing in synchrony with movement
- Speaking the language from the child's angle
- Talking before, during, and after the action
- Pausing for grammatical spaces or emphasis
- Transitioning beyond the comfort zone
- Connecting the familiar to the unfamiliar
- Recasting, expanding, and expatiating on the child's words
- Emphasizing actions, relations, and attributes
- Contrasting the meaning of words

GOAL 5: FACILITATE SPOKEN LANGUAGE AND COGNITION

Strategies
- Leaning forward with expectant looks
- Signaling with objects
- Providing self-statements
- Asking, "What did you hear?"
- Promoting auditory-verbal closure
- Waiting for the child's response
- Asking stage-appropriate questions
- Scaffolding for language production

GOAL 6: STIMULATE INDEPENDENT LEARNING

Strategies
- Pretending objects are something else
- Creating the unexpected
- Talking with imaginary friends
- Accepting and making mistakes

SIX GOALS

1. Create a Listening Environment
2. Facilitate Auditory Attention
3. Enhance Auditory Perception of Speech
4. Promote Knowledge of Language
5. Facilitate Spoken Language and Cognition
6. Stimulate Independent Learning

GOAL 1: Create a Listening Environment

Strategies

- Controlling the environment; setting the stage
- Speaking within earshot; leaning to the child's better hearing side

A child with a hearing loss may experience auditory deprivation dating from 3 months before birth (Yang, 2006). The length of sensory deprivation depends on the age of the child when he or she was first fitted with at least one effective hearing device. Once the child has access to sound, it is critical to help the child develop *focused auditory attention* so that the child *learns to listen* as quickly and efficiently as possible.

Listening improves when the child is *still* and attends to the adult who is talking (Schneider, Nelson, & Mooney, 2014). As the AV practitioner and parent help increase the child's auditory attention span (sustained attention), the child is more likely to discriminate between meaningful and nonmeaningful sounds, while "tuning out" irrelevant background sounds (Dalton & Fraenkel, 2012).

Controlling the Environment; Setting the Stage

Noise compromises speech perception and language learning (Newman, Chatterjee, Morini, & Remez, 2015). All children, especially those with hearing loss, benefit greatly from quiet environments with little reverberation (Smaldino & Flexer, 2014). Since AVT sessions may take place in the child's home, the AV practitioner informs parents of variables that create adverse listening conditions. Parents, subsequently, can create the most favorable listening and language learning conditions possible. Parents need to know that household appliances, televisions, music equipment, computers, and other electronic devices add to background noise and their use needs to be minimized. High ceilings and tile floors cause reverberation, so floor, window, and wall coverings are encouraged. Many AVT sessions, however, take place in clinical rooms where *controlling the environment* is more easily managed.

Speaking Within Earshot; Leaning to the Child's Better Hearing Side

A child with hearing loss has a reduced listening range (Anderson & Crowley, 2002). Within this range, adults need to speak clearly in a natural voice at normal conversational levels. The nearer the AV practitioner talks into the microphone of the child's hearing device, the more easily the child will understand the speech signal because the clarity of spoken language improves as the distance between listener and speaker decreases (Souza, 2014).

Speaking within earshot means that the person talking is close enough to the listener that all the sounds of speech are audible and/or intelligible. The best understanding of speech occurs in a *fairly quiet room* and typically where the person talking is within 3 to 12 inches of the microphone of the child's hearing device (Ling & Ling, 1978). This strategy may reduce listening effort for the child (Gustafson, McCreery, Hoover, Kopun, & Stelmachowicz, 2014).

When introducing new vocabulary and/or language patterns, the AV practitioner is positioned *up close and personal* to the child, approximately 3 to 12 inches from the child's microphone, with the person who is talking positioned on the side of the child's better ear (Holstrum, Gaffney, Gravel, Oyler, & Ross, 2008). To further minimize distortion of speech, the practitioner avoids having any obstruction between the speaker's mouth and the child's microphone.

GOAL 2: Facilitate Auditory Attention

Strategies

- Presenting a look of concentration with a verbal prompt
- Pointing to the ear and saying, "I heard something!"
- Using auditory hooks
- Using visual distractors
- Preparing the child to "listen first and last"

After the initial fitting of the hearing device(s) and while the child begins adjusting to newly acquired auditory potential, the AV practitioner focuses on helping the child to develop a *listening attitude* (Holstrum et al., 2008). Whether toddlers or preschoolers, children with hearing loss require the same opportunities for *learning to listen* as babies with typical hearing. The development of auditory attention is of prime importance (Gomes, Wolfson, & Halperin, 2007). To develop the *listening attitude*, the child learns that "listening must be a continuous activity" (Pollack, 1972, p. 29).

The child's attention *must* be directed to *focus on sounds* in order to develop listening skills. Auditory attention directs auditory learning (Halliday, Moore, Taylor, & Amitay, 2011). Therefore, for the child to develop a listening attitude, the AV practitioner repeatedly uses prompts to *direct the child's attention to sound* (e.g., "Listen!"). These prompts alert the child to *pay attention to what is heard*, and consequently learn that what he or she hears really matters. All adults need to expect that the child *will* attend to the sounds of life and, in particular, to what people say.

Presenting a Look of Concentration With a Verbal Prompt

Facial expressions can prime language acquisition, so they are important *cues* for young children (Woumans et al., in press). The AV practitioner often makes facial expressions to indicate anticipation or "listening," such as a furrowed brow, tilting of the head, or leaning forward to the sound source. These often capture the child's attention and signal that something is going to happen . . . and *then* a sound is made. *After the sound is made*, the practitioner points to his or her own ear and says, "I heard that!" or "Did you hear that?" or "I wonder what that was?" or "What did you hear?" Depending on the child's response, the practitioner may direct this strategy to the parent who, in turn, responds appropriately (e.g., with a head nod or pointing). The child typically follows the parent's cue by imitating what the parent just said or did.

Pointing to the Ear and Saying "I heard something!"

Pointing to the ear is a visual cue that alerts the young child to speech and environmental sounds that may be forthcoming. This gesture can also alert the child to the speech or an environmental sound that was just heard. Pointing to the ear facilitates auditory attention (Varghese, Ozmeral, Best, & Shinn-Cunningham, 2012). Pointing, along with the verbal cue (e.g., "Listen, I heard something!") is associated with word comprehension (Caselli, Rinaldi, Stefanini, & Volterra, 2012). Combining the gesture with the verbal cue facilitates joint attention that is important for both social interaction and language acquisition (Colonnesi, Stams, Koster, & Noom, 2010).

The AV practitioner *primes* the child to *get ready to listen* by saying, "Listen!" while pointing to his or her own ear. Used simultaneously with "Listen!" this gesture signals that some kind of sound will soon be coming. Sometimes referred to as a *set to listen* task, this strategy is used when the child is not expecting a sound. Immediately after hearing the sound, the practitioner says, "I heard that!"

Using Auditory Hooks

Auditory hooks are prompts that "hook the child on listening" and alerts him or her that something exciting is coming. Auditory hooks can be verbal encouragements that include a variety of words, phrases, and/or fillers, such as "Hmm" "uhm . . . " "Hey!" "Look!" "Wow!" "Listen to this!" "Oh my goodness!" "That's interesting" "That's cool!" "Mmmm, let's see." These *auditory hooks* direct the child's attention to either environmental sounds or spoken language, or to the joint activity itself and they can promote longer episodes of shared or joint attention (Flom & Pick, 2003).

Using Visual Distractors

Visual distractors refer to prompts used by the AV practitioner that direct or redirect the child's visual attention. Research findings show that when the child's visual attention is focused on a speaker's face, the act of listening may be compromised (Champoux, Lepore, Gagné, & Théoret, 2009). So, when a child persists in "reading" the speaker's face, visual distractors used by the practitioner include

- pointing to an item, toward the window, or to another person;
- placing a toy, book, or other interesting item in front of the child; or
- subtle postural shifting so that the child finds "reading" the speaker's face to be a bit more difficult.

The short-term objective *and* the child's level of auditory and linguistic functioning determine when and how visual distractors are used. For example, the AV practitioner introduces the sound "meow" associated with a cat during the first year of learning to listen:

- The child looks directly at the face of the practitioner when the practitioner says "meow."
- The practitioner makes a show of looking at a book on the desk that diverts the child's visual attention. (The book is the visual distractor.)
- The child momentarily looks at the book.
- The practitioner repeats "meow" before showing the toy cat, at which point the child's attention is reverted to the practitioner.
- The practitioner then presents the toy cat to the child.
- The child plays with the toy cat and the practitioner again says or sings, "meow."

Another visual distractor might be outside, for example, the AV practitioner points to the window and says, "Listen, I hear some birds. They're singing, tweet, tweet, tweet, tweet!" Following this, the practitioner presents a toy bird to the child.

When a child focuses more on watching faces than listening, another visual distractor may be when the practitioner moves his or her body so that the child's visual attention is partially obstructed. For example, the practitioner can bend down to the side of the child to retrieve a toy clock from the floor. The child watches the movement of the adult's body as she or he says "tick-tock, tick-tock, tick-tock." When the clock is placed on the table and the child plays with it, the child's visual attention is directed to the toy and the

adult can continue narrating. In all cases, the child's attention is diverted so that *hearing and listening happen before seeing.*

Preparing the Child to "Listen First and Last"

Listen First and Last refers to the presentation of information—first, in the auditory-only condition (at least twice and perhaps three times), followed by visual information, if required, and then ending the sequence with the auditory-only information again. This means the child first listens to the spoken language (auditory-only message). If the child does not understand the auditory-only message after a maximum of three presentations by the AV practitioner, then a visual reinforcer is used to help the child understand what was said. Once the child understands, the practitioner *always* returns to the auditory-only message (Estabrooks, 2006; Rhoades, 2011).

Aside from the practice of hearing the same message repeatedly (sustained auditory attentional focus), the process of *listening first and last* enables the child to fill in the missing pieces and then make accurate predictions based on the visual cues provided (Astheimer & Sanders, 2009). The practitioner makes every effort to help the child understand what was said and may implement other strategies such as *repetition* and *rephrasing*. If, after using these strategies, the child still does not understand, then the adult needs to use a visual cue such as speech reading, or a gesture, or a picture to enhance the child's understanding. Finally, when the child does comprehend the complete spoken message, the practitioner presents the message again in the auditory-only condition as it was initially presented.

GOAL 3: Enhance Auditory Perception of Speech

Strategies

- Speaking parentese
- Engaging in vocal play
- Associating sounds with objects and words
- Whispering
- Singing
- Stressing selected syllables, words, and phrases

Speech consists of segmental information (features that differentiate one sound or phoneme from another) and their suprasegmental properties (intensity, stress, intonation, rhythm). Auditory perception of speech is the process by which the sounds of a language are heard and understood. Newborn babies with typical hearing are able to detect some suprasegmental information and to differentiate between phonemes like /ba/ and /pa/ under certain conditions (McMurray & Aslin, 2005; Werker & Gervain, 2013).

Across the first few years of life, children's speech perception is shaped by their auditory system as well as their phonetic and linguistic knowledge (Brooks & Kempe, 2012; Houston, 2011; Johnson, 2012). We also know that children's speech perception is at least partially based on socially interacting with people who matter to them (Kuhl, Tsao, & Liu, 2003).

Early speech perception skills learned during typical infancy seem to be asso-

ciated with word learning by toddlers (Bosch, 2011; Cristia, Seidi, Junge, Soderstrom, & Hagoort, 2014). Even though today's hearing technology provides auditory access to all speech sounds at conversational levels, some children in AVT require further assistance to clearly hear some of these sounds. To increase the acoustic salience of spoken language, the AV practitioner uses appropriately selected *acoustic highlighting strategies* that enhance audibility of different sounds, words, or phrases and subsequently speech perception is made a little easier (Bedore & Leonard, 1995; Smith & Levitt, 1999).

Speaking Parentese

Parentese, also known as *infant-directed speech* or *motherese*, is a special speech mode that is higher-pitched, hyper-articulated, repetitive, rhythmic, and melodic and has a slower tempo than typical talking (Matsuda et al., 2011). This distinctive speaking style, characterized by exaggerated inflection and intensity as well as vowel prolongations, is universal and spoken by most caregivers in every culture, regardless of gender (van Heugten & Johnson, 2012). Parentese has inherent acoustic cues and consequently stimulates the young child's developing auditory system (Chang & Thompson, 2011). Children who hear parentese frequently become more efficient in understanding spoken language and have larger vocabularies as they mature (Weisleder & Fernald, 2013).

Children are more likely to attend to parentese (Ma, Golinkoff, Houston, & Hirsh-Pasek, 2011) and, in turn, parents tend to adjust their exaggerated inflectional and pleasant speech according to the child's developmental level. It is known that parentese facilitates both social interaction and language acquisition (Estes & Hurley, 2013; Xu, Chen, Cheng, & Ma, 2011); therefore, in different ways, the AV practitioner coaches parents to *speak parentese.*

Engaging in Vocal Play

Vocal play occurs during the prelinguistic or preverbal stage of early childhood, before toddlers say their first meaningful or recognizable words (Nathani, Ertmer, & Stark, 2006). During this stage, young children typically progress from intentional cooing and vowel utterances to "blowing raspberries" and making sounds with their lips and tongues (Kuhl & Meltzoff, 1996). It also progresses from simple babbling to more complex babbling that sounds more like the stress and intonation of their native language (Boysson-Bardies, 1999). Babbling happens when infants repeatedly alternate vowels with consonants such as "bababa" and "dadaboode" (Pettito, 2005). Finally, as children come to "know" their mother tongue, they use jargon that is babbling interspersed with some recognizable words (Saffran, Werker, & Werner, 2006).

Over the course of a year or so, vocal play results in increasingly complex, phonetically diverse, and speech-like vocalizations prior to speaking a language (Nathani et al., 2006). Because babies tend to match their vocalizations to those they hear, this vocal play becomes language-specific in that it varies from culture to culture (Kuhl & Meltzoff, 1996). The prelinguistic stage is important for building "internal phonological representations" (Narr, 2006). Adult feedback to infant babbling facilitates learning the speech patterns unique to their mother tongue (Goldstein & Schwade, 2008).

When appropriate vocal play is heard by children with cochlear implants, they perform like children with typical hearing in that they improve their own vocalizations (Ertmer & Stoel-Gammon, 2008). Research findings demonstrate that adults need to (a) reinforce and imitate their children's spontaneous vocalizations, (b) repeat the vocal play to help their children make associations between what was heard and what was said, and (c) vary their own vocal play in order to facilitate speech perception and production (Ertmer & Stoel-Gammon, 2008; Humes & Bess, 2014).

The sounds perceived and babbled by babies depend on the sounds they hear in their *linguistic environment* (Kokkinaki & Vitalaki, 2013). Therefore, as soon as hearing devices are fitted, it is important that adults provide many opportunities for the child to hear all the sounds used in their native language (Bass-Ringdahl, 2010).

Toward that end, the AV practitioner coaches parents on how to engage in vocal play with their children and, at the same time, parents learn the importance of delivering an "auditory phoneme schema" for specific sounds in their language (Pollack, 1972, p. 164). This means the child's brain receives a clear auditory imprint of those sounds that can be babbled directly into the child's ear while the parent carries the child and dances with him or her, all the while ensuring *speaking within earshot.* Playful babbling of isolated sounds can take place several times throughout the day, for a few minutes each time.

Subsequently, some children may babble and others may not (Jones,

2007). The child's babbling is not, however, the primary goal. The primary goal is to provide the child's brain with the experience of hearing native speech sounds in isolation (Sharma et al., 2004). The child is then much more likely to differentiate between sounds and to vocalize them in return (Werker & Gervain, 2013).

Associating Sounds With Objects and Words

Associative learning is one mechanism for enhancing speech perception (Kahana-Kalman & Walker-Andrews, 2001). For example, young infants learn the relationship between vocal affect and facial expressions (Kahana-Kalman & Walker-Andrews. 2001). Older infants learn to associate complex strings of speech sounds such as words with objects and actions; cognitive mechanisms affect their auditory perception of speech (Houston, 2011).

Sound-object association activities help infants and preschoolers to (a) strengthen auditory attentional focus, (b) develop an auditory imprint or brain schema for specific sounds, (c) recognize that these sounds or phonemes are different, and (d) maintain their interest while enhancing speech perception (Ertmer & Stoel-Gammon, 2008; MacKenzie, Graham, & Curtin, 2011). Furthermore, when children are repeatedly exposed to these activities, familiarity facilitates sound differentiation; this, in turn, enhances speech perception (Minagawa-Kawai, Mori, Naoi, & Kojima, 2006). Finally, this form of *symbolic learning* promotes language comprehension because the child learns to *associate meaning with each*

sound (Bernhardt, Kemp, & Werker, 2007; Monaghan, Shillcock, Christiansen, & Kirby, 2014).

For example, repeatedly saying "/b/b/b/" each time the child plays with a toy bus (the object) or sees a real bus, helps the child associate meaning with the phoneme /b/. Over a relatively short period of time, the child learns to differentiate /b/ from other phonemes such as /ah/ which was associated with a different object (an airplane). The AV practitioner can also associate particular sounds with actions that are particularly meaningful to the child, such as "/k/k/k/" with the act of coughing. Because many of these sounds can be easy for the young child to hear and say, they help the child to communicate as early as possible. These are often referred to as the *Learning to Listen Sounds* (Estabrooks, 2006) and/or *Sound-Object Associations* (Rhoades, 2007).

Rather than introducing sounds/objects in random order, it is helpful to group sound into similar categories, such as animal sounds versus vehicle sounds. Young infants categorize newly learned concepts (Hasegawa & Miyashita, 2002), and the earlier they establish a link between sounds or labels and categories, the more words they will learn; this important link facilitates cognition and furthers word learning (Ferguson, Havy, & Waxman, 2015).

Because the adult is *within earshot* every time specific sounds are associated with specific objects, the child is primed for verbal learning. The more sounds with which the child becomes familiar, the more quickly he or she will understand the words. The sounds selected need to be specific to the child's mother tongue and culture (e.g., the sound used for a barking dog varies from culture to culture). When the child spontaneously produces any of these sounds, it gives adults important information on how the sounds are perceived by the child.

Whispering

Babies and toddlers enjoy having adults *whisper* in their ears. Aside from the enjoyment, whispering can make certain sounds more acoustically salient (Kohlberger & Strycharczuk, 2015). Whispering a few inches from the child's microphone can be as loud as a shout from a distance of a few yards (Ling, 1976, p. 233). For example, whispering specific sounds, words, and/or phrases can help children hear them more easily, including high-frequency consonants such as /h/, /s/, /t/, /k/, /f/, /p/, /sh/, and /th/.

These high-frequency sounds tend to be more difficult to hear for some children who wear hearing aids (Narr, 2006), particularly those not wearing digital ones. Some children with hearing loss benefit from hearing these high-frequency consonants whispered in isolation and *within earshot*. First, consonants seem to have greater perceptual importance because they are essential to the intelligibility of words (Owren & Cardillo, 2006). Second, vowels, when voiced, carry more energy so they sound louder than high-frequency consonants, tending to mask those sounds. Third, when a sound/phoneme is not audible, the child cannot develop an auditory-based internal representation, and the likelihood of effortless phonemic production is diminished

(Narr, 2006). For these reasons, whispering select sounds and words is an important strategy in AVT.

Singing

Singing rhymes and songs is a universally pleasurable experience for children and their parents (Trehub, 2015). Singing facilitates listening skills, spoken language, speech and such cognitive skills as memory (Wang, Trehub, Volkova, & van Lieshout, 2013). Singing can also help lengthen the child's attention span and spontaneous imitation (Bergeson & Trehub, 2002) as well as facilitate parent-child interactions and social bonding (Cirelli, Wan, & Trainor, 2014).

The AV practitioner and parent encourage children with hearing loss to sing, even *when they cannot carry a tune*. The rhythmic nature of songs may play a vital role in speech fluency (Tierney & Kraus, 2015). Music can enhance the perception of pitch and the use of intonation (Marques, Moreno, Castro, & Besson, 2007). Young children in AVT can enjoy the rhythmic hand motions and gestures in such songs as "Twinkle, Twinkle, Little Star" and "The Wheels on the Bus" (Estabrooks & Birkenshaw-Fleming, 2003). Across the preschool years, listening to and rehearsing songs may help the child to memorize the words and subsequently remember all the verses while singing rhythmically. Restated, singing songs can facilitate language learning (Ludke, Ferreira, & Overy, 2014). Singing is typically integrated into AVT sessions where children can follow their parents' lead in singing and through cumulative practice they memorize the lyrics, similar to children with typical hearing (Driscoll, Gfeller. Tan, See, Cheng, & Kanemitsu, 2015).

Stressing Selected Morphemes, Syllables, Words, and Phrases

Stressed morphemes, syllables, words, and phrases are longer, louder, and higher pitched than those that are unstressed. Babies perceive stress as an acoustic cue to learning about word boundaries and figuring out the patterns of spoken language (Thiessen & Saffran, 2007). The AV practitioner refers to this strategy as another form of *acoustic highlighting* because it helps the child to hear particular features of language more clearly. This assigns "perceptual salience" to the morpheme, syllable, word, or phrase selected by the practitioner; the linguistic element is brought to the child's *focused auditory attention* (Pruden, Hirsh-Pasek, Golinkoff, & Hennon, 2006).

Examples of linguistic elements that AV practitioners often stress include

- the /s/ morpheme in Mario's to help the child learn about the possessive feature;
- the first syllable in *bron*tosaurus to help the child understand how this word differs from *brach*iosaurus;
- the word /*this*/ versus /*that*/ to help the child recognize the difference between the two articles within the same grammatical category; and
- the phrase /*no more*/ after the child has finished eating.

Just as stressing phonemes enhances speech perception (Narr, 2006), stressing linguistic features enhances language

learning and cognition (Mastropavlou, 2010; Pedale & Santangelo, 2015).

GOAL 4: Promote Knowledge of Language

Strategies

- Focusing on the "knowing" rather than the "using"
- Taking turns
- Imitating the child's early vocalizations
- Verbalizing in synchrony with movement
- Speaking the language from the child's angle
- Talking before, during, and after the action
- Pausing for grammatical spaces or emphasis
- Transitioning beyond the comfort zone
- Connecting the familiar to the unfamiliar
- Recasting, expanding, and expatiating on the child's words
- Emphasizing actions, relations, and attributes
- Contrasting the meaning of words

The goal of promoting familiarity with a spoken language can occur only if the child demonstrates focused auditory attention. Historically, parents were often given the generic advice of talking all the time to their children, but evidence shows this is not enough. *How* parents interact with their child also matters. The AV practitioner helps parents by supporting them in their child-directed verbal input—both in quality and quantity (Rowe, 2012). Likewise, knowing when *not* to talk is important. Adult-controlled pauses are known to structure and regulate language learning. Toward that end, the effective use of interactive silences is significant in AVT. The following strategies used by the AV practitioner are only part of an exhaustive list that might be shared with parents.

Focusing on the "Knowing" Rather Than the "Using"

Linguistic competence is typically attained by children between 3 and 4 years of age (Pinker, 1994). This means that very young children with typical hearing understand their native language by the time they are of preschool age. As long as the adult's vocabulary level is kept to the child's known vocabulary level, an adult can easily converse with preschoolers. Young children are able to independently detect and figure out the patterns of spoken language (Aslin & Newport, 2012), even when they might not have intelligible speech.

When a child *knows* a spoken language, he or she *comprehends* it. Typical 2-year-old children know about three times as many words as they actually say (Tomasello, 2003). The child who demonstrates linguistic competence is able to understand complex sentences and stories and to follow multistep verbal directions. Moreover, the preschooler with typical hearing intuitively understands the appropriate placement of grammatical categories having to do with pronouns, prepositions, adjectives, verb tenses, and articles (Arunachalam & Waxman, 2010). Day-to-day communication is possible. Of course, as children mature, their knowledge of grammar becomes more complex (Gao,

Zelazo, Sharpe, & Mashari, 2014). Rather than expressive language, early receptive language skills are good predictors of later language performance (Hay-McCutcheon, Kirk, Henning, Gao, & Qi, 2008).

Some children with hearing loss, however, are often unfortunately judged by what they say rather than by what they understand. Young children's comprehension of spoken language is far more important than their production of it (Duff, Reen, Plunkett, & Nation, 2015; Rescorla, 2009). *It is critical that the AV practitioner continuously guide parents to understand that "knowledge always precedes use" and that the number of words a child comprehends far exceeds the number of words produced.* In fact, a problem presents itself when a child says all that he knows; he or she will then have no *reservoir* of words from which to draw. Moreover, this reflects atypical, unnatural language development (Junge, Koojiman, Haggort, & Cutler, 2012). Children typically accumulate a considerable "storage bank" of word knowledge before they withdraw from it and start using it. Indeed, many children with typical hearing do not say more than a few words until they are 2 years of age, yet they "know" syntactic structure when listening to spoken language (Bernal, Dehaene-Lambertz, Millotte, & Christophe, 2010).

The AV practitioner ensures that parental expectations are high, realistic, and fair. In general, during the first year of hearing with hearing technology, children internalize the sounds of their native language and the rules of word order (Benasich, Choudhury, Realpe-Bonilla, & Roesler, 2014). During the second year, the child usually figures out the grammatical patterns of the language that is heard; this is when young children begin producing words combinations (Ferguson, Graf, & Waxman, 2014; Yang, 2006). When parents understand this, they are far more likely to focus on the "knowing" rather than the "using" of spoken language. Although this can be a difficult concept for some parents who are anxious to hear their child talk, the importance of this strategy cannot be overstated.

The AV practitioner and parent give voice to the child who has not yet developed a spoken language. Perhaps the practitioner noticed a subtle silent interaction that occurred between parent and child—that is, the child made a subtle eye or slight touch contact with the parent who automatically (perhaps unconsciously) responded to the child's cue by quietly doing something for the child. Because many parents new to AVT are not aware of these "wordless exchanges," the AV practitioner immediately informs the parents what he or she just observed and then demonstrates alternative ways of responding to the child, always using spoken language. Restated, the AV practitioner promotes change by bringing "wordless exchanges" to the parent's attention, in order to instill the habit of voicing each interaction with the child. Although the child does not yet talk, this enables parents to help their children "know" the spoken language.

Taking Turns

Turn-taking between the parent and child with typical hearing begins at birth (Gratier, 2003). When the parent talks, the newborn child stills and listens. When the parent stops talking,

the child moves. This turn-taking, measured in milliseconds, reflects mutual reciprocity or parent-infant coordination known as *interactional synchrony*. Taking turns gives the child *the power of being*, facilitates joint attention, and minimizes interruptions (Stanton-Chapman & Snell, 2011). This occurs across all cultures (Leclère, Viaux, Avril, Achard, Chetouani, Missonnier, & Cohen, 2014).

The child learns to embrace the turn-taking skill of listening, then talking, then listening, then talking. Taking turns is also one of the child's first steps toward attaining social competence (Stanton-Chapman & Snell, 2011). Even the toddler who does not have access to sound can take turns in all activities. The child learns to wait for his turn after the AV practitioner presents an item in a play activity. Equally important, the child also learns that when it is his turn, he will be able to freely manipulate the item for at least a few minutes.

Imitating the Child's Early Vocalizations

When the AV practitioner imitates what the young child says, he or she provides positive feedback by attending to the child and showing the young child that his communicative behavior is heard, acknowledged, and understood (Bovey & Strain, 2005). Imitating (echoing) what the child says, whether it is babbling or jargon, also promotes joint attention and turn taking, leading to social engagement (Farrant, Maybery, & Fletcher, 2011). Most importantly, because adult imitations reinforce what the child says, the child receives *auditory feedback* that encourages further vocalizations and further adult imitations. This ongoing turn-taking results in verbal expansions and is sometimes referred to as an expanding auditory-vocal spiral (Kuhl, 2004).

Interestingly, imitations can also facilitate language comprehension (Adank, Hagoort, & Bekkering, 2010). When parent-child verbal interactions are insufficient, the child may have a difficult time figuring out the patterns of language. In turn, this can lead to the child exhibiting language delays (Barker et al, 2009). So, it is important then, that the AV practitioner demonstrates ways to respond, *appropriately and often,* to the young child's attempts at communicating by *imitating early vocalizations.*

Verbalizing in Synchrony With Movement

The brain's mirror neuron system is tri-modal in that it integrates motor, visual, and auditory information. The processing of spoken language is linked to motor system activity in the brain (James & Maouene, 2009). Embedded in social interactions, the acquisition of spoken language is typically a layered process (Vigliocco, Perniss, & Vinson, 2014). Synchrony in the acquisition of information can facilitate more rapid learning (Lau & Salzman, 2009).

Because this cross-modal learning does not occur among young children without sufficient access to hearing, their brains are reorganized differently (Li et al,. 2012); hence, they learn differently (Marschark, Spencer, Adams, & Sapere, 2011). Lack of integration between seeing, hearing, and doing can affect language and social development as well as learning in general (Le Bel, Pineda, & Sharma, 2009).

When adults talk about what they do, children can learn language when *what they hear is time-synchronized with what they see,* particularly in terms of action-based behaviors (Macrae, Duffy, Miles, & Lawrence, 2008). This has been referred to as "language-action synchrony" (Rhoades, 2010). For example, when popping bubbles, the AV practitioner might say, "Pop!" at the same time that the child actually pops the bubble. Such synchronization may increase the child's attention to what was said in addition to facilitating a pattern of recognition of the acoustic event; this relates especially to action verbs (Bahrick & Lickliter, 2009; Gogate, Bahrick, & Watson, 2000).

Speaking the Language From the Child's Angle

Every child's behavior is a communicative message that the adult verbalizes for the child (Olson & Masur, 2013). To avoid having the child feel that spoken language is irrelevant, the parent's language needs to be meaningful, purposeful, and age-appropriate for the child.

The AV practitioner puts into words what the child's gestures, eye gazes, and vocalizations are trying to communicate. This *parallel talk*, found to be a predictor of later language functioning, means the adult talks about *what the child wants to say* rather than what the adult wants the child to say. It is important for the adult to try looking at the world through the child's eyes (Cruz, Quittner, Marker, & DesJardin, 2013).

By following the child's lead, the AV practitioner engages in "follow-in" speech and strives to understand what the child has seen, heard, and/or done and how the child feels. When the practitioner recognizes the child's interests, he or she talks about how the child is experiencing the world, using words that give rich meaning to the child's experiences (Yoder, McCathren, Warren, & Watson, 2001). As the child gains listening and spoken language skills, the parent listens closely to the child's utterances, and indicates that what he or she says is important. Parents learn not to interrupt when the child is talking, even if they do not understand what the child says. They also learn to imitate the child's sounds, actions, words, or sentences, and then to wait and see what the child does next.

During an AVT session, the child may point to an object that is somewhat related to the activity. Rather than ignoring what the child indicated, the AV practitioner takes advantage of the spontaneous diversion by verbally relating what was observed to the activity they are all doing. For example, during clean-up time, a feather in a box captures the child's interest and she says, "Bee!" Instead of ignoring the child's verbal attempt while cleaning up the toys and putting them in the box, the AV practitioner leans in and say, "Oh, you think this is a bee? No, it's not a bee; it's just a feather! Do you want to blow the feather out of the box?"

Talking Before, During, and After the Action

Lexical *knowledge* (the corpus of words understood by a young child) is associated with listening and word learning (Florit, Roch, Altoe & Levorato, 2009; Gray & Brinkley, 2011). The more words understood by a child, the more likely the child will rapidly learn new words

(Lederberg & Spencer, 2009). The size of a child's lexicon is a predictor of language and academic learning (Bishop & Adams, 2006). Therefore, practitioners and parents need to promote vocabulary expansion for children with hearing loss, as rapidly as possible.

Word learning, the process of acquiring a lexicon, is an indicator of the child's ability to understand or produce a word after repeated exposures in a supported learning context (Bobzien et al., 2015; Gray, 2004). Repetition, a feature of *parentese*, is integral to vocabulary acquisition (Newman, Rowe, & Ratner, in press). However, due to the effects of background noise, this feature may be even more important for children with hearing loss since their prior exposure to words may have been compromised (Blaiser, Nelson, & Kohnert, 2015).

The AV practitioner talks *before* the action. This allows the child to anticipate what the adult may be holding, what will happen, and when the activity will stop. Talking before acting encourages the child to listen to the adult's spoken language without attention being diverted elsewhere (Southgate, Chevalier, & Csibra, 2009). For example, the adult may have a toy in a paper bag and before opening it, says, "I have a toy in here." The adult looks in the bag without letting the child see it, and says, "Yes, my toy is in here. It's a wind-up monkey. Do you want to see it?" Then the child looks in the bag and can play with the toy while the practitioner narrates what the child is doing. The adult's repeated spoken language is given meaning. Similarly, the AV practitioner talks *after* the action is completed; this provides both repetition and support for the meaning of the message already heard. "We jumped up and down, up and down. Jumping was so much fun. But I'm tired now. No more jumping."

Pausing for Grammatical Spaces or Stress Markers

This refers to two specific types of deliberate adult-controlled silences known as the phrasal intraturn pause and the impact pause. Both pauses occur within a language-based activity, serving as listening prompts that cue the child to pay attention to the message of the spoken language. Both promote language learning by having silences effectively bracket meaningful language (Rowe & Rowe, 2006). In turn, this facilitates auditory attention, language growth, cognitive skills, and academic learning (Vassilopoulos & Konstantinidis, 2012). Neither type of pause is used to elicit vocal response from the child.

The first type of pause reflects a natural rest in the melody of spoken language to indicate *grammatical spaces* like the end of such linguistic units as phrases or sentences (Carey-Sargeant & Brown, 2003). The strategic placement of this pause cues the child to pay special attention to the word, phrase, or sentence that follows, or to think about what was just said. When deliberate silences serve as discourse markers, they can help the child understand what was heard (Yeldham & Gruba, 2014). Young children with hearing loss tend to require longer pause lengths to process linguistic information (Carey-Sargeant & Brown, 2003).

The second type of adult-controlled silence is the *impact pause*. Often used as a strategy when reading a story to children, this deliberate silence helps them recognize an important or new word or key phrase, or to wait in suspension for the next thought (Stahl, 1994). Impact pauses act as *stress markers* by giving the child time to think about what was or will be said. The child is not expected to provide a verbal response. Stressed words may help the child construct meaning from what was heard (Yeldham & Gruba, 2014).

The AV practitioner helps the child understand grammatical boundaries and promotes anticipation of a new word or linguistic unit just before verbalizing it (Read, Macauley, & Furay, 2014). For example, the practitioner tells the child, "This morning, I spilled my juice on the floor. (*pause*) I was so upset. (*pause*) The carpet was soiled (*stress new word and then pause*) and I did not know what to do. (*pause*) What do you think I did next?" This will be followed by a much longer pause. An incidental benefit of these pauses is that the child may use those moments of silence to offer suggestions or ask questions.

Transitioning Beyond the Comfort Zone

The child's *comfort zone* is the language level at which he or she currently *understands* with relative ease (Mercer, Ryan, & Williams, 2012). Parents typically talk within that comfort zone because it is safe, easy, and quick. In early sessions of AVT, the AV practitioner's language is also mostly tuned to the child's comfort zone. Shortly thereafter, however, the AV practitioner guides the parent to *raise the bar* or *up the ante* (Chaiklin, 2003; Wasik, Bond, & Hindman, 2006). Change forces growth. This means the language spoken to the child must become a bit more complex so the child can build his or her language knowledge. For example, when a child demonstrates understanding of a phrase like "Throw it away," the AV practitioner demonstrates using a different linguistic unit or phrase such as, "Please throw this in the can over there." This 1 plus 2 rule adds two new "bits" to the one "bit" that the child already knows.

If the child can remember two items when asked to get them from the basket across the room, the parent adds more to the mix, so that the child remembers even more. If the child can take two turns in conversation, the practitioner then demonstrates ways to take three turns. And if the child can identify an *item by description*, then the practitioner moves toward identification of an item with more attributes. The AV practitioner consistently encourages parents to transition beyond their usual ways of using language to reflect ongoing change and growth.

Connecting the Familiar to the Unfamiliar

The AV practitioner provides back-up support for the child's acquisition of new words by connecting the old with the new. Because the adult understands what the child already knows, the adult is the bridge between the known word and the unknown word and provides a "lexical hook." The parent provides a new word for an already-known one. For example, a father might say, "Let's go in my car (child knows this word). I got a new car. It's a convertible (new word to child). How about a drive in my convertible?" Adults clarify or 'bridge' new words with the old. This helps *expand* a child's vocabulary (Callanan & Sabbagh, 2004).

Recasting, Expanding, and Expatiating on the Child's Words

It is important that adults provide feedback in the form of good language models when young children produce their first words, phrases, and sentences. As long as the child's intended meaning is preserved, adults can recast, rephrase, paraphrase, or otherwise expand on the child's utterances to improve the child's knowledge and use of language (Proctor-Williams, Fey, & Loeb, 2001; Strapp & Federico, 2000). This means that adults do not tell children that their sentences are wrong (White, Livesey, & Hayes, 2015).

For example, the child says, "dada bye-bye." There are at least three ways to provide the child with feedback:

- *Recast:* restate the child's utterance into a different format, such as a question format, e.g., "Is daddy going bye-bye?"
- *Expand:* repeat the child's utterance but in a more grammatical and complete way without modifying the child's word order or intended meaning, e.g., "Yes, daddy is now going bye-bye."
- *Expatiate:* expand on the child's utterance, but with the addition of new information, e.g., "Yes, daddy is going bye-bye. Daddy has to go to work. Daddy will come home later. We'll miss him. See you later daddy!"

Feedback can be in the form of adding more information or just a word, or providing a complete grammatical structure (Cruz et al., 2013; Dunst et al., 2011; Wasik et al., 2006). Regardless, the adult provides a more complex form of language modeling than that of the child, without requiring the child to repeat anything.

Emphasizing Actions, Relations, and Attributes

Toddlers typically understand the grammar of their native language (Bernal et al., 2010). This means babies begin figuring out the grammatical rules so they later know how to put words together; this is often referred to as *connected language*. The three grammatical word categories that are critical for young children to understand are verbs, prepositions, and adjectives. These word types seem universal in that they interest babies across all cultures (Tomasello, 2003). Furthermore, these word types reflect language that emphasizes words and concepts needed for academic success (cognition), such as prepositions for spatial understanding and adjectives for categorical learning (Henninger, 2013; Weikart, Rogers, Adcock, & McClelland, 1971).

Action-based verbs are among the easiest category of words for young children to understand, especially when they are engaged in doing something (Twomey, Lush, Pearce, & Horst, 2014; Waxman, Fu, Arunachalam, Leddon, Geraghty, & Song, 2013). In AVT during purposeful play, the adults use sentences that include labeling the child's action while in progress (Syrett, Arunachalam, & Waxman, 2014). Because language tends to be action based, and the AV sessions are delivered through purposeful play, or real-life activities, the adults in the child's life have multiple opportunities to model many verbs (Bergen & Wheeler, 2010).

Grammatically speaking, adjectives tend to be dependent on nouns and verbs. Nevertheless, adjectives are descriptive words that can matter more to children, particularly when they are easily observable or experienced (Booth & Waxman, 2009). For example, the AV practitioner describes how things feel, sound, look, or move, for example, "Mmmmm, this feels so SOFT!" or "Wow, that is HOT!"

Prepositions, known as functional words, are typically understood before the end of infancy (Shi, 2014). The frequent use of prepositions occurs when adults talk about the relation of the child to something. This is referred to as spatial relations. The AV practitioner places a little more stress on prepositions when children are moving in, on, and around items, for example, "It's UNDER the chair."

When adults model spoken language for a child with hearing loss, both quality and quantity matter. Children learn by what they hear, remember, and recall, and they discover their native language by figuring out the rules and word order, like little investigators. Children determine the linguistic patterns when they hear the way adults use action verbs, prepositions, and adjectives (Tomasello, 2003). Toward that end, rather than stressing nouns, parents are encouraged to *acoustically highlight action verbs, prepositions, and adjectives* (Yin & Csibra, 2015).

Contrasting the Meaning of Words

Children come to understand the meaning of words more easily and precisely when *polar opposites* are brought to their attention (Bellon-Harn, Credeur-Pampolina, & LeBoeuf, 2013). In other words, a child can more easily understand the meaning of "hot" when contrasted to the word "cold" (Tomasello, 2003). To fully understand a word's meaning, it helps to understand what it is and what it is not. So, the AV practitioner makes concerted efforts to facilitate word learning by using words that contrast in meaning, for example, "This is so BIG; that one is NOT big. That one is little." and "My hair is STRAIGHT, but yours is CURLY."

GOAL 5: Facilitate Spoken Language and Cognition

Strategies

- Leaning forward with expectant looks
- Signaling with objects
- Providing self-statements
- Asking "What did you hear?"
- Waiting for the child's response
- Promoting auditory-verbal closure
- Asking stage-appropriate questions
- Scaffolding for language production

The AV practitioner uses a variety of strategies to elicit targeted verbal behaviors. Some strategies cited here consist of "actions" that are often referred to as prompting or prompts (see Goal 2). *Prompting* is the act of assisting or encouraging a child to perform an action such as giving a verbal response. In general, language prompts are used to initiate a series of interrelated language-based actions (Hayes, 2014). The selection of types of prompts and their

frequency of use, which decreases over time, depend on the child's stage of development and his or her responses to previously used prompts. Among these prompts is the use of interactive silences; the types of deliberate silences used as strategies for this goal specifically structure and regulate verbal interactions between adults and children (Damron & Morman, 2011).

Leaning Forward With Expectant Looks

Leaning forward to the child and/or parent and *looking expectantly* are nonverbal prompts used by the AV practitioner to model listening behaviors, encourage and establish joint attention, and signal the child and/or parent that a verbal response is expected. Leaning forward is a posture shift that is frequently used at the beginning of a conversation (Cassell, Nakano, Bickmore, Sidner, & Rich, 2001). If a child is looking at a book and points at a picture of a favorite toy and looks at the parent, the *parent leans in and looks as if he or she is waiting for the child to say something.*

This prompt is often used in conjunction with *eyebrow raising/lowering,* and *head nodding.* Guaïtella and colleagues (2009) found that eyebrow movements serve as an attention-getting device and play a role in turn-taking. Eyebrow raises also occur with questions, directions, and explanations, and signal that a verbal or nonverbal response is expected (Flecha-Garcia, 2010). The parent may say, "What happened to your shoes?" and wait. If the child does not respond, the parent leans forward, and looks expectantly at the child.

Adults make regular use of declarative questions such as, "Is this a ball?"

in their conversations with preschool children (Estigarribia, 2010). Typically, this question is initially accompanied by three features: (a) prosodic cues, such as the rising terminal pitch; (b) contextual cues, such as the object noted in the question; and (c) visual or facial cues such as raised eyebrows (Frota, Butler, & Vigário, 2014; Gunlogson, 2003; Srinivasan & Massaro, 2003). Without the presence of these three supplementary cues, preschoolers do not understand the question requires a yes/no response (Saindon, Trehub, Schellenberg, & Van Lieshout, in press). When the child responds appropriately to declarative questions with all features present, then the practitioner removes the visual cues. This facilitates the child's transition to listening for prosodic cues and comprehension of the question form.

Verbal fillers such as "hmm," "um," and "uh" may be used with facial or visual prompts. These "placeholders" or "unglossable syllables" seem to help children attend more to the words that immediately follow (Peters, 2001). These fillers also serve a grammatical function in conversation as well as benefit language comprehension (Barr & Seyfeddinipur, 2010). A verbal filler such as "um" can induce an anticipation effect, causing listeners to expect new information.

For example, the AV practitioner knows that the child wants to play with a particular toy in the therapy room because the child is looking at it with a look of anticipation. The AV practitioner rubs his chin and says, "Hmm" and waits expectantly. The child may then say, "Bubbles!" But if not, the AV practitioner may murmur "Um" again to get the child's attention and to let the child know that the practitioner is waiting for something to be said.

Signaling With Objects

As they learn language, young children are sensitive to the gestures of others in conversational situations (Iverson & Goldin-Meadow, 2005). This signaling strategy involves *using an object as a physical cue or prompt to signal the child that it is his turn to talk.* Some examples are toy microphones or symbolic representations such as cardboard tubes. This turn-taking prompt informs the child that a sound, word, or phrase needs to be imitated or initiated.

For example, the AV practitioner uses one of the aforementioned prompts, such as leaning forward and looking expectantly, to elicit a verbal response. But, if this is unsuccessful, the practitioner repeats the prompt with the addition of a physical item that is directed toward the parent, who models the targeted response. The physical item is then directed to the child who typically imitates the parent's model. Over time, signaling with objects decreases.

Providing Self-Statements

Verbal self-disclosure has been highlighted in the literature as an encouraging way for individuals to share their own thoughts and feelings, hence promoting verbal interaction between people (Ignatius & Kokkonen, 2007). In AVT, the child may make spontaneous statements in response to the AV practitioner's self-statements (Urry, Nelson, & Padilla-Walker, 2011). Simply described, the adult might begin the sentence with an "I" statement such as "I feel like singing."

For example, if a child points to a bottle of bubbles, and says, "Eh!", the AV practitioner may say, "You want those bubbles!" This provides a verbal model that matches the gesture and vocalization. Then the adult follows with a self-statement such as, "I want those bubbles too!" Or, at a slightly more advanced language level, the adult might say, "I have that at home, and it's one of my favorite toys!"

This strategy is dependent on the adult's willingness to trust that the child will continue the conversation by making an utterance. Increasing the use of self-statements, and moving away from direct questions, increases the child's willingness to converse with adults (Power, Wood, Wood, & Macdougall, 1990). Some children are passive communicators because they previously felt pressured to talk or because they felt like they were often being tested. This strategy, like all those in this chapter, helps the child become an *active communicator.*

The difference between modeling and providing self-statements is the tone of voice and the intent of the speaker, with self-statements sometimes sounding more humorously argumentative. When adults share their own thoughts and feelings, they promote the child's social skills (Moll & Meltzoff, 2011) and the child is encouraged to *think outside of the self* and to realize that others may have different perspectives.

Asking, "What Did You Hear?"

Sometimes the child with hearing loss quickly responds by saying, "What?" when an adult says something that the child does not fully understand. Rather than coaching the parent to automatically repeat the stimulus, the AV practitioner encourages the parent to ask, *"What did you hear?"* This encourages the child to *think about what was said,*

process the information, and then repeat those parts that were heard or understood. In turn, this can help the child use his or her linguistic knowledge to "fill in the missing pieces." This can help the child to develop listening skills that facilitate language comprehension, and make predictions based on key words he or she understood (Yeldham & Gruba, 2014).

Promoting Auditory-Verbal Closure

The development of spoken language is dependent on many factors, including cognitive skills, including working memory (Wingfield, & Tun, 2007). Cognitive skills play an even greater role for children with hearing loss because they often need to understand spoken language when the auditory input is compromised by background noise, conversations with people who speak very quietly, with imperfect diction or with a dialect. Prior knowledge of language and the topic of conversation are two factors that play a role in how well speech is understood within a sentence or longer linguistic units. These factors provide contextual and linguistic cues for understanding (Shafiro, Sheft, Gygi, & Ho, 2012).

The redundancy of language permits the child to engage in statistical learning—that is, to figure out what makes sense given that word order is based on rules where specific words are used repetitively. Practice in remembering sentences and then completing them when the sentences are incomplete can help the child's speech perception in noisy environments (Shafiro et al., 2012). Although this strategy enhances speech perception (Goal 3), it also facilitates spoken language and cognition in that the child is prompted to practice talking using a completed linguistic unit.

When the child is asked to infer missing words within sentences, the semantic and syntactic context provide cues to the missing words. This means the child is asked to complete the perceptual whole from incomplete language information (Gallun, Mason, & Kidd, 2007). This is a modified version of the cloze procedure used for the comprehension of printed language (e.g., Sharp, 2009). So, for purposes of this goal, the strategy to facilitate sentence completion is referred to as *auditory-verbal closure*: the child's ability to fill in missing portions of the spoken message based on prior knowledge and familiarity of the language and topic (Hannemann, Obleser, & Eulitz, 2007). This top-down processing strategy signals the child that it is his or her turn to finish the message,

Toddlers with typical hearing can be prompted with this *auditory-verbal closure* strategy in games such as "Peek-a-boo. I see ---!" Preschoolers can complete the last part of many well-known phrases, as in the story about the three little pigs: "He huffed and he puffed and he ---." Children who complete such tasks are able to predict the missing target word(s) or sound(s) based on context and prior knowledge of the spoken language (Pickering & Garrod, 2006).

Similarly the AV practitioner can sing a song familiar to the child, and then stop just before completing it. Concurrently, toward the end of the song, the practitioner *leans in toward the child and pauses*. If the child remembers the song, the child "fills in the blank." If the child does not complete

this task, then the practitioner redirects attention to the parent, repeats the rhyme or song in the same way, and the parent responds appropriately. The final step is that the AV practitioner repeats it with the child again. By this time, the child typically "gets it" and is able to complete the task. Both parent and child end up *feeling successful*. The AV practitioner can repeatedly use this strategy of *auditory-verbal closure* in relatively quiet environments. Over time, background noise can be gradually increased to make the task more difficult.

Waiting for Child's Response

Wait-time occurs after the AV practitioner asks a child a question. It is the length of undisturbed time that an adult waits for a child's response (Rowe, 1996). The child's response may come in the form of a single word, phrase, or connected language. Wait-times give the child opportunities to decode the meaning of the question (Stephenson, Carter, & Arthur-Kelly, 2011). Extended wait-times tend to be associated with positive responses and improved language learning (Brown & Wragg, 1993; Al-Balushi, 2009).

After a question is posed to the child with typical hearing, the undisturbed waiting time should *not* be less than 5 seconds (Gabel, 2004; Skinner, Pappas, & Davis, 2005). The wait-time, however, may need to be considerably longer for some children with hearing loss (Rowe & Rowe, 2006). The length of wait-time time is dependent on such factors such as linguistic complexity of the question and expected response, the child's developmental level, and auditory processing capacities as well as environmental noise level (Maroni, 2011). Because young children with hearing loss may not hear or understand the entire question, they may need more wait-time to fill in the missing pieces of the linguistic unit, known as "auditory perceptual restoration" (Winstone, Davis, & DeBruyn, 2012; Zekveld, Kramer, & Festen, 2011).

When the AV practitioner directs a question to a child, there is usually a prosodic cue (inflectional rise) at the end; this imposes a social obligation for the child to respond (Heeman, Lunsford, Selfridge, Black, & van Santen, 2010). A review of the literature shows that such self-controlled silences elicit many positive outcomes that include sustained auditory attention and increased linguistic-cognitive growth (Rhoades, 2013).

Asking Stage-Appropriate Questions

Questions can be viewed as either closed-ended or open-ended. An example of a simple closed-ended question is when an adult points at either a picture or object, and asks the child, "What is it?" Closed-end questions typically request one-word responses, such as the name of something, or a yes/no response. Adults who frequently ask closed-ended questions of children with hearing loss tend to take control of the verbal exchanges and the child often feels pressure, and subsequently is less likely to engage in conversations (Power et al., 1990).

Questions typically involve the prosodic cue of rising intonation (Maroni, 2011). Infants with typical hearing are sensitive to prosodic cues that differentiate questions from statements (Frota et al., 2014). Based on this information

as well as contextual and visual cues, children eventually learn when questions are being asked. When asking a question, the AV practitioner usually looks directly at the child (a sustained gaze). Children with hearing loss and well-programmed hearing devices can also learn to recognize questions as a vehicle for obtaining information early in the process of *learning to listen.*

The AV practitioner begins asking open-ended questions during story time at the 1- to 2-year age of language acquisition when the use of closed-end questions is considerably decreased. Open-ended questions require much more from the child in that they necessitate more thoughtful, descriptive responses. Parents typically ask questions to probe and, in doing so, seek to improve their child's thinking and language skills (Rowland, Pine, Lieven, & Theakston, 2003; Weizman & Snow, 2001). The more open-ended questions adults ask, the more likely there will be growth in the child's use of spoken language (Cruz et al., 2013).

For example, when the AV practitioner asks a preschooler an open-ended question such as, "Why is the wolf angry?" or "How did the frog get hurt?" or "What do you think will happen next?" the child is more likely to reply verbally in creative or descriptive ways than with a close-ended response.

When first using this strategy, parents may need to respond *for* their children. When an open-ended question is directed to the child, the child may look to the parent for help, and the parent will respond to the question. However, as soon as the child demonstrates improved language production, the parent needs to stop speaking for the child. The AV practitioner also coaches the parent to *avoid looking at the child* during such moments. Instead, the parent learns to visually focus on the practitioner and not to "rescue" the child unless requested to do so. Using this strategy, the child has time to think and respond, correctly or not.

Scaffolding for Language Production

Scaffolding is a process designed to promote a deeper level of learning. It is support tailored to each child's needs with the intention of helping that child achieve the session objectives and communication goals (Sawyer, 2006). Scaffolding involves interaction between the adult and child, whereby the adult can model and give subtle advice in helping the child build upon existing skills. Scaffolding can be in the form of verbal or nonverbal prompts; it is temporary in the provision of help and then in the gradual weaning of adult help. The goal is independent learning (Bransford, Brown, & Cocking, 2000; Reingold, Rimor, & Kalay, 2008).

Scaffolding takes place when the AV practitioner completes the first parts of a complex or long sequence of actions and then encourages the child to perform only the last action. After several turns at this, the practitioner begins doing less of the actions, encouraging the child to do a bit more each time until the entire sequence is completed by the child. For example, a child may attempt to put a multishaped puzzle piece back into its place but has difficulty lining the piece up with the shape of the space. The adult slowly turns the piece so that it matches up with the space, and waits for the child to push the piece into place. With the

next puzzle piece, the adult will put the piece next to the space with it turned askew. The child turns the piece slightly and pushes it into place. With the following piece, the adult places it next to the space, with the piece turned halfway around. The child then turns the piece around and pushes it into place. This process is repeated until the child gains the confidence to complete the puzzle independently. Restated, scaffolding is *the part that the adult does for the child* until the child is able to accomplish the task independently. This systematic strategy can occur on both verbal and nonverbal activities.

This strategy applies when the adult encourages the child to use longer utterances. If the child only verbalizes part of a message, the AV practitioner models the missing part. Over time, as the child gains more linguistic skills, there is a gradual decrease in adult modeling and in the amount of scaffolding and prompting.

GOAL 6: Stimulate Independent Learning

Strategies

- Pretending objects are something else
- Creating the unexpected
- Talking with imaginary friends
- Accepting and making mistakes

It is important that children *want* to participate in AVT sessions. Therefore, each AVT session includes activities that are playful, intentional, and intrinsically motivating for young children. In general, play stresses the means over the ends, tending to involve self-selective, variable, and nonstereotyped behaviors (Pelligrini, Dupuis, & Smith, 2007). Play is the "work" of children, and it is the fundamental means by which children gather and process information, learn new skills, and practice old ones (Ginsburg, 2007). Regardless of hearing status, play is enjoyable, meaningful, and goal oriented so that the child can discover solutions to problems (Conway, Bauernschmidt, Huang, & Pisoni, 2010; Tomasello, 2003). Through play, adults can implement many of the strategies cited here to facilitate listening and spoken language skills within the contexts of daily life.

Guided play is child-directed and planned learning; it lies midway between direct instruction and free play, presenting a learning goal, and scaffolding the environment while allowing children to maintain a large degree of control over their learning (Weisberg, Hirsh-Pasek, & Golinkoff, 2013). This is the means by which children *learn how to learn* during AVT sessions. As stated throughout this chapter, the AV practitioner uses and demonstrates strategies that facilitate goal-directed problem solving, referred to as *advanced cognitive capacities* (Blair & Razza, 2007; Bodrova & Leong, 2001).

Guided and pretend play provide wonderful opportunities for promoting positive parent-child interactions (Brown & Remine, 2004). The AV practitioner carefully observes how parents play with their children and guides them to adjust their play styles to match the needs and skills of the child. Parents learn to take advantage of spontaneous moments and are coached how to embed language learning strategies into playful interactions.

Pretending Objects Are Something Else

Symbolic play is the ability of children to use objects, actions, or ideas to represent other objects, actions, or ideas in their play activities. Symbolic play promotes cognitive development and is viewed as a precursor to literacy (Potter, 1996; Smith, 2007). A banana held up to the ear can be used as a make-believe telephone. A block being pushed around on the floor becomes a train. Running on a broom becomes horseback riding. A child makes noises with his baby toys by banging them together and shaking them.

The AV practitioner incorporates symbolism into shared play to promote joint attention, self-awareness, creativity, and spoken language (Lewis & Ramsay, 2004). When parents actively participate in pretending things are other things, higher levels of child pretend play tend to follow (Brown & Remine, 2004).

Creating the Unexpected

A novel item, activity or event that defies expectations or occurs in unexpected ways is easily remembered, encourages attentional focus, and is fun for the child (Mather & Plunkett, 2012; Stahl & Feigenson, 2015). The element of surprise, a violation of expectations, enhances learning and exploration. Experiencing something out of the ordinary can facilitate verbal language (Jarvis, 2005). The disappearing coin or ball is a simple magic trick that exemplifies how a toy elicits a surprise reaction from young children. The use of magic in play-based activities tends to facilitate cognitive growth (Woolley & Ghossainy, 2013).

For example, a child did not seem to understand the preposition "under" no matter what his mother did, so one day his father told him they were going to eat lunch *under* a table. When they did, the child was initially startled and, after his dad repeatedly noted they were eating *under* a table, the child learned the meaning of that preposition.

Some AV practitioners refer to facilitating the unexpected as *sabotage*, the "accidentally-on-purpose messing up of something" (Robbins, 2000). The AV practitioner observes if the child notices the error and then helps the child understand the violation of expectation as well as verbalizes the situation. Sabotage is simply one way to create the element of surprise for something that was unexpected.

For example, a preschooler may watch TV for an hour every day, while the parent is preparing dinner. One day, the parent decides to "create a language learning opportunity" by disconnecting the TV when the child is not looking. Later, the child anxiously runs into the kitchen saying, "TV! TV!" The parent responds, "Yes, the TV is in the living room. Go turn it on." The child frantically repeats what he just said, and the parent continues *faking it*, repeating what *she* just said. "I know, you said that. Turn the TV on. I know you want to watch it."

This exchange may occur a few times, but before the child becomes too frustrated, the parent says, "Hmmm . . . something must be wrong. Let's see what the problem is. OK, there's the TV. Now turn it on." The child turns it on and nothing happens. The parent says, "Oh, you mean the TV is *not working!* Oh my goodness, the TV is *not working!* Ah, I see the plug is *not* in the socket. Let's put the plug *in* the socket. Turn on the TV now. Is the TV *working?* Yes, the TV is *working* now. It's *not* broken."

Initially, the adult acts unaware of the problem, and waits for the child to react to it. When the child does make it known that something is wrong, a parent-child conversation takes place about the *problem* and how to fix it. Children enjoy exploring the potential outcomes of problems. Examples of parent-created novel situations or sabotage are as follows:

- Give the child a broken pencil.
- Pour cereal in a glass instead of a bowl.
- Forget where the book is at bedtime.
- Hide the child's coat.
- Give the child an empty lunch bag.

Talking With Imaginary Friends

Assigning roles to inanimate objects is a form of symbolic play. Most young children enjoy interacting with stuffed animals, dolls, or puppets as if they were alive; some preschoolers also create invisible friends who they know are not real (Taylor & Mottweiler, 2008). Children undergo significant growth in their understanding of invisibility during the preschool years (Woolley & Brown, 2015). Research findings show that children with imaginary friends tend to be less shy, more social, and more competent in starting and maintaining conversations as a result of practicing communication skills with these *special* friends (Roby & Kidd,

2008; Wooley & Ghossainy, 2003). The ultimate goal of this type of conversational play is for the child to eventually take the lead (Meltzer & Palermo, in press).

To promote conversational exchanges, the AV practitioner speaks for the doll, stuffed animal, or puppet. Having conversational turn-taking with imaginary friends in AVT enables the practitioner to incorporate different mental states into the activity. It is important for the child to understand how other people think and feel, and why these perspectives might be different. Children who do not yet understand another person's perspective have not acquired socioemotional competence (Lewis & Ramsay, 2004).

The AV practitioner has access to toys that include stuffed animals, puppets, or dolls wearing assorted hearing devices. There are many advantages to using such imaginary friends wearing hearing devices in AVT sessions: (a) hearing devices capture the child's interest, and hence, the imaginary friends serve as potential motivators; (b) they can be effectively used as prompts; (c) they can demonstrate or model a language target; (d) they can engage the child in verbal turn-taking; (e) they can provide opportunities for practicing conversational skills; (f) the child may feel less pressure in performing or talking; (g) imaginary friends can show that making mistakes is part of learning and thus are acceptable; and (h) imaginary friends can help children problem solve or work through some social or emotional conflicts (Stanton-Chapman & Brown, 2015).

The AV practitioner makes every attempt to use imaginary friends in creative ways. As a simple example, the practitioner can set up a situation where one puppet drops her food and cries because she has nothing to eat. Another puppet sees her crying and he says, "I'm sorry. What's wrong?" When he learns why she is crying, he shares half of his food with her and the child. The use of imaginary friends can also promote language and social skills when scenarios are scripted and practiced (Stanton-Chapman & Brown, 2015).

Accepting and Making Mistakes

A "fear of failure" established during early childhood can dramatically influence a child's motivation, negatively affecting the attitude toward learning (Mouratidis, Vansteenkiste, Michou, & Lens, 2013). It is crucial for the child to understand that making mistakes is a necessary part of the discovery process and learning.

The AV practitioner and parent must be sensitive to the child who demonstrates fear of providing the "wrong" response. The child is reassured that everyone makes mistakes, and that mistakes help us learn. At times, both AV practitioner and parent pretend to "not know" a word, an answer, or how to do something. Guessing activities further promote the idea that children and adults are not always "in the know."

CONCLUSION

This chapter presented the concept that an AV practitioner plans, delivers, and evaluates every AVT session with SIX GOALS as the central theme. For each of these SIX GOALS, a *select* number of evidence-based or evidence-informed strategies were delineated. The AV practitioner implements each of these effective strategies in isolation or in tandem with other strategies. Strategy selection is based on the knowledge, experience, and expertise of the individual practitioner, and influenced by the needs and skills of child and parent.

All strategies presented here are demonstrated by the AV practitioner for the parents, who are viewed as the primary client in AVT. Parents practice these strategies in AVT sessions and then use them to generalize the objectives and goals in everyday life to advance the child toward the expected outcomes of listening and talking.

In the future, research may be used to help analyze these strategies even more extensively (Brown & Fenske, 2011). It is hoped that researchers and AV practitioners will collaborate in studies that will further verify the effectiveness of these and other strategies that promote listening, talking and thinking in children with hearing loss.

REFERENCES

Adank, P., Hagoort, P., & Bekkering, H. (2010). Imitation improves comprehension. *Psychological Science, 21*(12), 1903–1909.

Al-Balushi, S. N. M. (2009). An investigation into how silent wait-time assists language learning. In S. Borg (Ed.), *Classroom research in English language teaching in Oman* (pp. 2–7). Muscat, Oman: Ministry of Education.

Anderson, K. L., & Crowley, D. J. (2002). When listening carefully is not enough: 12 steps to approaching speech language pathology services for a child who is hard-of-hearing. *Perspectives on Hearing and Hearing Disorders in Childhood, 12*(3), 33–36.

Arunachalam, S., & Waxman, S. R. (2010). Meaning from syntax: Evidence from 2-year-olds. *Cognition, 114*(3), 442–446.

Aslin, R. N., & Newport, E. L. (2012). Statistical learning from acquiring specific items to forming general rules. *Current Directions in Psychological Science, 21*(3), 170–176.

Astheimer, L. B., & Sanders, L. D. (2009). Listeners modulate temporally selective attention during natural speech processing. *Biological Psychology, 80*, 23–34.

Bahrick, L. E., & Lickliter, R. (2009). Perceptual development: Intermodal perception. In B. Goldstein (Ed.), *Encyclopedia of perception* (Vol. 2, pp. 753–756). Newbury Park, CA: Sage.

Barker, D, H., Quittner, A. L., Fink, N. E., Eisenberg, L. S., Tobey, E. A., Niparko, J. K., & The CDaCI Investigative Team. (2009). Predicting behavior problems in deaf and hearing children: The influences of language, attention, and parent-child communication. *Development and Psychopathology, 21*(2), 373–392.

Barr, D. J., & Seyfeddinipur, M. (2010). The role of fillers in listener attributions for speaker disfluency. *Language and Cognitive Processes, 25*, 441–455.

Bass-Ringdahl, S. M. (2010). The relationship of audibility and the development of canonical babbling in young children with hearing impairment. *Journal of Deaf Studies and Deaf Education, 15*, 287–310.

Bedore, L. M., & Leonard, L. B. (1995). Prosodic and syntactic bootstrapping and their clinical applications: A tutorial.

American Journal of Speech-Language Pathology, 4(1), 66–72.

Bellon-Harn, M. L., Credeur-Pampolina, M. E., & LeBoeuf, L. (2013). Scaffolded language intervention: Speech production outcomes. *Communication Disorders Quarterly, 34*(2), 120–132.

Benasich, A. A., Choudhury, N. A., Realpe-Bonilla, T. & Roesler, C. P. (2014). Plasticity in developing brain: Active auditory exposure impacts prelinguistic acoustic mapping. *Journal of Neuroscience, 34*, 13349–13363.

Bergen, B., & Wheeler, K. (2010). Grammatical aspect and mental stimulation. *Brain and Language, 112*, 150–158.

Bergeson, T. R., & Trehub, S. E. (2002). Absolute pitch and tempo in mothers' song to infants. *Psychological Science, 13*(1), 72–75.

Bernal, S., Dehaene-Lambertz, G., Millotte, S., & Christophe, A. (2010). Two-year-olds compute syntactic structure on-line. *Developmental Science, 13*(1), 69–76.

Bernhardt, B. M., Kemp, N., & Werker, J. F. (2007). Early word-object associations and later language development. *First Language, 27*(4), 315–328.

Bishop, D., & Adams, C. (2006). A prospective study of the relationship between specific language impairment, phonological disorders and reading retardation. *Journal of Child Psychology and Psychiatry, 31*, 1027–1050.

Blair, C., & Razza, R. P. (2007). Relating effortful control, executive function, and false belief understanding to emerging math and literacy ability in kindergarten. *Child Development, 78*, 647–663.

Blaiser, K. M., Nelson, P. B., & Kohnert, K. (2015). Effect of repeated exposures on word learning in quiet and noise. *Communication Disorders Quarterly, 37*, 25–35.

Bobzien, J. L., Richels, C., Schwartz, K., Raver, Sharon A., Hester, P., & Morin, L. (2015). Using repeated reading and explicit instruction to teach vocabulary to preschoolers with hearing loss. *Infants and Young Children, 28*, 262–280.

Bodrova, E., & Leong, D. J. (2001). The Tools of the Mind project: A case study of implementing the Vygotskian approach in American early childhood and primary classrooms. *INNODATA Monographs—7*. Switzerland: International Bureau of Education.

Booth, A. E., & Waxman, S. R. (2009). A horse of a different color: Specifying with precision infants' mappings of novel nouns and adjectives. *Child Development, 80*(1), 15–22.

Bosch, L. (2011). Precursors to language in preterm infants: Speech perception abilities in the first year of life. *Progress in Brain Research, 189*, 239–257.

Bovey, T., & Strain, P. (2005). Strategies for increasing peer social interactions: Prompting and acknowledgement. *What Works Briefs, 17*, 1–4.

Boysson-Bardies, B. (1999). *How language comes to children: From birth to two years*. Cambridge, MA: MIT Press.

Bransford, J., Brown, A., & Cocking, R. (2000). *How people learn: Brain, mind, experience and school*. Washington, DC: National Academy Press.

Brockmole, J. R., Davoli, C. C., Abrams, R. A., & Witt, J. K. (2013). The world within reach: Effects of hand posture and tool-use on visual cognition. *Current Directions in Psychological Science, 22*, 38–44.

Brooks, P. J., & Kempe, V. (2012). *Language development*. London, UK: Wiley.

Brown, G., & Wragg, E. C. (1993). *Questioning*. New York, NY: Routledge.

Brown, J., & Frenske, M. (2011). *The Winner's Brain*. Boston, MA: Da Capo Press.

Brown, P. M., & Remine, M. D. (2004). Building pretend play skills in toddlers with and without hearing loss: Maternal scaffolding styles. *Deafness and Education International, 6*(3), 129–153.

Callanan, M. A., & Sabbagh, M. A. (2004). Multiple labels for objects in conversations with young children: Parents' language and children's developing expectations about word meanings. *Developmental Psychology, 40*(5), 746–763.

Carey-Sargeant, C. L., & Brown, P. M. (2003). Pausing during interactions between deaf toddlers and their hearing mothers. *Deafness and Education International, 5*(1), 39–58.

Cassell, J., Nakano, Y. I., Bickmore, T. W., Sidner, C. L., & Rich, C. (2001). *Nonverbal cues for discourse structure.* Association for Computational Linguistics Joint EACL–2001 ACL Conference.

Caselli, M. C., Rinaldi, P., Stefanini, S., & Volterra, V. (2012). Early action and gesture "vocabulary" and its relation with word comprehension and production. *Child Development, 83*(2), 526–542.

Chaiklin, S. (2003). The zone of proximal development in Vygotsky's analysis of learning and instruction. In A. Kozulin, B. Gindis, V. Ageyev, & S. Miller (Eds.), *Vygotsky's educational theory in cultural context* (pp. 39–64). Cambridge, UK: Cambridge University Press.

Champoux, F., Lepore, F., Gagné, J-P., & Théoret, H. (2009). Visual stimuli can impair auditory processing in cochlear implant users. *Neuropsychologia, 47*(1), 17–22.

Chang, R. S., & Thompson, N. S. (2011). Whines, cries, and motherese: Their relative power to distract. *Journal of Social, Evolutionary, and Cultural Psychology, 5*(2) 10 20.

Cirelli, L. K., Wan, S. J., & Trainor, L. J. (2014). Fourteen-month-old infants use interpersonal synchrony as a cue to direct helpfulness. *Philosophical Transactions of the Royal Society Biological Science, 369*, 1658.

Colonnesi, C., Stams, G. J. M., Koster, I., & Noom, M. J. (2010). The relation between pointing and language development: A meta-analysis. *Developmental Review, 30*(4), 352–366.

Conway, C. M., Bauernschmidt, A., Huang, S. S., & Pisoni, D. B. (2010). Implicit statistical learning in language processing: Word predictability is the key. *Cognition, 114*(3), 356–371.

Cristia, A., Seidi, A., Junge, C., Soderstrom, M., & Hagoort, P. (2014). Predicting individual variation in language from infant speech perception measures. *Child Development, 85*, 1330–1345.

Cruz, I., Quittner, A. L., Marker, C., & DesJardin, J. L. (2013). Identification of effective strategies to promote language in deaf children with cochlear implants. *Child Development, 84*, 543–599.

Dalton, P., & Fraenkel, N. (2012). Gorillas we have missed: Sustained inattentional deafness for dynamic events. *Cognition, 124*(2), 367–372.

Damron, J. C. H., & Morman, M. T. (2011). Attitudes toward interpersonal silence within dyadic relationships. *Human Communication, 14*, 183–203.

Driscoll, V., Gfeller. K., Tan, X., See, R. L., Cheng, H-Y., & Kanemitsu, M. (2015). Family involvement in music impacts participation of children with cochlear implants. *Cochlear Implants International, 16*, 137–146.

Duff, F. J., Reen, G., Plunkett, K., & Nation, K. (2015). Do infant vocabulary skills predict school-age language and literacy outcomes? *Journal of Child Psychology and Psychiatry, 56*, 848–856.

Dunst, C. J., Raab, M., & Trivette, C. M. (2011). Characteristics of naturalistic language intervention strategies *Journal of Speech-Language Pathology and Applied Behavioral Analysis, 5*, 8–16.

Ertmer, D. J., & Stoel-Gammon, C. (2008). The conditioned assessment of speech production (CASP): A tool for evaluating auditory-guided speech development in young children with hearing loss. *The Volta Review, 108*, 59–80.

Estabrooks, W. (2006). Auditory-verbal therapy and practice. In W. Estabrooks (Ed.), *Auditory-Verbal Therapy and practice* (pp. 1–22). Washington, DC: A.G. Bell Association.

Estabrooks, W., & Birkenshaw-Fleming, L. (2003). *Songs for listening! Songs for life!* Washington, DC: A.G. Bell Association.

Estes, K. G., & Hurley, K. (2013). Infant-directed prosody helps infants map sounds to meanings. *Infancy, 18*(5), 797–824.

Estigarribia, B. (2010). Facilitation by variation: right-to-left learning of English yes/no questions. *Cognitive Science, 34,* 68–93.

Farrant, B. M., Maybery, M. T., & Fletcher, J. (2011). Socio-emotional engagement, joint attention, imitation, and conversation skill: Analysis in typical development and specific language impairment. *First Language, 31,* 23–46.

Fast, J. (2002). *Body language.* Lanham, MD: M. Evans.

Feldman, R., Magori-Cohen, R., Galili, G., Singer, M., & Louzon, Y. (2011). Mother-infant coordinate heart rhythms through episodes of interaction synchrony. *Infant Behavior and Development, 34*(4), 569–577.

Ferguson, B., Graf, E., & Waxman, S. R. (2014). Infants use known verbs to learn novel nouns: Evidence from 15- and 19-month-olds. *Cognition, 131,* 139.

Ferguson, B., Havy, M., & Waxman, S. R. (2015). The precision of 12-month-old infants' link between language and categorization predicts vocabulary size at 12 and 18 months. *Frontiers in Psychology, 6,* 1319.

Flecha-García, M. L. (2010). Eyebrow raises in dialogue and their relation to discourse structure, utterance function and pitch accents in English. *Speech Communication, 52,* 542–554.

Flom, R., & Pick, A. D. (2003). Verbal encouragement and joint attention in 18-month-old infants. *Infant Behavior and Development, 26*(2), 121–134.

Florit, E., Roch, M., Altoe, G., & Levorato, M. C. (2009). Listening comprehension in preschoolers: The role of memory. *British Journal of Developmental Psychology, 27,* 935–951.

Frischen, A., Bayliss, A. P., & Tipper, S. P. (2007). Gaze cueing of attention: Visual attention, social cognition, and individual differences. *Psychological Bulletin, 133*(4), 694–724.

Frota, S., Butler, J., & Vigário, M. (2014). Infants' perception of intonation: Is it a statement or a question? *Infancy, 19,* 194–213.

Gabel, D. (2004). Science. In G. Cawelti (Ed.), *Handbook of research on improving student achievement* (pp. 123–143). Arlington, VA: Educational Research Service.

Gallun, F. J., Mason, C. R., & Kidd, G., Jr. (2007). The ability to listen with independent ears. *Journal of the Acoustical Society of America, 122,* 2814–2825.

Gao, H. H., Zelazo, P. D., Sharpe, D., & Mashari, A. (2014). Beyond early linguistic competence: Development of children's ability to interpret adjectives flexibly. *Cognitive Development, 32,* 86–102.

Ginsburg, K. R. (2007). The importance of play in promoting healthy child development and maintaining strong parent-child bonds. *Pediatrics, 119*(1), 182–191.

Gogate, L. J., Bahrick, L. E., & Watson, J. D. (2000). A study of multi-modal motherese: The role of temporal synchrony between verbal labels and gestures. *Child Development, 71*(4), 878–894.

Goldstein, M. H., & Schwade, J. A. (2008). Social feedback to infants' babbling facilitates rapid phonological learning. *Psychological Science, 19,* 515–523.

Gomes, A., Wolfson, V., & Halperin, J. M. (2007). Is there a selective relationship between language functioning and auditory attention in children? *Journal of Clinical and Experimental Neuropsychology, 29*(6), 660–668.

Graham, S., Santos, D., & Vanderplank, R. (2011). Exploring the relationship between listening development and strategy use. *Language Teaching Research, 15,* 435–456.

Gratier, M. (2003). Expressive timing and interactional synchrony between mothers and infants: Cultural similarities, cultural differences, and the immigration experience. *Cognitive Development, 18*(4), 533–554.

Gray S. (2004). Word learning by preschoolers with specific language impairment: Predictors and poor learners. *Journal of Speech, Language, and Hearing Research, 47,* 1117–1132.

Gray, S., & Brinkley, S. (2011). Fast mapping and word learning by preschoolers with SLI in a supported learning context: Effect of encoding cues, phonotactic probability and object familiarity. *Journal of Speech, Language, and Hearing Research, 54,* 870–884.

Guaïtella, I., Santi, S., Lagrue, B., & Cavé, C. (2009). Are eyebrow movements linked to voice variations and turn-taking dialogue? An experimental investigation. *Language and Speech, 52,* 207–222.

Gunlogson, C. (2003). *True to form: Rising and falling declaratives as questions in English.* New York, NY: Routledge.

Gustafson, S., McCreery, R., Hoover, B., Kopun, J. G., & Stelmachowicz, P. (2014). Listening effort and perceived clarity for normal-hearing children with the use of digital noise reduction. *Ear and Hearing, 35,* 183–194.

Halliday, L. F., Moore, D. R., Taylor, J. L., & Amitay, S. (2011). Dimension-specific attention directs learning and listening on auditory training tasks. *Attention, Perception, and Psychophysics, 73*(5), 1329–1335.

Hannemann, R., Obleser, J., & Eulitz, C. (2007). Top-down knowledge supports the retrieval of lexical information from degraded speech. *Brain Research, 1153,* 134–143.

Hasegawa, I. & Miyashita, Y. (2002). Categorizing the world: Expert neurons look into key features. *Nature Neuroscience, 5*(2), 90–91.

Hay-McCutcheon, M. J., Kirk, K. I., Henning, S. C., Gao, S., & Qi, R. (2008). Using early language outcomes to predict later language ability in children with cochlear implants. *Audiology and Neurotology, 13*(6), 370–378.

Hayes, D. (2014). The use of prompting as an evidence-based strategy to support children with ASD in school settings in New Zealand. *Kairaranga, 14*(2), 52–56.

Heeman, P. A., Lunsford, R., Selfridge, E., Black, L., & van Santen, J. (2010). Autism and interactional aspects of dialogue. *Proceedings of SIGDIAL 2010: The 11th Annual Meeting of the Special Interest Group on Discourse and Dialogue* (pp. 249–252). University of Tokyo, September 24–25, 2010.

Henninger, M. L. (2013). *Teaching young children: An introduction* (5th ed.). New York, NY: Pearson.

Holstrum, W. J., Gaffney, M., Gravel, J, S., Oyler, R. F., & Ross, D. S. (2008). Early intervention for children with unilateral and mild bilateral degrees of hearing loss. *Trends in Amplification, 12*(1), 35–41.

Houston, D. (2011). Infant speech perception. In R. Seewald & A. M. Tharpe (Eds.), *Comprehensive handbook of pediatric audiology* (pp. 47–62). San Diego, CA: Plural.

Humes, L. E., & Bess, F. H. (2014). *Audiology and communication disorders: An overview* (2nd ed.). New York, NY: Lippincott Williams & Wilkins.

Ignatius, E., & Kokkonen, M. (2007). Factors contributing to verbal self-disclosure. *Nordic Psychology, 59,* 362–391.

Iverson, J. M., & Goldin-Meadow, S. (2005). Gesture paves the way for language development. *Psychological Science, 16,* 367–371.

James, K. H., & Maouene, J. (2009). Auditory verb perception recruits motor systems in the developing brain: An fMRI investigation. *Developmental Science, 12,* F26–F39.

Jarvis, M. (2005). *The psychology of effective learning and teaching.* Cheltenham, UK: Nelson Thornes.

Johnson, K. (2012). *Acoustic and auditory phonetics* (3rd ed.). New York, NY: Wiley.

Jones, S. S. (2007). Imitation in infancy: The development of mimicry. *Psychological Science, 18,* 593–599.

Junge, C., Koojiman, V., Haggort, P., & Cutler, A. (2012). Rapid recognition at 10 months as a predictor of language development. *Developmental Science, 15,* 463–473.

Kahana-Kalman, R., & Walker-Andrews, A. S. (2001). The role of person familiarity in young infants' perception of emotional expressions. *Child Development, 72,* 352–369.

Kohlberger, M., & Strycharczuk, P. (2015). ~~Voicing assimilation in whispered speech~~. Retrieved from https://www.internationalphoneticassociation.org/icphs-proceedings/ICPhS2015/Papers/ICPHS1016.pdf

Kokkinaki, T., & Vitalaki, E. (2013). Comparing spontaneous imitation in grandmother-infant and mother-infant interaction: A three generation familial study. *International Journal of Aging Human Development, 77,* 77–105.

Kotz, S. A., Opitz, B., & Friederici, A. D. (2007). ERP effects of meaningful and nonmeaningful sound processing in anterior temporal patients. *Restorative Neurology and Neuroscience, 25,* 273–284.

Kuhl, P. (2004). Early language acquisition: Cracking the speech code. *Nature Reviews Neuroscience, 5*(11), 831–843.

Kuhl, P. K., & Meltzoff, A. N. (1996). Infant vocalizations in response to speech: Vocal imitation and developmental change. *Journal of Acoustical Society of America, 100,* 2425–2438.

Kuhl, P. K., Tsao, F-M., & Liu, H-M. (2003). Foreign-language experience in infancy: Effects of short-term exposure and social interaction on phonetic learning. *PNAS, 100,* 9096–9101.

Le Bel, R. M., Pineda, J. A., & Sharma, A. (2009). Motor-auditory-visual integration: The role of the human mirror neuron system in communication and communication disorders. *Journal of Communication Disorders, 42,* 299–304.

Lau, B., & Salzman, C. D. (2009). The rhythms of learning. *Nature Neuroscience, 12,* 675–676.

Leclère, C., Viaux, S., Avril, M., Achard, C., Chetouani, M., Missonnier, S., & Cohen, D. (2014). Why synchrony matters during mother-child interactions: A systematic review. *PLoS ONE, 9*(12), e113571.

Lederberg, A. R., & Spencer, P. E. (2009). Word-learning abilities in deaf and hard-of-hearing preschoolers: Effect of lexicon size and language modality. *Journal of Deaf Studies and Deaf Education, 14,* 44–62.

Lewis, M., & Ramsay, D. (2004). Development of self-recognition, personal pronoun use, and pretend play during the 2nd year. *Child Development, 75*(6), 1821–1831.

Li, J., Li, W., Xian, J., Li, Y., Liu, Z., Liu, S., . . . He, H. (2012). Cortical thickness analysis and optimized voxel-based morphometry in children and adolescents with prelingually profound sensorineural hearing loss. *Brain Research, 1430,* 35–42.

Ling, D. (1976). *Speech and the hearing-impaired child: Theory and practice.* Washington, DC: AG Bell Association for the Deaf and Hard of Hearing.

Ling, D., & Ling, A. H. (1978). *Aural habilitation: The foundations of verbal learning in hearing-impaired children.* Washington, DC: AG Bell Association.

Ludke, K. M., Ferreira, F., & Overy, K. (2014). Singing can facilitate foreign language learning. *Memory & Cognition, 42,* 41–52.

Ma, W., Golinkoff, R. M., Houston, D., & Hirsh-Pasek (2011). Word learning in infant- and adult-directed speech. *Language Learning and Development, 7,* 209–225.

MacKenzie, H., Graham, S. A., & Curtin, S. (2011). Twelve-month-olds privilege words over other linguistic sounds in an associative learning task. *Developmental Science, 14*(2), 249–255.

Macrae, C. N., Duffy, O. K., Miles, L. K., & Lawrence, J. (2008). A case of hand waving: Action synchrony and person perception. *Cognition, 109*(1), 152–156.

Maroni, B. (2011). Pauses, gaps and wait time in classroom interaction in primary schools. *Journal of Pragmatics, 43*(7), 2081–2093.

Marschark, M., Spencer, P. E., Adams, J., & Sapere, P. (2011). Evidence-based practice in educating deaf and hard-of-hearing children: Teaching to their cognitive strengths and needs. *European Journal of Special Needs Education, 26*(1), 3–16.

Marques, C., Moreno, S., Castro, S. L., & Besson, M. (2007). Musicians detect pitch violation in foreign language better than nonmusicians: Behavioral and electrophysiological evidence. *Journal of Cognitive Neuroscience, 19*, 1453–1463.

Mastropavlou, M. (2010). Morphophonological salience as a compensatory means for deficits in the acquisition of past tense in SLI. *Journal of Communication Disorders, 43*, 175–198.

Mather, E., & Plunkett, K. (2012). The role of novelty in early word learning. *Cognitive Science, 36*(7), 1157–1177.

Matsuda, Y.-T., Ueno, K., Waggoner, R. A., Erickson, D., Shimura, Y., Tanaka, K., Cheng, K., & Mazuka, R. (2011). Processing of infant-directed speech by adults. *NeuroImage, 54*, 611–621.

McDonald, J. D. (1985). Language through conversation: A model for intervention with language-delayed persons. In S. F. Warren & A. K. Rogers-Warren (Eds.), *Teaching functional language: Generalization and maintenance of language skills* (pp. 89–122). Austin, TX: Pro-Ed.

McMurray, B., & Aslin, R. N. (2005). Infants are sensitive to within-category variation in speech perception. *Cognition, 95*, B15–B26.

Melzer, D. K., & Palermo, C. A. (in press). "Mommy, You are the princess and I am the queen": How preschool children's initiation and language use during pretend play relate to complexity. *Infant and Child Development.*

Mercer, S., Ryan, S., & Williams, M. (2012). *Psychology for language learning: Insights from research, theory and practice.* New York, NY: St. Martin's Press.

Minagawa-Kawai, Y., Mori, K., Naoi, N., & Kojima, S. (2006). Neural attunement processes in infants during the acquisition of a language-specific phonemic contrast. *Journal of Neuroscience 27*(2), 315–321.

Moll, H., & Meltzoff, A. N. (2011). How does it look? Level 2 perspective-taking at 36 months of age. *Child Development, 82*, 661–673.

Monaghan, P., Shillcock, R. C., Christiansen, M. H., & Kirby, S. (2014). How arbitrary is language? *Philosophical Transactions of the Royal Society B: Biological Sciences, 369*(1651), 20130299.

Mouratidis, A., Vansteenkiste, M., Michou, A., & Lens, W. (2013). Perceived structure and achievement goals as predictors of students' self-regulated learning and affect and the mediating role of competence need satisfaction. *Learning and Individual Differences, 23*, 179–186.

Musacchia, G. E., Sams, M., Nicol, T. G., & Kraus, N. (2006). Seeing speech affects acoustic information processing in the human brainstem. *Experimental Brain Research, 168*, 1–10.

Nappa, R., Wessel, A., McEldoon, K. L., Gleitman, L. R., & Trueswell, J. (2009). Use of speaker's gaze and syntax in verb learning. *Language Learning and Development, 5*(4), 203–234.

Narr, R. A. F. (2006). Teaching phonological awareness with deaf and hard-of-hearing students. *Teaching Exceptional Children, 38*(4), 53–58.

Nathani, S., Ertmer, D. J., & Stark, R. S. (2006). Assessing vocal development in infants and toddlers. *Clinical Linguistics and Phonetics, 20*, 351–369.

Nevo, I., & Slonim-Nevo, V. (2011). The myth of evidence-based practice: Towards evidence-informed practice. *British Journal of Social Work, 41*(6), 1176–1197.

Newman, R. S., Chatterjee, M., Morini, G., & Remez, R. E. (2015). Toddler's comprehension of degraded signals: Noise-vocoded versus sine-wave analogs. *Journal of the Acoustical Society of America Express Letters, 138*, EL311.

Newman, R. S., Rowe, M. L., & Ratner, N. (in press). Input and uptake at 7 months predicts toddler vocabulary: The role of child-directed speech and infant processing skills in language development. *Journal of Child Language.*

Olson, J., & Masur, E. F. (2013). Mothers respond differently to infants' gestural versus nongestural communicative bids. *First Language, 33,* 372–387.

Owren, M. J., & Cardillo, G. C. (2006). The relative roles of vowels and consonants in discriminating talker identity versus word meaning. *Journal of the Acoustical Society of America, 119,* 1727–1739.

Pedale, T., & Santangelo, V. (2015). Perceptual salience affects the contents of working memory during free-recollection of objects from natural scenes. *Frontiers in Human Neuroscience, 9,* 60.

Pelligrini, A. D., Dupuis, D., & Smith, P. K. (2007). Play in evolution and development. *Developmental Review, 27,* 261–276.

Peters, A. M. (2001). Filler syllables: What is their status in emerging grammar? *Journal of Child Language, 28,* 229–242.

Petitto, L. (2005). How the brain begets language. In J. McGilvray (Ed.), *The Cambridge companion to Chomsky* (pp. 84–101). Cambridge, UK: Cambridge University Press.

Pickering, M. J., & Garrod, S. (2006). Do people use language production to make predictions during comprehension? *Trends in Cognitive Sciences, 11,* 105–110.

Pinker, S. (1994). *The language instinct.* New York, NY: HarperCollins.

Pollack, D. (1972). *Educational audiology for the limited-hearing infant.* Springfield, IL: Charles C. Thomas.

Potter, G. (1996). From symbolic play to symbolic representation in early literacy: Clarifying the links. *Early Years, 16,* 13–16.

Power, D. J., Wood, D. J., Wood, H. A., & Macdougall, J. (1990). Maternal control over conversations with hearing and deaf infants and young children. *First Language, 10,* 19–35.

Proctor-Williams, K., Fey, M. E., & Loeb, D. F. (2001). Parental recasts and production of copulas and articles by children with specific language impairment and typical language. *American Journal of Speech-Language Pathology, 10*(2), 155–168.

Pruden, S. M., Hirsh-Pasek, K., Golinkoff, R. M., & Hennon, E. A. (2006). The birth of words: Ten-month-olds learn words through perceptual salience. *Child Development, 77,* 266–280.

Read, K., Macauley, M., & Furay, E. (2014). The Seuss boost: Rhyme helps children retain words from shared storybook reading. *First Language, 34,* 354–371.

Reingold, R., Rimor, R., & Kalay, A. (2008). Instructor's scaffolding in support of student's metacognition through a teacher education online course—A case study. *Journal of Interactive Online Learning, 7,* 139–151.

Rescorla, L. (2009). Age 17 language and reading outcomes in late-talking toddlers: Support for a dimensional perspective on language delay. *Journal of Speech, Language, and Hearing Research, 52,* 16–30.

Rhoades, E. A. (2007). Sound-object associations. In S. Easterbrooks & E. Estes (Eds.), *Helping children who are deaf and hard of hearing learn spoken language* (pp. 181–188). Thousand Oaks, CA: Corwin Press.

Rhoades, E. A. (2010, July 25). *Facilitating auditory-verbal learning for young children with impaired executive functioning.* Presentation at A.G. Bell Association Convention, Orlando, FL.

Rhoades, E. A. (2011). Listening strategies to facilitate spoken language learning among signing children with cochlear implants. In R. Paludneviciene & I. W.

Leigh (Eds.), *Cochlear implants: Shifting perspectives* (pp. 142–171). Washington, DC: Gallaudet University Press.

Rhoades, E. A. (2013). Interactive silences: Evidence for strategies to facilitate spoken language in children with hearing loss. *The Volta Review, 113*(1), 57–73.

Rigato, S., Menon, E., Johnson, M. H., Faraguna, D., & Farroni, T. (2011). Direct gaze may modulate face recognition in newborns. *Infant and Child Development, 20*(1), 20–34.

Robbins, A. M. (2000). Rehabilitation after cochlear implantation. In J. K. Niparko, K. I. Kirk, N. K. Mellon, A. M. Robbins, D. L. Tucci, & B. S. Wilson (Eds.), *Cochlear implants: Principles and practices*. New York, NY: Lippincott Williams & Wilkins.

Roby, A. C., & Kidd, E. (2008). The referential communication skills of children with imaginary companions. *Developmental Science, 11*(4), 531–540.

Rowe, K., & Rowe, K. (2006). *BIG issues in boys' education: Auditory processing capacity, literacy and behaviour*. Retrieved from http://research.acer.edu.au/boys_edu/2

Rowe, M. L. (2012). A longitudinal investigation of the role of quantity and quality of child-directed speech in vocabulary development. *Child Development, 83*, 1762–1774.

Rowland, C. F., Pine, J. M., Lieven, E. V., & Theakston, A. L. (2003). Determinants of the order of acquisition of wh- questions: Re-evaluating the role of caregiver speech. *Journal of Child Language, 30*, 609–635.

Saffran, J. R., Werker, J., & Werner, L. (2006). The infant's auditory world: Hearing, speech and the beginnings of language. In R. Siegler and D. Kuhn (Eds.), *Handbook of child development* (pp. 58–108). New York, NY: Wiley.

Saindon, M. R., Trehub, S. E., Schellenberg, E. G., & Van Lieshout, P. (in press). Children's identification of questions from rising terminal pitch. *Journal of Child Language*.

Sawyer, R. K. (2006). *The Cambridge handbook of the learning sciences*. New York, NY: Cambridge University Press.

Schneider, D. M., Nelson, A., & Mooney, R. (2014). A synaptic and circuit basis for corollary discharge in the auditory cortex. *Nature, 513*(7517), 189–194.

Shafiro, V., Sheft, S., Gygi, B., & Ho, K. T. N. (2012). The influence of environmental sound training on the perception of spectrally degraded speech and environmental sounds. *Trends in Amplification, 16*, 83–101.

Sharma, A., Tobey, E., Dorman, M., Bharadwaj, S., Martin, K., Gilley, P., & Kunkel, F. (2004). Central auditory maturation and babbling development in infants with cochlear implants. *Archives of Otolaryngology-Head and Neck Surgery, 13*(5), 511–516.

Sharp, A. (2009). Reading comprehension in two cultures. *International Journal of Learning, 16*, 281–292.

Shi, R. (2014). Functional morphemes and early language acquisition. *Child Development Perspectives, 8*(1), 6–11.

Skinner, C. H., Pappas, D. N., & Davis, K. A. (2005). Enhancing academic engagement: Providing opportunities for responding and influencing students to choose to respond. *Psychology in the Schools, 42*, 389–403.

Smaldino, J., & Flexer, C. (2014). Acoustic accessibility: Room acoustics and remote microphone use in home and school environments. In J. R. Madell & C. Flexer (Eds.), *Pediatric audiology: Diagnosis, technology, and management* (2nd ed., pp. 255–267). New York, NY: Thieme.

Smith, L. Z., & Levitt, H. (1999). Consonant enhancement effects on speech recognition of hearing-impaired children. *Journal of American Academy of Audiology, 10*(8), 411–421.

Smith, P. K. (2007). Pretend play and children's cognitive and literacy development: Sources of evidence and some lessons from the past. (pp. 3–19) In K.

Roskos & J. Christie (Eds.), Play and literacy in early childhood: Research from multiple perspectives (2nd ed., pp. 3–19). Mahwah, NJ: Lawrence Erlbaum Associates.

Snyder, P. A., Rakap, S., Hemmeter, M. L., McLaughlin, T. W., Sandall, S., & McLean, M. E. (2015). Naturalistic instructional approaches in early learning: A systematic review. *Journal of Early Intervention, 37*(1), 69–97.

Southgate, V., Chevallier, C., & Csibra, G. (2009). Sensitivity to communicative relevance tells young children what to imitate. *Developmental Science, 12*(6), 1013–1019.

Souza, P. (2014 June 29). Improving audibility: The foundation for speech understanding. In *Maximizing Brain Adaptability*. Presented at the A. G. Bell Association 2014 Research Symposium, Orlando, FL.

Srinivasan, R. J., & Massaro, D. W. (2003). Perceiving prosody from the face and voice: distinguishing statements from echoic questions in English. *Language and Speech, 46*, 1–22.

Stahl, A. E., & Feigenson, L. (2015). Observing the unexpected enhances infants' learning and exploration. *Science, 348* (6230), 91–94.

Stahl, R. J. (1994). Using "Think-Time" and "Wait-Time" skillfully in the classroom. *ERIC Digest*, ED370885. Retrieved from http://www.ericdigests.org/1995-1/think.htm

Stanton-Chapman, T. L., & Brown, T. S. (2015). Facilitating commenting and requesting skills in 3-year-old children with disabilities. *Journal of Early Intervention, 37*, 103–118.

Stanton-Chapman, T. L., & Snell, M. E. (2011). Promoting turn-taking skills in preschool children with disabilities: The effects of a peer-based social communication intervention. *Early Childhood Research Quarterly, 26*(3), 303–319.

Stelmachowicz, P. G., Pittman, A. L., Hoover, B. M., Lewis, D. E., & Moeller, M. P. (2004). The importance of high-frequency audibility in the speech and language development of children with hearing loss. *Archives of Otolaryngology-Head & Neck Surgery, 130*, 556–562.

Stephenson, J., Carter, M., & Arthur-Kelly, M. (2011). Professional learning for teachers without special education qualifications working with students with severe disabilities. *Teacher Education and Special Education, 34*(1), 7–20.

Strapp, C. M., & Federico, A. (2000). Imitations and repetitions: What do children say following recasts? *First Language, 20*(60), 273–290.

Syrett, K., Arunachalam, S., & Waxman, S. R. (2014). Slowly but surely: Adverbs support verb learning in 2-year-olds. *Language Learning and Development, 10*(3), 263–278.

Taylor, M., & Mottweiler, C. M. (2008). Imaginary companions: Pretending they are real but knowing they are not. *American Journal of Play, 1*, 47–54.

Thiessen, E. D., & Saffran, J. R. (2007). Learning to learn: Infants' acquisition of stress-based strategies for word segmentation. *Language Learning and Development, 3*(1), 73–100.

Tierney, A., & Kraus, N. (2015). Evidence for multiple rhythmic skills. *PLoS ONE, 10*(9), e0136645.

Tomasello, M. (2003). *Constructing a language: A usage-based theory of language acquisition*. Cambridge, MA: Harvard University.

Trehub, S. E. (2015). Cross-cultural convergence of musical features. *Proceedings of the National Academy of Sciences, 112*(29), 8809–8810.

Twomey, K. E., Lush, L., Pearce, R., & Horst, J. S. (2014). Visual variability affects early verb learning. *British Journal of Developmental Psychology, 32*(3), 359–366.

Urry, S. A., Nelson, L. J., & Padilla-Walker, L. M. (2011). Mother knows best: Psychological control, child disclosure, and maternal knowledge in emerging adulthood. *Journal of Family Studies, 17*, 157–173.

van Heugten, M., & Johnson, E. K. (2012). Infants exposed to fluent natural speech succeed at cross-gender word recognition. *Journal of Speech, Language, and Hearing Research, 55*(2), 554–560.

Varghese, L. A., Ozmeral, E. J., Best, V., & Shinn-Cunningham, B. G. (2012). How visual cues for when to listen aid selective auditory attention. *Journal for Research in Otolaryngology, 13*(3), 359–368.

Vassilopoulos, S. P., & Konstantinidis, G. (2012). Teacher use of silence in elementary education. *Journal of Teaching and Learning, 8,* 91–105.

Vigliocco, G., Perniss, P., & Vinson, D. (2014). Language as a multimodal phenomenon: implications for language learning, processing and evolution. *Philosophical Transactions of the Royal Society Biological Sciences, 369*(1651).

Wang, A. T., Lee, S. S., Sigman, M., & Dapretto, M. (2006). Developmental changes in the neural basis of interpreting communicative intent. *Social Cognitive and Affective Neuroscience, 1*(2), 107–121.

Wang, D. J., Trehub, S. E., Volkova, A., & van Lieshout, P. (2013). Child implant users' imitation of happy- and sad-sounding speech. *Frontiers in Psychology, 4*(351), 1–8.

Wasik, N. A., Bond, M. A., & Hindman, A. (2006). The effects of a language and literacy intervention on Head Start children and teachers. *Journal of Educational Psychology, 98,* 63–74.

Waxman, S., Fu, X., Arunachalam, S., Leddon, E., Geraghty, K., & Song, H-j. (2013). Are nouns learned before verbs? Infants provide insight into a long-standing debate. *Child Development Perspectives, 7*(3), 155–159.

Weikart, D. P., Rogers, L., Adcock, C., & McClelland, D. (1971). *The cognitively oriented curriculum.* Urbana, IL: ERIC-NAEYC.

Weisberg, D. S., Hirsh-Pasek, K., & Golinkoff, R. M. (2013). Guided play: Where curricular goals meet a playful pedagogy. *Mind, Brain, and Education, 7,* 104–112.

Weisleder, A., & Fernald, A. (2013). Talking to children matters: Early language experience strengthens processing and builds vocabulary. *Psychological Science, 24*(11), 2143–2152.

Weizman, Z. O., & Snow, C. E. (2001). Lexical input as related to children's vocabulary acquisition: Effects of sophisticated exposure and support for meaning. *Developmental Psychology, 37,* 265–279.

Werker, J. F., & Gervain, J. (2013). Speech perception in infancy: A foundation for language acquisition. In P. D. Zelazo (Ed.). *The Oxford handbook of developmental psychology, Vol 1: Body and mind* (pp. 909–925). New York, NY: Oxford University Press.

White, F. A., Livesey, D. J., & Hayes, B. K. (2015). *Developmental psychology from infancy to adulthood* (3rd ed.). Frenchs Forest NSW, Australia: Pearson.

Wingfield, A., & Tun, P. A. (2007). Cognitive supports and cognitive constraints on comprehension of spoken language. *Journal of American Academy of Audiology, 18,* 548–558.

Winstone, N., Davis, A., & De Bruyn, B. (2012). Developmental improvements in perceptual restoration: Can young children reconstruct missing sounds in noisy environments? *Infant and Child Development, 21,* 287–297.

Woolley, J. D., & Brown, M. M. (2015). The development of children's concepts of invisibility. *Cognitive Development, 34,* 63–75.

Woolley, J., & Ghossainy, M. (2013). Revisiting the fantasy-reality distinction: Children as naive skeptics. *Child Development, 84*(5), 1496–1510.

Woumans, E., Martin, C. D., Bulcke, C. V., Assche, E. V., Costa, A., Hartsuiker, R. J., & Duyck, W. (in press). Can faces prime a language? *Psychological Science.*

Xu, W., Chen, A., Cheng, F., & Ma, H. (2011). A study on the prosodic features of infant-directed speech in Mandarin Chinese. *Proceedings of the ICPhS XVII,* 2177–2180.

Yang, C. D. (2006). *The infinite gift: How children learn and unlearn the languages of the world*. New York, NY: Scribner.

Yeldham, M., & Gruba, P. (2014). Toward an instructional approach to developing interactive second language listening. *Language Teaching Research, 18*, 33–53.

Yeung, H. H., & Werker, J. F. (2013). Lip movements affect infants' audiovisual speech perception. *Psychological Science, 24*, 603–612.

Yin, J., & Csibra, G. (2015). Concept-based word learning in human infants. *Psychological Science, 26*, 1316–1324.

Yoder, P. J., McCathren, R. B., Warren, S. F. & Watson, A. L. (2001). Important distinctions in measuring maternal responses to communication in prelinguistic children with disabilities. *Communication Disorders Quarterly, 22*(3), 135–147.

Zangl, R., Klarman, L., Thal, D., Fernald, A., & Bates, E. (2005). Dynamics of word comprehension in infancy: Developments in timing, accuracy, and resistance to acoustic degradation. *Journal of Cognition and Development, 6*, 179–208.

Zekveld, A. A., Kramer, S. E., & Festen, J. M. (2011). Cognitive load during speech perception in noise: The influence of age, hearing loss, and cognition on the pupil response. *Ear and Hearing, 32*, 498–510.

11

PARENT COACHING STRATEGIES IN AUDITORY-VERBAL THERAPY

Ellen A. Rhoades and Karen MacIver-Lux

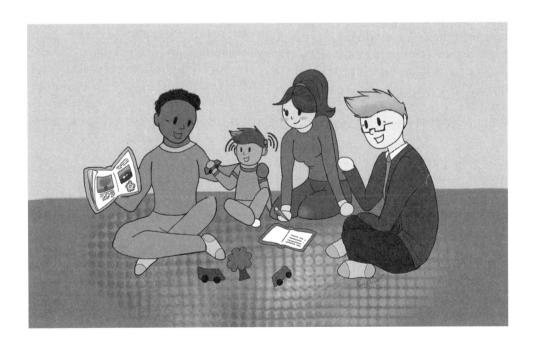

INTRODUCTION

Parent coaching is an *evidence-based interactive and developmental process* that facilitates adult learning and competencies (Friedman & Woods, 2012; Hanft, Rush, & Shelden, 2004). In Auditory-Verbal Therapy (AVT), as in other family-based early intervention models, this is a collaborative effort between practitioner and parent, helping parents discover their own strengths and enabling them to become confident parents of children with hearing loss (Rush & Shelden, 2005).

Coaching practices are used in multiple contexts and across numerous settings, and there is typically a predicable sequence to the process that includes (a) setting the stage which is either center or home based, (b) applying opportunities and feedback for adult learning, and (c) mastery whereby the parent generalizes and problem solves the effective use of strategies to encourage listening and talking as detailed in Chapter 10 (Friedman & Woods, 2012).

THE NEED FOR PARENT COACHING

Speaking parentese, known as infant-directed speech (see Chapter 10), is an imperative for effective parent-child interactions. Soderstrom and colleagues (2007) note that the nature and content of this speech input to preverbal children involves great variability. Relative to typical adult-adult speech, parentese involves exaggerated intonation and prosodic characteristics, reduced lexi-cal complexity, along with shorter and more simplified syntax that is not necessarily grammatically correct. In addition to incorporating such phonological differences as lengthened vowels and pauses, parentese tends to be repetitive, fluent, melodic, and rhythmic.

As reviewed by Golinkoff, Can, Soderstrom, and Hirsh-Pasek (2015), parentese occurs during parent-child interactions that, in turn, promote language learning. In addition to parentese, exchanges of eye gaze and affection are important features of parent-child interactions. These positive parent-child interactions foster social bonding while familiarizing children with their mother tongue. It is important that parents be consistently and appropriately responsive to their children on verbal and social levels.

Parent-child interactions that involve young children with hearing loss and limited language skills are at risk for poor communication (Barker et al., 2009; Quittner et al., 2010). Therefore, *the AV practitioner needs to focus on the nature and extent of parent interactions with their child, and hence the need for highly effective parent coaching strategies.*

POSITIVE OUTCOMES OF PARENT COACHING IN AVT

Kemp and Turnbull's (2014) review of the evidence indicates that there are many positive outcomes of parent coaching, and the most frequently occurring one is parental mastery of strategies that facilitate the child's development of communication skills. In addition to demonstrating greater progress in child development, other outcomes are

- improved parental perception of their child's abilities,
- more positive responsiveness to their child,
- decreased stress,
- more self-confidence, and
- a stronger alliance with the practitioner.

The AV practitioner promotes the parents' ability to reflect on their actions, and coaches them in developing and refining them to promote the child's listening and spoken language skills and general developmental outcomes. Parent coaching provides supportive learning situations so that parents can problem solve in order to effect behavioral change (ASHA, 2008).

In AVT, parent coaching strategies tend to involve a three-way relationship —the AV practitioner, the child with hearing loss, and the parent, all of whom are present during the AVT session. In AVT, because the parent actively participates in every session, the opportunities are great for the AV practitioner to focus on his or her skills in the development of parent coaching strategies.

STRENGTHS-BASED PARENT COACHING

Implementing *strengths-based coaching*, in general, is a compelling goal for AV practitioners. Strengths-based parent coaching requires that the practitioner note the perceived positive characteristics of the parent, the child, and their interaction style, and it is essential

to facilitate positive outcomes (Dunst, 2000). Across *all* parent coaching strategies, parents are encouraged to engage in strengths-based self-reflection. Outcomes of strengths-based coaching are parents who are more competent, confident, and insightful as well as children who participate more effectively in family life (Dunn, Cox, Foster, Mische-Lawson, & Tanquary, 2012).

AV practitioners often ask open-ended questions that promote parental reflection (Rush & Shelden, 2008) and/or make self-reflective statements and encourage parents to do the same. Open-ended questions may be as follows:

- "How will you know when your child understands?"
- "Why might that be hard for your daughter?"
- "How did you feel about what you just accomplished?"
- "What made that a worthwhile exercise?"
- "How was this beneficial to you or your child?"

When asking such questions, the AV practitioner is comfortable with moments of silence as they give parents time to think and respond. This is, indeed, similar to "waiting" strategies outlined for children in Chapter 10. Self-reflective statements of parents may be as follows:

- "My son did more than I hoped for."
- "It doesn't seem so difficult now."
- "I saw what I did that made it hard."
- "Wow, I'm surprised that my daughter responded so well to what I did!"

■ "Now that I understand it, I'll make sure to —."

■ "Hmmm . . . interesting . . . so I can use that as a guideline for planning goals."

■ "That's do-able for me."

When using parent coaching strategies, the AV practitioner engages in strengths-based observations (verbalized statements) and questions. Table 11–1 provides examples of how questions can be worded in a strengths-based manner.

Such questions facilitate *strengths-based self-reflection* as well as positive parental responsiveness (Steiner, 2011).

TOP FIVE PARENT COACHING STRATEGIES

Although the literature reflects differences in what constitutes coaching strategies (Artman-Meeker, Fettig, Barton, Penney, & Zeng, 2015; Kemp

Table 11-1. Strengths-Based Questions for Self-Reflection

Examples
• Were parents better able to self-regulate their displays of negative emotions (disapprovals, impatience, frustration)?
• Did they provide comfort when the child seemed frustrated or insecure?
• Did they demonstrate more flexibility?
• Did the parents use a variety of listening and language facilitative strategies?
• Which language facilitative strategies did parents most effectively use?
• Did they use those strategies consistently?
• Which of those strategies do the parents express most comfort in using?
• Did they seem more attuned to their child's feelings, needs, and wants?
• Were parents better able to refrain from controlling behaviors?
• Did parental engagement with the activity or their child seem more enjoyable and more sustained?
• Did the parents feel like the activity and child's performance met their expectations?
• Do parents feel more comfortable about doing the next activity with their child?
• Do parents seem to better understand their child? Were parents able to show more positive affect?
• In what ways were positive affect displayed to the child?
• Did the child seem to feel safe, secure, comfortable, and free to explore and play?
• Did the child seem more positive and responsive to the parent? How so?
• Did the parents seem especially pleased when their own behaviors produced desired child outcomes?
• Did they verbally express those feelings or in any way demonstrate more confidence as a result of the child outcomes?

& Turnbull, 2014), the following five parent coaching strategies suggested here are similar to most:

1. Having Conversations and Sharing Information
2. Collaborating in Setting Goals and Planning Activities
3. Demonstrating
4. Guiding Practice with Feedback
5. Providing Video-Feedback

The extent and degree to which AV practitioners use each parent coaching strategy varies considerably, depending primarily on parental characteristics, needs, and context (Friedman & Woods, 2012).

Parent Coaching Strategy #1: Having Conversations and Sharing Information

Having conversations and sharing information is a critical learning process that involves at least the parent and practitioner (Fitzpatrick, Graham, Durieux-Smith, Angus, & Coyle, 2007). Both adults are actively engaged in multipurpose bidirectional conversations (Friedman & Woods, 2012) and, in fact, the child with hearing loss may or may not be present.

Each participant comments, asks, and responds to questions. For example, when the AV practitioner first meets parents, questions may be asked about the child's daily routines, the child's interests and skills, the family's current stressors and needs, the parents' goals for the child, the family's current schedule, and the extent to which each member can participate in the AV process. This fact-finding conversation helps the AV practitioner to support the parent's perspectives and cultural practices (Rhoades, 2007). The practitioner endeavors to learn what the parent already knows and understands; this facilitates parental learning of new information when it fits within the parent's existing mental framework (Rush & Shelden, 2008).

Having a concrete but flexible approach is integral to the sharing of information (Kaiser & Hancock, 2003). This means the practitioner simplifies complex issues to help the parents understand them as quickly as possible while simultaneously demonstrating respect for the parent's level of competence. Parents want *practical* information (Knowles, Holton, & Swanson, 2005), so sharing information is presented in the context of the child. For example, understanding the importance of audiological testing is more likely to occur when the practitioner discusses implications of specific tests for the child. Likewise, the practitioner may observe the child engaging in disruptive behaviors while the parent is reading a story; this might precipitate a discussion about specific evidence-based strategies that effectively minimize or prevent children's inappropriate behaviors.

The practitioner continually acquires knowledge pertaining to all issues and all domains related to AVT and typical child development. For example, the AV practitioner strives to facilitate "parental reflective functioning" (understanding the child's behavior in light of underlying mental states and intentions). This parent coaching strategy of having *conversations and sharing information*, then, may involve a discussion on different perspectives (Slade, 2005).

Knowledge can be shared through individual and/or group parent meetings (Glanemann, Reichmuth, Matulat, & am Zehnhoff-Dinnesen, 2013; Henderson, Johnson, & Moodie, 2014). Sometimes books, DVDs, and other materials are loaned to parents or a single page of information may be given to them along with a 10 to 15-min discussion after each AVT session. When information is shared with more than just one adult in the child's family, this can strengthen the parent's supportive network (Jackson, Wegner, & Turnbull, 2010). Sometimes, expanding a parent's resources necessitates information sharing beyond the usual workday. Some family-based early intervention programs encourage flexible hours so that practitioners can accommodate the needs of families unable to attend AVT sessions during typical work hours (Bernstein & Eriks-Brophy, 2010).

After each information-sharing episode, the AV practitioner can ask the parent questions such as the following:

- "Do you feel like this meeting was helpful?"
- "Would you like more information on this subject?"
- "Which part do you feel was most helpful?"
- "Are there other ways we could have exchanged information?"
- "Did the video/booklet make sense when you reviewed it?"

Parent Coaching Strategy #2: Collaborating in Setting Goals and Planning Activities

Collaborating in setting goals refers to the act of parent and practitioner

exchanging information, and then making decisions about which long-term goals and short-term objectives will be targeted within a certain time frame (Palisano, Snider & Orlin, 2004); this has an added advantage of facilitating practitioner-parent rapport (Wolf, Launay, & Dunbar, in press).

Parents are provided with the results of all assessment outcomes that represent the baseline for their child's progress; this includes informing them about their child's current level of development relative to peers with typical hearing. Sharing typical developmental milestones is essential in that these are typically used as referents for determining goals, objectives, and progress. Then, the AV practitioner asks parents to talk about their desired long-term listening and spoken language outcomes.

The AV practitioner engages the parent in discussions and/or joint evaluations of the child's current skills, and the daily needs of family members. They collaboratively select age-appropriate long-term goals and/or short-term objectives that can be targeted in the AVT sessions and, most importantly, in the child's daily activities and interaction with others. Parents who participate in this process are usually better able to follow through on the use of relevant strategies such as those referred to in Chapter 10 (Rone-Adams, Stern, & Walker, 2004). These parents tend to be more motivated and active in the generalization of targeted skills than those who did not collaborate in goal planning (Øien, Fallang, & Østenja, 2010).

Collaborating in planning activities refers to the parent and practitioner jointly selecting or planning follow-up home activities. Typically, parents know their child's interests better than anyone else, but the AV practitioner is prepared to suggest at-home activities that can reinforce the session activities. Some practitioners share a plan of activities with the parents prior to every AVT session; this can help parents better understand the purposes of each activity as well as the general flow of the session. Regardless, the AVT plan will be adjusted throughout the session based on the child's level of responsiveness and demonstrated skills.

At the end of each AVT session, the practitioner and parent jointly evaluate outcomes of each activity and collaboratively develop a plan to incorporate the newly learned strategies and short-term objectives into the family's daily routines. Collaborative planning helps give parents a sense of control over their child's services, supports, and resources that contribute to the child's, the parent's, and the family's well-being (Coyle & McKee, 2015).

As parents develop skills and rapport, the practitioner can ask the parent the following:

■ "What would you like to focus on between now and our next visit?"
■ "Based upon what we've done today, what is your plan for the next week?"
■ "What do you want to accomplish between now and the next time that we talk?" (Rush & Shelden, 2008).

Parent Coaching Strategy #3: Demonstrating

Prior to the initiation of AVT sessions, there is an assessment and fact-finding period; the purpose of this is to help the AV practitioner to understand both child and family. This includes observing how the parent interacts with the child. The practitioner makes notes as to whether the parent was sufficiently and positively responsive to the child, and may share some of those observations with the parent.

In subsequent AVT sessions, the practitioner may provide a few *demonstrations* of play activities with a child without the parent being actively engaged. This means the parent just observes and makes written notes. If the practitioner chooses, this demonstration can help the parent "see" the child from a different perspective (e.g., to realize that the child can hear or can vocalize with a bit of encouragement). The practitioner can use this opportunity to comment on the child's strengths, on the purposes of the practitioner-demonstrated activities, and on the strategies used by the practitioner during interactions with the child.

Demonstrating without actively involving parents may be a viable option for some parents who are initially uncomfortable being put "on the spot" and who have not yet developed rapport with the AV practitioner. Some parents may seem "guarded" or withdrawn, and they may want to become more familiar with what is expected in the AVT session prior to actively jumping in to participate. Some parents do not respond well if they sense they are "in the hot seat."

When parents are "new" to AVT, they may look to the AV practitioner as "the expert" who creates a safe and supportive environment for learning (Kaiser & Hancock, 2003). In most family-based early intervention models, however, the practitioner disavows the expert position simply because the practitioner is *not* the agent of change (Espe-Sherwindt, 2008). Instead, the parent is the agent of change, and it is the job of the practitioner to enable the parent to act on that perspective (Rhoades, 2010). Fortunately, a basic adult learning principle is that parents can and do learn by observation (Knowles et al., 2005). Even though the AV practitioner demonstrates a high degree of expertise in applying the strategies outlined in Chapter 10, the "expert" role is to be shared with parents (Bæck, 2010; Dunst, Boyd, Trivette, & Hamby, 2002).

As soon as possible, a transition is made to having parents *actively* participate in AVT sessions. Transitioning to "guided practice with feedback" (coaching strategy #4) is discussed with parents prior to the actual transition.

Parent Coaching Strategy #4: Providing Guided Practice With Feedback

Providing guided practice with feedback involves opportunities for parents to practice implementing strategies, to obtain feedback from the practitioner, and to refine those skills that are critical for optimal parent-child interactions. This interactive triadic coaching strategy results in transformative learning because it creates a *continuous cycle of action* that involves parental reflection upon action (Dexter, Dexter, & Irving, 2011). A realistic goal is to have parents internalize and master implementation of all appropriate strategies (Brown & Woods, 2015).

The practitioner and parent jointly create and implement structured activities that are preplanned, focused on targeted short-term objectives, and different from one AVT session to the next. Suggestions and rationales that are provided to the parent (ahead of each activity as well as during and after each activity) are easy to understand, such as the following:

- "Did you see how I leaned in closer to her microphone when I said the /s/ sound? That helped Akisha hear the sound more clearly."
- "What I'm hoping to show you is how we can get your son to vocalize if he wants the jack-in-the-box to pop out."
- "It's your turn to _____."
- "Let's see if we can prompt your daughter to move that bus when we sing the song."

When the parent takes turns participating in an activity, the practitioner provides verbal transitions such as the following:

- "That was so much fun, Ali! Do that with daddy!"
- "Let's give mommy another turn!"
- "Uncle Jeremiah, can you guess what is in the box?"
- "I want a turn, too!"

The parent is encouraged to practice a number of specific strategies while the AV practitioner remains quiet and observes the interaction. When the parent gains more confidence, the practitioner becomes engaged as the "guide on the side," and coaches in his or her own personal style.

The practitioner's coaching is built on what the parent already knows, so it is scaffolded, both guided and broken down into smaller, manageable sections for easier recall and comprehension (Hanft et al., 2004). The practitioner's feedback is direct and formative in that it is nonjudgmental, timely, supportive, and specific (Shute, 2008). Such feedback may be as follows:

- "Did you see what happened when you whispered that?"
- "Wow, Juan so enjoyed doing that with you!"
- "Were you as thrilled as me to see that?"

The practitioner facilitates self-reflection by asking open-ended questions that are positive and nonthreatening:

- "How do you feel you did?"
- "What do you think was the best part of that activity?"
- "Why did that work so well for Dosa?"

The practitioner recognizes that making mistakes is part of the learning process. With the practitioner's targeted and positive feedback, parents learn to self-correct and to continually adjust their strategies as they practice new skills when interacting with their children (Girolametto & Weitzman, 2006). The practitioner helps parents in this process, for example, "I noticed that when you waited a bit longer, your son vocalized!" The AV practitioner also encourages them to reflect upon what they did and upon the feedback they received, for example, "That was awesome the way you got your daughter to listen for softer sounds. Why did you decide to increase your distance from her?" In addition, the practitioner records and maintains clinical notes

during and after all AVT sessions, including all observed successes and stated parental concerns (Kaiser & Hancock, 2003).

Parent Coaching Strategy #5: Providing Video-Feedback

Providing video-feedback, also known as *video interaction guidance*, is an evidence-based means of coaching for optimal interaction between parents and children with hearing loss (Lam-Cassettari, Wadnerkar-Kamble, & James, 2015; Pilnick & James, 2013; Quittner et al., 2013). This systematic intervention is based on a review of video segments taken during parents' interactions with their children.

Prior to initiating each video, parents with the practitioner their goals for the activity in a goal-setting conversation (see parent coaching strategy #1). The practitioner then video records the 15 to 20-min activity, and the video is replayed in a later *shared viewing*. During the shared viewing session of approximately 45 min, parent and practitioner analyze the behaviors observed. The AV practitioner focuses on the parent's strengths, targeting those behaviors that meet the activity goals. The parent's *successful moments of interacting* with the child are highlighted, thus helping the parent to self-reflect.

An advantage of this joint video analysis is that parents may be more objective in viewing their own behaviors, and coaching may be more effective. In fact, researchers find that improvements in parent-child interactions happen after just a few short sessions of video-feedback intervention (Kemppinen, 2007; Lam-Cassettari et al., 2015).

Videos may not capture the parents' typical communicative styles, but they can be a reliable indicator of the *interactions occurring during specific activities* involving children with hearing loss (Glanemann et al., 2013; Kemppinen, 2007). Particularly with high-risk and low-socioeconomic families and with families who have children with special needs, providing video-feedback is typically effective in facilitating parent-child interactions (Juffer & Steele, 2014; Negrão et al., 2014; Poslawsky et al., 2014; Yagmur et al., 2014).

Video analyses can be especially helpful for those parents who are unable to participate effectively in AVT in the presence of the AV practitioner, or are uncomfortable with receiving praise and direct feedback during AVT sessions via guided practice (Kaiser & Hancock, 2003). Video-recorded sessions can also reveal whether there is a need for further intensive intervention from the AV practitioner (Lawrence, Davies, & Ramchandrane, 2012).

ATTRIBUTES OF AN EFFECTIVE COACH IN AVT

Certain traits and skills are needed to effectively communicate with parents (Geldard & Geldard, 2008). The communicative attributes considered here provide the underpinning for all coaching strategies suggested above and in general need to guide the behaviors of the AV practitioner. His or her "professional persona" needs to embrace the following: creating *a trusting alliance, a supportive relationship, a genuine communicative style, reflective listening and a problem-solving approach.*

A Safe, Confidential, Trusting Alliance

This involves building rapport between practitioner and parent. Warmth can be facilitated when the practitioner appropriately and selectively imitates the parent's unique conversational mannerisms, sometimes known as *mimicry* (Leander, Chartrand, & Bargh, 2012). The practitioner does not demonstrate cultural or religious preferences. When discussing issues of culture, the practitioner shows an ease and respect for those issues, including race and poverty. The family's privacy is assured at all times and the practitioner demonstrates behaviors that facilitate a trusting alliance.

An Attentive and Supportive Relationship

This signifies demonstrating unconditional positive regard and nonjudgmental acceptance (even when the AV practitioner does not approve of the parent's behaviors, providing the child is safe). The AV practitioner treats each child and parent with dignity and respect, building upon each person's strengths. Every parent comes to the practitioner with considerable experience of his or her own, and the AV practitioner ensures parents that all their thoughts are welcomed, listens actively, and pays close attention to what the parent shares (Geldard & Geldard, 2008).

A Genuine Communicative Style

The AV practitioner shows a genuine interest in the parent and the child's family life and demonstrates *authenticity, sincerity, honesty*, and a friendly sense of humor. Just as the AV practitioner is sincere about the positive progress of both child and parent, he or she is honest when *bad news* needs to be shared (Geldard & Geldard, 2008). The AV practitioner is able to recognize when he or she and the parent may not be a "good fit" with each other and know when it might be better to have another practitioner work with the parent, and be demonstrative in facilitating a transition with ease and professionalism.

A Reflective Listening and Problem-Solving Approach

The AV practitioner engages in reflective listening and a problem-solving approach with parents. *Reflective listening* is the mirroring of emotional communication, both in tone and feeling (affective responses) as well as in content and meaning (behavioral and cognitive responses). Also known as *echoing*, it involves active listening and interpretation, empathy, and open-ended questioning (Hodge & Chantler, 2010).

For example, the parent might say, "I'm sad today" and the practitioner responds by saying, "Sorry to hear that. Sorry to hear that you are sad about something." Without any further questioning, this may encourage the parent to say more. Reflective listening signals to the parent that he or she is being heard and the deeper meaning of the message is being sought. Such reflective responses from the AV practitioner give parents opportunities to elaborate on what they said.

The AV practitioner as a reflective listener might also say the following:

- "If I'm hearing you correctly, you're really frustrated that the MRI appointment is 2 months away."
- "Do you mean that you would like to have your mother come to some AVT sessions?"
- "I want to make sure I understand; I'm hearing that you want your husband to be more involved in the IEP process. Is this right?"

Demonstrating *a problem-solving approach to conversing* with parents is very important. The practitioner makes suggestions rather than gives directions or recommendations (Flasher & Fogle, 2011). A simple suggestion may be embedded in questions such as the following:

- "Have you considered that maybe this . . . or that . . . might be tried?"
- "Did you try . . . ?"
- "Hmm, I wonder if the child . . . ?"
- "Do you think that the strategy of . . . might work?"
- "Have you thought about . . . ?"
- "Is it possible that . . . ?"

These guided questions can suggest to parents that there are new ways of looking at an old problem (Friedman & Woods, 2012).

CONCLUSION

In addition to appropriate and consistent audiological management at an early age, a high level of parent engagement in AVT is the best predictor for developing age-appropriate listening and spoken language skills in children with hearing loss (Glanemann et al., 2013; Reichmuth et al., 2013). The AV practitioner, therefore, needs to be knowledgeable and comfortable about implementing effective parent coaching strategies this can help ensure that desired listening and spoken language outcomes will be achieved as quickly as possible (e.g., Fitzpatrick, Grandpierre, Durieux-Smith, & Sallam, 2016). In conjunction with the strategies for developing listening and talking presented in Chapter 10, the AV practitioner uses these parent coaching strategies to optimize parent-child interactions that, in turn, will help close the listening and talking gap created by the child's hearing loss.

REFERENCES

American Speech-Language-Hearing Association (ASHA). (2008). *Core knowledge and skills in early intervention speech-language pathology practice* [knowledge and skills]. Retrieved from http://www.asha.org/policy

Artman-Meeker, K., Fettig, A., Barton, E. E., Penney, A., & Zeng, S. (2015). Applying an evidence-based framework to the early childhood coaching literature. *Topics in Early Childhood Special Education, 35*, 183–196.

Barker, D. H., Quittner, A. L., Fink, N. E., Eisenberg, L. S., Tobey, E. A., Niparko, J. K., & The CDaCI Investigative Team. (2009). Predicting behavior problems in deaf and hearing children: The influence of language, attention, and parent-child communication. *Development and Psychopathology, 21*, 373–392.

Bæck, U-D. K. (2010). "*We are the professionals*": A study of teachers' views on parental involvement in school. *British Journal of Sociology of Education, 31*, 323–335.

Bernstein, A., & Eriks-Brophy, A. (2010). Supporting families. In E. A. Rhoades & J. Duncan (pp. 225–257). *Auditory-verbal practice: Toward a family-centered approach*. Springfield, IL: Charles C. Thomas.

Brown, J., & Woods, J. (2015). Effects of a triadic parent-implemented home-based communication intervention for toddlers. *Journal of Early Intervention, 37*, 44–68.

Coyle, J., & McKee, D. (2015). A comparison of the beliefs and priorities of early intervention providers and the families they serve. *Journal of Education and Social Policy, 2*(2), 1–9.

Dexter, J., Dexter, G., & Irving, J. (2011). *An introduction to coaching*. Thousand Oaks, CA: Sage.

Dunn, W., Cox, J., Foster, L., Mische-Lawson, L., & Tanquary, J. (2012). Impact of a contextual intervention on parental competence and children's participation for children with Autism Spectrum disorders (ASD): A pretest posttest repeated measures design. *American Journal of Occupational Therapy, 66*, 520–528.

Dunst, C. J. (2000). Revisiting "Rethinking early intervention." *Topics in Early Childhood Special Education, 20*, 95–104.

Dunst, C. J., Boyd, K., Trivette, C. M., & Hamby, D. W. (2002). Family-oriented program models and professional help giving practices. *Family Relations, 51*, 221–229.

Espe-Sherwindt, M. (2008). Family-centred practice: Collaboration, competency and evidence. *Support for Learning, 23*, 136–143.

Fitzpatrick, E., Graham, I. D., Durieux-Smith, A., Angus, D., & Coyle, D. (2007). Parents' perspectives on the impact of the early diagnosis of childhood hearing loss. *International Journal of Audiology, 46*, 97–106.

Fitzpatrick, E., Grandpierre, V., Durieux-Smith, A., & Sallam, N. (2016). Children with mild bilateral and unilateral hearing loss: Parents' reflections on experiences and outcomes. *Journal of Deaf Studies and Deaf Education, 21,* 34–43.

Flasher, L. V., & Fogle, P. T. (2011). *Counseling skills for speech-language pathologists and audiologists* (2nd ed.). San Diego, CA: Singular.

Friedman, M., & Woods, J. (2012). Caregiver coaching strategies for early intervention providers: Moving toward operational definitions. *Infants and Young Children, 25,* 62–82.

Geldard, K., & Geldard, D. (2008). *Personal counseling skills: An integrative approach.* Springfield, IL: Charles C. Thomas.

Girolametto, L., & Weitzman, E. (2006). It Takes Two to Talk®—The Hanen Program® for parents: Early language intervention through caregiver training. In R. McCauley & M. Fey (Eds.), *Treatment of language disorders in children* (pp. 77–103). Baltimore, MD: Paul H. Brookes.

Glanemann, R., Reichmuth, K., Matulat, P., & Zehnhoff-Dinnesen, A. (2013). Muenster Parental Programme empowers parents in communicating with their infant with hearing loss. *International Journal of Pediatric Otorhinolaryngology, 77,* 2023–2029.

Golinkoff, R. M., Can, D. D., Soderstrom, M., & Hirsh-Pasek, K. (2015). (Baby)Talk to me: The social context of infant-directed speech and its effects on early language acquisition. *Current Directions in Psychological Science, 24,* 339–344.

Hanft, B. E., Rush, D. D., & Shelden, M. L. (2004). *Coaching families and colleagues in early childhood.* Baltimore, MD: Brookes.

Henderson, R. J., Johnson, A., & Moodie, S. (2014). Parent-to-parent support for parents with children who are deaf or hard of hearing: A conceptual framework. *American Journal of Audiology, 23,* 437–448.

Hodge, N., & Chantler, S. (2010). It's not what you do; it's the way that you question: That's what gets results. *Support for Learning, 25,* 11–14.

Jackson, C. W., Wegner, J. R., & Turnbull, A. P. (2010). Family quality of life following early identification of deafness. *Language, Speech, and Hearing Services in Schools, 41,* 194–206.

Juffer, F., & Steele, M. (2014). What words cannot say: The telling story of video in attachment-based interventions. *Attachment and Human Development, 16,* 307–314.

Kaiser, A. P., & Hancock, T. B. (2003). Teaching parents new skills to support their young children's development. *Infants and Young Children, 16,* 9–21.

Kemp, P., & Turnbull, A. P. (2014). Coaching with parents in early intervention: An interdisciplinary research synthesis. *Infants and Young Children, 27,* 305–324.

Kemppinen, K. (2007). *Early maternal sensitivity: Continuity and related risk factors.* Doctoral dissertation retrieved September 30, 2015, from http://wanda.uef.fi/uku-vaitokset/vaitokset/2007/isbn978-951-27-0672-3.pdf

Knowles, M. S., Holton, E. F., & Swanson, R. A. (2005). *The adult learner: The definitive classic in adult education and human resource development* (6th ed.) London, UK: Elsevier.

Lam-Cassettari, C., Wadnerkar-Kamble, M. B., & James, D. M. (2015). Enhancing parent-child communication and parental self-esteem with a video-feedback intervention: Outcomes with prelingual deaf and hard of hearing children. *Journal of Deaf Studies and Deaf Education, 20,* 266–274.

Lawrence, P. J., Davies, B., & Ramchandani, P. G. (2012). Using video feedback to improve early father-infant interaction: A pilot study. *Clinical Child Psychology, 18,* 61–71.

Leander, N. P., Chartrand, T. L., & Bargh, J. A. (2012). You give me the chills: Embodied reactions to inappropriate amounts of behavioral mimicry. *Psychological Science, 23,* 772–779.

Negrão, M., Pereira, M., Soares, I., & Mesman, J. (2014). Enhancing positive parent-child interactions and family functioning in a poverty sample: A randomized control trial. *Attachment and Human Development, 16,* 315–328.

Øien, I., Fallang, B., & Østenja, S. (2010). Goal-setting in paediatric rehabilitation: Perceptions of parents and professional. *Child Care Health Development, 36,* 558–565.

Palisano, R. J., Snider, L. M., & Orlin, M. N. (2004). Recent advances in physical and occupational therapy for children with cerebral palsy. *Seminar in Pediatric Neurology, 11,* 66–77.

Pilnick, A., & James, D. M. (2013). "I'm thrilled that you see that": Guiding parents to see success in interactions with children with deafness and autistic spectrum disorder. *Social Science & Medicine, 99,* 89–101.

Poslawsky, I. E., Naber, F. B. A., Bakermans-Kranenburg, M. J., De Jonge, M. V., Engeland, H. V., & van IJzendoorn, M. H. (2014). Development of a video-feedback intervention to promote positive parenting for children with autism (VIPP-AUTI). *Attachment and Human Development, 16,* 343–355.

Quittner, A. L., Barker, D. H., Cruz, I., Snell, C., Grimley, M. E., & Botteri, M. (2010). Parenting stress among parents of deaf and hearing children: Associations with language delays and behavior problems. *Parenting, 10,* 136–155.

Quittner, A. L., Cruz, I., Barker, D. H., Tobey, E., Eisenberg, L. S., & Niparko, J. K. (2013). Effects of maternal sensitivity and cognitive and linguistic stimulation on cochlear implant users' language development over four years. *Journal of Pediatrics, 162,* 343–348.

Reichmuth, K., Embacher, A. J., Matulat, P., Am Zehnhoff-Dinnesen, A., & Glanemann, R. (2013). Responsive parenting intervention after identification of hearing loss by Universal Newborn Hearing Screening: The concept of the Muenster Parental Programme. *International Journal of Pediatric Otorhinolaryngology, 77,* 2030–2039.

Rhoades, E. A. (2007). Setting the stage for culturally responsive intervention. *Volta Voices, 14*(4), 10–13.

Rone-Adams, S. A., Stern, D. F., & Walker, V. (2004). Stress and compliance with a home exercise program among caregivers of children with disabilities. *Pediatric Physical Therapy, 16,* 140–148.

Rush, D. D., & Shelden, M. L. (2005). Evidence-based definition of coaching practices. *CASEInPoint, 1*(6), 1–6.

Rush, D. D., & Shelden, M. L. (2008). Tips and techniques for effective coaching interactions. *BriefCASE, 1*(2), 1–4.

Shute, V. J. (2008). Focus on formative feedback. *Review of Educational Research, 78,* 153–189.

Slade, A. (2005). Parental reflective functioning: An introduction. *Attachment and Human Development, 7,* 269–281.

Soderstrom, M. (2007). Beyond babytalk: Re-evaluating the nature and content of speech input to preverbal infants. *Developmental Review, 27,* 501–532.

Steiner, A. M. (2011). A strength-based approach to parent education for children with autism. *Journal of Positive Behavior Intervention, 13,* 178–190.

Wolf, W., Launay, J., & Dunbar, R. I. (in press). Joint attention, shared goals, and social bonding. *British Journal of Psychology.*

Yagmur, S., Mesman, J., Malda, M., Bakermans-Kranenburg, M. J., & Ekmekci, H. (2014). Video-feedback intervention increases sensitive parenting in ethnic minority mothers: A randomized control trial. *Attachment and Human Development, 16,* 371–386.

12

BLUEPRINT OF AN AUDITORY-VERBAL THERAPY SESSION

Warren Estabrooks, Karen MacIver-Lux,
Louise Hönck, and Rosie Quayle

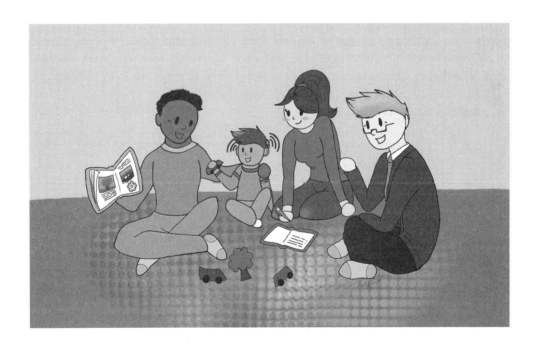

INTRODUCTION

The *blueprint* of an Auditory-Verbal Therapy (AVT) session is driven by the principles of AVT (see Chapter 1) and the evidence generated from current research in hearing and speech science, child development, and family-centered intervention. A blueprint is "a plan, template, guide, prototype or sample" (Oxford Advanced Learning Dictionary, 2015). In terms of AVT, this blueprint is a plan that shows what can be achieved and how it can be accomplished. It is individually tailored to meet the needs of the child with hearing loss and his or her family and follows a composition or organization that may be used by the AV practitioner to simplify his or her workload and to accommodate the practitioner's individual therapy style. For the most part, depending on the age and stage of development in AVT of the child, the blueprint for all AVT sessions contains components that forward the SIX GOALS of the AV practitioner (Chapter 10) and the Parent Coaching Practices in AVT (Chapter 11). This chapter is an opinion piece of the authors based on many years of experience, and outlines suggested components of an AVT session:

- Pre-session (Figure 12–1)
- AVT Session in Action (Figure 12–2)
- Post-session (Figure 12–3)

PRE-SESSION

Review the Child's Current Progress Summary and Long-Term Objectives

Study the child's chart (the record) and review (a) the child's current skills as demonstrated in the previous session; (b) the "homework" or take-home messages generated by the parents (carry-over targets, planned visits and/or communication with other members of the family's team, etc.); (c) the practitioner's additional notes on any topic pertaining to the child and his or her family; and (d) recently received reports from other professional partners (Chapter 16) (e.g., reports from audiologic assessments, etc.).

Set Short-Term Objectives

Set short-term objectives based on the child's hearing age, chronological age and stage of development, and the

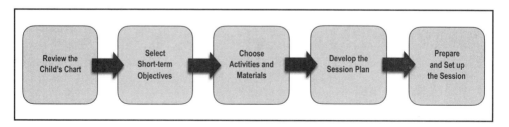

Figure 12-1. Pre-session.

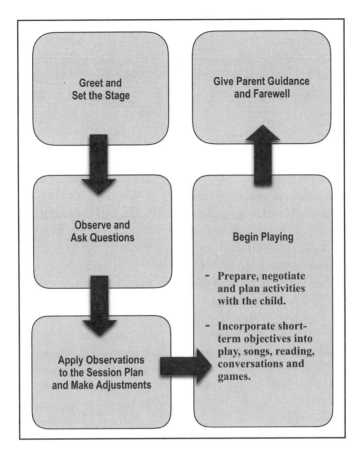

Figure 12–2. AVT session in action.

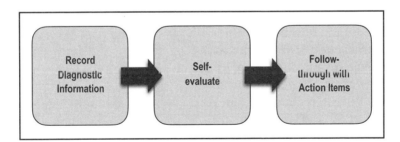

Figure 12–3. Post-session.

child's *zone of proximal development* (Vygotsky, 1997) demonstrated in previous sessions including those that parent(s) are eager to help their child learn. Short-term objectives are those that can be accomplished in one to four AVT sessions and need to cover audition, speech, language, communication, and cognition. Some families may also have "behavior" objectives if they are shaping positive behaviors during the therapy session and at home. Set the short-term objectives on professional performance of the practitioner (skills you want to improve) and the short-term objectives of the parent (skills the parent needs to improve).

Choose the Materials and Activities

Choose activities that (a) are age and stage appropriate, (b) can stimulate and hopefully measure the short-term ob-jectives, (c) hold the child's interest but will not be too distracting, (d) suit the family's culture, (e) encourage the child's sense of self by supporting his or her thinking and problem-solving skills, and (f) contain intrinsic and extrinsic rewards (feeling excited about making cookies (intrinsic) and eating the cookies after baking them (extrinsic).

Develop the Session Plan

List all the short-term objectives and selected activities. Plan how each one will be delivered and how the transition will happen from one activity to another; cite the strategies planned (Chapter 10); determine the questions you might ask the parents; collect resources (hand-outs, books, etc.); and anticipate the "homework" that might be required or the possible take-home messages that might arise from the session.

Prepare Session and Set It Up

Ensure that all toys, books, and other therapy materials are within reach and

in good condition. Select appropriate seating for all participants (unless you plan to play only on the floor) and check the acoustic environment so that it is as free from extraneous noise as possible.

AVT SESSION IN ACTION

Greeting and Setting the Stage

An AVT session begins when the family comes through the door or when the practitioner enters the child's home, depending on the location of the session. The practitioner asks leading questions, states objectives, models the activity, and passes it to the parent who practices with the child, coaches the parents to help them achieve the expected outcome of each activity, and provides feedback on how both the child and the parent are doing.

Greeting the Child

- Greet the child in a calm, friendly, and enthusiastic manner, getting down to his or her level, smiling and making eye contact. This sets up the expectation of interaction and conversation for the entire session.

Greeting the Parents

- The AV practitioner asks, *"How are things going?"* and listens carefully to the parents' response as it may change the plans. The child may only observe the conversation or may join in.

- The practitioner's second leading question might be, *"How can I help you most today?"* or *"What do you want me to help you with today?"* or *"What would you like to get from the session today?"*
- The AV practitioner follows the parents' answers to ensure that the short-term objectives based on the current level of functioning of the child, actually address needs of the parents' and the child makes adjustments when necessary.
- The practitioner may say, *"It sounds as if it might be useful to . . . "* *"Based on what you have told me, it might be a good idea to . . . ,"* or *"Let's begin with the end in mind,"* or *"Keep your eyes on the prize."* We do not set up nor encourage unrealistic expectations.
- Sometimes the parent may not have a lot to say, but with cumulative experience in AVT they will come to know that these questions are asked every session and will be prepared. It is only in the first few sessions that that may feel they are in the "hot seat," but it is they who are the primary "client."
- Sometimes, the practitioner can follow the session exactly as he or she planned it in advance, following the lead of the child and the parents and simply adapting the session as it proceeds following the Auditory-Verbal Therapy Session Cycle (AVTSC). Sometimes all the objectives can be met in one activity, one scenario, or one unexpected event.

Hearing Technology Check

That AV practitioner may or may not include this as part of each session. After a few sessions, the parents know how to do this and will have done it either in the waiting room or just before the practitioner arrives for the session.

Observation

Diagnostic AVT involves knowing the child's current stage of development in listening, talking, thinking, and problem solving and the next steps to move forward so that we do not "teach things the child already knows." Sometimes it is good to observe the parent and child begin the session by playing together (they are the best playmates), by doing a puzzle, blowing bubbles, or reading a book. The practitioner is the "fly on the wall," observing the parent-child interactions to informally determine current skills in audition, speech, spoken and receptive language, play, gross and fine motor development, sensory skills, and so on. The practitioner observes these behaviors based on clinical experiences, their knowledge of each child and family, and by using his or her clinical intuition (Chapter 10).

The interactions are particularly important and can reveal the following among other things:

- How do the parents get their child's attention?
- In the parents' initiations, do they "tune in, talk more, and take turns" (Suskind, 2015)?
- Do the parents require a little or a lot of coaching or should the

child's listening and language levels be adjusted?

- Are the parents able to engage actively in play by modeling, narrating, and scaffolding?
- Are the parents' expectations for their child to be part of the conversation or do the parents rescue the child when anticipating an error?

The practitioner can then apply the results of the observation to the session plan and make adjustments as required.

Discussing the Plan for the Session

Based on the observations of the child and parent during their interactions, the AV practitioner and parent discuss the short-term objectives and the parent restates them.

The AV practitioner discusses the strategies the parent most likely requires based on the parent-child interaction.

Begin the Session by Playing

Prepare, Negotiate, and Plan Activities With the Child

The AV practitioner or parent explains the plan in language that is appropriate for the child and talks about the activity and what is going to happen, and how many steps it might involve, such as one step (Let's do drawing!), two steps (We're going to do drawing and then read a book!), or three steps (first we'll draw, then we'll read, and then we can go outside!). The practitioner may offer a choice of activities or the order in which they might occur.

- By using play as the cornerstone of the AVT session, the AV practitioner incorporates short-term objectives into each activity from early sessions of *Beginning Sounds* (Chapter 10) to higher-level sessions where the demands on auditory-cognitive skills are great.
- During each activity, the AV practitioner incorporate the suggested Auditory-Verbal Therapy Session Cyle (AVTSC) (Figure 12–4) using the following steps:

1. State the objectives to the parent(s) (e.g., *"Today we're thinking about building Mary's repertoire of two word sentences, and we're going to focus particularly on using 'No' to reject and to mark absence."*),

2. Explain the activity (e.g., *"As you said you love to cook at home, we're going to make little cereal cakes in a moment, but we'll forget to get a plate out for you. We can then go round and say 'She has a plate, you have a plate, but Mummy has __," and help Mary fill in the gap 'no plate.' Then have a good giggle when the cup and a spoon are forgotten and see if she tells you there is "no spoon" herself."*).

3. Demonstrate the activity (one to three times) (e.g., *"Did you see how I leaned in closer when I said the /s/ sound? This will help Susie to hear it." "Did you see how she filled in the*

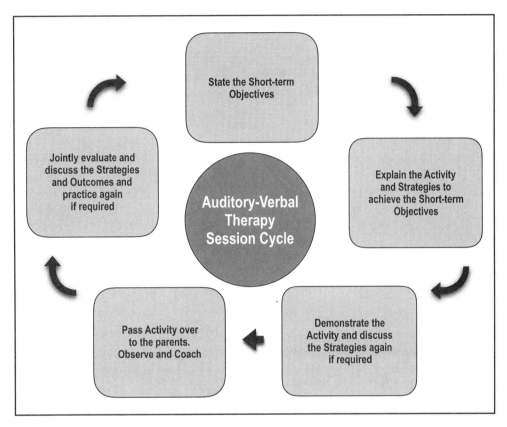

Figure 12–4. Auditory-Verbal Therapy Session Cycle (AVTSC).

gap with 'no spoon' when you waited a bit longer and gave her a look of expectation?").

4. Pass the activity to the parent(s) and observe as the parent practices (e.g., *"Look how he is enjoying it. Why don't you try it now?"* or *"That was so nice Mary! Why don't you do this with Daddy?").*

5. The AV practitioner and the parent(s) jointly evaluate the outcomes of the activity and talk about ways to generalize the outcomes of this at home during the

family's daily routines (e.g., *"I've noticed that when you waited a little longer there, he vocalized! How do you think you can do this more at home?").*

Parent Guidance and Farewell

The auditory-verbal practitioner ensures that parents do not leave the session wondering what they are supposed to do during the following week. The final 10 to 15 min of the AVT session are reserved for discussing the child's and parent's progress; reviewing the short-term objectives and how they can be incorporated into the family's daily routines and extended to life in the community; and identifying key strategies to develop listening and spoken language (Chapter 10). Parents might write these down in their "parent book" or add them to the child's "experience book." Each parent, like each child, is unique, and one size does not fit all. So, depending on their learning style and what works best for them, the AV practitioner and parent will reach an agreement as to how all that will work best for them.

Sample Questions to Parents

- *What happened during the AVT session that surprised you?*
- *What happened that was new today?*
- *Which short-term objective do you think was accomplished with ease or was challenging?*
- *How do you think you will handle . . . during the next week at home?*
- *What strategies might you use?*
- *Did you see or hear how (name of child) did/said during . . . ?*
- *Are you feeling encouraged by today's session?*
- *Do you have any other concerns that I can help with at this time?*

Finally, the child, practitioner, and parent say goodbye in ways that create excitement for the week ahead and for the next session. The session ends on a high note with the child feeling successful and the adults feeling prepared for the next stages. The farewell is simply another routine that is common in real life, in which the child hears and uses the social language of saying goodbye and includes some of the objectives in the session plan.

POST-SESSION

1. Record the diagnostic information in all the domains obtained from the session into the child's chart. Evaluate and note the strategies that did or did not promote success.
2. Self-evaluate performance considering appropriateness of the short-term objectives and use of strategies.
3. Note action items and follow through on any collaboration with other professionals.

REFERENCES

Degangi, G. (2000). *Pediatric disorders of regulation in affect and behavior: A therapist's guide to treatment and assessment.* San Diego, CA: Elsevier.

Department for Education. (2012). *Statutory framework for the early years foundation stage: Setting the standards for learning, development and care for children from birth to five.* United Kingdom: Author.

Fidishun, D. (2000) Teaching adult students to use computerized resources: Utilizing Lawler's keys to adult learning to make instruction more effective. *Information Technology and Libraries, 19*(3), 157–158.

Guardian Newspaper. (2013, July). An open letter by Christine Blower *NUT*, Kevin Courtney *NUT*, Max Hyde *NUT*, Malorie Blackman *Children's laureate*, Michael Rosen, Alan Gibbons, Andy Seed, John Coe *National Association Primary Education*, Dr Terry Wrigley *Leeds Met Uni-*

versity, Dr Clare Kelly *Goldsmiths University,* Sara Tomlinson *Lambeth NUT,* Jess Edwards *Primary charter co-ordinator,* Dr John Yandell *Institute of Education,* Alex Kenny *NUT Inner London,* Sarah Williams *Downhills campaign,* Debra Kidd *AST for Teaching and Learning.*

Mahoney, G., & Perales, R. (2005). The impact of relationship focused intervention on young children and children with disabilities. *Topics in Early Childhood and Special Education, 18*(4), 206–221.

Oxford Advanced Learner's Dictionary (9th ed.). (2015). Oxford, UK: Oxford University Press.

Pollack, D., Goldberg, D., & Calleffe-Schenck, N. (1997). *Educational audiology for the limited hearing infant and preschooler: An auditory-verbal program.* Springfield, IL: Charles C. Thomas.

UNICEF. (2003). *Happy Learning! A guide to best practises for achieving the potential of children.* New York, NY: UNICEF, South Asia.

Vygotsky, L. (1978). *Mind in society; development of higher psychological processes.* Cambridge, MA: Harvard University Press.

13

AUDITORY-VERBAL THERAPY IN ACTION: STEP-BY-STEP SESSION PLANS

Warren Estabrooks, Louise Hönck,
Sally Tannenbaum-Katsaggelos,
Maria Emilia (Mila) de Melo,
Becky Crow Clem, David Sindrey, Lisa Katz,
Karen MacIver-Lux, and Pamela Steacie

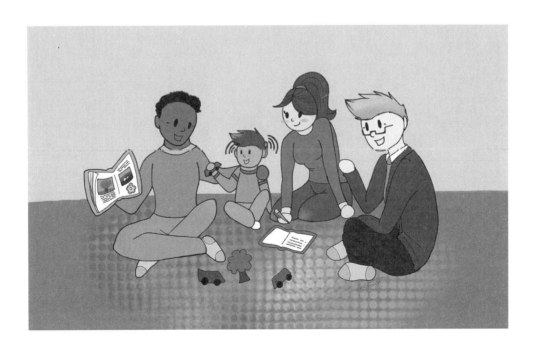

INTRODUCTION

This chapter showcases a variety of *sample session plans* for children from infancy through age 6 in Auditory-Verbal Therapy (AVT). All AVT *sample session plans* were developed and delivered by highly experienced AV practitioners. These *sample session plans* outline the background of the child; the current progress summary; short-term objectives to be accomplished in one to four sessions; a step-by-step presentation of exactly what happened in the session using many of the strategies outlined in Chapters 10 and 11, and the session outcome analysis. Names, places, and some dates have been excluded to respect the privacy of the families.

An AV practitioner who has a very busy caseload does not have the time, or the need, to write such detailed session plans. But, these *sample session plans* may be of great value to students, aspiring AV practitioners, and AV practitioners who teach, train, and/or mentor others, and to those who desire to "raise the bar," on their professional performance.

Many AVT sessions take on a life of their own, and a creative AV practitioner may not follow a written script, but the practitioner does aspire to achieve the short-term objectives. These *sample session plans* demonstrate the artful applications of AVT based on the evidence-based and evidence-informed knowledge that guides clinical practice.

Session Plan 1: The Ten-Month-Old

<table>
<tr><td colspan="2">AV PRACTITIONER
Louise Honck (as reported by Rosie Quayle)</td></tr>
<tr><td>NAME OF CHILD
Charlotte</td><td>ETIOLOGY
Unknown</td></tr>
<tr><td colspan="2">DEGREE & TYPE OF HEARING LOSS
Moderate—severe ski-slope bilateral HL</td></tr>
<tr><td>CHRONOLOGICAL AGE (CA)
10 months</td><td>HEARING AGE (HA) 7 months</td></tr>
<tr><td>AUDITORY-VERBAL AGE (AVA)
2 months</td><td>HEARING TECHNOLOGY HISTORY
• Fitted with bilateral hearing aids at 3 months</td></tr>
<tr><td colspan="2">INTERVENTION HISTORY
• First AVT session at 7 months of age
• Fortnightly AVT sessions started at 8 months</td></tr>
<tr><td colspan="2">DEVELOPMENTAL HISTORY
• Born following emergency caesarean section at 39 weeks' gestation as she was breech and stopped moving in utero.
• Spent 12 days in NICU.
• No family history of hearing loss.
• Cytomegalovirus results were negative.
• Diagnosed with a bilateral hearing loss following Newborn Hearing Screening.
• Repeated ABR indicated a moderate to severe sloping loss.
• Absent otoacoustic emissions.
• Fitted with bilateral digital hearing aids at 3 months.
• Charlotte is an attentive, engaging 10-month-old with two older siblings.</td></tr>
</table>

continues

	PROGRESS SUMMARY Based on developmental norms, the child is able to:	**SHORT-TERM OBJECTIVES** To be accomplished in one to four AVT sessions
AUDITION	• Detect all 6 sounds of the Ling Six-Sound Test at 1 m • Associate environmental sounds with their source, including looking at the door when there is a knock and looking for her dog when he barks. • Discriminate duration and pitch by looking at correct toy when hearing "up up up" (for the stairs on a slide game) versus "round and round" (for a merry-go-round) • Sustain auditory attention when she hears an animated voice or singing. • Turn consistently when someone calls her • Localize to talking on both sides	• Localize sounds presented at both sides at 1 m by turning her head toward the source. • Respond to auditory hooks (Uhoh! Look! Yuck!) when attending to another toy. • Associate more Learning to Listen Sounds to objects ("ss" for snake and "oo" for train). • Discriminate between songs, showing differing actions for different songs (hand movements for "Wheels on the Bus").
SPEECH	• Vocalize when she wants to be picked up by using the correct vowel and number of syllables associated with the action (e.g., "up up up"). • Imitate the pattern for an elongated sound when she is eating and wants more. (e.g., "mmm"). • Imitate features of duration (e.g., broken sound when she wants to be picked up and a longer sound when she wants her food). • Use reduplicated babble in bilabial-vowel combinations (e.g., "bababa," "mamama").	• Use longer strings of repeated syllables (bababababa) in turn-taking games. • Start to monitor her voice by shaping sounds that are similar to an adult model (e.g., quack-quack).

	PROGRESS SUMMARY Based on developmental norms, the child is able to:	**SHORT-TERM OBJECTIVES** To be accomplished in one to four AVT sessions
LANGUAGE	• Rock back and forth when she hears singing. • Vocalize "aaah" when a space is left at the end of "Row, row, row your boat." • Understand "no" when spoken with an angry voice. • Use vocalizations to attract attention. • Demonstrate understanding of routines (e.g., puts her arms up to be picked up when she hears "up up up," Look to her stroller where she naps when hears "shhh"). • Associate some Learning to Listen Sounds with meaning.	• Increase repertoire of Learning to Listen Sounds to 20. • Follow simple requests ("Give it to me," "Can you give me a kiss?"). • Respond with appropriate arm gestures and vocalizations to words "bye-bye" and "clap-clap-clap." • Increase "protowords" to request objects ("quack quack," "bounce bounce"). • Fill space in songs with the appropriate vocalization (three little ducks "quack quack", wheels on the bus "round and round").
COGNITION	• Enjoy looking at herself, and familiar adults in a mirror. • Imitate actions such as banging. • Try to imitate actions of songs. • Play simple hiding and finding games. • Point to familiar faces and toys when she wants something or when something falls.	• Joint attention for 3–4 min when looking at and acting on pictures of baby faces. • Begin pretend-play when acting on the book. • Demonstrate object permanence by following an object that falls.
COMMUNICATION	• Track people talking by looking from one to another. • Take part in verbal turn-taking games in singing and reduplicated babble. • Imitate blowing raspberries. • Point and vocalize to request. • Refuse objects/actions. • Play anticipation games. • Vocalize during games.	• Increase nonverbal communication to greet by waving, and holding her hand out to request. • Begin book sharing by pointing to pictures in a book and looking back to the adult. • Wave bye-bye to toys to indicate that she has finished something.

continues

AV PRACTITIONER GOALS

- Use the "Getting to the room" activity to coach the parent more effectively.
- Guide and coach parents to listen carefully to Charlotte's vocalization and predict what her best effort will be at home.

PARENT GOALS

- Use auditory hooks to establish and maintain auditory attention.
- Create simple pretend play scenarios.
- Improve ability to wait for Charlotte to vocalize.

STEP-BY-STEP SESSION PLAN **ORIENTATION**

- Charlotte arrives with her mother, and I ask, "How are things going?" This allows her time to talk about the successes and challenges in a casual and comfortable way.
- I listen and comment and then ask:
  - "What do you want from the session?" We start the session with this question so that the parent can talk about an area of development or part of the day that she needs help with.
  - Mother says that she finds it is hard to get Charlotte's attention, particularly to books.
  - Dad will join the session half way through. I use this information to plan the session with the parent incorporating all the objectives.

INTRODUCTION

- Charlotte sits in a well-adjusted high chair.
- Toys are visible around the room so that Charlotte can request them and so I can check her understanding of their labels.
- I greet Charlotte and Mother at the door.
- Charlotte smiles when I bend down to see her in her pram.
- I ask Mother to bend down so she is at her ear level and points toward her as she says "Hello," in an animated tone. I wait until Charlotte vocalizes and then say, "Hello Charlotte" and smile.
- Mother bends down to check Charlotte's nappy. I coach Mother to tell Charlotte the plan first before doing the action, "Let me check your nappy." (Charlotte will become accustomed to listening first about what will be happening next.)

- Mother leans in close and says "Do you want some milk? "mmm mmm," let's give you some milk, "mmm," "mmm." Charlotte's eye gaze shifts to the bottle on her stroller. Mother says "mmm" again and waits for Charlotte to vocalize.
- Charlotte is very excited and waves her arms around. She stops and says "mmm" and Mother smiles while she gives her the bottle. I encourage mother by letting her know how well she did (talking ahead, using sounds, and waiting for vocalizations).

ACTIVITY #1. GETTING INTO THE ROOM

- On the way to the window of the therapy room, I coach mother to continue to talk ahead, telling Charlotte what she will hear, see and do. As Mother pushes the stroller, she says, "I think we'll see a car! Brmmm!" and waits for Charlotte to vocalize to carry on the conversation.
- Mother gets down to Charlotte's level, and says 'look!' when Charlotte's gaze shifts, she points to direct her attention outside. Charlotte's eye gaze follows mother's pointing. Charlotte smiles when she sees a bus. I coach Mother to say "bu bu bu" a few times and to wait for a response. Charlotte gazes to her mother and turns back to the window.
- I coach Mother to point out other things with words she knows. She then says, "Look! I see a train that goes "oo-oo" (without pointing). She waits and Charlotte gazes toward a train that passes by. Mother say, "Oh, I love that you see that train! Father goes on the train!"
- I tell Mother that the slow pace of presentation and plenty of wait time helped Charlotte to discriminate the two sounds. Mother says "oo-oo" again and pauses. The baby spontaneously vocalizes while she is looking at the train. Mother gives her a big kiss!
- A woman walks past with a dog and Charlotte vocalizes. Mother spontaneously points and says, "Look! It's a dog, woof woof!"
- Another bus stops and they start singing "the wheels on the bus." I coach Mother to start singing first and to look for stilling of movement to indicate that Charlotte recognizes she is singing before she starts the actions.
- Charlotte smiles, stills, and turns to her mother. Mother and I then do the simple actions to the song.
- After the song, Charlotte vocalizes. Mother interprets it as a request for "more!" I coach Mother to say "you want more!" and acoustically highlight "more." After some repetitions, I coach mother to tell Charlotte the plan "We're going to play!" and they move off toward the therapy room.

continues

357

ACTIVITY #2. TECHNOLOGY CHECK

- Mother asks Charlotte if she wants to come "up up up" using a singsong voice. Charlotte looks up and holds out her arms. I coach her to wait with outstretched arms, to see if Charlotte vocalizes. Charlotte frowns and moves her arms up and down. Mother smiles and repeats the instruction.

- Charlotte vocalizes and Mother moves closer, saying again "up up up." Charlotte vocalizes "u/u/u/." Mother says, "I heard you saying up up up," and she picks up the baby.

- Charlotte reaches for a spinning toy that is on the table. I stand a meter behind Charlotte to the right hand side and coach Mother, who is now sitting next to the baby to say, "Do you want the toy that goes round and around and around?" While Charlotte reaches for the toy, I present the Ling sound /ah/ using a soft voice. Charlotte stills and turns her head towards the right side.

- Mother says, "You heard that /ah/" and I show her a toy that corresponds with the Ling sound just heard (airplane). Mother says "Look at the toy that goes round and around and around." When Charlotte looks at her, she points to the toy in front of her on the table and the baby's attention shifts to the toy on the table.

- I move to the left to present the /ah/ on the other side. Before I present the sound she waits to make sure the baby is not looking for the airplane anymore or tracking my movement to a different side. This way there can be no false-positive responses.

- When Charlotte responds, by turning to where the sound is coming from, she is handed the airplane to play with for a few seconds.

- I repeat the routine for "ee," "sh," and "s." ("m" and "oo" were verified at the window).

- Charlotte vocalizes and reaches for the toy and I coach Mother to lean in, use acoustic highlighting to say, "Do you want the round and around and around?" and then point. Charlotte points and vocalizes /ow/ow/. Mother reinforces "round and around and around" and hands her the toy.

- I return to the table, and says, "We need to say bye bye," with highlighting and points at the toy. She says, "bye bye" again and then waves.

- Charlotte frowns. She does not want to say goodbye to the toy. I move the toy toward her mother, and coach her to say "bye-bye" and then wave. Charlotte reaches for it, and Mother moves closer and models "bye-bye," while taking her hand and showing her how to wave to the toy. Charlotte starts crying when the toy goes away.

- I point to the table and say "Oh don't cry, because right here we are going to get the snake that says "ss-ss." Charlotte stills a bit and mother repeats "ss" as a snake appears. Mother exclaims, "Oh look Charlotte! It's that snake that says "ss-ss." Mother repeats this as I move the snake closer.
- I tell mother to keep pointing at the snake, to wait and see if Charlotte will call the snake. Charlotte points to the snake, then bangs on the table and reaches for the toy. Everyone waits. Charlotte bangs again and says "uh." They move the snake closer. Mother points to the snake and models "ss" again. Charlotte bangs on the table and says "uh" then vocalizes an extended vowel sound. Mother gives the snake to her. She squeals with delight. I move the snake toward Mother, saying "ssssss," pretending to bite her. Mother says "no-no-no" and then waits and says "no-no-no" again, as she wags her finger. The snake moves backward. After a repetition, I move the snake toward Charlotte, and she tries to grab it.
- Mother leans across and says "no no no." to the snake. I tell Charlotte's mother to hold her finger, look expectantly and wait.
- Charlotte wags her finger at the snake. Mother models "no-no-no" and waits. Charlotte vocalizes "uh" three times with the correct intonation.

ACTIVITY #3. DUCKS

- Plastic ducks are on a shelf within Charlotte's view. They are very interesting to her and give her something to talk about.
- I remind Mother to talk ahead "we're going to get those ducks! Ducks say, "Quack quack quack!" (Mid-frequency contrast to the low-frequency "brmm" and "bu bu.")
- I say, "Let's get those ducks. Quack, quack quack!" and look around. Charlotte gazes towards the ducks. I ask, "Did you see how she gazed toward the ducks?" Mother calls the ducks over (like the snake previously). Charlotte vocalizes /a/ and Mother moves the duck closer. I coach Mother to do this to develop the auditory feedback loop
- Charlotte begins to produce two syllables a/a/. Once the duck reaches her, she reaches out for it.
- I demonstrate it again and hand it over to Mother; Charlotte vocalizes "a/a/" again.
- To call the third duck over, I coach mother to wait to see if Charlotte will vocalize an approximation of "quack quack" rather than imitate it. Mother tells Charlotte that she is going to get some ducks, she gets them out and waits.
- Charlotte uses the "a/a/" pattern by herself and gets the duck!
- I suggest they get water for the ducks (to build Charlotte's associations of water with ducks).

continues

ACTIVITY #3. DUCKS *continued*

- However, as she is explaining this, Charlotte drops her duck. Her mother goes to pick it up, but I explain that this is a great listening and language opportunity. I say "uhoh!" to indicate the problem and then point down to the duck. The baby begins to move her arm to point to the duck. I say, "you can call it up up up!" (another context to use up up).

- Each time Mother calls "up up up" I move the duck a little until it is back on the table.

- Mother then "accidentally" knocks her duck on the floor and they repeat the strategy; after some waiting, Charlotte says "u/u/" to call the duck back up.

- I introduce the song "Three Little Ducks."

- Everyone needs a duck, so I say to Charlotte, "Give it to me!" Charlotte doesn't respond. I say it again and then hold out my hand.

- Charlotte's mum tries this herself and comments that she usually holds her hand out right away; she says she will practice saying it first before holding out her hand.

- I manipulate the ducks to pretend to kiss each other after the command, "Give me a kiss!"

- The first time Charlotte's mum says it, Charlotte leans in to give her a kiss, and Charlotte gets a big kiss. I demonstrate the ducks kissing and saying "Mwah!" Charlotte copies the "mmm" sound.

- I sing, "Three Little Ducks went swimming one day, over the hills and far away, Mummy duck said . . . " And Mother fills in the blank by saying, "quack quack quack quack"; Mother takes her turn and leaves a blank; Charlotte vocalizes but does not approximate "quack quack."

- After repetitions, Charlotte vocalizes two syllables "e-e" but not yet "a-a."

- There is knock at the door and we move on to the next activity.

ACTIVITY #4. KNOCKING ON THE DOOR

- There is a knock at the door. Charlotte stills a bit and stops playing.

- Father knocks again. Charlotte stills again and mother points to her ear and says, "You heard Father go knock-knock-knock."

- She turns Charlotte toward the sound and he knocks again. Charlotte looks towards the door and Mother points to the door and says, "Come in!"

- I coach Father to stand at the door and say, "You heard me knocking— knock-knock-knock, He knocks on the door again and says, "I brought you a duck—quack-quack-quack."

- Father goes out and knocks again. Charlotte immediately turns to the door and Mother says, "Come in."

- Everyone waits. Charlotte looks from one adult to the other and points to the door. Mother models it all again.

- Charlotte points to the door and vocalizes. Father comes in with a big smile and he gives her a duck.

ACTIVITY #5. BABY FACES BOOK

- I comment that Charlotte has shown early understanding of labels for sound-object associations, so the next goal is understanding early instructions.

- The stimulus is a book of photographs of babies.

- Father tells Charlotte the plan: "We're going to get a book!" He pauses but Charlotte does not show any understanding. I tell her with acoustic highlighting on the final syllables, "It's a book about a baby who goes wa-wa-wa!" Charlotte smiles when she hears this. Father models it following my model and again she smiles. Father takes out the book and says, "Look!" and then points to the baby who is crying.

- I coach him to say "wa wa wa!" and then wait. Charlotte imitates "a-a" with similar intonation.

- Father then acts out the scenario with a dolly and gives the dolly some milk.

- I get a milk bottle, a wipe, and a hairbrush and put them on the table. Charlotte starts to reach for the hairbrush, and through coaching Father says, "Let's give baby some milk, mmm mm."

- Charlotte shifts her gaze to the milk bottle but doesn't start to pick it up.

- Father asks again and this time she reaches for it, but puts it into her own mouth. He takes her hand and shows her how to feed the baby with it. She smiles and imitates feeding the baby.

- Baby cries again "Wa-wa!" Through coaching, Mother highlights the phrase, "We need to wipe wipe!"

- Charlotte pauses when she hears this new sound pattern but does not look towards the wipe. She goes back to feeding the baby with the bottle. Mother repeats this but they do not see understanding.

- I coach mother to point to the wipe; so Charlotte reaches out for it and wipes the table with it. (She demonstrates understanding of its functional use.)

- Father models wiping the baby and again she imitates.

- She looks away from the book and starts reaching for Mother, who captures her attention using an auditory hook, points to the book and says, and says "Uhoh! Baby's crying wa-wa-wa!"

- Through coaching, her mother says, "Let's give her a kiss!"

- This time, the baby leans towards the book and pushes her face into it. Mother narrates, "You kissed her! Kiss kiss!"

- This routine is repeated for "brush brush."

continues

	SESSION ANALYSIS
AUDITION	• Detection and localization to all six Ling sounds at 1 m. • Detection and localization to an environmental sound while engaged. • Responded to auditory hooks (e.g., "Look!"). • Identified Learning to Listen sound for objects on the street and singing. • Filled in the blank with the correct syllables in singing three little ducks.
SPEECH	• Copied syllable pattern (e.g., "No-no-no" and "oo-oo") • Monitored own voice by shaping sounds similar to an adult model when calling over toys (e.g., "Quack-quack").
LANGUAGE	• Vocalized to greet (e.g., "Bye), to request an action (e.g., toys to come up), for recurrence (e.g., more singing), to call toys (e.g., "quack quack), to refuse (e.g., "No-no-no"), to call people to come in (e.g., "Come in"), and give instructions (e.g., "up up") • Understood sounds associated with objects. • Demonstrated understanding of "up up up" (stretched her arms out to be picked up) and "quack-quack-quack" (looked over at the ducks), "mmm," "oo" and "kiss."
COGNITION	• Interest in pretend scenario with the snake. • Object permanence (e.g., ducks that fell to the floor). • Imitated arm movements in singing (e.g., wheels on the bus). • Imitated simple actions during play (e.g., brushing the baby and giving it a kiss).
COMMUNICATION	• Imitated a wave to say bye. • Vocalized the pattern for "quack quack" after a number of models. • Pointed and vocalized to attract attention (e.g., dog passing in the street). • Vocalized to call father to come in. • Interested in book sharing with an adult.

- Come close to the microphone of the hearing technology; use a clear highlighted presentation of the Learning to Listen Sounds; comment, followed by a pause and a point to direct her attention.
- Point out everyday objects on their walk to the clinic room and do this on their daily walks to the park using Learning to Listen sounds to associate them with the objects.
- Wait after the comments to see if Charlotte discriminates (e.g., looks at the correct object or puts her hands up to be picked up).
- Use auditory hooks and singing.
- Check for understanding before pointing to direct attention or doing actions to songs.
- Give words to Charlotte's vocalizations and thoughts, e.g., when she wants more, by saying, "Do you want more?" using acoustic highlighting and putting "more" at the end of the sentence.
- Wait for vocalization before picking up Charlotte. After she vocalizes, model the target sound again to help her to develop her auditory feedback loop to begin shaping the sound so that it matches the adult model; wait again to give the baby another opportunity to shape her vocalization. Say " bye-bye" and show Charlotte how to wave to transition from one activity to the next.
- Model the utterance using acoustic highlighting, then point to direct the baby's attention; use an expectant look and wait for a vocalization that matches the adult model when she calls toys over.
- Call toys at home before they are taken down to play with or hide them around the room, call them and find them.
- Use incidental things that happen like items falling to add language by showing her how "up up" is used in another context when toys are called up when they fall down.
- When singing "Three Little Ducks" leave a blank at the end of the song and have an adult model filling in the blanks.
- Use sounds in a meaningful way by knocking on doors or ringing the bell so that you can use your voice to call people to come in.
- Use pretend play to extend and expand listening and language.
- Introduce Learning to Listen Sounds in playful scenarios like we did with the snake game.
- Pretend to make a baby sleep and when they call "wake-up."
- Use books and action words in everyday routines to show her how to do actions on others (e.g., wipe, brush, kiss); say the target phrase and then demonstrate it with the object.
- At the end of the session, the parents and I talk about what they feel the key learning was and this forms the basis for the "take home messages" that parents take away with them.
- I ask the leading question, "I wonder how we could do that at home?" and the parents think about the objectives and generate their own plans for how they might incorporate the new learning into their everyday life.

continues

CONCLUSION
The parents and I obtained diagnostic information during and following the session. I recorded it in the child's chart and it is used to plan the next sessions.

REVIEW OF PRACTITIONER TARGETS
I used the "Getting to the room" activity to coach parents to use spontaneous opportunities to check understanding (e.g., the train) and checked detection "mm" and "oo" ahead of the Ling sound check.
I "seized the moment" (e.g., ducks falling and father coming later) to demonstrate how unplanned events can be turned into useful, fun and purposeful play!
I coached the parents how and when to accept 'best effort' for their child's vocalizations. In the next session, I will wait for the parents to make the judgement for themselves first.

Session Plan 2: The Fourteen-Month-Old

AV PRACTITIONER	
Sally Tannenbaum Katsaggelos, M.Ed., DT-H, LSLS, Cert. AVT	
NAME OF CHILD Omar	**ETIOLOGY** Cochlear Nerve Deficiency
DEGREE & TYPE OF HEARING LOSS Profound sensorineural	
CHRONOLOGICAL AGE (CA) 14 months	**HEARING AGE (HA)** 10 months
AUDITORY-VERBAL AGE (AVA) 2 weeks	**HEARING TECHNOLOGY HISTORY** • Received right side cochlear implant at 13 months • Scheduled for left side cochlear implant at 18 months
INTERVENTION HISTORY • Enrolled in Early Intervention Program at 4 months and currently receives: ○ Weekly speech therapy, physical therapy, social work services, developmental therapy by a hearing specialist	
DEVELOPMENTAL HISTORY • Born full term, after an unremarkable pregnancy. • No family history of hearing loss. • Diagnosed with a bilateral hearing loss following Newborn Hearing Screening. • Sedated ABR indicated a bilateral, profound, sensorineural hearing loss. • CT scans revealed bilateral cochlear nerve deficiency. • Vision evaluation came back within normal limits. • PE tube placement at 11 months.	

continues

	PROGRESS SUMMARY Based on developmental norms, the child is able to:	SHORT-TERM OBJECTIVES To be accomplished in one to four AVT sessions

AUDITION	• Wear his CI throughout his waking hours although he has some difficulty with magnet retention.
	• Demonstrate some sound awareness to environmental sounds and loud speech.
		• Demonstrate the absence or presence of sound.
		• Associate a specific environmental sound with an occurrence (hears knocking will look toward the door).
		• Detect the Ling 6 Sounds (ah, oo, ee, m, sh, s) at a distance of 12 inches.
		• Respond to the following:
		  ◦ parent's voice (with varied intonation).
		  ◦ variety of vowels and pre-speech sounds.
		  ◦ his name (by movement or smiling).
		  ◦ the learning to listen sounds.
		  ◦ music/singing by dancing, singing, or clapping

SPEECH	• Vocalize u, and eh during play.
	• Blow raspberries.
		• Imitate the following:
		  ◦ prosodic features of speech (duration, intensity, pitch).
		  ◦ pre-speech sounds (tongue click, raspberries).
		• Make approximations of the learning to listen sounds.
		• Make playful sounds (coos, yells, laughs).

LANGUAGE	• Attend to a speaker's face. • Vocalize sounds other than crying.	• Listen to someone talking and anticipate the next events. • Vocalize in response to talking and singing. • Share in vocal turn-taking. • Respond with appropriate actions when common words are used (bye-bye, all gone, how big is the baby, peek- a- boo, where's mama).

	PROGRESS SUMMARY Based on developmental norms, the child is able to:	SHORT-TERM OBJECTIVES To be accomplished in one to four AVT sessions
COGNITION	• Smile and laugh during games such as peek-a-boo and a tickling game. • Imitate actions such as banging. • Play simple hiding and finding games. • Play appropriately with toys.	**Build a two to three-block tower.** • Imitate actions (fly airplane, put arms up in the air and lower them down). • Sustain interest in desired object for two minutes or more. • Demonstrate functional use of objects (stirs with a spoon). • Look at pictures in a book.
COMMUNICATION	• Vary cries to indicate his needs. • Make appropriate eye contact. • Look at the person who is talking. • Point to what he wants.	• Respond to simple verbal requests when accompanied by gestures (bye-bye, give it to mama). • Vocalize when greeting a familiar adult. • Attend to an object or person. • Recognize early words such as Mama, bye-bye, more. • Take initiative in vocalizing and enjoy adult interaction. • Vocalize to make something happen, for attention and to have needs met. • Initiate interaction (point to something and then look at person, give something to person). • Request using vocalizations or gestures (puts hands up to be picked up).

continues

Session Plan 2: The Fourteen-Month-Old *continued*

AV PRACTITIONER GOALS

- Use wait time to make sure Mom is really a partner in therapy; give her time to ask questions, to comment on her observations, and to develop her interactions with Omar.
- Guide and coach mom effectively, while engaging the other children in the family.

PARENT GOALS

- Call attention to a variety of sounds including environmental sounds and speech.
- Respond by narrating what Omar is doing.
- Respond in ways that build his language in routines such as mealtimes, getting dressed, cleaning up, and diaper changes.

| STEP-BY-STEP SESSION PLAN
ORIENTATION |
| --- |

This is the third auditory-verbal session with Omar and his family. The session takes place in Omar's home. It is summer and some of his siblings are at home. An interpreter who speaks Arabic attends all sessions and today meets me outside the building. The session begins as soon as I knock on Omar's apartment door.

ACTIVITY #1. ENTERING THE HOME and KNOCKING GAME

- I ring the doorbell outside the building and Mom buzzes the interpreter and me into the building.
- We walk up the stairs and see that the door is ajar indicating that we should enter. One of Omar's goals is to associate an environmental sound with an occurrence so I seize the moment, peek in and tell Mom that we want Omar to make the connection between the sound of knocking and a person appearing at the door.
- I let Mom know that I am going to close the door and knock on it, and coach Mom to point to her ear and then to point out the sound to Omar. Then, with Omar in her arms, she'll come and open the door.
- I close the door and knock several times. I hear Mom telling Omar that she hears knocking.
- Mom opens the door with Omar. She smiles but is quiet.
- I greet Omar and Mom using an excited voice and give him a kiss on his cheek; then I encourage Mom to wave and say hello to me.

- Mom waves and says, *"Hi,"* and Omar smiles.
- I explain that this *knocking game* will help Omar associate a specific sound with something that happens next; (when he hears a knock on the door, he will know that someone is there).
- I knock on the open door and say to Omar, "You heard me knocking, knock, knock, knock."
- I suggest trying this activity again, and coach Mom to get excited when she opens the door to help make learning to listen interesting.
- I coach Mom to wave and take Omar's hand to wave, if he doesn't do it alone. I wave and say, *"Bye-bye."*
- Mom waves and says, *"Bye-bye,"* then she waves Omar's hand, and closes the door.
- I wait and silently count to 20 (to help Omar listen for the onset of the sound) before I knock on the door.
- Mom opens the door and says in a soft but excited voice, *"Hi Sally,"* and she waves.
- I guide Mom to wave Omar's hand, which Mom does.
- I ask her how Omar responded to the knocking.
- Mom reports he started to kick his legs when he heard the knocking.
- I let Mom know that Omar is telling her that he heard the knocking by kicking his legs.
- Two of Omar's siblings, Cyrus and Ali, walk into the room and Omar is happy to see them.
- After greetings, I suggest repeating the activity with the brothers. Cyrus goes outside and knocks softly on the door.
- I do not see a response from Omar so coach the older brother, through the closed door, to knock a little louder.
- Cyrus knocks again and Omar kicks his legs.
- Mom and Omar open the door and Mom says *"Hi,"* and waves to Cyrus.
- I coach Cyrus to wave and say hi to Omar, who is clearly happy to see him.
- Cyrus says, *"Hi,"* and gives Omar the high five.
- I coach Cyrus and Ali to use their voices when they give high fives and everyone goes around giving high fives and saying, *"High five."*
- I explain the objective that Omar will respond with appropriate actions when he hears a common phrase; saying *"High five,"* ahead of time.
- Mom asks Ali if he wants a turn and he says he does.
- Before Ali goes into the hall I coach him to count to 10 slowly and silently, and then knock on the door.
- I explain to everyone that the wait time indicates to Omar that when there is no sound, nothing is happening, but that sound makes things happen. In this case, the knocking causes Mom to open the door.
- Ali waits for about 10 seconds and then knocks on the door.
- Omar looks around and then Mom opens the door and greets Ali.
- I share my observation that Omar looked like he was anticipating a knock during the wait time and when he heard it he turned his head.

continues

ACTIVITY #1. ENTERING THE HOME and KNOCKING GAME *continued*

- Mom agreed and said that since he received his cochlear implant he seems to be more tuned in to his environment.
- I remark that this is exciting
- I ask Mom if she has any questions about this activity and if it is something that they can continue working on.
- Mom doesn't have any questions and says that she will let family members and others know that they need to knock on the door and not just walk inside the apartment, so that Omar can work on this objective every day.

ACTIVITY #2. FREEZE DANCE

- I ask Mom and the siblings if they have any music in the home.
- They don't, but they do have some noisemakers and musical instruments.
- While Cyrus and Ali are collecting them, I check Omar's cochlear implant and ask Mom how the week went.
- Mom reports that Omar is not taking off his cochlear implant, but she is concerned that the magnet keeps falling off.
- I check the site on Omar's head where the magnet is placed and observe that it does not look red. I offer to speak to the audiologist about switching to a stronger magnet, although I let Mom know that this is not always possible with a young child.
- I suggest trying a longer cord that may help with retention. I also offer to bring a pilot cap next week.
- The siblings come back with Moroccan shakers and start to give them out.
- I coach them to call Mom's name and look around for her in order to help Omar learn his Mom's name.
- Cyrus says, *"Mama."*
- I coach him to say it a little louder which he does.
- I also call, *"Mama,"* and put out my hands as I ask, *"Where is Mama?"*
- Omar does not glance in Mom's direction so I ask again, *"Where's Mama?"*
- Then Ali points to Mama and with my help, says *"Here's Mama."*
- Cyrus gives Mama a shaker and the process is repeated with Ali.
- Mom holds Omar in her arms and has a Moroccan shaker; each of the brothers also has a Moroccan shaker.
- I explain when I say, *"1-2-3 GO,"* everyone shake the instrument and dance and when I say, *"STOP,"* everyone freezes in place.
- I say, *"1-2-3 GO."* Everyone dances and I point to my ear, nod my head, smile and say, *"I hear the music,"* while I am dancing to the music.
- Mom dances with Omar in her arms and the siblings dance too. Everyone is smiling, including Omar.
- I say, *"STOP,"* and I wait a few seconds, then say, *"Shhh—I don't hear the music. The music stopped,"* and I shake my head to indicate the music has stopped.

- Mom freezes along with the siblings.
- I coach Mom, who is very close to Omar's ear, to say, *"Shhh,"* to indicate the music stopped.
- *"Omar, shhh, the music stopped. Do you want more?"* asks Mom.
- I ask who wants a turn to say, *"1-2-3 GO,"* and suggest waiting a few minutes before saying it to see what might happen.
- Omar's brothers are still feeling shy, so Mom takes a turn.
- Mom waits a few seconds and then says, *"1-2-3 GO,"* and everyone starts to dance.
- Omar does not respond to Mom's voice, but he does kick his feet and smile when the dancing begins.
- I coach Mom to say, *"STOP,"* and everyone freezes.
- Omar vocalizes soon after the music and dancing stop.
- I say, *"I heard you—you want more music,"* and coach everyone to dance to Omar's request.
- I explain that the goal is for Omar to use his voice to make things happen, so in the beginning everyone needs to respond to any of his vocalizations, and that over time these vocalizations will change and match more closely what they are saying. Omar is just beginning to learn to listen and it is exciting to hear him use his voice to make things happen
- Everyone dances to Omar's request.
- I explain to Mom that if they don't have musical instruments available they can sing a song and dance to it.
- I ask the family members if they have a favorite song that they could sing.
- Ali suggests a song from their country.
- I coach them to dance to the song and then freeze when someone shouts out, *"STOP."*
- The family begins to sing a child friendly song and everyone dances to it.
- About halfway through the song, Mom says, *"STOP."* Everyone is quiet and stops dancing.
- Mom says, *"Shhh, I don't hear the song. It stopped."*
- When the dancing and singing stop, Omar starts to move his body in Mom's arms and begins to vocalize.
- Mom immediately tells Omar that she heard him and acknowledges that he wants more singing, and the singing and dancing resume.
- When the activity ends, Mom lets me know that she needs to change Omar's diaper.

ACTIVITY #3. DIAPER CHANGE

- I share with Mom that learning to listen and talk is a way of life and that the best activities are the ones that take place routinely, so I ask Mom if I can participate in the diaper change.
- Mom agrees and lets me know that we need to go into the bedroom to change his diaper.

continues

ACTIVITY #3. DIAPER CHANGE *continued*

- Mom looks at Omar and says; *"Phew,"* while she waves her hand in front of her nose. Then she takes Omar by the hand to walk him to the bedroom.
- I coach Mom to be at Omar's level and to talk about what they are going to do.
- Mom kneels next to Omar and says, *"You have a dirty diaper. We need to change your diaper—phew. Let's go to the bedroom to change your diaper. Phew."*
- After several *"Phews,"* Omar appears to understand that he is going to the bedroom to have his diaper changed.
- Mom encourages Omar to lie down on the carpet in the bedroom and starts to take off Omar's diaper.
- I coach Mom to continue to talk about what she is doing.
- Mom tells Omar, *"Phew—you have a very dirty diaper. I need to change your diaper!"*
- To encourage Mom I explain that she is using the repetition strategy which helps Omar hear keys words such as diaper, dirty, and phew over and over again.
- I also share that by narrating what she is doing Omar is hearing *the language of changing his diaper.*
- Mom continues and says, *"You have a dirty diaper and I am taking it off. Now I have to wipe you and put on your new diaper."*
- While Mom is talking, I am nodding my head in encouragement.
- I point out how many times Omar heard the word *"diaper,"* and *"dirty,"* and ask Mom to think about how many times in a day he will hear these words, if she continues to narrate the activity.
- While he is on the rug Omar is making a few sounds, so I coach Mom to use this opportunity to babble the sounds back to him.
- I share that sometimes I hear the most talking from kids while they are having a diaper change. I fondly call this "potty-talk."
- Omar has been the most vocal while he is having his diaper changed.
- With my guidance Mom repeats the sounds that Omar is making.
- I coach Mom to wait after she repeats the sounds to let Omar have a turn. I explain that turn taking begins at a very young age and is the foundation for conversations. I ncourage Mom to *have a conversation* with Omar.
- Mom waits a few seconds and Omar says, *"Eh."*
- Mom repeats the sound and waits.
- Omar says, *"U, u."*
- Mom repeats the sound and it continues back and forth until Mom bends over and blows raspberries on Omar's tummy.
- Omar cracks up laughing
- Mom says, *"You like that. Do you want more?"* and blows raspberries again.

- I encourage Mom by letting her know this is a really fun game, and point out what great eye contact Omar is making with her and what a terrific laugh he has.
- I ask her to wait a few minutes to see if Omar will vocalize to indicate he wants more. I guide her to lean in and give Omar an expectant look to indicate that it is his turn to talk.
- Omar blows raspberries and both Mom and I get so excited that we give a little cheer. Then Mom leans over and repeats the sounds to Omar.
- Mom finishes dressing Omar, narrating as she puts his pants back on. She pulls him up on his feet.
- I clarify that another goal is for Omar to respond with actions to everyday phrases, and that *"Stand up,"* is one of these common phrases. Each time you want him to perform an action you need to use the *matching language.*
- We take a few minutes to talk about other phrases that are important to them.
- Mom says, *"Sit down and stand up are phrases that Omar hears a lot."* She also includes *all gone, bye-bye, give me, and let's walk.*
- As we start to walk back into the living room where Cyrus and Ali are waiting, Omar stops walking and raises his arms to be picked up.
- Before Mom has a chance to pick him up I coach her to talk about what Omar wants.
- Mom says, *"Oh, you want me to pick you up? Ok, I can pick you up."*
- When I suggest adding this phrase to the common phrases, Mom nods in agreement.
- Cyrus and Ali are waiting in the living room and I greet them when I see them, and ask if they will help out with one more game.

ACTIVITY #4. CALLING GAME

- I tell Mom to hold Omar with his back on her chest so they are both facing the same direction.
- I stand about a foot behind them and, using a sing song voice, call *"Omar!"*
- I tell Mom to turn around with Omar in her arms, point to his ear and say, *"I hear that. I heard Sally say Omar."*
- I am very enthusiastic when Mom turns him around, and along with his brothers, wave and say, *"Hi Omar."*
- I give him a small toy to play with so that he learns that responding to his name has a *payoff.*
- After saying hello, we all wave and say, *"Bye-bye."*
- This time, as Mom and Omar wait, I ask one of his siblings to call his name.
- I explain that Omar seems very much attached to his brothers so it will be more motivating and meaningful for him to turn to their voices.
- They both want to do it, so together they call his name.
- Mom waits a few seconds to see if Omar reacts. When he moves in her arms, she immediately turns him around.

continues

ACTIVITY #4. CALLING GAME *continued*

- I guide Ali to face away from Mom and Omar so that they can call his name.
- I coach Mom to count to 10 silently before she calls Ali's name to see if Omar will vocalize.
- Omar reaches out to his brother but does not vocalize, so I point to the brother's ear, shake my head, shrug my shoulders and tell Omar, *"Ali doesn't hear you."*
- Omar is quiet and after about 10 seconds Mom calls the brother's name. Ali immediately turns around and tells Omar, *"Hello."*
- The game continues a few more times with each brother taking a turn.
- At one point Omar does vocalize, but not to get his brother's attention. He wants to get down and starts to complain.
- I guide the brother to turn around immediately in response to this vocalization.
- I encourage the family to respond to any vocalization that Omar makes to show him that his voice makes things happen.
- Cyrus and Ali both want to go, so I thank them, tell them that they were a huge help and coach them to say good-bye to Omar before leaving.

ACTIVITY #5. LEARNING TO LISTEN SOUNDS AND EVERYDAY PHRASES

- I pick up Omar's toy airplane, which is lying on the rug, and place it in a brown paper bag that I brought with me.
- Next, I point to my ear and say, *"Listen, ahhh. I hear an airplane."*
- I bring out the bag with the airplane inside, and fly it as I say, *"Ahhh."*
- I explain to Mom that by keeping the airplane in the bag I am helping Omar focus on the sound rather than the object.
- I stop vocalizing and then stop moving the bag with the airplane.
- I coach Mom to vocalize *"Ahhh,"* and I move the airplane to match Mom's vocalizations.
- Next, I hold the bag near Omar and wait for him to say the sound.
- Omar is quiet.
- I shake the bag, point to my ear, and say, *"I hear that, it is an airplane, ahhh."*
- I shake the bag near Mom's ear, who points to her ear and says, *"I hear ahhh, it is an airplane."*
- I give the bag to Mom.
- Mom shakes the bag next to Omar's ear and he reaches for it and opens the bag and finds the airplane.
- While he is playing with it Mom says the airplane sound again. She varies her pitch, with my help; while it is flying high she makes the sound high and as the airplane comes down she lowers her voice.
- When the airplane stops flying, Mom says, *"Shhh I don't hear it, it stopped."*

- When it is time to put the airplane away, I ask Mom to put the airplane back in the bag.
- Everyone says, *"Bye-bye,"* to the airplane including Omar who waves his hand.
- Since they live near an airport, I coach Mom to point out airplanes in the sky.
- While Mom and I are talking, Omar picks up a teddy bear and starts to fly it around vocalizing, *"Ahhh."*
- Both Mom and I laugh and then point to our ears to let Omar know that we hear him.
- Mom shares that this is the longest vocalization she has heard from Omar.
- I encourage Mom by telling her that this is a very insightful observation.
- Mom has a copy of the learning to listen sounds and common phrases that I review with her as Omar is *flying his bear.*
- I suggest adding *"Phew,"* to the list since this is what Mom says when Omar has a dirty diaper.
- Mom looks at the list and reports that they have been playing with a big toy car, and asks if she should get it from the other room.
- I ask Mom to tell Omar what she is going to do.
- Mom turns to Omar and says, *"Listen, brrr, beep- beep. I hear your car. I am going to go get your car, brrr beep- beep."*
- Mom leaves the room to get the car.
- Omar looks a little suspicious being left alone in the room with me so I repeat the car sound to Omar and tell him that Mom will be right back.
- Mom walks back into the room and I coach her to call Omar's name.
- Mom calls Omar's name but Omar does not turn instead he is looking at me.
- I point to my ear and then to Omar and say, *"I hear Mama calling Omar"* and then ask Mom to call his name again.
- Mom calls his name again and Omar still does not turn.
- Then Mom makes the raspberry sound and Omar turns. He climbs off the sofa and starts to crawl toward the car.
- Both Mom and I take turns saying the car sound while Omar explores the car.
- He indicates that he wants to go in the car.
- I coach Mom to knock on the door and open the car door before putting Omar in the car.
- Mom vocalizes, *"Knock, knock, knock,"* as she knocks on the car door.
- Everyone takes turns knocking on the door.
- As Omar opens the door Mom says, *"Open the door."*
- Mom tells me that Omar blows raspberries on his own but not in association with the car.
- I reinforce that blowing raspberries is an important pre-speech skill. The next step is sound-object association between the raspberry sound and the car.
- Omar is busy playing in his car so I re-visit the learning to listen sounds and everyday phrases with Mom.

continues

ACTIVITY #5. LEARNING TO LISTEN SOUNDS AND EVERYDAY PHRASES *continued*

- I explain that it is helpful to find sounds in the home and that they can be incorporated into Omar's daily routines.
- Mom looks at the list and says there is a cabinet door in the bathroom that Omar keeps getting his finger stuck in and she could use this as a chance to say, *"Ow! That hurts!"*
- I let Mom know it is a great activity because it is meaningful and I suggest walking Omar to the bathroom.
- Both Mom and I say, *"Bye- bye,"* to the car.
- As soon as Mom stands up Omar puts his arms up asking to be picked up.
- I tell Mom to give him the words to match what he wants.
- Mom says, *"Oh, you want me to pick you up,"* and she picks him up.
- As we walk to the bathroom I say, *"Walk, walk, walk, we are walking to the bathroom."*
- I reach for the cabinet door and pretend to get my finger stuck and cry out, *"OW, that hurts,"* and then pretend to cry, *"Waaa waaa."*
- Mom takes a turn and says, *"OW,"* and then tells the door, *"No no no,"* as she shakes her finger at it.
- Omar starts to laugh and sticks his finger out and then pulls it back.
- I give Omar a kiss on his finger and suggest that Mom present the sound to Omar the next time they are in the bathroom. It is a very meaningful interaction.
- I let Mom know that if Omar looks in the direction of the cabinet door then he is letting her know that he is making the association between the sound and the object, but that it will probably take a lot of repetition before he makes the association.
- I suggest showing Omar a book that I brought that has photographs of babies crying on one side and babies laughing on the other side.
- When I return with the book I call Omar's name before I come inside the bathroom and this time he looks up at Mom.
- I tell Mom to say, *"Sally called you!"* and then to point to me.
- Clearly intrigued by the book, Omar grabs it and stares at the crying babies, and as he looks at the book both Mom and I pretend to cry.
- Omar looks very concerned.
- I turn the book over to show him the happy babies. Then I smile and say, *"Ha Ha Ha, I am feeling happy now."*
- Both Mom and I continue talking in ways that build Omar's receptive language.

ACTIVITY #6. LING SIX-SOUNDS

- Mom has had some experience with the Ling six-sounds from the previous two sessions and understands that one of Omar's objectives is to detect all of the Ling six-sounds at a close range.
- Omar has lost interest in the book so I take my index finger and hold it above Omar.
- I vocalize, "Sssssssssss," and move my finger to the snake sound until it gets to Omar's belly and starts tickling him with my finger.
- I coach Mom to repeat the activity.
- Mom holds her finger up and moves it as she says, "Sssssssss," and then starts to tickle Omar with her finger.
- I ask Mom if she thinks he heard the sound.
- Mom replies that Omar got excited when he saw her finger move, but she couldn't tell if he heard the sound.
- I coach Mom to say the sound first, wait a few seconds, and then move her finger.
- Mom holds her finger up and without moving it says, "Sssssssss," and then moves her finger toward Omar.
- Omar eyes shift and he starts to giggle at the onset of the vocalization before Mom moves her finger, indicating that he heard it! I let Mom know that this is awesome!

ACTIVITY #7. SAYING GOOD-BYE

- I ask Mom is she has any questions about anything we did.
- Mom asks if it is okay if she plays with a toy snake and to match it with the sss sound.
- I tell her absolutely and explain that I showed her how to use her finger as a snake in case she didn't have the toy available.
- I explain that a variety of objects such as puzzles, books, photos, real objects, toy objects and even t-shirts can be used to reinforce the learning to listen sounds.
- I suggest that on my next visit we play with Omar's toy snake.
- I wave bye to Omar and Mom, and tell Omar, "Bye-bye Omar, see you later."
- I also give Omar a hug and kiss him on his cheek.

continues

	SESSION ANALYSIS The child did the following:
AUDITION	• Demonstrated the presence of sound. • Responded to music/singing by movement/dancing. • Associated a specific environmental sound with an occurrence. • Detected the Ling sounds /ah/ and /s/ at 1 foot • Responded to parent's voice (with varied intonation). • Responded to vowel variety and pre speech sounds. • Responded to his name by movement. • Responded to the learning to listen sounds (airplane and car).
SPEECH	• Imitated duration. • Imitated pre-speech sound (raspberries). • Played at making sounds. • Imitated physical actions in preparation for speech imitation. • Imitated vowel (ah). • Imitated approximations of learning to listen sounds—airplane and car sounds.
LANGUAGE	• Appeared to listen to the person who was talking and anticipate certain events. • Vocalized in response to speech and singing.
COGNITION	• Copied actions. • Sustained interest in desired object for two minutes or more. • Demonstrated functional use of objects. • Looked at pictures in a book.
COMMUNICATION	• Responded to simple verbal requests when accompanied by gestures. • Attended to object or person. • Vocalized to make something happen, and for attention. • Initiated interaction. • Requested through vocalizations and/or gestures goods/services.

- Omar's Mom and I reviewed the session and Mom shared how she would incorporate the activities from the session into Omar's daily routines.
- We discussed using the context of everyday activities and routines to help Omar make sense out of what he is hearing.
- Mom stressed the importance of saying "Phew," each time he needs a diaper change so Omar will understand it is time for a diaper change.
- To help Omar make the association between environmental sounds and an occurrence the family will continue with the knocking game.
- Mom said she would need to do the following :
- Each time they go into the bathroom, talk about the cabinet door before Omar sees it to help him anticipate certain events.
- Point to her ear and tell Omar what she is hearing, and then point to the object to help Omar make sound-object associations.
- Talk about the airplanes flying near their apartment and vocalize the "Ahhh" sound each time they see one.
- Talk about his toy car, and her own car, and say the car sound before she brings out his car or before they go to her car.
- Play with his toy snake and/or her finger and vocalize the "Ssss" sound.
- Provide appropriate spoken language to match Omar's gestures.
- Use wait time, to check sound awareness by looking at Omar's physical signs, such as body movement, eye shifts and a possible smile, and to wait for vocalizing and turn-taking.
- Continue to use an excited voice.
- Use repetition to give Omar a lot of exposure to everyday sounds and language.
- Talk about objects, before showing them to Omar.
- Continue to sing songs.

continues

CONCLUSION

I am really pleased that I "seized the moment" and introduced the knocking game in a meaningful context.

My wait time was adequate. In my next session, however, I will wait for Mom to comment before I make a recommendation. In addition, I will ask Mom leading questions such as, "I wonder what would happen if you . . . ? Coaching Mom during the diaper change helped her incorporate spoken language and listening strategies into this daily routine.

Mom called attention to environmental sounds and speech and reported on how Omar responds to sound. She responded to Omar's gestures with spoken language and appeared more comfortable talking about things before they happened.

Omar is diagnosed with cochlear nerve deficiency, so I was very encouraged to see some auditory responses from him.

I noted that although Mom tended to speak softly, she was great about staying within earshot.

Omar appeared much attached to Mom and Mom acted very loving with Omar.

Mom appeared a little confused about the strategy of wait time so I noted to review this in the next session.

The next session will include looking at Omar's response to all six of the Ling six-sounds.

I made a note to: ensure that Mom understands the meaning of receptive language, expressive language and speech and what is developmentally appropriate given Omar's listening age and auditory verbal age; ask Mom what a typical day looks like including naptime, mealtime, and bedtime; to ask Mom if she would wait to get Omar dressed so we can go through this daily routine together; to check with the audiologist regarding a stronger magnet and bring in a pilot cap for Omar to help with retention.

Session Plan 3: The Sixteen-Month-Old

<table>
<tr><td colspan="2">AV PRACTITIONER
Maria Emilia (Mila) de Melo, S-LP, Aud(C), Reg. CASLPO, LSLS Cert. AVT</td></tr>
<tr><td>NAME OF CHILD
Beatriz (Bea)</td><td>ETIOLOGY
Unknown</td></tr>
<tr><td colspan="2">DEGREE & TYPE OF HEARING LOSS Congenital bilateral severe to profound sensorineural hearing loss</td></tr>
<tr><td>CHRONOLOGICAL AGE (CA) 1 year, 4 months</td><td>HEARING AGE (HA) 4 months post activation of both cochlear implants</td></tr>
<tr><td>AUDITORY-VERBAL AGE (AVA)
1 year</td><td>HEARING TECHNOLOGY HISTORY
• received behind-the-ear hearing aids at 3 months of age
• received bilateral cochlear implants at 11 months
• CIs activated at 12 months</td></tr>
<tr><td colspan="2">INTERVENTION HISTORY
• First AVT session at 4 months of age (2.5 weeks after diagnosis)
• Weekly 1-hour AVT sessions since August 2014</td></tr>
<tr><td colspan="2">DEVELOPMENTAL HISTORY
• Born full-term, at 40 weeks' gestation
• Received a "refer" result on newborn hearing screening
• Following discharge, further test results consistent with diagnosis of bilateral severe to profound sensorineural hearing loss. Diagnosis confirmed at 3 months of age
• Five days after diagnosis, received behind-the-ear hearing aids (worn during all waking hours)
• Diagnostic sessions revealed Bea had minimal access to speech sounds with hearing aids
• Good eye contact, joint attention, and attention span during therapy sessions
• Demonstrates age-appropriate non-verbal cognitive skills and fine and gross motor skills
• Explores and manipulates toys and objects appropriately
• An only child of a young couple and at home with mother, a music teacher</td></tr>
</table>

continues

	PROGRESS SUMMARY Based on developmental norms, the child is able to:	SHORT-TERM OBJECTIVES To be accomplished in one to four AVT sessions
AUDITION	• Indicate when she hears something by searching, smiling or pointing to her ear • Localize people talking and a variety of noisemakers • Become quiet or excited in response to novel sounds • Respond appropriately to meaningful sounds (e.g., music by swaying) • Recognize primary caregivers' voices • Discriminate between harsh and soothing voices • Look at the family member when named (e. g., Where's mommy?) • Respond to her name by searching for the person calling her • Associate some Learning to Listen (LTL) sounds with the corresponding toys or objects • Select one item out of a small set of toys when she hears the corresponding LTL sound (i.e., aa for the airplane, quack for the duck) • Recognize a few songs (e.g., "If you're happy and you know it" and "Head & Shoulders")	• Demonstrate detection of all speech sounds • Begin to perform conditioned play audiometry tasks with help • Turn to name when called from a distance of 12–18 feet • Localize people talking and noisemakers from side to side, upper and lower right/left angles, and from behind at distances up to 3 feet • Respond to music and finger plays by swaying, making a few hand or finger motions, and attempting to sing or talk • Imitate more LTL sounds (auditory memory) • Identify LTL sounds and labels by pointing to corresponding pictures and toys, for example. • Demonstrate auditory closure by "filling in the blank" with the last word approximation or sound in song or rhyme
SPEECH	• Imitate suprasegmental features (intensity, duration, and pitch). • Produce a variety of vowel sounds and some early developing consonant sounds ("ah", "oo" /b/, /m/, /n/, and /d/) • Imitate and spontaneously produce consonant-vowel combinations (e.g., consonant (C)-vowel (V), CVCV, and VCV). Babble two syllables together (e.g., mama, baba)	• Use appropriate intonation to scold, state, respond, exclaim, and greet • Imitate inflectional speech patterns • Use word approximations: highly motivating words and commonly heard (stereotypic) phrases • Produce (/m/, /d/, /b/, /p/, /h/) in babble and word approximations • Expand production of consonant (C)-vowel (V) combinations CVC and VC

	PROGRESS SUMMARY Based on developmental norms, the child is able to:	SHORT-TERM OBJECTIVES To be accomplished in one to four AVT sessions
LANGUAGE	• Vocalize and gesture to request, protest, and comment • Vocalize in response to speech • Understand and respond to "no" (e.g., stops action • Look at some objects and a few named people • Participate in speech routine games (e.g., vocalizes for "go" in "1, 2, 3 . . . " games) • Respond to early-developing yes/no questions (e.g., smiles back when asked: Do you want more?) • Follow one-step directions with contextual cues (e.g., open the door, wave bye-bye, give a kiss, come with me, and stop).	• Respond to early negation (no, stop, don't touch) by stopping the activity • Use word approximation for "no" in appropriate context; for example, when protesting. • Look at common objects and toys when named. • Understand and follow simple directions with minimal then no contextual cues (e.g., "Wave bye-bye!," "Blow a kiss"). • Use interjections (e.g., oh no!) and approximation of words to express observations, wants, and needs.
COGNITION	• Search for hidden objects. • Use more than one object in play (e.g., feeds a baby toy). • Demonstrate appropriate use of objects in play.	• Demonstrate functional and symbolic use of objects. • Request or get adults to activate toys (means–end). • Know a few body parts, foods, and clothing items.
COMMUNICATION	• Demonstrate age-appropriate eye contact and attention span. • Maintain attention to pictures. • Enjoy nursery rhymes and finger plays.	• Take turns in playful verbal exchanges. • Respond verbally to adults talking. • Use word approximations to request, initiate pretend play, comment or tell information, acknowledge or respond.

AV PRACTITIONER GOALS

• Speak at a regular voice volume.
• Improve Active Listening skills.

PARENT GOALS

• Obtain Bea's attention through listening first.
• Pause/wait after presenting information through listening (e.g., asking Bea a question) to allow her to process the information and respond.
• Encourage her to use her voice to make something happen (vocalize with intent).

continues

ACTIVITY #1. GREETING

The session typically begins with greetings in the waiting room, where there are puzzles, books, and a few toys. I encourage parents to arrive at least 10 minutes before their session to allow the child time to settle in.

I come to the waiting room and see Bea sitting on her mother's lap following a book. Out of Bea's sight, about 16 feet away, I sing Bea's name and observe her ability to discriminate my voice with little or some background noise. Singing Bea's name makes it more acoustically salient and attractive to her. Bea reacts by looking at her mother.

After waiting for about 10 seconds, I call her for the second time and she looks around, but not look in my direction.

Vanessa (mother) points to her ear and says, "I hear Mila. Where is she?"

Without moving or changing my position, I sing Bea's name for the third time and she looks in my direction and smiles. I smile back and sing her name for the last time and say, "You heard me! Welcome sunshine!"

Mother says, "It is Mila! Hi Mila!" without waving.

I say hello to mother and then look at Bea and say, "Hi Bea!"

Mother looks at Bea and says, "Would you wave hi-hi to Mila?" Bea smiles, waves and says "ah-ba" in excitement.

I wave and say, "Hi Bea!"

She jumps out of her mother's lap and walks towards me to give me a hug.

On the way to the room, we review the strategies we have already worked on:
- obtain attention through listening first
- draw attention to the sounds
- encourage Bea to find the source of the sound
- put meaning to sound ("I hear Mila")
- use body language or posture that facilitates listening (leaning in to hear, pointing to ear)
- pause or wait after talking to allow Bea time to respond
- talk before giving a visual or tactile cue and then say the message again (Listen First and Last)
- give a maximum of three opportunities to respond, then model the expected response with another adult (if the situation permits).

PARENT GUIDANCE

- Call Bea's name for a reason with no visual or tactile cues. If you call simply to test, she may learn to ignore you. If you constantly prompt her visually, it will not encourage her to learn to listen.
- When helping Bea to localize the sound, help her to find the source without moving it.
- Create the most favorable listening environment by turning off the TV, radio, and other sources of noise.

- Help Bea identify sounds she hears: a knock at the door, the dishwasher, a barking dog, a fire truck, etc.
- Take Bea on a Listening Walk in the neighborhood to listen to all the sounds: soft or loud, close or far, high or low-pitched ones.
- In your book, keep a record of the sounds that you know she responds to and the ones she doesn't.

ACTIVITY #2. INTO THE THERAPY ROOM AND PARENT REPORT

Mother always brings a video camera and tripod to record the session, so that father can watch it. She also records notes, reports, goals, and ideas in her parent book.

I sit on Bea's high chair and say, "This is my chair!"

Bea smiles, shakes her head, vocalizes a combination of vowels and a few consonant sounds and tries to push me off the high chair.

I ask her, "Isn't it MY chair? "

Bea continues vocalizing and shaking her head, then looks at her mother and points to me.

Mother says, "Mila, don't be silly. This is Bea's chair! (pause) This chair's too small for you!"

I sit on my chair and say, "This is MY chair!" Bea smiles, claps her hands, and vocalizes.

Mother gets close to Bea and says, "Let's sit on your chair."

Bea raises her arms quietly.

I coach mother to ask the question again, look at Bea and wait for a verbal response.

Mother follows and Bea responds verbally while keeping her arms up.

Mother says "up-up-up" and then "down-down-down" for each corresponding movement.

Bea is comfortably seated on the high chair with good support under her feet.

The adults sit on either side of Bea.

Since mother has already checked Bea's cochlear implants and the batteries just before the session, I do not need to double check.

I give Bea a big baby doll and some accessories, so she can happily play by herself while I talk with mother, about the previous week. Mother gets my undivided attention and I listen to her carefully, since this information is often significant for the theory session.

PARENT GUIDANCE

- Keep your language short and simple and use complete sentences with correct grammar.
- Try to provide new information that is just slightly above Bea's current language level.
- When necessary, acoustically highlight key words (This is MY chair!) to enhance comprehension and emphasize the critical element.

continues

PARENT GUIDANCE *continued*

- Talk about everything you and Bea are doing as well as the things you see. Narrate her routines.
- Wait for her to take her turn.
- Help Bea contently play while you are doing tasks that don't involve her.

ACTIVITY #3. THE PARENT REPORT

Mother opens her parent book and shares information about future appointments with other professionals (checkup with an optometrist), and outcomes of appointments attended (hearing assessment with the audiologist), Bea's responses during the week, and questions she or her relatives have. Then, we discuss the short-term objectives for this session and strategies we may use.

She records most of my "online guidance" in her parent book.

During our conversation, Bea looks at us on some occasions when we say her name.

Mother says she consistently recognizes her name in different contexts, including when she is not talking directly to her.

I review the importance of incidental language learning.

PARENT GUIDANCE

- Continue to bring the parent book to every therapy session.
- Continue to take notes at home and during the therapy session.
- Share objectives, goals, and progress with family members and professionals involved in Bea's development.
- Observe Bea when she is playing by herself.

ACTIVITY #4. TRANSITION FROM ONE ACTIVITY TO ANOTHER

"We will help Bea to transition from playing with the doll to the next activity. How do you think we can do that?"

Mother suggests that we join Bea and play a little with her, then sing the "Clean Up" song to give her a cue of what is about to happen.

She also suggests that Bea clean up the toys by identifying and selecting a few items after hearing the related label.

Mother says "Ssshh" and Bea stops what she is doing and looks at her mother.

Mother repeats the sound and whispers, "Ssshhh, the baby is sleeping" and waits to observe Bea's reaction.

Bea holds the baby in her arms and sways.

Mother says, "You're right! Ssshhh, the baby is sleeping."

After a while, she says, "Wake up!" and Bea makes the doll stand up.

We repeat this well-known "wake-up" game once more.

Then, mother and Bea feed the baby. Mother says, "Mmm, do you want more?." She wipes the doll's face, saying, "Wipe, wipe, wipe."

I coach her to label and reinforce the vocabulary of clothing items, and body parts by saying, "The baby is cold, let's put her shoes on" "The baby is hungry, give her something to eat!" "Mommy is thirsty (pause), how about something to drink?"

When Bea doesn't understand a direction, mother models the expected response with me and then asks Bea again.

I ask Bea to give the baby a hug. "Ah, baby," we say and Bea says, "Ah beebee."

Mother asks Bea to give the doll a kiss.

We change the doll's diaper, saying, "Pee-oo!"

We hand the dirty diaper to Bea and wait for her verbal reaction.

Then we put the doll to bed, whispering, "Ssshhh, the baby is sleeping. Ssshhh."

We sing "Rock-a-Bye Baby" and sway.

As soon as mother starts singing the "Clean Up" song, Bea looks at her, smiles and produces vowels in alternation and melody similar to the model presented.

Mother gets the big red bucket and asks for different items, one at the time; "Bea, would you give me the baby's shoe?," "I wonder… Where's the baby's ball?," "How about the spoon?"

When mother says "spoon," Bea is puzzled and does not select the item.

I suggest that mother say something related to the spoon, such as, "Humm, we use the spoon to eat yummy soup."

Right away, Bea grabs the spoon, brings to her mouth, says "mmm," puts is in the bucket, and claps her hands saying "Yeah!"

She is proud of herself. We all join in celebrating everyone's accomplishment.

PARENT GUIDANCE

- If Bea does not understand the noun, use a synonym, different segmental features, or an onomatopoeic sound.
- Give her up to three opportunities to respond before modeling the correct response.
- Find fun ways to transition from one activity to the next.
- Predictable actions may help Bea to self-regulate, keep her content and willing to play, and prevent challenging behaviors.
- Provide good reasons for listening and talking.
- Having fun during purposeful play is the best way to learn to listen and talk.
- Put meaning to all parts of speech (nouns, verbs, adjectives, prepositions, and interjections)
- Help Bea follow single-step directions in daily routines. For example, "Give it to me."
- Occasionally, depending on the context, use soft speech or whisper a simple and well-known message. We want Bea to be responsive to all sounds in life and to prepare her to respond to soft sounds when being assessed by the audiologist.

continues

PARENT GUIDANCE *continued*

- When bathing Bea, keep the cochlear implants on (protected by water resistant cover) and talk about her body parts and action words (e.g., rub, wipe, and dry) and about smells and feelings. When going for a walk, facilitate opportunities for Bea to respond to sounds at a distance, but be close to her when providing directions, making comments, or any verbal interaction.
- When dressing her, be silly and encourage Bea to protest by saying "no" when, for example, trying to put her socks on her hands.
- Engage in pretend play with dolls, animals and puppets.
- Read books like "Little Red Hen" (Galdone, 2011), which was Vanessa's favorite book when she was about Bea's age, "The Napping House" (Wood, 1996) and "Moo, Baa, La La La" (Boynton, 1982). Encourage Bea to take her turn verbally.

ACTIVITY #5. LING SIX-SOUNDS

Bea is responsive to speech sounds, understands cause and effect, has a good attention span and fine motor skills and coordination.

Mother and I have introduced a conditioned play game in the last few sessions. Mother tells me that Bea enjoys this activity and has just begun to wait longer and respond more reliably to at least two of the Ling Six-Sounds. I acknowledge that and explain to her that Bea is ahead of the game as children may master conditioned play activities when they are older than 24 months. Thus, it is appropriate that she may be a little impatient after two or three sounds.

Sometimes mother models the targeted responses to the "test" and other times I do it.

For example, I may ask her to hold a stacking ring or plastic block to her ear, attend as though anticipating a sound, and, upon hearing it, put the ring on the stacking toy or the block in a pail.

We want Bea to demonstrate that she has optimal access to all sounds of the speech spectrum. This activity also prepares Bea for pure-tone testing, detects changes in the functioning of cochlear implants, and determines the effects of distance on the audibility of speech.

I introduce and model this activity as early as possible, if the child is developmentally ready.

Before I take out a colorful plastic stacking toy, I lean towards mother and say, "Guess what I have?"

She says, "What?" I respond by saying, "I have a stacking toy. Do you want to see it?"

Bea's mother nods and enthusiastically replies "Yeah."

I turn to Bea and ask the same question.

She smiles and vocalizes "Yeah!"

I bring out the toy and place it on the table.

We encourage Bea to approximate the word "up-up" as each ring is taken off the peg and "doowwn" as each ring is put on the table.

Bea approximates the sounds of up and down.

After all the rings are on the table, I give one to Bea's mother and say, "Listen!" as she places it by her ear and waits.

I say "Ah," and mother enthusiastically places the ring on the peg.

I offer the next ring to Bea, who just puts it on the peg. Because she does not hold it to her ear, we help her do this. As she does not wait for the sound and puts the ring again on the peg, mother and I continue to model it, and from time to time, offer Bea a turn.

Mother says, "I wish she would show you how she can do it so beautifully for at least one sound."

Mother and I make jokes about how kids can perform so differently in distinct situations or settings.

I say, "Bea may have not done this as she does at home, but I see that every time one of us said one of the Six-Sounds, Bea consistently looks in the direction of the person who is talking, which tells us that she is detecting and localizing at a short distance."

Once all the rings have been placed on the peg, we wave "bye-bye" and put the toy away.

PARENT GUIDANCE

- Use creative ways of doing conditioned-play tasks.
- Conditioned play activities are just a very small portion of the carryover activities. Tests are tests and have a specific purpose.
- Focus on Bea's auditory-verbal development by taking advantage of daily life situations to learn to listen and talk in a fun and meaningful way.

ACTIVITY #6. LTL TOYS, SONGS, AND GAMES: THE SNAKE

While Bea is looking at me I say, "Vanessa, would you introduce the next LTL toy?"

Mother says "Ssss" and Bea looks at her.

Mother smiles and says, "You heard the snake!" (pause) "The snake goes sss."

From a bag on the table, she takes out a rubber snake and repeats her last sentence.

While still holding the toy and keeping Bea's eye contact, mother says, "Mila (pause), what does the snake say?"

I say "Sss" and Bea looks at me.

I point to my ear and say, "You heard the snake! (pause) It goes ssss."

Mother asks Bea the same question: "What does the snake say?"

Bea says "Oww!" and hides her finger.

"Is the snake going to bite your finger?" says mother.

She puts the snake close to Bea's finger and pretends to bite it.

"Ouch! No, no, no, don't bite me!" says mother.

continues

LTL TOYS, SONGS, GAMES: THE SNAKE *continued*

We wait for Bea's vocal attempts and then put the toy on the table in front of her. She plays with it.

We narrate other things about the snake, such as, "It has a big (low pitch voice) mouth," "The snake is so looong," and "Ouch, it has sharp teeth! (pause) Let me see if you have sharp teeth!"

Then I pick up the basket, and say, "Let's put the snake in the basket. Wave bye-bye?"

We wait and look expectantly for Bea's response.

I repeat the direction and as Bea does not respond again, I lean towards her mother, and am about to give her the direction when Bea says "A-ba" and waves.

Mother hugs Bea and then says, "Bye-bye, snake"!

I present the basket and Bea puts the snake inside it, waves and says "Ba-ba" and we move on to the next activity.

PARENT GUIDANCE

- Always present the message for listening first, then present the visual reinforcement associated with the sound. (Listen First and Last!)

- There is not a magic number of seconds that one needs to wait for the child's response. Considering the child has optimal access to all speech sounds, I usually count to 10 silently. Sometimes children need more time to process the information and organize their responses. Other times they may be using the silence to control other people's behavior, or finally, they just don't know what or how to respond. This is the reason modeling the expected response is more effective than over repeating the message.

- Present the key word in final position. Occasionally, present a word Bea is familiar with in the middle of the sentence.

- Without visual cue, present the sound when she is distracted but not too focused on another activity.

- Change the pitch, duration, and loudness of your voice. Be animated and play with the suprasegmental features of speech.

- There are (a) sounds that are age appropriate for her to identify and (b) sounds that are age appropriate for Bea to produce. For example, with 4 months of optimal listening experience, expect Bea to be able to identify all sounds of the speech spectrum, including /s/; however, it is not (chronological) age appropriate for her to produces some sounds, including /s/. So it is expected that she identifies /s/ as the snake sound but it is not expected that she produce the last sound on "Yes." At this point, it is acceptable that she says yeah for "yes."

- Read books like "Brown Bear" (Martin, 2010) and "I Hear, Sounds in a Child's World" (Ogle & Thoburn, 1970).

- Make a snake with recycled materials, such as toilet paper rolls, small cereal boxes, empty plastic water bottles, or plastic bottle tops and put them together with yarn.

- Go to the zoo or pet store and visit the snakes.

Mother tells me that Bea got a clown toy from her aunt and it's in her bag.

I coach that before she shows it, she introduces it in an auditory-verbal way. "How would you do it, Vanessa?" I ask.

She says, "Maybe singing the song and observing her response. Let's try that!"

Mother sings the "Funny Little Clown" song (Estabrooks & Birkenshaw-Fleming, 1994).

Bea turns in the direction of a clown on the shelf, finds it, and says "A-a-a." (an approximation for the LTL sound similar "ha-ha-ha")

Mother provides positive reinforcement by smiling and saying, "You found a clown!"

Mother brings it to the table and we sing the song again.

While we're singing, Bea is babbling, dancing and playing with the clown, making it jump up and down, and then upside down, as we usually do.

"I have another clown! It's in my bag." Mother takes Bea's clown out of the bag.

Before mother gives the toy to Bea, I say "One of the language goals is to encourage Bea to verbally request, so I wonder how you could use this opportunity to do that?"

Mother holds the toy and asks, "Do you want the clown?"

Bea smiles and tries to grab the toy.

Mother points to her ear and says "Listen."

Once she gets her attention mother says, "Do you want the clown?"

Bea smiles and says "ah! A-a-a".

I coach mother to give Bea the clown now because she vocalized to request. I also indicate that mother might ask me to provide a higher-level of verbal response. "You know Bea the best, we don't want her to get frustrated and lose the momentum."

Still holding the clown, mother decides to do the latter. She looks at me and asks the question to which I say, "Yes please, yes!"

Mother looks at Bea and asks the question again and Bea says "Yeah!"

Mother gives the toy to her then gives her a big hug! "It was worth it to try!" says mother, satisfied for seizing the moment to raise the bar.

We all play with the clown toys for a few minutes and I say, "It's time to put the clown away. Would you blow it a kiss?"

Bea looks at me and remains quiet.

I wait and then repeat the question and wait again.

Bea does not respond, so I pick up the bucket and ask again.

Bea blows a kiss, produces some babbling sounds and waves bye.

When she is putting the clowns in the bucket, one of them falls down on the floor without her noticing it.

I look at mother who says, "Oh-oh, it fell down!"

continues

THE CLOWN *continued*

Bea looks at her mother and says "oh-oh."

As soon as mother repeats the sentence, Bea looks at the floor but cannot find what her mother is talking about.

"Oh no, the clown fell on the floor!," I say and point to the toy to reinforce that Bea's understanding.

I wait to see if she comments on the happening.

As she remains quiet, I say, "What should we do, mom?"

Mother says, "We better pick it up."

I lift the toy just a little from the floor, and say "Up," stop, and look at Bea.

She says "a" and I bring the toy higher and stop. Every time Bea vocalizes, I move the toy higher until it is on the table.

Bea gets the toy, I hold the bucket and ask her, "Would you give the clown to mommy, please?"

Bea looks at her mother and gives her the toy.

Mother says, "Good job!"

While Bea is smiling at her mother, I say, "High five!"

Bea turns to me and I repeat the phrase. She holds her hand up and gives me five.

"Oh, it's a new thing her dad has been doing, but it's the first time I've seen it!" says mother.

PARENT GUIDANCE

- Use some sabotage (I held the bucket up and asked her to give the toy to you).
- Expect Bea to use her voice to indicate her wants and needs.
- Listening is learned, it is not a test, so if Bea does not understand what you say, use auditory and verbal strategies to help her put meaning to words and sounds (e.g., Listening First and Last).
- Listen attentively when she talks and respond in a way that shows you understand. Repeat back what she says.
- Change your facial expressions to amusingly and dramatically reflect your mood.
- Encourage Bea's imagination while you play with her and her puppets, dolls, and stuffed animals.
- Think about questions such as, What is the next step in Bea's development?, How can I help her to get there?, Why am I doing it?
- Toddlers in particular may lose interest quickly, so keep the pace up and change activities when you need to do so.

When mother is putting the clown back to her bag, I say, "Vanessa, how about we read a book now?"

She explains that she has been reading a lot of books with Bea. She usually offers her two books and encourages her to vocalize to request one of them. She also reads the same book many times. "You said that repetition helps her to anticipate what comes next and I want to see her filling in the blanks as she has begun to do it when we're singing songs." She says that she makes comments about the pictures and encourages Bea to show that she understands what her mother is talking about by pointing to a picture upon hearing the related label or onomatopoeic sound.

I ask mother what Bea's favorite books are and I select two of them from my library: "The Wheels on the Bus" (Wickstrom & Raffi, 1998) and "Where's Spot?" (Hill, 2003).

Mother demonstrates how she reads the book at home. I coach her to keep three things in mind. (1) "good ear contact," so hold the book in front of both of you and sit beside Bea. (2) Talk about what is on the page and about what will come next, before turning the page. (3) Sometimes present the key word or sound in the middle of the sentence.

Mother says, "Bea, let's read a book! Which one would you like? The Wheels on the Bus or Where is the Doggy?."

Bea tries to grab the book about the dog. "Oh you would like to read Where's the doggy?,"says mother.

I coach mother to wait for Bea's verbal response.

She pauses and few seconds later she asks again.

Bea gets impatient and vocalizes in a protesting tone.

I suggest that mother proceeds to put meaning to Bea's vocalization. "Oh, you want me to read the book about the doggy!"

Mother reads the book to Bea and with some online parent guidance, she asks questions, makes comments, gives directions, pauses, and waits as per the following:

- Doggy, where are you?
- Do you think the little dog is in the closet?
- Is this a dog?
- I think I see a snake! Can you find it?
- Ee-ee-ee, listen I hear a monkey!
- I see the monkey's eating!
- I wonder what animal is under the stairs.
- Oh, no! It's not a dog.
- The big dog's bowl is empty. It's all gone!
- The little dog's bowl is full. What's it doing?

continues

ACTIVITY BOOKS *continued*

When mother finishes reading the book, I ask her to give the book to Bea so she can go over it again if she wants.

Bea opens the book on the page where the snake is in the closet, makes the natural gesture for "no," and with a frown on her face she says "Da-da-da" with similar suprasegmental features used by adults when we say, "No, no, no (don't bite me!)."

Mother interprets this speech production and says, "You found the snake! No, no, no (pause) don't bite me!"

Bea says, "Dow-dow-dow (pause) Oww" and hides her finger.

Bea closes the book and, without visual cues, mother asks Bea to give it to me, and she does.

PARENT GUIDANCE

- Add details to what she says. "Yes, that's a snake. It's a long snake. It's really big!"
- When Bea vocalizes, you may imitate her production and also may provide the correct model. This is a good way to reinforce development of the auditory-feedback loop.
- Acoustically highlight key words if necessary (Do you want a cookie?)
- After playing with a toy or reading a book, give her some time to explore the object by herself. We can observe valuable information about her auditory, language and cognitive development when we just follow her lead or are quiet beside her.
- Wait a little bit longer and try not to answer your own questions.
- Draw auditory attention to the size of objects and model accordingly; for example, "Daddy's shoes are so biiig" (elongated and low pitch sound).
- Continue to provide choices by using nouns, verbs and other parts of speech as such as: "Would you like an apple or an orange?," "Do you want to wear your red shirt or your yellow one?," "Shall we read 'Goodnight Moon' (Brown & Hurd, 2007) or 'But Not the Hippopotamus' (Boynton, 2012), and "Would you like something to eat or to drink?" In the beginning, you have visual and contextual cues associated with the verbal message. Later on, you may present the options through listening only.

CLOSING

Mother gets a container with healthy snacks from her bag and gives it to Bea by using the same procedure that we follow when introducing all parts of the session: listening first and last.

Mother and I need each other's full and undivided attention during this wrap up. We talk about "what" (diagnostic information collected), "how" (strategies used and discussed) and "why" (the rationale behind every action and decision) of what we did during the therapy and make plans for the following week.

I guide the mother to understand Bea's responses and auditory-verbal potential.

By guiding mother in identifying Bea's progress, she comes to recognize her daughter's achievements and her own. By guiding her, I hope to help her to continue the great work she's been doing for her child and to keep her eyes on the next skills and steps.

I guide her with questions such as:

What do you think the next step is since Bea can follow simple directions?

What strategies could we use to promote that?

How do you think you might do that at home?

My partnership with mother is also focused on empowering her with questions that encourage her thinking about where we are, where we believe we can be, and how to get there.

We spend 5 to 10 minutes in conversation so that mother knows what to do at home. Not often, she may wait until the last moment to tell me about significant concerns. I accommodate these by scheduling ample time between the therapy sessions.

continues

	SESSION ANALYSIS
AUDITION	• Turns to name when called from a distance of 16 feet. • Localizes speakers from side to side and from behind at distances up to 3 feet. • Detects speech with the presence of moderate background noise (figure-ground discrimination). • Recognizes and discriminates her name in incidental language contexts. • Demonstrates detection and localizes all sounds of the Ling Six-Sound-test. Identifies by imitating the following ones: "m," "ah." • Identifies soft high pitch speech sound ("sh") when attention is not brought to the sound. • Responds to /s/ without attention be brought to the sound and when she is slightly distracted. • Identifies onomatopoeic sounds, interjections and early developing words presented in the beginning and middle of the sentence; e.g., "Humm, we use the spoon to eat <u>yummy</u> soup," "Would you give the clown to <u>mommy</u>, please?" • Imitates a word presented in the middle of a sentence (up). • Responds to whispered speech. • Imitates suprasegmental features of speech: "ah, beebee" (ah, baby), Clean Up song, short and repetitive versus elongated sound (Auditory Memory). • Recognizes "Clean Up," "Rock-a-Bye Baby," and "The Funny Little Clown" songs. • Associates the song with corresponding toy. • Selects one item upon hearing related noun or sound out of a set of nine items. (Activity #4) • Recalls listening games (auditory memory) played before (e.g., "Ow" for Ouch). • Identifies the labeled toy (down) among others on the shelf. • Improves speech production after hearing corrected model (i.e., from "ah" to "aba" and then to "ba-ba" for "bye-bye," and from "da-da-da" to "dow-dow-dow" for "no-no-no").
SPEECH	• Uses appropriate intonation to exclaim, greet and complain. • Vocalizes diphthongs; i.e., "aaaeeaaw" and vowel-consonant-vowel (VCV) and CVCV combinations; i.e., aabaadaa, dadaba. • Uses early developing consonant and vowel sounds (e.g., b, m, and d). • Produces "baba" for bye-bye and "ow" of ouch. • "Babble-sings" a known song. • Says "beebee" for baby, "eeaa-eeaa" for clean up, clean up, "a-a-a" for "ha-ha-ha," "a" for up, and "oh ow" for "oh no."

	SESSION ANALYSIS
LANGUAGE	• Understands stereotypical messages and phrases and follows simple directions without visual cues, e.g., high five, give _ to mommy, "Wake Up" game, "blow a kiss," wave "bye-bye" or "hi," and "oh-ow, it fell down." • Understands early developing words; e.g., no and mommy. • Shakes head "no." • Vocalizes, babbles, and points to express her wants, needs, make a comment or protest. • Uses a verbal interjection in appropriate context (i.e., Yeah!). • Understands a few phrases; such as, "oh ow, it fell down."
COGNITION	• Enjoys following a book with an adult. • Understands silly games that are part of the routine (early demonstration of sense of humor development). • Demonstrates functional and symbolic use of objects. • Explores toys appropriately for her chronological age. Plays with a toy in different ways. • Places one object inside another (e.g., puts toys in a bucket upon request). • Imitates actions she can see be performed. • Points to face parts on the baby doll, on her and other people's faces (i.g., eyes, mouth, and nose): matches what are identical. • Puts six rings on pegs. • Overcomes simple obstacles. • Builds a tower of three rings. • Anticipates and initiates games that are part of her routine.
COMMUNICATION	• Vocalizes with communication intent. • Looks at mother for support. • Maintains attention on task. • Uses vocalizations more frequently during interactions. • Takes turn in verbal interaction. • Initiates verbal games that are part of her repertoire. • Demonstrates joint attention. • Looks from one person to the next. • Participates in reading age-appropriate books and nursery rhymes, singing songs, and playing games.

continues

CONCLUSION

- Mother was able to achieve most of the goals. She was able to: obtain Bea's attention through listening first; pause and wait after presenting information through listening; give her three opportunities to respond appropriately, model the expected response, and then ask Beatriz again; and encourage her to vocalize with communication intent.

- I was able to self-monitor the intensity of my speech, which can be louder than ideal especially when I'm excited about the child's and parent's achievements. I was able to practice "Active Listening" with more awareness. I attended to the mother fully, made sure there weren't misunderstandings, and encouraged her to share her questions and concerns. Mastering these skills, continuously improving my professional performance and keeping myself updated are commitments on a collaborative journey during which parents, caregivers and practitioners work towards the expected outcome: a happy child who listens and talks in kind, respectful and compassionate ways.

References

Boynton, S. (1982). *Moo, baa, la la la*. New York, NY: Little Simon.

Boynton, S. (2012). *But not the hippopotamus*. New York, NY: Simon & Schuster.

Brown, M. W., & Hurd, C. (2007). *Goodnight moon*. London, UK: HarperCollins.

Estabrooks, W., & Birkenshaw-Fleming, L. (1994). *Hear & listen! Talk & sing!* Washington, DC: Alexander Graham Bell Association for the Deaf and Hard of Hearing.

Galdone, P. (2011). *Little red hen*. Boston, MA: Harcourt Brace and Company.

Hill, E. (2003). *Where's spot?* London, UK: Penguin Books.

Martin Jr., B., & Carle, E. (2010). *Brown bear, brown bear, what do you see?* New York, NY: Holt & Company, Henry.

Ogle, L., & Thoburn, T. (1970). *I hear, sounds in a child's world*. American Heritage Press, ISBN-10:007047544X ISBN-13: 978-0070475441.

Wickstrom, S. K., & Raffi. (1998). *The wheels on the bus,* New York, NY: Random House Children's Books.

Wood, A. (1996). *The napping house*. New York, NY: Red Wagon Books/Harcourt Brace & Company.

Session Plan 4: The Two-Year-Old

AV PRACTITIONER	
Becky Crow Clem, M.A., CCC-SLP, LSLS Cert. AVT	
NAME OF CHILD Annie	**ETIOLOGY** Congenital Anomaly of Inner Ear per ENT diagnosis—similar to Enlarge Vestibular Aqueduct

DEGREE & TYPE OF HEARING LOSS Bilateral Sensorineural Hearing Loss—moderate

CHRONOLOGICAL AGE (CA) 2 years, 1 months	**HEARING AGE (HA)** 23 months
AUDITORY-VERBAL AGE (AVA) 20 months	**HEARING TECHNOLOGY HISTORY** • Bilateral behind-the-ear hearing aids at 2 months of age

INTERVENTION HISTORY

- First AVT evaluation at pediatric medical center at 5 months of age with intervention initiated 2 weeks later.
- Participated in AVT with at least one parent, sometimes both, for one 60-minute session once a week.
- Starting at 18 months of age attended a toddler program with peers with typical hearing.
- At age 2 years, started a pre-school program with peers with typical hearing.
- At age 3 months of age participated in Kindermusik program.

DEVELOPMENTAL HISTORY

- Born full-term, at 40 weeks' gestation. Mild torticollis at birth. Treated by physical therapist and discharged with good results.
- Genetic testing was negative for familial hearing loss.
- Two MRIs at age 6 months showed evidence of inner ear abnormality. Pediatric otolaryngologist diagnosed this as "Congenital Anomaly of Inner Ear." Personal communication with him revealed that it is a similar abnormality to Enlarged Vestibular Aqueduct (EVA)
- Motor and cognitive milestones reported and observed as developmentally appropriate.

continues

	PROGRESS SUMMARY Based on developmental norms, the child is able to:	SHORT-TERM OBJECTIVES To be accomplished in one to four AVT sessions
AUDITION	• Identify all Ling Sounds by repeating them • Identify and name at least 15 learning to listen sounds • Demonstrate auditory memory for familiar requests (open the door, wave bye-bye) • Follow two-part related directions (i.e., go get your shoes and socks; put your cup in the sink;) • Understand language given about events as they are happening • Identify nursery rhymes and finger plays by making the motions/body movements that accompany them • Demonstrate the beginning of conditioned play audiometry activities.	• Complete a known linguistic message from a familiar song or predictable book • Demonstrate understanding of two critical elements (e.g., big truck, little car; under the table; on the chair)
SPEECH	• Use suprasegmentals consistently • Produce all vowels and dipthongs with some accuracy • Use question inflection • Produce consonants /m/ /b/ /d/ /g/ /k/ /h/ /wh/ /y/ /l/ • Approximate /s/ and /sh/	• Imitate consonants varying by manner cues (e.g., mama bebe; nono dada) • Sing some words in known songs with approximate pitch and intonation
LANGUAGE	• Use one to two words with emerging three words • Begin to tell about past events with one to two words when asked (i.e., what did you get for your birthday? Shoes! Crocs!) • Understand familiar information in a frequently read picture book • Relate specific people to events/actions/objects (i.e., Mom tells her, "we are going to see Miss Becky," Annie responds "baby baby" because we play with baby dolls in therapy); I am leaving this because it is a good example.	• Use two to three words together to request an action or object, or to comment Demonstrate use and understanding of at least 10–12 new words weekly • Follow along in book reading about a familiar subject with pictures

	PROGRESS SUMMARY Based on developmental norms, the child is able to:	SHORT-TERM OBJECTIVES To be accomplished in one to four AVT sessions
LANGUAGE *continued*	• Spontaneously use 70–80 words including, nouns, modifiers, verbs, prepositions • Answer yes/no questions appropriately • Use jargon with many true words when trying to tell family something	
COGNITION	• Look for hidden objects • Point to pictures of people and objects she knows • Pretend to play schemes of daily living, to do conditioned play activities with baby dolls, and to read books saying a few familiar words • Assert independence • Attempt to fix something that's broken • Demonstrate curiosity about new experiences/activities/toys	• Expand make believe skills to include more than one activity in a pretend play scheme • Take turns in a play scheme with a friend, parent, and/or AV practitioner
COMMUNICATION	• Engage in communication with family • Initiate communication during play activities in therapy sessions • Use greetings and farewells (hi and bye bye) • Use common responses with prompting (please, thank you, sorry)	• Take at least two turns in communicative attempts.

AV PRACTITIONER GOALS

• Speak more slowly with the child and during my parent guidance and coaching
• Turn the activity over to the parent more consistently
• Explain goals and activities to parent in advance
• Explain and model strategies to parent
• Provide encouragement to parent as to what they do and the impact it has on the child

continues

PARENT GOALS

- Use rich vocabulary in conversation replacing generic words with more specific words (i.e., instead of "Where is it?" use "Where is the bouncy ball?"
- Use comments and open-ended remarks in lieu of yes/no questions to facilitate expressive language

ACTIVITY #1. GREETING

- I greet Annie and her mom in the waiting room and we walk back to the therapy room.
- We do a walking routine.
- Mom and I hold Annie's hand and say "walk, walk, walk, wheeeeee"—as we swing her up . . . then we repeat it two to three times. The third time we say "walk, walk, walk" . . . and pause—and wait for Annie to say "wheeeee."
- She looks up at us and smiles and says "wheee" . . . and we perform the routine of lifting her up and swinging her.
- This routine continues until we reach the therapy room.
- The door is closed intentionally so that Annie will initiate telling us to open the door.
- Her mom looks at her expectantly as Annie knocks on the door.
- Annie smiles, looks at mom again, and knocks.
- Mom uses an expectant look and this time Annie says "open open!"
- We open the door and talk about where to sit.
- The toys are in a large box covered with a sheet to maximize the use of audition throughout the session.
- Annie sits in the cut-out part of the u-shaped table, mom sits on one side and I sit on the other. We place all toys at the front of the table. We are seated slightly behind Annie.
- There is an "occupying toy" on the table for Annie to play with while I visit with mom.
- Mom and I talk about what has worked well this week at home based on the goals and strategies of the last session.
- Annie plays with the Peek-a-Blocks and calls attention to them by telling mom "look!"
- She names some of the animals along with the correct learning to listen sounds.
- She holds the block up to mom and says "open."
- Mom says, "It doesn't open Annie, see? The top doesn't come off."
- Annie says "Becky?" and hands it to me.
- I say, "The block won't open. The horsey is inside. See the horsey moves inside the block."
- Annie says "Inside?"

- We sing the clean up song and Annie sings a little and begins to put the toys away.
- I check Annie's equipment with a listening kit (both hearing aids are working and sound clear).
- I tell mom and Annie that it's time to listen.
- Mom says, "I'm ready to listen."
- Annie imitates "listen."
- I place a clear empty container on the table and tell Annie to listen.
- We use Halloween erasers and bouncy balls.
- She places the bouncy ball by her cheek and waits.
- Mom presents each sound at 3'.
- Annie imitates all of them and places the ball in the container each time.
- She holds a ball up to mom's cheek and makes the sound "ahhhh" and tells mom to "listen."
- Mom says "I hear ahhh" and drops the ball in the container.

PARENT GUIDANCE

- Do a quick Ling Six-Sound check in the morning, afternoon, and evening to ensure the hearing technology is working throughout the day.
- Present sounds at conversational level at various distances. Present short sounds similar to how quickly they occur in speech. (instead of ahhhh, say ah; instead of uuuuuuuu, say u). (Annie is skilled at identifying Ling sounds and developing her conditioned play responses quite well).
- Encourage Annie to pretend to do the Ling Six-Sound Test as she attempted today.

ACTIVITY #2. TRANSITION TO SPEECH GOAL

- As mom and I are talking about Ling sound check at home, Annie picks up a pumpkin and attempts to say "Halloween."
- Mom comments about the pumpkin and Annie drops it on the floor.
- Annie says, "uh oh Halloween."
- Mom models "pick up Halloween" (I encourage mom).
- Annie says "Halloween" (approximation).
- Mom models separately "pick up _____ Halloween."
- I coach her about using full phrases with acoustic highlighting.
- Mom does this 2 more times and Annie repeats, "Pick it up."
- I model—"Yes, pick up the Halloween pumpkin."
- (Because she is still interested in the Halloween erasers, we continue to use these for speech babble).

continues

ACTIVITY #3. MAGIC WORDS

- Mom reports that Annie is doing well on imitating consonants by manner.
- (She's beginning to use those targets in functional phrases such as" bye mama, my daddy, my puppy, no no Caleb) (brother).
- I tell Annie, "It's time for Magic Words!"
- She imitates an approximation for "magic words" and holds up an eraser and makes silly sounds to the pumpkin eraser.
- We do several repetitions of consonants varying by manner using the Halloween erasers and dropping them in the bowl.
- Annie repeats up to three to four consonants varying by manner with the same and different vowels.
- Mom and I discuss that this goal is completed.
- I explain that our next goal is to say consonants that vary by voicing cues.
- We talk about some examples such as: be po be po; ta ko ta ko; and functional phrases—my cookie, go Caleb (brother), bye Caleb.
- Mom shares some words that are Annie's favorite things that we can use at home (bye puppy, go car, tea cup).

PARENT GUIDANCE

- Goal met for consonants varying by manner. Encouraged mom to introduce consonants varying by voicing cues. Coached mom to write down the targets and examples discussed.
- Talked about how speech babble facilitates natural sounding speech.
- I counseled mom that Annie's speech is developing very naturally and accurately.

ACTIVITY #4. LET'S PLAY BABIES

- As Mom and I finish talking about speech targets, Annie says "baby?" (She is communicating that it is time to transition to something else. She wants to play with the baby dolls).
- I say, "I think I found a baby! I hear a baby crying! Whaa Whaa."
- Mom says, "Uh Oh, I hear baby crying. I wonder why she's crying."
- Annie says "Bath Bath."
- Mom replies, "Oh she needs a bath?"
- I pull out the baby and Annie says "wawa (water), wawa." I tell Annie that first we have to get the baby undressed. She can't take a bath with her clothes on. While Annie is exploring the baby doll with clothes, I explain the goal, activity, and strategies to mom.
- (We will try to expand Annie's vocabulary and not use some 'tired' or frequently used words. We will model longer phrases for her to use in requesting. We will work toward the goal of increasing her sentence length from 1–2 words to 2–4 words. We will use modeling, repetition, and acoustic highlighting to do this).

- I tell mom that it's like 'being a thesaurus." Once a child knows and uses a word quite well, it's time to teach new words (e.g., Annie already knows 'take clothes off' so today we introduce "undressed." We use "take clothes off" as we introduce undressed.)
- We use the words: undress, scrub, wipe, washcloth, clean, messy, sticky, bathtub, squeeze, shampoo, throughout the bathing activity.
- We use modeling, expansion, parallel talk, expectant look, and waiting.
- Mom uses several yes-no questions in conversation attempts.
- I demonstrate commenting and pass the activity to mom who follows my model.
- Annie imitates the new words bathtub, shampoo (poo), clean, messy.
- She consistently uses one word to comment with three occurrences of independent two word use.
- We model expansion to two to three words with about 30% success.
- Annie is very busy playing.
- We use the words, "Listen Annie" to help her attend to the expanded model.

PARENT GUIDANCE

- I ask mom to talk about activities the family could do at home that to carry over this goal.
- We brainstorm about:
  - Laundry activities—(Annie likes to help her with the laundry.)
  - Dressing activities—(Bring your socks AND shoes.)
- Use complete sentences if Annie misses a word rather than repeating just the portion she misses.
- Demonstrate how you can use the whole phrase with highlighting the missing part.
- Use expectant look and waiting.

ACTIVITY #5. THE BABY IS HUNGRY

- We continue to play with the baby and change some of the materials to address the critical elements goal.
- I explain to mom that critical elements are key pieces of information presented through audition. We want Annie to process and remember those. For example, we can give Annie a group of items and ask her to choose some or act on them. For example, we give her a baby doll, toy dog, toy cat, brush, washcloth, soap, water, and bathtub. We ask her to brush the dog. The two critical elements are "dog and brush." We might also ask her to "put soap on the washcloth." The two critical elements are "soap and washcloth."
- We add two more babies so that each of us has a baby.
- I explain that we will try to help Annie remember two critical elements in the message.

continues

ACTIVITY #5. THE BABY IS HUNGRY *continued*

- I tell mom, "I want to be sure I've done a good job explaining critical elements. How will you share this with Annie's dad?"
- She gives me good examples of critical elements in a message. This confirms that she understands the goal.
- (We will use repetition, acoustic highlighting, slow rate of speech, wait time, and expectant look.)
- We use actions and objects related to feeding. We add a toy bear and a toy dog to the feeding routine. The feeding toys include apple, cookie, milk bottle, juice bottle, and banana.
- Before starting the activity, we do a vocabulary check. When working on critical elements, we use known vocabulary.
- The feeding toys and animals are in a box.
- We sing, "What's inside the box? What's inside the box? Open up the top and see (pause and knock on the box), what's inside the box.
- We wait and Annie knocks on the box.
- We sing the song one more time and pause for the "knocking" on the box. Annie knocks on the box top when we pause.
- I tell Annie that we are going to feed the baby. I tell her that we will feed a bear and a dog, too.
- I take off the top and show the toys to Annie and Mom.
- I tell mom to find the bear and she does.
- I tell Annie to find the dog and she does.
- We complete the vocabulary check by selecting the toys by name.
- Mom and I take turns saying which toy to select.
- Annie takes a turn and tells mom "apple" to select an apple. (this is a "role reversal")
- Next, I say, "The baby, dog, and bear are hungry! They want to eat some lunch!"
- Mom says, "Yes they are hungry! It's time for lunch. They want to eat."
- Annie says, "Eat, hungry" (word approximation for hungry is "hun-gee").
- First we model the activity.
- I tell mom, "The bear wants to eat the apple." (Mom gives the bear the apple and pretends to feed it to him.)
- Mom tells me, "Miss Becky, the baby wants to drink some milk." (I give the baby the milk bottle and pretend to give her a drink.)
- Annie says, "My baby!"
- I say, "Oh your baby is hungry? Your baby wants to eat a banana." (Annie gets the banana and pretends to feed the baby doll.)
- I tell Annie, "Listen. The dog wants to drink some juice."
- (Annie gets the juice bottle and moves toward the baby)

- I say "Listen Annie. The dog (highlight) wants to drink some juice." (Annie moves toward the dog and pretends to have the dog drink the juice."

- I say, Yes Annie, the dog wants to drink some juice.

- I explain to Mom that we need to practice listening first and last (Chapter 11) so that she hears the whole phrase again. I share that it reinforces her correct response and helps her develop her auditory memory for two critical elements.

- At mom's request, I complete one more example of two critical elements with Annie. I point out how to highlight the critical element she misses by saying the whole phrase again. Annie says, "Cookie! Cookie?"

- Mom expands by saying, "Oh you want to feed someone a cookie? Who wants a cookie?

- Annie says, "Doggie cookie."

- Mom says, "The doggie wants a cookie. Let's feed the doggie a cookie."

- Annie says, "Doggie cookie."

- Mom says, "The doggie eats a cookie. It's yummy!"

- (Mom follows Annie's lead by expanding Annie's language. She gives Annie an opportunity to verbalize and comment. Mom models longer phrases and Annie comments using two-word phrases.)

- Mom says , "Listen Annie. The bear is thirsty. The bears wants to drink some milk."

- Annie takes the milk and pretends to give the bear a drink.

- Mom says "Yes, you are giving the bear a drink of milk. The bear is drinking his milk" (she reinforces Annie's response for two critical elements).

- I encourage mom to follow Annie's lead.

- By taking a few minutes to follow her lead with the cookie, Annie used two words to comment.

- Mom tells Annie, "Listen Annie, Let's feed the baby some banana. The baby wants to eat some banana."

- Annie says, "nana? Eat nana? "

- Annie picks up the banana, puts it in her mouth and laughs.

- We all laugh and say, "That's funny Annie!"

- Mom says, "Annie, the baby is hungry. The baby wants to eat the banana." Mom highlights "baby."

- Annie pretends to feed the banana to the baby doll. Annie says, "yum yum, mmmm, nana.'

- I say, "Yes, that banana is yummy. The baby's eating a yummy banana."

- Mom asks Annie if she wants to feed someone else. Annie answers No!

- Annie is engaged in the activity again.

- Mom does the critical elements activity two more times with Annie. She effectively highlights the missed elements with complete phrases following my modeling and encouragement.

continues

PARENT GUIDANCE AND CARRYOVER

- I ask mom how using two critical elements could be used at home in routines.
- We talk about doing the following at home:
- Ask her to take things to her brother or dad (take Caleb his shoes; Give Daddy a book).
- Have Annie help set the table (get the fork and plate).
- Target two critical elements when reading books (find the mouse eating the cookie).

ACTIVITY #6. IT'S BETTY BEAR'S BIRTHDAY!

- We transition to reading a book about a little bear's birthday. (Annie recently celebrated her second birthday.)
- Annie is geting restless and her mom does an excellent job of redirecting her through audition and getting her attention by saying, "Look Annie, it's Betty Bear's birthday."
- I tell mom that we are working on following along with the book and allowing Annie to talk and fill it what she knows from familiar information about birthdays.
- (We will also sing the Happy Birthday song to see if she can sing along with us and complete some of the song when we stop.)
- I begin reading in an animated voice, "Look Betty Bear is waking up. It's my birthday it's my birthday!"
- Annie pushes me away and tells me NO!
- Mom again engages using an auditory hook (Wow!) and a visual distractor (the book).
- She reads, "She got up and washed her face and brushed her teeth. She put on her birthday dress! Annie had a birthday dress."
- Annie looks at mom, points to her dress and says, "dress," then turns to me and says "Kecky" and touches my dress.
- Mom expands by saying, "Yes. You have a dress and mommy has a dress, and Becky has a dress."
- Annie looks back at the book.
- Mom continues reading using acoustic highlighting, and an animated voice to emphasize parts of the book that Annie will like.
- At one point mom reads, "And her (bear) daddy gives her a big kiss and says Happy Birthday."
- Annie says "to you!" (Demonstrates she can complete a known linguistic message.
- I say, "And Happy Birthday to You Annie!"
- Annie turns to mom and says, "Got Shoes Crocs" (meaning that she got Croc brand shoes for her birthday).

- Mom says, "Yes, you got Crocs for your birthday."
- Annie says, "Shell" (meaning that her friend Rachelle was at her birthday party).
- Mom comments, "Yes Shell was at your birthday party, too."
- (The book ends with the Betty Bear and her friends around a cake).
- We sing Happy Birthday. Annie joins in.
- We stop before the end of the song and Annie fills in "to you."
- Mom tells Annie to blow out the candles and Annie leans over and blows on the cake in the book.

PARENT GUIDANCE

- I shared my observation of Annie's attempts at conversation related to her birthday party.
- I asked mom to share what she observed during the book reading: Annie's use of three words together "got shoes Crocs," recalling who attended her birthday party, how she followed along with the words from the book and imitated some of them.
- Mom and I talked about how to facilitate conversation at home about the birthday party book.
- Mom stated that would make an experience book about Annie's birthday and read it together.
- Annie could 'read' the book to her dad and her brother, too.

PARENT GUIDANCE SUMMARY

- I identified 12 new words Annie used.
- Pointed out how Annie is attempting conversation with mom—using inflection and expecting mom to answer. When mom answers, Annie imitates her response or has an appropriate answer.
- Coached mom on reducing her number of yes-no questions.
- Mom was able to describe how Annie responds with specific words when she makes comments versus yes-no questions.

continues

	SESSION ANALYSIS The child demonstrated the following:
AUDITION	• Demonstrated identification of all Ling Six-Sounds • Beginning to understand two critical elements. 100% with one critical element; about 60% on two critical elements on first attempt, 80% on second attempt after highlighting • Completed known linguistic message from familiar content
SPEECH	• Used a variety of consonants in conversation attempts • Production of three-syllable words • Sang some of the words to a familiar song • Imitated consonants differing by manner • Attempted imitating consonants by voicing cues
LANGUAGE	• Used one word consistently to communicate multiple meanings. • Used one to two words for about 50% of communication attempts. (Occurs more often in spontaneous speech while playing or reading a book versus in response to comment or question.) • Used 12 new words. • Attempted to use two to three words after repetition and modeling from mom and practitioner. • Readily imitated new words heard in conversation. • Commented on information in a book as it related to past event (birthday).
COGNITION	• Took turns in play activity. • Expanded play to include others. • Requested more objects and actions to expand the activity. (When she was finished bathing the baby, she communicated that she wanted the baby to eat without needed to be prompted.)
COMMUNICATION	• Initiated conversation about her birthday. • Had conversational exchange twice with mom on birthday subject. • Initiated new words heard in conversation readily. • Listened and commented on a story,

REFLECTING ON THE PRACTITIONER TARGETS

- I used a slower rate of speech throughout the session.
- I pointed out a mistake I made to mom. I showed the toy before telling Annie about it. Mom was able to identify Annie's visual interest in the toy instead of attending to listen to what I said about it.
- I encouraged mom by telling her that what she did helped to improve Annie's use of longer phrases.
- I asked mom to demonstrate what she understood about critical elements.
- I followed the child's lead to allow her to initiate requests and use one- to two-word phrases independently.
- I responded to the child's requests and modeled expansions to work toward the goal of two to four word phrases.
- I guided mom to highlight a missed critical elements in a message.
- I made quick effective transitions between activities to keep Annie's attention.
- I quickly turned over the book to mom.

CONCLUSION

- Annie's session centered on short-term goals designed to facilitate growth and development in speech, language, listening, cognition, and conversation. By focusing on reducing yes-no questions and using rich vocabulary, Annie's mom saw improvement in Annie's responses and use of longer phrases.
- Annie loved the baby doll activities and she stayed engaged for most of the session. When she was distracted or fidgety, we could redirect her through audition.
- Using songs and predictable messages is effective in determining her ability to use auditory closure
- She is consistently imitating consonants varying by manner and advancing to imitating consonants varying by voicing cues. Varying consonants by manner is occurring in functional phrases.
- Use of 2+ word phrases is progressing. She uses these more often when playing with other children or with her brother.
- Because Annie verbalizes often during book reading we can plan for more reading activities and follow up at home to facilitate new vocabulary and increasing phrase length.

Reference

Fujikawa, Gyo. (1977), *Betty bear's birthday*. Grosset & Dunlap.

Session Plan 5: The Three-Year-Old

AV PRACTITIONER	
David Sindrey, M.Cl.Sc. LSLS Cert. AVT	

NAME OF CHILD	ETIOLOGY
Dylan	Unknown

DEGREE & TYPE OF HEARING LOSS Bilateral profound sensorineural hearing loss identified at birth.

CHRONOLOGICAL AGE (CA)	HEARING AGE (HA)
3 years 2 months	2 years 11 months

AUDITORY-VERBAL AGE (AVA)	HEARING TECHNOLOGY HISTORY
2 years 5 months	• Fitted with bilateral digital hearing aids at 3 months of age. • First implant surgery at age 13 months. • Implant processor mapped at age 14 months. • Bimodal technology used until second implant surgery at age 2 years 4 months. • Mapped and binaural cochlear implant use on at age 2 years 5 months.

INTERVENTION HISTORY

• Home visiting sessions with Teacher of the Deaf/Hard of Hearing. General oral language and listening training and parent training since aided at 3 months of age.

DEVELOPMENTAL HISTORY

• Full-term pregnancy.
• No family history of hearing loss.
• Cytomegalovirus results were negative.
• Diagnosed with a bilateral hearing loss following Newborn Hearing Screening.
• Absent otoacoustic emissions.
• Repeated ABR indicated a profound bilateral loss.
• Fitted with bilateral digital hearing aids at three months.
• Sitting unaided at 5 months, walking at 13 months
• Dylan is an active and talkative preschooler with no siblings.

	PROGRESS SUMMARY Based on developmental norms, the child is able to:	SHORT-TERM OBJECTIVES To be accomplished in one to four AVT sessions
AUDITION	• Identify all six-sounds and silence when presented the Ling Six-Sound Test at 1 m and 2 m • Enjoy listening to and singing familiar songs. • Follow commands using two different prepositions (e.g., "on" and "in"). • Attend to speaker at a distance/ speaker in noisy situations • Identify two items when named in a sentence presented in a large set of same syllable words (≥20 items) • Discriminate rhyming words by initial manner in a small set (≤6 items) • Discriminate minimal pairs different in word endings (manner) in a small set (≤6 items) • Identify objects based on description of their appearance, use or locative information such as, "Do you see something you use to cook?," "Can you see an animal that is black and white?," and "Show me who is in the tree."	• Follow commands using two unrelated steps (e.g., "Take your plate to the kitchen and then find us a book to read") • Try to overhear interesting comments made by others • Follow three-step directives • Identify three items when named in a sentence presented in a large set of familiar and acoustically dissimilar words (≥20 items) • Discriminate the following: ○ rhyming words by initial manner in a medium set (≤12 items), minimal pairs different in word endings (manner) in a medium set (≤12 items) and /p/ versus /t/ in repeated syllables (e.g., "puhpuhpuh" versus "tuhtuhtuh").

SPEECH	• Vocalize with good vocal quality and normal use of intonation and volume
	• Produce the following:
	  ○ vowels and diphthongs
	  ○ final consonants in some contexts (esp. "p," "m" in new words)
	  ○ syllables including those unstressed in most contexts
	  ○ nasals "m," "n," and "ng" in words.
		• final consonants "p," "m," and "n"
		• fricatives "f," "s," and "sh" in final word position in some targeted words.
		• /k/ in isolation

continues

	PROGRESS SUMMARY Based on developmental norms, the child is able to:	SHORT-TERM OBJECTIVES To be accomplished in one to four AVT sessions
SPEECH *continued*	○ glides "w" as in "wall" and "y" as in "yes" ○ stops and plosives "p," "b," "t," and "d" in beginning and middle word positions (the sounds "k" and "g" are fronted as "t" and "d," respectively). ○ fricatives "f," "s," "h," and "sh" in initial word position. ○ affricate "ch" in initial word position.	

LANGUAGE	• Understand and use:
	  ○ common questions such as, "What's your name?," "How many?," "What color?"
	  ○ "What" and "Where" questions.
	  ○ prepositions "in," "on," "under," "up," "down," and "in back of"
	• Express the following:
	  ○ pronouns "I," "you," and "me"; possessive pronouns "my" and "mine"; time concepts such as yesterday (although that may be used to indicate yesterday and events past), today, and tomorrow (although that word may be used to indicate tomorrow and all future events)
	  ○ present progressive "ing" with verbs
	  ○ simple 2, 3, and sometimes 4-word sentence forms (MLU = 2.4)
		• Respond appropriately to "Who" versus "What," and "Where" questions.
		• Use the following:
		  ○ prepositions "in front of," "beside," and "next to"
		  ○ possessive pronouns "your" and "yours."
		  ○ uncontractable copula "is" with well known adjectives (e.g., "The cow is dirty")
		• the negative "not" instead of "no" (e.g., "Daddy's not little" versus "Daddy no little")
		• Understand both "s" and "es" as plural marker for regular plural nouns
		• Understand the pronouns "it," "us," "we," "them," "this," "that," "he," and "she."
		• Produce sentences using the conjunction "and"

	PROGRESS SUMMARY Based on developmental norms, the child is able to:	**SHORT-TERM OBJECTIVES** To be accomplished in one to four AVT sessions
COGNITION	• Understand "one" and "all" • Identify the basic shapes (square, triangle, and circle) • Match primary colors • Understand concept of size as which is "smallest" or "largest." • Sort by color, size or shape • Count out loud and is able to answer to "How many?" (for up to five items) • Complete a six-piece puzzle • Initiate and maintain pretend play using themes from daily activities	• Demonstrate understanding of descriptive/size (e.g., tiny/hug, short/tall, etc.) • Identify words that begin with letters ("s" for Start, "t" for Time) such as those on the oven. • Demonstrate ability to identify first/number one, second/number two, etc. • Sequence and plan out steps for baking activity and list the items needed for the activity.
COMMUNICATION	• Take a turn in play but may have trouble when turns are shared in groups of three or more participants • Adapt to change in topic • Use a variety of communicative intents • Show understanding of other's needs or feelings • Initiate conversation with others	• Complete three turns in conversations. • Request repetitions to repair communication breakdowns • Use word approximations to request, initiate pretend play, comment or tell information, acknowledge or respond.

AV PRACTITIONER GOALS

• I recognize that I often rescue activities by being animated in order to regain Dylan's attention. Therefore, I need to coach mother to use strategies that will engage her child and rescue activities on her own.
• Discuss the need to involve father.
• Guide mother to promote skills that will engage both father and her mother-in-law in daily interactions with Dylan.

PARENT GOALS

• Use pausing, negative assertions, and sabotage to allow Dylan to become more conversationally active.
• Replace direct questions with self-statements.
• Read more books
• Engage Dylan in pretend play in an animated way.
• Repeat back what Dylan says (in correct form) and highlight key words (eg., "You are right Dylan, the cow IS dirty")

continues

**STEP-BY-STEP SESSION PLAN
TECHNOLOGY AND ORIENTATION**

- I meet Dylan and his mother in the "Get Ready" room, where a CDA (communicative disorders assistant) has helped the parent to do the Ling Six-Sound Test at the level (identification) and distance (1 meter) following my recommendation. Dylan's mother conducts the test for each CI and then again with both devices at 1 meter. She is guided to expect Dylan to vocally respond to the sound presented while he points to a picture associated with the sound (e.g., Doctor looking in mouth for "ah," ghost for "oo," vacuum cleaner for "ee," baby sleeping for "sh," snake for "s," ice cream cone for "mm," and blank space for nothing). The CDA knows to watch that Dylan's mother randomizes the presentation so that he cannot predict the sound. Mother still needs coaching to vary the pause time between presentations. The room has a video feed to the therapy room so that if necessary I can observe the Ling Six-Sound Test administration from there and make further recommendations.

Then I do the following:

- I talk with mother while Dylan puts away the Six-Sound Toys (The CDA keeps him entertained until both parent and practitioner are ready to head for the therapy room).
- I open the conversation by asking. "How are things going this week?" and then "Do you want to focus on something in particular today?"
- We review the successes and challenges of the past week in stimulating language and listening
- We briefly problem solve and then I adjust the session plan to deal with this particular parent's need.
- Mother reports that Dylan was very interested in talking with his older cousins who had come to visit and that everyone was thrilled with what he could do.
- I discuss the short-term objectives for the session and prompt mother to think of a two step direction to give Dylan as they enter the room.

ACTIVITY #1. EXPERIENCE BOOK OR PAGE SHARE

- As she enters the room, Mother visually scans it and says "Dylan, can you close the door and then show Dave your Experience Book?" Dylan follows her directions and the AV practitioner praises them and points out that the more often Dylan demonstrates these types of directives, the stronger his understanding will become.
- (Dylan's mother creates a new Experience Page each week based on a favorite recent event or experience. She uses the inside half of a file folder and draws enough to represent the event and glues in mementos that will bring the event to Dylan's mind. This week's Experience page is about going on Grandpa's boat to catch fish for breakfast)

- I wait for Dylan to show the page and say "Wow!" I then wait. Dylan points to the character in the boat and says "Poppa," the name for Grandpa. I explain to mother that the extra pause time is very important as a way to give Dylan time to think of what to say on his own.
- Then I ask, "Wow Dylan. How many fish did you catch?" (Mother has drawn three fish to the left of the boat). Dylan is not familiar with this question but he begins to count "One, two three . . . Three!" and I expand by saying, "Three! Three fish. Three big fish!"
- (There is a bloody Band-Aid taped to the page and Dylan eagerly shows his finger and says "Ouch").
- I encourage Dylan to provide more information and mom provides more too. I compliment them on the page as a great conversational starter.
- I guide mother to add to the page at home in order to integrate some of Dylan's objectives (There could be tiny fishing rods for pretend play. There could be paper fish to be caught (held in a pocket on the folder). The fish could be different colors (new ones include black, purple, white and pink and/or different sizes). Photos of cleaning and cooking the fish could be a great addition. The photos could be a simple three step sequence story Dylan's conversational partner can use them to retell the story using new words such as catch, clean, cook).
- Once Dylan's experience page is exhausted, (in some AVT sessions, the experience book may be used for the entire session), I bring out my own page to share, a traditional activity at the start of AVT as it is effective in modeling different ideas for displaying experiences within the file folder format. As the folder is retrieved from the shelf, I coach mother on how to practice wait time and how to expand any utterances Dylan makes.
- I say, "This is a sad story," and then hand the folder to mother. Mother opens it and says, "What happened?" in a concerned voice as they look at the items. She gives Dylan lots of time to respond. I praise her and she continues to expand Dylan's language throughout the conversation about the demise of a pet turtle.

ACTIVITY #2. THE TIPPY BOAT

- (I had prepared an inexpensive activity by using a plastic ice cube tray and a circle of sturdy cardboard (the diameter is the same length as the ice cube tray). The cardboard was cut into two halves and then glued inside the grooves along the edge of each side of the tray. The end result is what I call a "Tippy Boat" with the ice cube tray sections used as the "deck" of the boat. Small toys can be piled on the tray until, the boat finally tips over and the items fall out.)
- I introduce it as "Poppa's boat" to link it to the previous discussion.
- I pass the boat to mother.
- She looks confused about what is expected.
- I coach her by asking her, "Is that Poppa's boat?"

continues

ACTIVITY #2. THE TIPPY BOAT *continued*

- She then talks in a Grandpa voice and says, "Come on Dylan. Let's go catch some fish. I'm really hungry!" and pushes the boat slowly around the table saying "puh puh puh puh."

- She then gives Dylan a turn to push the boat and imitate the sound. "Poppa's boat is slow!" she adds.

- I place the tippy boat just out of reach and then place 20 familiar items on the table around it. (Dylan knows the names of the objects). The names of the objects are acoustically different from one another and are from familiar categories such as furniture, food, clothing, and vehicles.)

- I explain the objective again. (Dylan will demonstrate memory for three items). I tell mother that it should be easy as Dylan knows the words. (Later we need to discuss how to move to the next level).

- I hold out my hands and ask mother, "Can you give me the hat, the sheep and the airplane?"

- Mother starts to pick up everything and I coach her to only pass two of the items which she does.

- I look at the two items and say, "Something's missing."

- Mother asks me to repeat the question.

- She adds the missing item.

- I explain that this is a way to model for Dylan how to ask for clarification and also provide another auditory experience.

- I carefully place all three items on the tippy boat, while using an animated voice to say "Oh oh! Don't fall down!" and "Careful!" The tippy boat does not tip and the turn is passed to the mother.

- Mother asks Dylan for three items.

- I coach mother to speak slowly and to emphasize the conjunction "and" while naming the three items.

- (Dylan was successful at times with only one presentation but typically needed to ask for clarification and at least one repetition.

- Dylan takes his turn and demonstrates his understanding of the activity by placing his hands in front of him and asking the practitioner for three items.

- (After all of the items are selected, the tippy boat does not tip.)

- I bring out a toy shark and pass it to the mother who says, "Num, num, nummm" as she pretends the shark is attacking the boat.

- I say that this sound is good for practicing final /m/. Dylan takes a turn to say, "Num num num" with the shark.

- (All of the items are pushed off the boat by Dylan's shark and I comment that the game can be played again, but that it is better to move onto something else and that they could take the tippy boat home.)

- (The toys are put away according to category.)

- I model how to ask for "one" versus "all" as part of the task (e.g., "Give me one of the animals" versus "Give me all of the clothes").

- A big plastic mixing bowl is placed in front of Dylan. The instant chocolate pudding box is passed to the mother under the table.
- She peeks at the box and then looks to the AV practitioner for guidance.
- I remind her to talk ahead and she replies by saying, "I love this. This is great pudding. Mmmmmmm! Yummy Yummy pudding."
- I compliment her for using a self-statement rather than asking a question.
- I explain that in making the pudding, one objective is to practice taking turns among three people and that both adults can each model the language for turn-taking. Mother has been using both sabotage and failure to anticipate needs as ways to promote expressive language over the past few sessions. I do not mention these strategies and hopes to see them used spontaneously during this activity.
- I slide the container holding milk, a big spoon, scissors, and cups with small spoons under the table to mother. (One of the cups is broken.) I coach mother to say familiar phrases using lots of animation in her voice and to talk about what she is doing and before she shows it.
- Mother says, "Ooooo, what do we have here? I have some cooold milk!"
- Then, she brings out the milk and holds it to her cheek and says, "Brrrr . . . This milk is cold!"
- I coach her to do the same to Dylan and to say the phrase again.
- Mother says what she is going to do before she does it. "I'm going to open the pudding with the scissors, cut, cut, cut."
- She opens the pudding and says "Shake shake shake" as she shakes some of the chocolate powder into the bowl.
- I model, "My turn!" and the mother passes him the pudding box.
- I repeat the phrases and he takes his turn.
- Mother says, "My turn!" and waits for Dylan to say the same phrase, which he does. Mother hands him the box.
- Mother models ("Pour it! Pour it!" and "Stir, Stir, Stir," and "Round and round and round and round").
- Dylan has many chances to wait and then take a turn using phrases modeled by the two adults.
- He begins to spontaneously say, "My turn."
- When the pudding is ready, I hand the cups to Dylan and say, "Give one to Mommy and give one to me."
- Dylan follows this and then I hand him a broken cup, without comment, as though the fact that it is broken was not noticed.
- Mother begins to mention the cup but the practitioner cues her to wait.
- Dylan responds "Oh Oh!" as the pudding is being served.
- Mother says, "What's wrong?" and pauses to wait for Dylan to respond.
- He does so by holding up the cup and saying "Broken." I expand this phrase "Oh . . . your cup is broken!" and replace the cup.

continues

ACTIVITY #3. CHOCOLATE PUDDING *continued*

- Dylan eats the pudding and I ask mother why the broken cup was a good idea.
- She recognizes the strategy as sabotage.
- I ask her to think about other ways to use sabotage within the same activity.
- She comes up with the idea of only giving him a little pudding compared to everyone else and also by "forgetting" to give him a spoon.
- I point out that this activity is good for giving Dylan a meaningful opportunity to use the possessive pronoun "yours."
- Mother makes note in her therapy journal (parent book).
- As the pudding is finished I get everyone's attention by placing a big spoonful of chocolate pudding right in the middle of the table.
- This sets things up for the next activity.

ACTIVITY #4. SIMPLE STORY

- I announce, "We are going to read a book!" (The book cover is described first and then shown (it is a printable book that can he can inexpensively with the parent. The book has no printed text and parents are expected to adjust their language to suit the needs of the child who is listening.) "There is a cow, a pig, a sheep, and a big muddy pond."
- I pretend to smell the mud on the book cover and say "Peeeuuuuu!"
- I repeat the same action with the pile of chocolate pudding on the table to help everyone understand it represents the mud puddle.
- Then, I talk about each animal in the story and produce them one at a time.
- I open the book to the first page so that only I can see.
- I describe the scene in simple sentences, highlighting the conjunction "and." "The cow AND the sheep AND the pig see some dirty, dirty mud."
- I prompt mother to listen and she responds by lining up the animals in front of the "pudding."
- Then I show the page and say the sentences again.
- I pass the book to mother who needs a reminder to hold it hidden and to talk about what she sees before showing the page.
- As the animals each jump in the mud there are many opportunities to use the copula and auxillary "is" (e.g., "the pig is bad," "the cow is jumping," the sheep is dirty").
- Mother, Dylan and I each take a turn reading and acting out the story as it progresses.
- The story ends with the farmer appearing and catching the animals playing in the mud.)
- Mother and I model many simple sentences using "is" in sentences like "the farmer is mad."
- We wash all the animals in a basin and modeled sentences such as "the cow is clean," "the sheep is happy," etc.

- Mother and I ask several simple questions about the story, including a "Who" question ("Who was mad?").
- He responded correctly and then I talk about the next level of questions.
- Dylan's mother comments that they could do the same story at home in the sandbox with real mud!
- We pack the animals into a bag so the mother will have props for the story at home.
- We also talk with Dylan while cleaning up the table.

ACTIVITY #5. "FIVE-IN-THE-BOAT"

- I start singing, "There were five in the boat and the little one said . . . Move over! Move over!" (sung to the tune of "There were five in the bed").
- I produce a garden glove with a drawing of a boat glued to the palm, and five different drawings of children glued to each finger (the smallest on the thumb). The four fingers are cut through below the characters so that they can come off the hand and be used as finger puppets. On the back of the glove is a "cheat sheet" card for the parents with the following lyrics . . .

> *There were five in the boat and the little one said . . .*
> *Move over! Move over!*
> *So . . . they all moved over and one fell out!*
> *SPLASH! The boy (girl) is wet!*
> *How many?* (Help your child to count) . . . *1, 2, 3, 4, . . . 4*
>
> *There were four in the boat and the little one said . . . (continue)*
> (For last child) . . . *There was one in the boat and the little one said . . .*
> *Ahhh, that's better. This boat is mine!*

- I tell Dylan the plan: "We're going to sing a song! Let's give Mommy the glove."
- Dylan doesn't understand, so I say, "Give it to Mommy!" and Dylan follows the direction.
- I coach mother to start singing and she sings along.
- When the first chorus ends, one child falls out and I demonstrate it by taking a child puppet off mother's finger and say "SPLASH" as I place the figure on the table.
- Then I say, "Oh no! The boy is wet!," and follow by pointing to the remaining children in the boat and say to Dylan, "How many are left?"
- Through coaching, mother pauses after they sing "Move over . . . " and I model by filling the pause with the next line, "Move over!"
- I move back a little from the activity and mother takes over the song.
- I note that mother waits for Dylan to complete "Move over" on the chorus and gives him the opportunity to count the characters after another falls off the boat.
- I point out how talkative Dylan has been without the need to ask him direct questions.

continues

	SESSION ANALYSIS
AUDITION	• Demonstrated identification of all six Ling sounds and silence at 1 meter with each CI device and both together. • Recognized a negative assertion made by the mother. • Demonstrated understanding of words and phrases without context Good spontaneous listening behaviors. • Demonstrated ability to fill in the correct word during a pause in singing, "Five in the Boat."
SPEECH	• Some practice with final /m/ and final /p/ within activities ("up goes the cow," "cup" for the pudding and "numm nummm" for the shark). Speech production was not a focus of the session as Dylan's mother is being encouraged to avoid correcting and use more modeling strategies to encourage productions.
LANGUAGE	• Used possessive pronoun "your" • Used uncontractable copula "is" with well-known adjectives (e.g., "The cow is dirty")
COGNITION	• Demonstrated some understanding of "one" versus "all" in putting away the toys in the Tippy Boat game • Sorted objects by category • Counted out loud and is able answer to "How many?" for "5 in the boat" song. • Followed a simple sequence story while acting that story out with small objects
COMMUNICATION	• Demonstrated appropriate turn-taking with three participants. • Used "My turn" within a structured activity in order to gain his turn. • Responded by using language in response to negative assertions, sabotage, and pausing

REVIEW OF PRACTITIONER TARGETS

- I coached the parent to add interest to the activity in order to keep Dylan engaged rather than do it myself.
- I helped mother to better engage Dylan in pretend play and use an animated voice.
- I was able to brainstorm ways to involve Dylan's father and grandmother.

REVIEW OF PARENT TARGETS

- Mother will add new colors to the Experience book.
- Mother will emphasize the conjunction "and" within the story and the tippy boat task and throughout the day.
- She learned to take longer pauses to give Dylan the chance to take a conversational turn.
- She used a few spontaneous "negative assertions" and saw that this gave Dylan the chance to consider the meaning of what was said.
- She made a plan to include both the father and grandmother as described in the conclusion.

CONCLUSION

Mother and I will invite Dylan's grandmother to attend the next AVT session.

They will plan a number of strategies for building the successful partnership discussed.

Mother will ask Dylan's father to watch some videos about strategies used in the AVT. They will watch them together to help her highlight different language goals. She will try to avoid correcting what he does and give sincere thanks for his input. She will discuss the idea of him attending AVT sessions, observing sessions by Skype, and/or participating in some of the telepractice sessions.

I ask mother what was the most important thing that she learned and would like to have as a more established skill by the next appointment. She believes the need to better engage Dylan and keep his attention in play was by far the most important skill to learn.

I give mother the book, the tippy boat, and the garden glove puppet for use at home. I promised to send links to YouTube videos that show the song.

I mention another link that leads to an explanation of the strategy "Model and Expand" for both parents to watch and share with Dylan's grandmother. These are very simple explanations videotaped by myself with an iPad and then uploaded to YouTube under a private link.

Mother and I discuss the benefits of each activity in terms of objectives for both the parent and the child and she makes notes of strategies to use for each of the activities she would take away. So that Dylan's mother leaves with focus on engaging Dylan in play, I ask her to think about different ways to play with the same activities at home. She comes up with a great idea about singing the "Five in the Boat" song with playschool figures and an empty margarine container floating in a wash basin. Dylan's mother leaves saying she is most excited about acting out the Cow, Pig, and Sheep story with real mud in the sandbox. I tell her that's a fantastic plan.

Session Plan 6: The Four-Year-Old

AV PRACTITIONER	
Lisa Katz, M.H.Sc., SLP(C), Reg. CASLPO, LSLS Cert. AVT	
NAME OF CHILD	**ETIOLOGY**
Emma	Progressive hearing loss due to bilateral Mondini malformations
DEGREE & TYPE OF HEARING LOSS Bilateral Profound Sensorineural	
CHRONOLOGICAL AGE (CA)	**HEARING AGE (HA)**
4 years, 6 months	1 year, 6 months post activation of cochlear implants
AUDITORY-VERBAL AGE (AVA)	**HEARING TECHNOLOGY HISTORY**
2 years	• Received a pass result on her newborn hearing screen.
	• At two and a half, her preschool teacher expressed concern about delayed speech and language skills.
	• Audiologic testing was conducted and Emma was diagnosed with a bilateral moderate to severe sensorineural hearing loss.
	• Emma was immediately fitted with bilateral behind-the-ear hearing aids, which she wore during all waking hours.
	• Over the next 6 months, she exhibited a decline in hearing.
	• At 3 years, thresholds had dropped into the profound range.
	• Diagnosed with bilateral mondini malformations.
	• Received bilateral cochlear implants

INTERVENTION HISTORY

- Began attending weekly Auditory-Verbal therapy following the diagnosis.
- During her first 6 months of therapy, she made maximum use of her aided residual hearing.
- Heard differences in auditory patterns and was able to detect low- and mid-frequency speech sounds.
- Quickly learned many Learning to Listen Sounds and some stereotypical phrases, such as "Uh-oh!" and "It's all gone."
- Could perform closed-set selection type test tasks and was highly motivated to communicate by using words, phrases, and gestures.
- Drop in hearing prevented her from adequately monitoring her speech.
- Following activation of the CIs, listening and communication developed very well.
- At this session (1 year, 5 months post activation) she was receiving Auditory-Verbal therapy intervention every other week.

DEVELOPMENTAL HISTORY

- Born full-term following a normal pregnancy.
- Other than delayed speech and language skills secondary to progressive hearing loss, developmental history is unremarkable.
- Presents as bright and curious.
- Attends kindergarten at her local school and is doing well.

continues

	PROGRESS SUMMARY Based on developmental norms, the child is able to:	**SHORT-TERM OBJECTIVES** To be accomplished in one to four AVT sessions
AUDITION	• Follow directions containing four to five critical elements. • Identify objects based on hearing a related description in a closed set. • (Open set identification is emerging.) • Demonstrate auditory sequential memory for four items.	• Follow multielement directions (I would like three scoops of chocolate ice cream with blue sprinkles in a small cup). • Identify objects based on a related description in an open set (I have something that is the same color as a lemon). • Demonstrate auditory sequential memory for five items. (Recite back the items—ball, shoe, fish, hat, apple—in the order in which they were presented.)
SPEECH	• Produce all consonant sounds appropriate for her hearing age. • Produce /l/ in syllables, but not in words. • Produce /s/ in isolation but omits in blends and in the word final position. • Attempt to sing some simple songs and nursery rhymes.	• Produce /l/ at the word level in all positions (lion, silly, ball). • Produce /s/ in the final position of words (socks, trucks). • Sing with appropriate imitation of the suprasegmental (duration, intensity, and pitch) features.
LANGUAGE	• Answer "what," "where," and "who" questions. • Ask questions when prompted. • Produce the present progressive verb form. • Inconsistently produce plurals and possessives. • Inconsistently use articles in spontaneous conversation.	• Use regular past-tense verbs (walked, dressed, jumped). • Use plurals consistently (socks, cows, houses). • Use articles (a, an, the) and conjunctions (and, or, but) consistently.

	PROGRESS SUMMARY Based on developmental norms, the child is able to:	SHORT-TERM OBJECTIVES To be accomplished in one to four AVT sessions
COGNITION	• Rote count to 20 (skips numbers when continuing beyond). • Identify some letters of the alphabet. Sound-letter association is not yet developed. • Generate an opposite when given a target word.	• Expand counting to 30. • Identify letters and recite the alphabet. • Begin to understand sound-letter association (/s/ is for snake, /p/is for popcorn, etc.). • Understand various age-appropriate concepts (some, a few, except). • Understand the concept of rhyming and generate rhyming words (e.g., bat, hat, mat, cat).
COMMUNICATION	• Take a turn in a conversation, but occasionally requires prompting. • Initiate a verbal interaction with a familiar partner. • Use polite vocabulary such as "please" and "thank-you" in conversation without prompting. • Ask for clarification when prompted.	• Take several turns in a conversation. • Ask for clarification from the person who is talking (e.g., child asks, "Can you say that again please?). • Respond to requests for clarification (e.g., child repeats statement if asked to do so by the adult).

AV PRACTITIONER GOALS

• Guide and coach the parent effectively in language that is easily understood.
• Use acoustic highlighting appropriately.
• Use leaning and waiting more effectively.

PARENT GOALS

• Create opportunities for Emma to engage in conversation during daily routines.
• Improve ability to wait for Emma to initiate and respond.
• Ask Emma, "What did you hear?" rather than automatically repeating.

continues

ACTIVITY #1. INTRODUCTION

- I greet Emma and her mother in the waiting room.
- I inquire if Emma has recently had her hair cut and comment on the doll's house with which she is playing.
- On the way to the therapy room, I talk to her mother about events of the past week and about how Emma is doing in school.
- Emma's mother expresses that she seems happy to go to school each day but is unsure how she is adjusting socially.
- I ask about the possibility of arranging some play dates with her peers.
- When we are seated at the table, I follow up on the objectives from the previous session.
- I also assess Emma's mother's comfort with the suggested carryover activities. Her mother says she attempted some but not all of the activities.
- I then initiate a conversation about the weekend.
- At first, Emma is not forthcoming, but she eventually becomes chatty.
- This session helps evaluate Emma's development toward conversational competence.

LING SIX-SOUND TEST

- I place 10 small plastic cups on the table.
- Emma's mom or I make one of the sounds.
- I incorporate additional sounds such as "f," "t," and "th."
- Upon hearing the sound, Emma repeats it (identifies each sound) and puts a scoop of ice cream (made of colored pompoms) into a cup.
- Prior to giving her each scoop, I ask Emma to guess its color by providing her with an association (e.g., "This scoop is the same color as the snow").

PARENT GUIDANCE

- Begin each day with a quick sound check to ensure that the cochlear implants are functioning properly. Say each of the Six-Sounds at normal conversational volume and expect Emma to repeat them.
- Since she is beginning to learn sound-letter association, try to generate a word beginning with each sound ("sssss" is for summer, "mmmm" is for monkey etc.).
- Visit an ice cream store. Talk about all the flavors.
- Use the word favorite. Emma can survey friends and family members about their favorite flavors.

TRANSITION

- I ask Emma about her favorite ice cream store and tell her that we are going to take a make-believe trip there and prepare some tasty treats.
- I ask Emma if we should ride our bikes or walk there.

ACTIVITY #2. SENSATIONAL SUNDAES

- I tell Emma that we are going to make ice cream sundaes (a new word) and show her a finished product.
- I introduce the materials needed (colored pompoms for the various flavors of ice cream, small brown beads for chocolate sprinkles, brown confetti for nuts, red beads for cherries, and colored bowls).
- I begin by asking Emma to prepare a sundae with three scoops of strawberry ice cream, chocolate sprinkles, and two cherries. I add that I would like my sundae served in the blue bowl.
- We then switch roles for Emma to place her order.
- Emma requires prompting to express herself in complete sentences.
- When talking about her desired toppings, Emma omits /s/. I coach her mother to acoustically highlight /s/ or /z/, and Emma produces the words correctly.
- Her mom and I incorporate such concepts as some, or, a few, and except.

PARENT GUIDANCE AND CARRYOVER

- I ask Emma's mother how we might reinforce the goals of this activity at home. Together we decide on the following:
- Make real ice cream sundaes and talk about toppings. Emma can take orders from other family members and help prepare the treats.
- Emma can order her own meal at restaurants.
- (In these contexts, she will be able to practice important conversational skills such as asking for clarification and responding to requests for clarification.)
- Help Emma develop auditory memory skills in daily routines (setting the table and cleaning up after dinner, folding laundry, making a shopping list).
- Reinforce the concepts some, a few, and except.
- Acoustically highlight /s/ or /z/ in the final position of words in games and books.

TRANSITION

- I ask Emma if she knows any songs about ice cream.
- She immediately responds that she does not.
- I ask her to ask her mother, which she does.
- Her mother is unable to come up with anything.
- I tell them that I know a song and ask if she wants to hear it.

continues

ACTIVITY #3. I LIKE ICE CREAM

- I sing the song "I Like Ice Cream" (Estabrooks & Birkenshaw-Fleming, 2003) while snapping my fingers and clapping my hands alternately.
- Emma and her mother join in.
- Next, we listen to the song on the CD.
- I take out a set of cards depicting a variety of food items and select a card.
- I sing the song again, substituting the item on the card for the word ice cream, and then place it face down on the table.
- Emma and her mother follow my model.
- We continue singing until five items have been presented.
- I ask Emma to recall the items, verifying the responses by revealing the corresponding picture.
- If Emma has difficulty remembering an item, I provide a brief description ("It's a fruit that a monkey likes to eat").
- Emma's mom encourages her to remember the items in the correct order and to sing the song.
- We sing the song several times, and Emma enjoys it.

MUSICAL SUGGESTIONS

- In addition to clapping and snapping fingers to the beat, you can clap or play the rhythm pattern of the words on the drum, tambourine, wood block, or an upended plastic ice cream tub.
- Each person in the session can have a different percussion instrument. One plays the rhythm of measure one, another plays the rhythm of the second measure, the third person plays the rhythm of the third measure, and then all play for the "all day long" measure.
- The lyrics of the song can be changed to discuss things that children don't like: thunder, hail, bullies, liars, turnips.

PARENT GUIDANCE AND CARRYOVER

I provide her mother with the following information about singing.

- Singing helps to improve voice quality and refine the suprasegmentals of speech.
- Songs are useful for the expansion of auditory memory and the development of auditory sequencing. We rely on memory throughout the day, from remembering telephone numbers to recalling directions.
- Memory skills are important for success at school, as children are typically required to store a substantial amount of auditory information prior to performing a task ("Before you turn to page five in your books, make sure that you have handed in your field trip money and you have thrown away all the scraps of paper from the art activity").

- Singing this song helps Emma arrange items into categories. The category food can be subdivided into fruits and vegetables, snack foods, breakfast foods, and so forth.
- Practice categorizing and subcategorizing objects to help increase vocabulary.
- This song can also be sung alphabetically or by phoneme—an excellent way to incorporate speech targets and practice sound-letter association.
- Avoid modeling the correct production while Emma is singing. A better time to model and acoustically highlight the final /s/ or /z/ is when Emma is recalling the items.
- Clapping and/or finger snapping reinforces the beat and rhythm of the song.
- Although this song can be used to introduce new vocabulary, Emma's inability to recall new words may be due to a lack of familiarity with the vocabulary as opposed to a problem remembering the items.

ACTIVITY #4. RULES FOR THE KITCHEN AND BAKING

- I ask Emma how many flavors of ice cream she has tasted.
- I tell her that I have a poem called "Eighteen Flavors" that I would like to read with her.
- "I bet you can't think of eighteen?" I challenge.
- Emma is excited by the competition and thinks of another one.
- We turn to her mother to come up with several more, and I offer some suggestions.

A DECADENT LIGHT

- I conclude the session by reading the poem "Eighteen Flavors" (Silverstein, 1974, p. 116).
- I pause after each line and prompt either Emma or her mother to repeat it.
- We talk about the meaning of new vocabulary words (luscious, scrumptious) and provide synonyms for them.
- We discuss the colors and ingredients of each flavor (mocha contains chocolate, rocky road has marshmallows).

PARENT GUIDANCE AND CARRYOVER

I ask her mother how she thinks she might use the above to follow up at home and together we decide on the following:
- Read this poem over and over to reinforce the new vocabulary.
- Discuss flavors and help Emma recall the ones mentioned in the poem.
- Learn the ice cream rhyme: "I scream, you scream, we all scream for ice cream."
- Talk about synonyms and antonyms for words commonly used.
- Use other written materials of interest to Emma to practice auditory tracking.

continues

	SESSION ANALYSIS
AUDITION	• Identified all sounds of the Six-Sound Test. • Inconsistently identified objects (colors) based on hearing a related description in the open set (difficulty with "same color as snow" and "same color as lettuce"). • Consistently demonstrated auditory memory for four items. • Consistently sequenced four items but exhibited difficulty sequencing five items. • Followed directions containing four to five critical elements.
SPEECH	• Produced /l/ in words when provided with the auditory model, /lllllll/ (lengthening the phoneme and occasionally, the verbal cue, "lift your tongue up"). • Frequently omitted /s/ in the word final position (primarily for production of plurals and possessives). • Demonstrated appropriate pitch and rhythm during singing activities. • Attempted to match suprasegmentals with the adult model.
LANGUAGE	• Produced some irregular past tense verbs (e.g., "went") but required prompting and modeling to generate regular past tense. • Inconsistently produced plurals and possessives in a structured activity. • Required modeling to produce articles and conjunctions both in a structured activity and in conversation.
COGNITION	• Counted to 25 and then began skipping numbers. • Identified letters of the alphabet. • Sound-letter association is emerging but not yet mastered. • Did not understand the concepts "some," "a few," and "except." • Beginning to understand rhyming and was able to generate some rhyming words following a model.
COMMUNICATION	• Took a few turns in conversation following a model. • Required prompting to ask for clarification. • Reluctant to respond to requests for clarification.

CONCLUSION

- Emma's session consisted of targets from which diagnostic predictions can be made for the development of long-term goals.
- The activities were enjoyable and age appropriate.
- The song activity was used to extend auditory memory, evaluate Emma's ability to arrange objects into categories, and further develop the suprasegmental and prosodic features of speech inherent in song.

Reflecting on the practitioner targets:

- Specific parent guidance suggestions were provided online as well as following each activity.
- I encouraged Emma's mother to write down the carryover activities and ideas in her parent book.
- I made sure that her mother was often the primary adult who was involved in each activity.
- I made sure to avoid using too much professional jargon when guiding and coaching and to confirm that her mother understood everything well.
- I pointed out what I was looking for during each activity and when the outcomes happened, I pointed them out at the time, so that Emma's mother was able to understand the objective and outcome of each activity.
- In my use of acoustic highlighting, it was necessary to emphasize the plural morpheme, which Emma frequently omitted.
- I often used leaning and waiting in our conversations when Emma was reluctant to offer a response. These strategies worked well.
- Following my guidance, her mother used the strategy of asking, "What did you hear?" Prior to the session, she reported that Emma has been saying, "huh?" a lot.
- Based on the outcome of using this strategy, it appeared that Emma heard the message but did not comprehend it.
- Emma's mother was frequently the model and offered the desired response when Emma was unable to come up with the correct response independently.
- Following the session, her mother and I discussed the use of all strategies and whether she felt comfortable using them at home.
- I encouraged Emma's mother to provide feedback in the subsequent session.

References

Estabrooks, W., & Birkenshaw-Fleming (Eds.). (2003). *Songs for listening! songs for life!* Washington, DC: Alexander Graham Bell Association for the Deaf and Hard of Hearing.

Silverstein, S. (1974). *Where the sidewalk ends.* New York, NY: Harper Collins.

Session Plan 7: The Five-Year-Old

AV PRACTITIONER: Karen MacIver-Lux, M.A., Aud(C), Reg. CASLPO, LSLS Cert. AVT	

NAME OF CHILD: Michael	**ETIOLOGY:** Unknown

DEGREE and TYPE: Right ear: Severe sensorineural; Left ear: Moderate to severe sensorineural (Diagnosed at 3 months of age); Bilateral Auditory Neuropathy Spectrum Disorder (ANSD) (Diagnosed at 5 years, 5 months of age)

CHRONOLOGICAL AGE (CA): 5 years, 10 months	**HEARING AGE (HA):** 3 months post activation of right CI (5 years, 7 months with bilateral hearing aids)
AUDITORY-VERBAL AGE (AVA): 5 months	**HEARING TECHNOLOGY HISTORY** • Bilateral behind-the-ear hearing aids (4 months of age) • Right cochlear implant activated at 5 years, 7 months

INTERVENTION HISTORY

• First AVT session at a community based early intervention program, at 7 months of age; discharged at 15 months of age due to limited progress and suspected autism.

• Received speech-language therapy for motor speech issues, receptive and expressive language, delay for 4 years.

• Enrolled in AVT program with Karen following diagnosis of ANSD and determination of candidacy for CI in right ear at 5 years, 5 months of age

DEVELOPMENTAL HISTORY

• Born full-term. No complications at birth.

• Received weekly support (academic and language) from a teacher of the deaf.

• Psychological consult/assessment at 4 years of age, to investigate if autism is present. Results were negative, however, some evidence of emotional and sensory regulation dysfunction/challenges.

• Another audiologist seen for second opinion at 5.5 years of age; sedated ABR results—presence of bilateral ANSD; behavioral audiometry—profound hearing loss in right ear and severe hearing loss in the left ear.

• Approved for cochlear implant candidacy and first cochlear implant activated at 5 years, 7 months.

• Referred by CI team for diagnostic AVT to monitor development with CI, and to address delays in audition, speech, language, cognition, and communication.

• Pre-implant expressive vocabulary tests showed age equivalency of 3.8 years, but results of receptive and language tests showed age equivalency of 3.0 years (receptive) and 3.2 years (expressive). Speech intelligibility judged to be poor.

• Genetic testing was negative for familial hearing loss.

	PROGRESS SUMMARY Based on developmental norms, the child is able to:	SHORT-TERM OBJECTIVES To be accomplished in one to four AVT sessions
AUDITION	• Detect all sounds of the Six-Sound Test; identifies /s/ "sh" (/i/ "ee") but misidentifies (/u/ "oo") and "mm" occasionally. • Demonstrate auditory memory for two items and for single-step directions (open the door, wave bye-bye). • Respond consistently to his name in a quiet room. • Maintain auditory attention when engaged in activities that involve multitasking (e.g., listening to directions while drawing a picture). • Follow directions when the key word is in the initial or final position of phrases.	• Identify all sounds of the Ling's Six-Sound Test • Demonstrate auditory memory for three items, to follow single directions containing two to four critical elements, and follow two-step directions. • Respond to his name when called from a different room. • Identify any "alerting" sounds such as the oven timer. • Respond consistently to his name when called from a distance (e.g., from another room). • Demonstrate comprehension of directions or questions when the key word is in the medial position of phrases. • Demonstrate ability to perform auditory close tasks (in final position of phrases)
SPEECH	• Imitate suprasegmental features (intensity, duration, and pitch). • Produce some vowel sounds (/ah/, /oo/) in CVC words, and some early developing consonant sounds (/ah/, /oo/ /b/, /m/, /n/, /d/, /p/, /k/) in initial position of words consistently and final position of words inconsistently. • Produce approximations of known words and phrases.	• Imitate inflectional speech patterns with yes/no questions, consistently. • Produce (/m/, /d/, /b/, /p/, /h/, /t/, "sh," /k/, and /g/) in initial, medial, and final positions of words (e.g., mommy, cookie, baking, sheet, etc.), consistently, and in medial position of words inconsistently. Produce clearer approximations of words and phrases.
LANGUAGE	• Understand early forms of negation but does not use them consistently • Use three to four word utterances from time to time, but prefers to use one to two words. • Recognize and use names of family members, familiar people, and commonly used items such as utensils. • Refer to self by name	• Use "not" appropriately (e.g., I'm not, It's not) • Expand length of utterances to four to five words • Look at or get objects appliances and baking items when named (e.g., refrigerator, baking sheet, cookie dough, spoon). • Demonstrate use of pronouns "I" and "you" and understanding of "me" when others make request.

continues

	PROGRESS SUMMARY Based on developmental norms, the child is able to:	SHORT-TERM OBJECTIVES To be accomplished in one to four AVT sessions
LANGUAGE *continued*	• Demonstrate understanding of Wh- questions such as "What __?" and "Where __?" • Use many early verbs such as "go" "run" "walk" "drink" "eat" and some adjectives (big, small) and adverbs (quickly, slowly).	• Answer "Where __?" questions using prepositions or positional phrases. • Answer Why questions (e.g., Why does the mouse need a glass of milk?). • Expand receptive and expressive vocabulary to include more verbs (e.g., roll, pat, squeeze), adjectives (cool, hot) and adverbs (softly, carefully).
COGNITION	• Identify letters by sound (sound-letter identification). Identifies letters in some words (spoken and print). Identifies sight words (print) upon request. • Understand some opposites (e.g., big/small, long/short, on/off). • Counts to 100.	• Demonstrate understanding of descriptive/size (e.g., tiny/hug, short/tall, etc.). • Identify words that begin with letters ("s" for Start, "t" for Time) such as those on the oven. • Demonstrate ability to identify first/number one, second/number two, etc. • Sequence and plan out steps for baking activity and list the items needed for the activity.
COMMUNICATION	• Demonstrate age-appropriate eye contact and attention span. • Initiate some conversations, but loses ability to continue taking turns. • Demonstrate some greetings by saying "Hi" and introduces himself by saying "I Michael!" • Argue or plead and often uses "I be good!" or "I behave!" • Sing when encouraged	• Complete several turns in conversations. • Request repetitions to repair communication breakdowns. • Use word approximations to request, initiate pretend play, comment or tell information, acknowledge or respond.

AV PRACTITIONER GOALS

• Speak at regular volume.
• Demonstrate an activity no more than three times, and then pass activity over to the parent.
• Ask the child, "What did you hear?" instead of repeating.
• Ask Mom what she would do next, based on the short-term objectives.
• Have Mom start an activity, and guide from the side for the duration of it.

PARENT GOALS

- Use two-step directions.
- Expand vocabulary by using synonyms.
- Pause/wait after presenting information to allow time for processing and to respond.

ACTIVITY #1. GREETING

- The session begins when the doorbell rings at my house, (where the therapy sessions are usually conducted). I walk to the door and ask, "Who is it?" and wait.
- Michael knocks on the door again.
- I sing, "Who is it?"
- Michael shouts, "Michael!"
- I open the door and it appears that Michael is alone.
- Michael giggles and says, "Mommy not here!"
- I reply, "No? Where is Mommy?"
- Michael put his finger to his lips.
- I look expectantly at him, lean forward and wait.
- "Shh. Mommy hide outside!" he says.
- I laugh quietly and whisper, "Okay, I'll be quiet. Is Mommy in the car?"
- Michael looks at the car, nods his head, and points to the car. Michael says, "Mommy in car!"
- I reply, "Oh there she is!" I give Mom a signal to take her time. "I wonder what's taking Mommy so long. She's so slow! We should tell her to hurry!" I say. Michael shouts, "Mommy, hurry! Come!"
- I crouch down and pretend to whisper in his right ear but use my voice, "We're going to bake some cookies!"
- Michael looked at me and says, "Huh?"
- I wait for two three seconds and then say, "We need to bake cookies."
- Michael says, "Cookie(s)?"
- "Yeah, we're gonna bake some cookies today! Tell Mommy to hurry!"
- Michael runs to his Mom and says, "Mommy come! Cookie(s)!"
- Mom laughs and says, "Cookie(s)? What's this about cookies?"
- Michael says, "Karen ha(ve) cookies! Michael eat cookie(s)!" (Mom knew that the personal pronoun "I" is a short-term goal, and she has been working on it. It appeared, however, that Michael was falling into the habit of referring to himself by his name.)
- She waits, and furrows her eyebrows, shakes her head and says, "I want to eat cookies. I will eat them all!"
- Michael smiles and shout, "No, I eat cookie(s). I eat cookie(s)!"

continues

ACTIVITY #1. GREETING *continued*

- I hold my thumbs up, to signal to Mom that it was a great strategy to use. The three of us walk to the door arguing about who is going to eat all of the cookies, using the personal pronouns, "I" and "You" and negative form of "not" and the phrase "eat all of the cookies."

- Mom and I take turns arguing and acoustically highlighting target words, "You are not going to eat all of the cookies. I will eat all of the cookies!"

- Michael replies, "No, I eat all of the cookies!"

- (Mom says that she's been working on "You" and "I" for a week but it seems that while Michael uses it after models, he still uses "Michael" often.)

- I explain that this may take some time, and that we will use it for the next three weeks. I explained that if he doesn't learn to use "I" or "You" spontaneously, we will return to it later. I ask her how things are going at home as Michael takes his shoes off and dances toward the stairs leading to the basement where the therapy room is located.

- Mom reports that Michael's teachers are thrilled with the positive changes in Michael's behavior, and that they think Michael's speech is becoming easier to understand. Mom also reports that Michael is now saying "Mommy" perfectly, and asks if I notice. I reply that I do. (Previously, he called his Mom "Bobby.")

- "I'm so happy he can say Mommy with the cochlear implant! I love it!" Mom adds.

- We see Michael go down the stairs to the basement, and before Mom could call him for his attention, I said, "Let him go, I want to see if I can get his attention when he's in the therapy room which is pretty far away."

- Mom nods and we wait until Michael disappears into the therapy room. I nod my head and upon seeing this, Mom calls, "Michael!" and waits. After five seconds of waiting, she calls again. Michael comes out of the room and stands at the bottom of the stairs.

- "Michael, we need to go to the kitchen. We got cookies to bake!" We wait for Michael to request repetition, as this was another short-term objective. Michael looks at me. I look at Mom and say, "Pardon? What did you say?" and I lean in to listen.

- Mom says "We need to go to the kitchen. We got cookies to bake."

- "Oh! The kitchen. That's right. We're not going downstairs." I reply.

- Michael calls impatiently, "Come! Come down!"

- Mom says, "Nope. The kitchen is where we need to go. Come up Buddy, we're going to the kitchen!" and we wait.

- Michael hesitantly begins coming up the stairs. Mom smiles, and nods. "Yeah, we're going to bake cookies in the kitchen. Not the play room."

- As we walk into the kitchen, Mom and I agree that kitchen and other rooms of the house would be good vocabulary for Michael to learn.

PARENT GUIDANCE

- Make the most of any opportunity to call for Michael's attention at (a) extended distances and (b) when he's in another room. Make sure that when you call him, there's a reason otherwise he will learn to ignore you.

- Ensure that the kitchen (or room) is acoustically friendly by ensuring that there is little reverberation (carpets and area rugs), and that the radios/stereos and appliances in the kitchen are off. Michael is in the early stages of listening, and any noise or reverberation will make it difficult for him to hear and process auditory information. He is learning to listen in noise already in his kindergarten classroom.

- Use of hearing aid for the first several months of cochlear implant use is discouraged so that his progress with the cochlear implant can be monitored. It's best to eliminate any chance of "amplified distortion" from the ANSD and hearing aid of non-implanted ear interfering with the clearer signal that the CI provides. We can slowly introduce the hearing aid to see if he can adjust to processing speech with two different types of speech signals in the next month.

- Talk about the different rooms of the house and what they are used for.

ACTIVITY #2. REVIEW THE SESSION PLAN, SHORT-TERM OBJECTIVES & STRATEGIES

- Michael waits patiently as Mom sits down at the kitchen table and retrieves her parent book so she can write down the short-term objectives and the strategies we plan to use.

- I get down to Michael's level and look at him as if I were talking to him and not his mother. I say, "Michael, to help you use 'I' instead of 'Michael,' Mom and I will use self statements to model 'I.' We will do this because you usually copy what we say."

- I provide guidance to mom "through Michael" because I wanted him to feel included in the discussion of strategies that we are going to be using. This also helps him to maintain focus and attention.

- I use auditory closure with numbers to pair them with words such as "first," "second," "third," and "last." For example, "The first strategy is number one on the list. Mom and I are going to talk about what we do before we do it!

- The second strategy, is number ___" and I wait for his response.

- He doesn't respond, so I look over at Mom and she says, "two."

- Michael catches on to the pattern and says "three" for the third strategy.

- I use acoustic highlighting strategies to help Michael improve his speech production during numbers such as producing the "w" and "n" in one, "oo" as in two, "ee" as in three, etc.

- Mom writes these down as we go through the list of strategies.

- When we get to fifth strategy, Mom takes over and describes another strategy. After number six, we finish, and prepare for the next part of the session. This was done quickly so that we can move on with the session.

continues

PARENT GUIDANCE

- Record Michael's progress in listening and comprehension with his cochlear implant.
- Record sounds and words that he can say correctly
- Take a language sample at home once a day this week. Write down what he actually says, not what you think he is saying. Take note of missing words or missing grammatical markers. You could mark those with a "red pencil" in the actual text. Use acoustic highlighting to encourage the use of the correct model.
- If Michael doesn't understand respond correctly to a model it with his older brother, Dad or an adult.
- Expand on first, second, and third by creating a page in the Experience Book to review what happened in today's session.

ACTIVITY #3. RULES FOR THE KITCHEN AND BAKING

- Michael and I approach the island of the kitchen and I tell him that I have a footstool.
- He looks at Mom.
- Mom looks at me and replies, "You have a footstool? How cool!"
- Michael looks at me and says, "Cool!"
- I look at Mom and she says, "Where is the footstool?"
- I look back at Michael and he says, "Where?"
- I tell Michael it's behind the island, and we make our way there so that he finds it. He gleefully climbs it and is delighted to see that he is almost as tall as me.
- We practice going "up" and "down" the stool, and seeing how Mom and I become "tall" or "short."
- After this, I tell Michael that there are rules for the kitchen and baking cookies. (This gives us the opportunity to discuss the importance of rules of the kitchen.)
- "First, (number one) we need clean hands to bake cookies."
- Mom says, "Why?"
- "Because baking with dirty hands might make us sick."
- "What do we do to get our hands clean?"
- "We wash our hands with soap and water."
- "Second, (number two). No eating the cookie dough!"
- "Why?"
- "Because we won't have any cookies to eat."
- "What do we do with the cookie dough?"
- "Put on a cookie sheet."
- Mom takes over. Third, (number three) only Karen opens the oven.
- "Why?"
- "Because it's hot!"
- "Next, (number four) use a spatula to pick up cookies, not your hands."
- Why? (And so on.)

- I explain the rules of the session or an activity before it starts. This helps Michael to: (a) know what's expected of him, (b) manage his emotions and prepare mentally if a rule is "challenging" to follow, (c) initiate any negotiation to request any change to the rules or come to a compromise, and (d) remain safe in an environment that could potentially be unsafe Follow Michael's lead, but be sure to take advantage of any new opportunity to target the short-term objectives.
- Identify potential problems (e.g., safety hazards, etc.) and talk about possible solutions helps to promote theory of mind development.

ACTIVITY #4. BAKER'S LING RAP

- To check that Michael is identifying all the sounds of the speech spectrum, I incorporate my version of Ling's Six-Sound Test by doing the "Baker Ling's Rap." I already know he can detect the sounds, because Mom reported she did a listening check that morning.
- I put on my baker's hat, apron and use the spatula as my microphone. I close my eyes, dance like a rapper saying, "Ah, ah, ahh! Don't touch, it's hot!"
- Michael laughs as Mom dances and sings, "Ah, ah, ahh!"
- I dance around the island in the kitchen and continue with "Ooo, it's hot!"
- Mom follows saying "Ooo!" Michael follows mom and says, "Oo" and laughs.
- I continue with "Cookies bake and say, sssss!"
- By this time, Michael and his mom follow me around the kitchen as if we're doing a Congo dance.
- Mom repeats the sounds, and Michael follows her model.
- Michael reaches for my spatula to have a turn and says, "Michael's turn!"
- I look at Mom and she says, "My turn!" which Michael repeats.
- I give him the spatula Michael says the sounds and dances.
- He struggles to match the timing patterns but Mom and I allow him time to listen, process and self-correct his movements and approximations. He identifies and produces the Ling Six-Sounds accurately.
- I explain to Mom that incorporating movement and singing into the Ling Six Sound Test helps me to determine which sounds of the speech spectrum Michael has access to in the kitchen (where it's harder to hear because of the reverberations caused by the high ceilings and tile floor) while he is "multi-tasking" (dancing and concentrating on imitating body movements). Movement helps Michael get the sensory input to engage fully in the activity that requires him to focus, pay attention, and self-regulate.
- I explain to Mom that when children are encouraged to listen, dance and sing at the same time, it provides the brain with opportunities to process, sequence and execute information sent from several areas of the brain to the muscles of various parts of the body. In other words, listening, singing, and dancing together will Michael to strengthen and develop auditory processing skills that contribute to good listening behaviors, particularly in school. Michael learns by using all of his senses.

continues

PARENT GUIDANCE

- When children have ANSD, we need to ensure that they can not only detect the sounds of the speech spectrum consistently, but can identify them and match various patterens, rates, voicing aspects of speech. In cases of ANSD, audibility does not always mean intelligibility.
- Continue to do the Ling Six-Sound Test daily, and make sure there are plenty of opportunities for Michael to demonstrate what he understands through listening alone.
- Consider involving Michael in music and movement activities (movement and music play a key role in the development of effective auditory processing skills).

ACTIVITY #5. FINDING THE INGREDIENTS FOR BAKING

- I ask Michael, to tell Mom to close her eyes.
- Michael says, "Close your eye!" and Mom closes both eyes. (She understands that plural /s/ is not a an objective that we are concerned about at this time.
- I tell Michael the items we need for baking, before we locate them.
- I say, "We need cookie dough, and the cookie dough is in the fridge" and then we walk to the fridge.
- Before I open the fridge door I say, "We're going to take a "quick peek" at the cookie dough. Just a quick peek!"
- Michael provides a good approximation of "quick peek!"
- I quickly open the door and point out the cookie dough and then close the door. "What did you see?" I ask.
- Michael says, "Cookie dough!"
- Then, I say, "We need a baking sheet. The baking sheet is in the cupboard beside the fridge" and then we walk to the cupboard and take a "quick peek" at the baking sheet and so on.
- After we take a "quick peek" at all the items for baking, I tell Michael that he can ask his mom to open her eyes.
- Michael says, "Huh?" I wait and lean and then say, "What did you hear?"
- Michael says, "Open" and points to the fridge.
- "Yes, open. But don't open the fridge. Tell Mommy to open her eyes."
- Michael then asks his mom to open her eyes.
- I guide Mom to talk through what one needs to bake cookies and ask where they are so she can retrieve them.
- Mom says, "First, we need the cookie dough. I wonder where the cookie dough is?"
- Michael runs to the fridge and opens it to reveal the cookie dough.
- I model, "Here it is!" and Michael repeats an approximation of "Here it is!"
- Mom takes the bowl of cookie dough out and places it on the countertop.

- Mom says, "Awesome! Now, I think we need the baking sheet!" and Michael runs to retrieve the baking sheet and he says, "Here it is!"
- Because we know that Michael is familiar with the word "spoon," I guide Mom to ask where the spoon is with the word in the middle of the question.
- I help her by whispering, "And the spoons, where are they?"
- After Mom repeats the question, Michael hesitates. I guide Mom to wait.
- "Spoon?" Michael asks?
- Mom excitedly says, "Yeah! Where are the spoons?" and Michael runs to the drawer where the spoons are.
- I suggest to mom that she go over to the oven and ask Michael push the buttons to turn the oven on.
- He knows his numbers in print, and so Mom tells Michael to push the numbers 3, 7 and 5."
- Michael pushes three and five.
- We reset the oven and remind Michael that it's 3, 7, 5 and we put emphasis on the number 7.
- Michael pushes three, seven, and five.
- I explain to Mom that this is a way to extend and check auditory memory; which for single items or numbers is three-item memory.
- Mom asks Michael to point to a word that begins with the letter B.
- Michael finds the word, "Bake."
- She tells him to push the "Bake" button.
- Michael does it easily.
- I say, "He follows single step directions with familiar vocabulary really well. What do you think we can do next to raise the bar?" Mom replies, "Maybe I can ask him to push the bake button and then push the start button."
- I nod and say, "That's a great idea."

PARENT GUIDANCE

- Start any activity/daily routine with directions that are familiar and can be followed easily. It creates a foundation for success.
- Ensure that you pick your "language correction/modeling" battles wisely. We need to be highly responsive to Michael's communication attempts, even when they are not grammatically correct.
- Choose to provide models or corrections that are hearing age and stage appropriate.
- Keep your language short enough to be easily understood, but just long enough to "raise the bar" in stimulating listening and language development.
- Use new phrases (e.g., take a quick peek) often.
- If a word is familiar within a simple direction, raise the bar for listening, by putting the key word in the middle of the sentence.
- If Michael has difficulty with three-item memory, then go back to two-item memory but make the phrase longer or say it at a faster rate.

continues

ACTIVITY #6. BAKING COOKIES

- I explain to Mom that in order to help Michael maximize his newly acquired listening potential, we need to talk about objects before we show them, or talk about what we are going to do before we do it.
- I demonstrate by saying, "I'm going to take a spoon, and scoop up some cookie dough" and then I scoop up the cookie dough with the spoon.
- I explain that if a goal is to assess what he can comprehend, then it's best to first use language that incorporates a lot of what he knows. It gives him a successful start. Then add language that he doesn't know. This helps him learn new words and grammatical structures.
- I demonstrate this by saying, "Michael, can you get the spoon?" and then I wait.
- This is easy and he passes me the spoon quickly.
- Mom nods and says, "That was easy for him. So great, Buddy! You're listening!"
- A few seconds later, I ask, "Can you pass me the spoon?"
- Michael grabs the spoon and uses it to scoop out dough himself.
- I say, "Hey!" and look at Mom, "Can you pass me a spoon?"
- Mom nods and gives me her spoon.
- I scoop out some cookie dough, put it on the baking sheet, and then put the spoon down.
- Mom then says, "Buddy, can you pass me the spoon?"
- Michael picks up the spoon and passes it to Mom.
- Mom tries this a few times again with other items.
- Then I suggest that we use new verbs to expand his vocabulary so we roll, pat, squeeze and cut the cookie dough.
- Then we add other elements to the directions, by asking Michael to make a big cookie and a small cookie and add synonyms such as "huge" and "tiny."
- By this time, Mom is confidently adding new words and directions.
- I write the directions and new words in the parent book because Mom is busy providing Michael good language while they cover the sheet with cookie dough.
- Once we are done with putting the cookie dough on to the cookie sheet, I say, "Ugh, my hands are dirty. I don't like it."
- Mom says, "Me neither! I hate it when my hands are dirty."
- We both look at Michael and he repeats, "Hand dirty! Don't like it!"
- I then sigh and look at my hands and remained quiet.
- Michael looked at his mother and back at me. After five seconds, I say, "Ugh! What a mess! What am I gonna do?"
- Mom says, "You can wipe your hands with a paper towel. Do you have a paper towel?"
- I reply, "Yeah I do. Where did I put it?" and I look around for it.
- Michael points to the paper towel by the kitchen sink.

- "Ah, yes, there it is!" I exclaim, and I pull a sheet of paper towel and wipe my hands.
- "Look!" I say, "My hands are still dirty!"
- Michael says, "Wash hand. Water and soap."
- Mom says, "That's a great idea Michael!"
- Michael reaches up to turn the faucet on and says, "Michael wash hand!"
- I playfully bump into Michael and say, "I want to wash my hands!"
- Mom playfully bumps into me and says, "No, I want to wash my hands first."
- I lightly bump into her again and say, "No, I want to wash my hands first."
- Michael bumps into me and says, "No, I want to wash my hands!"
- We laugh and let Michael be the first to wash his hands.
- Once our hands are dried, I say, "Okay, I'm going to open the oven door and put the cookies in."
- Michael says, "I want open oven!"
- Mom smiles and says, "Michael, remember the rules? Karen opens the oven door. Not you."
- Michael pleads, "No, I want open oven. I be careful. I be good boy."
- I reply, "I know you will be very careful, and yes, you're doing so well, but I must open the oven. It's dangerous and very ____" and I pause. Michael looks forlorn and says, "Hot."
- I continue, "I don't want you to burn yourself. If you burn yourself, you'll have an ____" and I pause.
- Michael says, "owie."
- Mom continues, "Yeah, and when we call the police, the ambulance will have to take us to the ____" and pauses.
- "Michael says, "hospital."
- Mom says, "And when we get to the hospital, we see the ____" and Michael says, "Doctor."
- I say, "I don't want to go to the hospital."
- Mom says, "I don't want to go to the hospital either. What about you, Michael?"
- Michael says, "No. I don't want hospital."
- I take the baking sheet, put it in the oven, and close the oven door.
- Michael quickly arrives at my side and says, "I want push button."
- I smile and look back at Mom and I see her pumping her fists.
- We share a quick and non-verbal celebratory moment because Michael is spontaneously using "I" instead of his name.
- (It's important for the therapist to acknowledge success and share it with the parents as this promotes and nurtures the partnership.)
- "Okay" I say, "You need to find a word that begins with the letter 'T' and then push 1 and 2."
- Michael looks and finds the button that says, "Time" and pushes it, and then he pushes, 1, and hesitates.
- "Two?" he asks.

continues

Session Plan 7: The Five-Year-Old *continued*

ACTIVITY #6. BAKING COOKIES *continued*

- "Yes!"
- And after you push 2 you need to push a button that starts with the letter 'S.'"
- Michael pushes 2 and then the Start button.
- Mom is elated and says, "Great job Michael! I gotta do this more at home. I had no idea he would be so great in the kitchen. He loves this!"

PARENT GUIDANCE

- Talk about everything you and Michael are going to do before and/or during what you do or see. Narrate life!
- Once Michael understands a phrase, then say it another way. Do the same with known words; use synonyms! Play the name game where you name as many different words that mean the same thing (e.g., cat, kitty, kitten, feline, etc.).
- Use auditory closure to monitor comprehension of language, and to help Michael develop auditory processing skills that will help him to listen to and understand speech that is hard to hear (e.g., degraded speech, accents, noisy environments, etc.).
- When necessary, acoustically highlight key or new words (I want to bake cookies) to enhance comprehension and help him to pay attention to the word so that it's easier to hear, learn and say.
- Use playful sabotage or arguing.

ACTIVITY #7. MILK AND COOKIES

- While the cookies are baking, we sit at the table to read the book "When You Give A Mouse A Cookie."
- Mom reviews her parent book to quickly consult the list of today's short-term objectives. She knows that it's important to ensure that short-term objectives are not abandoned or forgotten, and she also knows that they can be incorporated into any activity.
- Mom sees that answering "Why?" questions and having conversations that consist of several turns remain on the list.
- She also reads that we need to be mindful about facilitating theory of mind (ToM) development.
- She admits she's not sure if she remembers what it means to have a conversation consisting of several turns.
- I thank her for letting me know this so that I know what to focus on.
- I remind her, that I am the one that needs to explain things in a way that is easy to understand, and that I am still working on improving this skill.
- Mom shakes her head and smiles and says, "You're fine!"

- I smile and reply, "Uh huh. I know, but you can't leave here not knowing what to do and what we are trying to help Michael accomplish, right?" Mom laughs and says, "I think I have a pretty good idea after today's session, but you're still going to tell me about the conversational turn right?"
- I reply, "I'll do you one better, by demonstrating what I mean. So let's get started."
- I ask Mom to begin reading the book.
- She reads, "If you give a mouse a cookie, he's going to ask for a glass of milk" and waits upon seeing my hand signal.
- I tap my chin and Michael looks at me.
- I look at Mom and say, "Why does the mouse want a glass of milk?"
- Mom says, "Maybe because he's thirsty."
- "Oh, right!" I reply, "But I don't like milk. I like apple juice."
- And I look expectantly at Michael. Michael says, "I like chocolate milk."
- I say, "You do? Me too! I love chocolate milk."
- Mom says, "Lilli loves chocolate milk too. It's her favorite drink."
- I say, "Really? I love chocolate milk. But apple juice is my favorite drink."
- There are a few seconds of silence. Michael says, "Nicholas like chocolate milk."
- I nod at mom and whisper, "This is the conversational turn I was talking about and hoping for. So, when I start a conversation, that's initiating a conversation. When you respond, you're taking a turn. Then I respond to keep the conversation going. Books are not just for reading. They are conversational starters."
- Mom nods and says, "Okay, got it! Makes sense. It's just amazing to see that he can express himself and have a conversation. Finally, after so many years of very little."
- I reply, "I can imagine and I'm happy to see this as well. He is picking up so quickly and I'm so glad that Michael can benefit from this cochlear implant." Mom continues the book until the timer indicates the cookies are done baking.

PARENT GUIDANCE

- Try to read as many books as you can. Reading aloud stimulates many areas of the auditory and language centers of the brain, and promotes success at school and beyond. Reading aloud will grow Michael's emerging literacy skills.
- Initiate conversations from books, events, photo albums and family videos. Lean in, listen, wait, and look expectantly at Michael for his input.
- Create an Experience book to document what happened in the session and share with the extended family members.
- Make your own book. "If You Give Daddy a Cookie!" Talk about what will happen if Daddy eats a cookie. Will he want a glass of milk too? Would he want to cut his hair? Would he make a mess? Create and share!

continues

PARENT GUIDANCE DURING MILK AND COOKIES

As Michael enjoys his cookies and milk, Mom and I review our notes. We review what was accomplished as the session unfolded, and the short-term objectives that we targeted. We spend 2 minutes jointly evaluating Michael's functioning in audition, speech, language, cognition and communication. We also review the strategies that were used to help Michael learn and generalize the short-term objectives. At the end of the session Mom had written the following in her parent book:

1. talk about what you're going to do, and then do it
2. use language in synchrony with actions to facilitate language learning
3. use opposites to expand knowledge and use of vocabulary and concepts
4. use body language or posture that facilitates listening (leaning in to hear, pointing to ear) and talking
5. pause or wait after talking to allow Michael time to respond. Use the 5-second rule!
6. talk before giving a visual or tactical cue and then saying the message again (Listen First and Last)
7. give a maximum of three opportunities to respond, then model the expected response with another adult (if the situation permits) (three strikes and I'm out!)
8. use sabotage to get Michael to use spoken language to solve problems
9. use self-statements to model use of the target/correct language
10. sing out phrases to make target language structures easier for Michael to hear, remember and use
11. use each other (adults) to model the expected listening behaviors, responses and/or target language
12. use strategies such as elongating, putting stress on key words to make them more acoustically salient (acoustic highlighting)

- Then, we talk about ideas of how we can reinforce the short-term objectives using the strategies learned during the family's daily routines.
- Mom replies right away by saying, "This guy is helping me to cook and bake from now on! I'm not a fan of baking, but seeing how much he enjoyed this, and how much he learned today was so motivating! I just have to do more baking from now on!"
- We discuss the importance of finding things to do that they BOTH enjoy, such as crafting or making experience books, decorating seasonal items like Easter Eggs or playing games the family likes to do together.
- Mom closes the session by saying, "I bet I can get Michael's Dad to get him involved in washing the cars. That will be so fun to watch!" Michael pipes up and says, "Yay! I want help Daddy wash cars!"

PARENT GUIDANCE

- Continue to take notes at home and record your observations about Michael's auditory functioning and development in listening and spoken language. (These are helpful to the CI team in validating the programming of the cochlear implant.)
- Share objectives, goals and progress with family members and professionals involved in Michael's development.
- Observe Michael when he plays with his brother and sister. Does he share? Does he request a turn with a toy? Does he use his language to solve problems as they occur? Does he listen and comprehend the spoken language as provided by his brother and sister? Does he play with them, or beside them with little interaction?
- Having fun during purposeful play or activities that involve cooperative play or work is the best way to learn to listen and talk.
- Put meaning to all parts of speech (nouns, verbs, adjectives, prepositions, and interjections), and repeat these in various contexts.
- Occasionally, depending on the context, use soft speech or whisper a simple and well-known message to help Michael to hear and comprehend all intensity levels of speech, especially soft speech.
- Read recipe books or instructional manuals written for children. Building toy models from printed instructions would be beneficial for Michael's spoken language and literacy development.

SESSION ANALYSIS
The child demonstrated the following:

AUDITION

- Demonstrates identification of sounds of the Six-Sound Test accurately
- Turned to name when called from a distance of 12–18 feet, when he was in the therapy room in the basement and adults upstairs.
- Followed single-step directions with 100% consistency when vocabulary/language was familiar (e.g., Put it in the garbage, push the button, etc.).
- Followed two-step directions with 80% accuracy with familiar vocabulary/language (e.g., Cut the cookie and then give Mommy the knife).
- Demonstrates auditory memory for three items 50% of the presentations (e.g., remembered T, 1, 2).
- Demonstrates auditory memory to follow single or two-step directions containing two to four critical items. (Give *me* the *big* cookie and *Karen* the *small* cookie, etc.)
- Detected the timer when the cookies were finished, without any assistance from the adults.

continues

	SESSION ANALYSIS The child demonstrated the following:
SPEECH	• Imitated inflectional speech patterns with yes/no questions. • Used word approximations: highly motivating words and commonly heard (stereotypic) phrases. • Matched, intensity and pitch (suprasegemental) aspects of speech, but had difficulty with rate and/pattern. • Produced (/m/, /d/, /b/, /p/, /h/, /t/, "sh," /k/, and /g/) in initial, medial and final positions of words (e.g., mommy, cookie, baking, sheet, etc.).
LANGUAGE	• Responded appropriately to negation (no, stop, don't touch) by stopping the activity. • Said "not" in context; for example, when protesting or disagreeing (e.g., It's not a __, I'm not). • Looked at or got objects and appliances found in a kitchen, and baking items when named (e.g. refrigerator, baking sheet, cookie dough, spoon). • Followed simple to two-step directions within familiar contexts ("Put it down" "Push the button, etc.) (see Audition). • Demonstrates understanding and use of expressive use of new vocabulary that included (e.g., cookie dough/batter, spatula, etc.), and verbs (e.g., roll, pat, squeeze). • Used personal pronoun "I" when making requests or self-statements instead of referring to himself by his name towards end of session. • Expanded length of utterances to four to five words (e.g., "No, I want open oven."). • Answered Why questions (e.g., Why does the mouse need a cookie? "Because mouse hungry." • Used the phrase "eat all of the cookies" after several models.
COGNITION	• Used descriptive/size adjectives (e.g., tiny/hug, short/tall, etc.). • Identified words that begin with letters ("s" for Start, "t" for Time) such as those on the oven. • Identified ordinals such as first/number one, second/number two, third/number three. • Sequenced and planned out steps for baking activity and the items that we need to accomplish the activity with adult assistance.
COMMUNICATION	• Took three turns in playful verbal exchanges. • Initiated and took turns in conversations. • Greeted appropriately at the door; answer "Who's there?" by saying his name. • Requested repetitions to repair communication breakdowns due to mishearing by saying "Pardon?" • Used word approximations to request, initiate pretend play, comment, or tell information, acknowledge or respond.

CONCLUSION

- Michael's mom was able to see how short-term objectives could be targeted during an activity that commonly takes place in the home. She was able to see that when Michael is engaged in activities that happen in real-life, he paid attention for longer periods of time. The rules and boundaries, along with the extrinsic and intrinsic rewards embedded in the baking activity, were strong motivators that helped Michael to self-regulate and learn.

  I worked hard at encouraging Mom to take over activities once she had seen me demonstrate once or twice. I also met my objective of letting Mom initiate an activity and coaching her from the side. This was a new experience for me that resulted in positive outcomes for Mom, Michael, and me.

Reference

Numeroff, L. J., & Bond, F. (1985). *If you give a mouse a cookie.* New York, NY: Harper Collins.

Session Plan 8: The Six-Year-Old

<table>
<tr>
<td colspan="2">AV PRACTITIONER
Kelley as reported by Pamela Steacie, Dip. Ed., M.Sc., LSLS Cert. AVT</td>
</tr>
<tr>
<td>NAME OF CHILD
Tanya</td>
<td>ETIOLOGY
Unknown</td>
</tr>
<tr>
<td colspan="2">DEGREE & TYPE OF HEARING LOSS
Bilateral severe to profound sensorineural</td>
</tr>
<tr>
<td>CHRONOLOGICAL AGE (CA)
6 years, 2 months</td>
<td>HEARING AGE (HA)
4 years, 7 months</td>
</tr>
<tr>
<td>AUDITORY-VERBAL AGE (AVA)
4 years, 7 months</td>
<td>HEARING TECHNOLOGY HISTORY
<ul>
<li>Fitted with hearing aids at 18 months old, just 3 weeks after her moderately-severe to severe, sensorineural hearing loss was initially diagnosed.</li>
<li>At 25 months her hearing had decreased to severe to profound levels and her parents decided to proceed with cochlear implantation.</li>
<li>Right side, Nucleus 5 cochlear implant was activated, at 32 months.</li>
<li>Left side, Nucleus 5 device was activated at 43 months.</li>
</ul>
</td>
</tr>
</table>

INTERVENTION HISTORY

- At this centre, audiology, auditory-verbal therapy and ENT services are all provided in one department thereby ensuring seamless service.
- The same day that Tanya's hearing loss was identified, she was seen by one of the ENT physicians. The hearing loss was diagnosed as a permanent, sensory/neural loss and an order for blood tests was made to investigate genetic causes.
- One of the audiologists took earmold impressions.
- The family was introduced to an Auditory-Verbal practitioner to describe the therapy services. (Because Tanya's family is from Quebec, they didn't qualify for or follow the Infant Hearing Program of Ontario protocol.)
- Tanya's audiologist and AV practitioner fit her hearing aids together.
- During subsequent AV therapy sessions, hearing threshold checks and immittance testing were always booked as back-to-back appointments.
- It was possible to manage Tanya's frequent middle ear infections effectively as ENT physicians work closely with the AV practitioners. Tanya, as a hearing aid user, was seen the same day as her AV therapy session whenever middle ear issues made that necessary.
- When Tanya's hearing thresholds worsened, her family was introduced to the cochlear implant audiologists and cochlear implant surgeon. The entire team (hearing aid audiologist, cochlear implant audiologist, AV practitioner, CI team leader, and CDA) discussed Tanya's case history.
- After it was determined that Tanya was a CI candidate, her name went on the surgery list and her CI audiologist and Kelley counselled and prepared the family and Tanya for the surgery and activation.
- Despite her age Tanya and her parents have been permitted to attend weekly AVT sessions during her single kindergarten year, as her school board in another region, provides very limited services and no direct therapy of any kind for children with hearing loss. AVT services will be discontinued upon her entry to grade 1.

DEVELOPMENTAL HISTORY

- Born at term.
- Unremarkable pregnancy and delivery.
- No family history of hearing loss.
- Parents self-referred to because of concerns that Tanya was not talking.
- Today, Tanya is independent, tempestuous, strong-willed, persistent, and creative.
- Receptive language and vocabulary within the average range.
- Expressive language and vocabulary is delayed.
- Tanya is very self-conscious and can act out when she knows a task is challenging.

continues

	PROGRESS SUMMARY Based on developmental norms, the child is able to:	SHORT-TERM OBJECTIVES To be accomplished in one to four AVT sessions
AUDITION	• Identify all Ling sounds ("m," "ah," "oo," "ee," "sh," and "s") "ba," whispered "p," "t," and "k," and "f," at a distance of 6 feet in quiet. • Recall four facts from a short, open-set story. • Recall four unrelated words. • Recall four critical elements in a sentence. • Discriminate words whose initial or final consonants vary by voicing, manner, and place. • Perform some phonological awareness skills (rhyming, word-initial consonants). • Follow age-appropriate conversations in open set. • Identify 100% of the Phonetically Balanced Kindergarten (PBK) list with monitored live voice during an audiologic assessment. • Can repeat sentences with 81% accuracy, when presented with monitored live voice.	• Recall five facts from a story in bridge set (a bridge set is one where the items/topic is known but not seen.) • Perform the phonological awareness skills: syllable clapping—closed then open set; • Segmentation—closed then open set. • Process five to six critical elements of information.
SPEECH	• Produce all age-appropriate phonemes in words. • Produce all age-appropriate phonemes in short sentences, if speaking slowly.	• Speak more slowly during conversations in order to improve speech intelligibility.

	PROGRESS SUMMARY Based on developmental norms, the child is able to:	SHORT-TERM OBJECTIVES To be accomplished in one to four AVT sessions
LANGUAGE	• Demonstrate comprehension of vocabulary typical for her age, although expressive vocabulary is delayed. • Comprehend age-appropriate conversation. • Understand: pronouns: "I, me, my, you, your, he/his/him, she/her/hers, they, their, we"; prepositions: "in, out, on, off, under, behind, beside, between"; questions: "who, what, where, when, why, how"; simple present, present progressive, simple past and simple future tenses. • Express herself in five- to seven-word sentences that contain some grammatical errors. Use the following: pronouns: "I, me, my, mine, you, your, he/his, she/her" in conversation; prepositions: "in, out, on, off, under, behind, beside" in conversation; questions: "who, what, where, why" in conversation; simple present, present progressive, simple past, and future progressive tense in conversation.	• Expand receptive/expressive vocabulary such as words from the book "Going on a Bear Hunt" and camping vocabulary. Demonstrate the following: story-telling grammar: combine three to four sentences in a logical way to re-tell a story; • Past progressive verb tense; • Expressive use of the pronoun "they" • Comprehension and expressive use of the preposition "through".
COGNITION	• Count to 100. • Perform simple addition/subtraction to five in her head. • Recognize and identify by name and sound, all of the alphabet. • Read some sight words.	• Provide reasons during problem-solving by responding to What would you do if? or What do you think X will do?
COMMUNICATION	• Express herself appropriately for her age, in terms of pragmatics. • Get along well with friends at school.	• Play board games by the rules.

continues

AV PRACTITIONER GOALS

- Do a continuous assessment of Tanya's functional hearing.
- Guide dad to use the slow down cue as effectively as possible
- Guide dad to use auditory highlighting to focus on specific grammatical targets, such as pausing briefly and emphasizing the preposition "through" and the pronoun "they."
- Utilize a printed schedule to manage behavior.

PARENT GOALS

- Use slow-down cue.
- Practice being a commentator.
- Practice acoustic highlighting of targeted words "through" and "they" as well as words that Tanya has said incorrectly.

STEP-BY-STEP SESSION PLAN ORIENTATION

In our center, the AV practitioners like to coach and guide parents using themes as often as possible. The practitioners find it is a very advantageous way to introduce new vocabulary that doesn't just happen during daily routines and in addition, the children find the themes engaging.

- Tanya has just been to a week-long, sleepover camp, so Kelley has chosen a camping theme for this AVT session.
- Tanya arrives with her dad, and when Kelley greets them in the waiting room, her dad mentions that Tanya has been asking for repetitions more often of late.
- As they walk to the therapy room, they chat about the equipment troubleshooting that he has tried at home. He has already tried everything that Kelley can think of, so they make a note to double check her hearing during the session and to make an appointment with the CI audiologist if needed.
- As Tanya settles in her chair, she excitedly tells Kelley about the frog that she had found at camp and brought home. (First she put it in her pocket and then she took off her sock and kept it in there!)
- Tanya is speaking very quickly so, first Kelley uses a cue to slow down (she holds up a flat hand and lowers it down). When that doesn't work, she asks Tanya to tell her again and to "slow down" Tanya is a bit "put out" by the request, and refuses to repeat it.
- Kelley asks Dad how the slow-down cue has been going at home and he sheepishly admits that he hasn't been remembering to use it.

- To help Tanya feel that she has some control over the session and to have a sense of what she can expect, Kelley devised a visual schedule they can use. She has already drawn four circles on a page and has the four activities that she has planned set up on a nearby shelf. Upon completion of each activity Tanya will draw a face in one of the circles. She knows that she can pick any one of the four activities, in any order, but that she has to complete all four activities before she gets to pick a reward game at the end. A simple structure like this has been very successful in reducing Tanya's pouting and task refusals.

ACTIVITY #1. "THROUGH"; VOCABULARY ("STOMP, SQUELCH, WHOOSH, STUMBLE, FOREST")

- Just before they start the activity, Kelley asks Dad to stand by the door and perform the Ling Six-sound test. Dad does so and Tanya easily repeats all six-sounds plus "p, t, k," and "f."
- Tanya picks the book *We're Going on A Bear Hunt* by Michael Rosen and Helen Oxenbury (Walker Books, 1989) as her first activity. She is very excited, exclaiming, "I did it at camp!," and launches into the chant, "Going on a bear hunt, going on a bear hunt." Kelley has all of the props that go with the book and asks Tanya to set them up while she explains to Dad, "We're going to be practicing the preposition word 'through' and some unusual verbs (stomp, squelch, whoosh) with this book. I'll start and then halfway through, you get to take over"
- As Tanya is clearly familiar with the book, the practitioner does not pre-teach the vocabulary, as she had initially planned.
- They chant the song in call and respond style, with Kelley calling and Tanya and her dad responding, "Going on a bear hunt./Going on a bear hunt . . . " When they get to an obstacle, the practitioner says, "We can't go over it. We can't go under it. We have to go . . . " She then stops and looks at Tanya with eyebrows raised clearly indicating that she should fill in the ending.
- Tanya looks confused the first time, so the practitioner looks at Dad to prompt him to fill in the ending. Dad says, "through it." They both look expectantly at Tanya and she says, "through it."
- They do this for each obstacle and Tanya, after the second try, is able to provide the preposition "through" every time.
- Unfortunately, as they get further into the book it becomes evident that Tanya doesn't know the vocabulary, and she is so engaged by the props that she is not able to slow down sufficiently.
- As Kelley turns the page to approach the next obstacle, she deliberately slows the pace of the activity. She turns the book over and says, "Oh no! A river! I will go first!" She takes her figurine and makes it do the action and says "Swish, swish, swish. Hear that sound I make as I go through the water? Dad, your turn!" Tanya's dad takes his figurine and walks it through the water but he doesn't say anything.

continues

ACTIVITY #1. "THROUGH"; VOCABULARY ("STOMP, SQUELCH, WHOOSH, STUMBLE, FOREST") *continued*

- Quietly, she coaches Dad, "Say 'swish, swish, swish' as your person goes through the water and then explain it." Dad follows her instructions. Then the practitioner says, "Tanya, it's your turn. Make your girl SWISH through the water. Say, 'swish, swish, swish.'" Tanya plays along well now that the activity has been slowed down.

- They continue to follow the same routine for each of the obstacles until they reach the cave and meet the bear. At that point, Kelley says, "Oh no! The bear is going to chase us. We have to run back home. Dad, you lead the way." Tanya's dad puts his figurine at the last obstacle and very nicely models, "The forest! Stumble, trip. Stumble, trip. Ok, Tanya, your turn." Tanya takes her figure and laughs and makes her figure stumble and trip but says nothing.

- The practitioner waits for a few moments, then when Dad just laughs along, she quietly coaches him, "Say it again and then tell Tanya that it's her turn to say it too." Dad does so and this time, Tanya repeats the words.

- They continue backward through all the obstacles. Tanya tries to rush ahead a few times, but Kelley keeps control of the story props to help keep her on task.

As they clean up the toys after finishing the book, the practitioner chats with Dad about books, the rich language used in them and how the vocabulary often consists of words that we rarely use in day-to-day conversation so they may need to be explicitly taught. Tanya used the preposition through quite well, but Kelley emphasizes that her use of it in a structured setting isn't the same as having full, expressive control of the word. She asks Dad if he can think of any times that they could practice that word over the next few days at home. "When we drive the four-wheeler through the field and then through the woods," is his suggestion.

ACTIVITY #2. PHONOLOGICAL AWARENESS (SYLLABLES); VOCABULARY: FLASHLIGHT, LANTERN, TENT, SLEEPING BAG, AXE, SHOVEL, WHISTLE, MARSHMALLOW

- When the props for the book are all put away, the practitioner hands Tanya a marker and the paper with the circles and says, "You can make a happy face." Tanya draws a face and hands it back to Kelley. "I make bear face," she says. Kelley acoustically highlights and says, "Yes, I see. You MADE A bear face. Look dad!" Tanya's dad looks and says, "Yup, you made a bear face." Quietly, the practitioner coaches Dad, "Remember to highlight the words that she said incorrectly." Dad repeats his sentence, this time using the highlighting strategies they just discussed.

- The next activity that Tanya chooses is a box filled with camping toys. Kelley quickly explains to Dad that they will be reviewing the camping vocabulary (they had looked at these toys just before she went off to camp) and then they will be clapping the syllables. The adults have already talked about phonological awareness, its importance for reading and its great application to listening. In previous sessions they have worked on rhyming words, clapping words in sentences and identifying the first sound in a word.

- The practitioner hands Dad the box of toys and each time he takes one out he waits for Tanya to name it. Tanya is very quick to say, "I don't know," with a shrug. Dad tells Kelley that "I don't know" and "I don't know how" are two of Tanya's favourite avoidance strategies of late. She asks Dad what they do when this happens. Dad shrugs and says, "We usually ask her again and then just give up and tell her." The practitioner nods and says, "I want to figure out if she knows the word or if this is a behavioral issue. Let's try a couple of things."

- After Dad pulls out the next toy and Tanya says yet again, "I don't know," Kelley provides a couple of clues: "Tanya, it's something that starts with "t" and rhymes with 'lent'." Tanya shrugs. So then she tries another strategy: "Let's try this. Is it a bed, a tent, or a car?" Tanya grins and says, "Tent." She acknowledges that this is the correct word, and then says to dad, "I am pretty sure the problem is that she doesn't know the vocabulary. Try the 'pick from 3 words' strategy, just like I did, if she says she doesn't know."

- Dad takes over for the rest of the items and is able to apply the "pick the word from a choice of 3" strategy when it is needed. This strategy is a selection from a closed set of probable responses.

- With all the toys in view on the table, the practitioner then says, "Let's clap the syllables in tent" and claps once as she says, "Tent. Your turn, Dad." Dad claps once and says, "Tent. Your turn Tanya." Tanya claps once, says "tent" and they all cheer.

- Kelley directs Dad to pick a toy, say the name of it and and clap the syllables. He does so and encourages Tanya and her to take their turns.

- Then it's Tanya's turn to lead. Dad and the practitioner wait for her to choose a toy. She points and says, "I want that one." Dad reaches to give her the toy and Kelley quietly coaches, "Offer her a choice." Dad then says, "Do you mean the sleeping bag, the marshmallow, or the axe?" Tanya replies, "The marshmallow." Dad hands her the marshmallow and she easily claps the 3 syllables.

- They continue the activity in the same manner, with Tanya accurately clapping the syllables to each word.

- With the activity goals completed, they spend a few minutes playing with the toys, chopping wood, and making a pretend fire. The practitioner notices that Dad is making a real effort to be a commentator as he plays.

- She then says, "I'm going to make s'mores, now." Tanya excitedly starts describing the s'mores she had when she was at camp. She is talking too quickly and Kelley is having difficulty understanding her, so she uses the cue for Tanya to slow down. This time, she does slow down, and describes making s'mores in good detail and in order!

- They finish playing with the toys and the practitioner hands Dad the box to do the clean-up routine. She suggests that he ask for one item because she is not sure that Tanya knows the vocabulary well enough to do a more difficult task. Tanya accurately chooses each item, showing that she has established comprehension.

- The adults chat briefly about how to reinforce this vocabulary at home. They aren't camping people and don't have any of these toys. Kelley suggests that they borrow some books from the library.

continues

ACTIVITY #3. MAKING A SNACK: RECALLING A SEQUENCE OF EVENTS; TELLING A SEQUENCE OF EVENTS USING 3 TO 4 CONNECTED SENTENCES

- The practitioner hands Tanya the paper circle to make her second face. She draws a face and announces, "I do two more." Kelley looks over to Dad, and he says, "Yup, you have two more games and then you get to pick."

- Tanya chooses the snack activity next. (Tanya enjoys food preparation and does lots of baking and cooking with her mom. Kelley frequently incorporates snacks in to her sessions because it is an activity that appeals to Tanya and there are short-term objectives that can be targeted.)

- The practitioner quickly explains to dad that she is going to describe the snack preparation procedure, similar to how she did it in the previous AVT session and tell Tanya how to make it without her seeing the ingredients. Then, as Tanya recalls each step, Kelley will reveal the item. After making and eating the snack, Dad will film her on his mobile phone as she explains to her mom how she made the snack. Then they will e-mail the clip to her mom so they can use it for review at home this evening.

- Today's snack activity is called fish in the pond. Kelley says, "Listening hands, please, Tanya. Remember last week we made a cookie snack we called 'Bear in the Mud?' Now I'm going to tell you how to make a snack called 'Fish in the Pond'. I am going to tell you all the steps and then you get to tell me." The steps Kelley tells her are:

  1. Put some icing in the bowl.
  2. Get the blue food dye.
  3. Stir the five drops of food coloring into the icing.
  4. Get one cookie and spread the icing on the cookie.
  5. Get five fishy crackers and put them on the blue icing.

- Tanya is not able to remember each step accurately, so to make the activity a bit easier, Kelley put all the items out on the table. With the ingredients in view, Tanya listens to all the instructions, and then tells how to make the snack in the right order and proceeds to do so.

- Before eating the snack, Tanya's dad gets out his phone and prompts her to tell how she made the snack while he films her. Tanya speaks quickly and, without Kelley's guidance, dad gives her the slow down cue and it works! Tanya's speech, when she slows down, is very intelligible. Dad and the practitioner are now able to understand her better and it is evident that she is telling the steps in the correct order.

- As they clean up, they talk about using the slow down cue more at home. Kelley asks Dad what reminders he could use to help him to remember to use it. He suggests that, because they have an open concept house, posting a few signs in key places would likely work.

- Kelley gives Tanya the paper circle and she draws in a face. Then, reluctantly, she points to the last activity. (Tanya doesn't care for board games but Kelley hopes that she will find this one engaging.)

- The game is "Bears," by Dave Sindrey (Word Play). The premise of the game is that the characters (Kelley uses boy and girl figures so they can practice they) have gone for a walk and while standing on top of a cliff overlooking their camp ground, they see a bunch of mischievous bears heading for their camp site. They have to find all the things they need to get past a variety of obstacles and get back to their campsite before the bears destroy everything.

- Kelley hides the game cards under the stimulus they cards, while explaining the game to Tanya and Dad. When a game card is discovered, Tanya and her dad need to discuss whether it will solve the current obstacle or if it needs to be kept for a later obstacle.

- In spontaneous conversation, Tanya substitutes she or he for they so Kelley and Dad take turns modeling they, using acoustic highlighting. Tanya's self-consciousness makes her irritable when the adults focus on a pronoun that she doesn't know.

- Kelley reflects to herself that targeting a structure that Tanya finds difficult, in a game situation that she doesn't like, is a bit too demanding. She decides to make the game move along more quickly by abandoning the figures and only using the stimulus pictures to elicit they.

- Tanya gives very good reasons for why each card can solve an obstacle or not. Kelley comments to Dad about the the good problem-solving skills Tanya demonstrates, but that her sentences contain many grammatical errors, for example, "She need flashlight for seeing in dark." Kelley then coaches Dad to acknowledge and then repeat Tanya's sentence, with the correct grammar, and to highlight the target structure they. "Yeah, THEY need a flashlight to see in the dark."

- Though it is a target for Tanya to learn to play board games by the rules, Kelley elects to finish the game as quickly as possible, in order to finish the session on a good note.

- Tanya hurriedly draws her last face.

- Tanya chooses a toy to play with for a few minutes while her Kelley and Dad discuss the session.

- Kelley asks Dad to reflect on how he well he achieved his goal, Be a commentator, for the session. He says he feels like he has done a bit better and Kelley agrees. They discuss reading books as a strategy for talking more and he volunteers that he could probably read more with Tanya. Kelley suggests that they get the *Going on a Bear Hunt* book because Tanya liked it so much and because it would provide an opportunity for them to review the vocabulary. As an added extension activity, she suggests that they all try to use those words and the preposition through while they do outdoor activities together.

continues

ACTIVITY #4. "THEY"; GIVE REASONS/EXPLANATIONS; PLAY A BOARD GAME BAKER'S LING RAP *continued*

- Kelley and Dad talk about the strategy of repeating Tanya's sentences back to her while emphasizing the correct grammar. Dad acknowledges that this is a challenge for him. They decide that practicing that will be his goal during the week and for the next AVT session. In the meantime, he will focus on modeling they.

- Finally, they talk about the slow down prompt. Dad reiterates that they haven't been using it very much at home because they understand everything that Tanya says. He agrees that they will try to use it more often. Tanya will have more practice speaking slowly so that teachers and friends will be able to understand her easily.

- Throughout the entire session, Kelley has been monitoring Tanya's responses to what was said and has listened to her imitations in order to assess her functional listening. Tanya appeared to be hearing well. She made no mistakes and her imitations were all correct. There were no instances when she asked "What?" Kelley makes this observation to Dad. He agrees that Tanya was hearing well in this AVT session. Kelley asks him for his thoughts. He reflects and replies that Tanya probably heard well in the AV session because it is quiet in the therapy room and she was focused on the activities.

- Kelley agrees and wonders aloud how that might influence what is done at home. Dad answers that they don't typically have background sound sources on at home. Kelly recalls that their house is open concept, and suggests that they keep in mind the arms-length rule (staying within earshot) and move closer to Tanya when talking to her.

- Kelley checks Tanya's chart, and notices that it has been 5 months since her last CI mapping, so she recommends booking an appointment with Tanya's CI audiologist just to make sure that all the equipment is functioning optimally and to ensure that her map is providing optimal access to all frequencies.

- As the session comes to a close, Kelley asks Tanya to clean up and they then go to find her CI audiologist to book an appointment.

- Kelley's final good-bye is a variation on "See you later, alligator!" She has a wonderful list of these sayings posted on her door and they have been picking new ones to learn weekly. It's a fun rhyming activity and a fun way to say good-bye. ("See you later, alligator. Pretty soon, baboon. Got to swish, jellyfish. Ciao ciao brown cow.")

	SESSION ANALYSIS The child demonstrated the following:
AUDITION	• Recalled five facts from a story (the sequence of the story events) in a bridge set (a familiar book). • Demonstrated phonological awareness of syllable counting. • Recalled five elements in closed set but not in open set (she needs to practice at the bridge set level).
SPEECH	• Spoke more slowly, and thereby more intelligibly, when prompted with the slow down prompt.
LANGUAGE	• Retained comprehension of new vocabulary (squelch, swoosh etc.) from camp (but not expressive mastery). • Demonstrated understanding of the camping vocabulary but hadn't mastered it expressively. • Produced the preposition through accurately during structured practice. • Demonstrated the ability to imitate the pronoun "they" during structured practice.
COGNITION	• Gave good explanations for what she would need to solve an obstacle to the "Bears" game.
COMMUNICATION	• Completed a board game, with lots of support.

continues

PARENT GUIDANCE SUMMARY

- Use highlighting to emphasize through and new vocabulary.
- Plan opportunities to use and model they.
- Acknowledge and repeat Tanya's sentences back to her with correct grammar.
- Be a commentator.
- Choose books to introduce new, unusual, and infrequently used words and to expose Tanya to different ideas, and concepts.
- Use the slow down prompt to help Tanya remember to speak more slowly.
- Post reminders around the house to use the slow-down prompt.
- Use visual props such as numbered cards on which Tanya can draw a face upon completion of each activity, or magnetic numbers which Tanya can put up on the fridge or other nearby magnetic surface, a to help Tanya learn to manage her expectations and her behavior.
- Modify the difficulty level of activities to stay just ahead of Tanya's ability level to help manage her frustration and to provide a positive learning experience.
- Plan to incorporate the preposition through into regular activities so that Tanya transfers it from structured activities to the to open set.
- Give a first letter or a choice of 3/4/5 words for her to identify a word that she knows receptively but doesn't use expressively.

CONCLUSION AND NEXT STEPS
Review of practitioner targets:

- The AV practitioner assessed Tanya's hearing acuity using the Ling Six-Sound Test and by observations throughout the session.
- She coached Tanya's dad to use auditory highlighting to emphasize the new vocabulary and grammatical targets they and through.
- The AV practitioner coached and guided Tanya's dad to use the slow down prompt to encourage Tanya to speak more slowly and intelligibly.
- The AV practitioner utilized strategies to manage behavior, such as slowing down the pace by turning the book upside down during the *"Bear Hunt"* book; modifying the difficulty level during the snack and the board game; and using the visual schedule.

Review of parent targets

- Dad learned to use the slow down cue, effectively employing it several times.
- Dad was able to utilize auditory highlighting of targeted grammatical structures.
- Dad practiced being a commentator during play and made a plan of how he can talk more while reading books at home.
- Both Kelley and Dad agreed that using the visual schedule to help Tanya know what was coming next was very effective for managing her behavior and that the slow-down cue was effective in helping Tanya speak more intelligibly.

SUMMARY

- At the point of discharge from AVT, Tanya's auditory skills are developing nicely. Word and sentence discrimination are excellent. She is able to recall five elements from a familiar story or in a closed set. Future targets could involve recalling facts from unfamiliar content and/or in an open set.
- Tanya's speech is usually intelligible, expecially when prompted to slow down. Next steps involve reduction of prompting.
- Receptive language and vocabulary have kept pace with that of her peers but expressive language is a little delayed.

I would like to acknowledge with immense gratitude my colleague Kelley Rabjohn, who prepared and conducted this session.

APPENDIX 13-A

LEARNING TO LISTEN SOUNDS

Karen MacIver-Lux and Warren Estabrooks

Learning to Listen Sounds (Estabrooks, 1994, 2006) is a term used by many auditory-verbal (AV) practitioners and parents to describe a selection of onomatopoeic sounds, ideophones, words, and/or phrases. Many of the *Learning to Listen Sounds* imitate or resemble the source of the sound or are associated with their referents such as "moo" for the cow and "choo choo" for the train (onomatopoeic sounds), are words or phrases that depict sensory information ("swish" for sudden movement of a fish) and feelings such as "ouch" for pain (ideophones), or are words and/or phrases that describe what animals and/or objects do such as "hop" for the bunny "round and round" for the spinning top. Some *Learning to Listen Sounds,* however, have been adapted from commonly used onomatopoeia, such as the *Learning to Listen Sound* for the bus ("bu bu bu" instead of "beep beep beep") or the car ("brr beep beep" instead of "vroom") so that sounds of the child's native language are represented during playful experiences with the *Learning to Listen Sounds.*

Learning to Listen Sounds, however, are *not* represented the same in all languages. They are, however, for the most part, shaped by the linguistic system of the family and used in the child's everyday environment (Bredin, 1996). For example, the Learning to Listen Sound for a clock may be *tick tock* in English, *dī dā* in Mandarin, *katchin*

katchin in Japanese, or "tik-tik" in Arabic.

Learning to Listen Sounds have specific acoustic properties. Some consist of vowels and diphthongs that have their first formants in the low- to mid-frequency range; other *Learning to Listen Sounds* consist of consonants that contain bursts of energy clustered in the mid- to high-frequency range (Estabrooks & Marlowe, 2000). By observing the child's response to each of these sounds, the AV practitioner gains valuable information about the child's functional auditory access across the speech spectrum using hearing aids, a cochlear implant, or both (see Chapter 14). The *Learning to Listen Sounds Audiogram* (Figure 13–1) and the *Acoustics of LTLS Chart* (Figure 13–2) are suitable references for auditory-verbal practitioners, audiologists and parents. The icons on the *Learning to Listen Audiogram* represent *some* of the *Learning to Listen Sounds* and are placed *according to the location of their first and second formants/band of energy.* The child's detection and identification responses to the *Learning to Listen Sounds* can be plotted on the *Learning to Listen Sounds Audiogram* to indicate at which frequencies the child has auditory access. The *Learning to Listen Sounds* need to be presented at the intensity level of conversational speech, at a distance of one meter from the microphone of

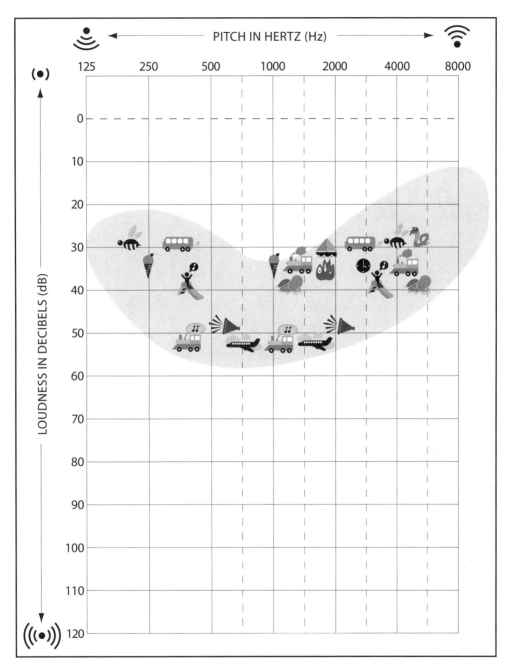

Figure 13–1. Learning to Listen Sounds Audiogram

the hearing technology in order to predict auditory access on the ***Learning to Listen Sounds*** Audiogram as accurately as possible. Most children, if provided with appropriately selected and programmed hearing devices, should find these sounds easy to hear (Estabrooks, 2006).

LEARNING TO LISTEN SOUNDS (LTLS) IN ENGLISH	1ST FORMANT OR BAND OF FREQUENCY	2ND FORMANT OR BAND OF FREQUENCY
/m/ "mmm" — ice-cream ("make")	250 - 350 Hz @35 - 40 dB HL	1000 - 1500 Hz @35 - 40 dB HL
/u/ "ooo" — train ("true")	430 -460 Hz @55 dB HL	1105 - 1170 Hz @55 dB HL
/tʃ, tʃ, tʃ/ "ch, ch, ch" — train (chicken)	1500 - 2000 Hz @35 - 40 dB HL	4000 - 5000 Hz @35 - 40 dB HL
/wi/ "whee" — slide (three)	370 -437 Hz @40 dB HL	2761 -3200 Hz @40 dB HL
/ɑ/ "ahh" — airplane ("on")	768 - 1030 Hz @55 dB HL	1370 - 1551 Hz @55 dB HL
/e/ "ey!" — call out ("hay")	536 - 610 Hz @50 dB HL	2530 - 2680Hz @50 dB HL
/bʌ, bʌ, bʌ/ "buh buh buh" — bus ("bubble")	300 - 400 Hz @30 dB HL	2000 - 3000Hz @30 dB HL
/h/ "h!" — hot ("hat")	1500 - 2000 Hz @35 dB HL	
/p, p, p/ - "p, p, p" — boat ("peek")	1500 -2000 Hz @30 dB HL	
/ʃ/ "shh" — sleeping baby ("show")	1500 - 2000 Hz @40 dB HL	4500 - 5500 Hz @40 dB HL
/z/ "zzz" — bee ("zoo")	200 - 300 Hz @30 dB HL	4000 - 5000Hz @30 dB HL
/t, t, t/ "t, t, t" — ticking clock ("top")	2500 - 3500 Hz @35 dB HL	
/s/ "sss" — snake ("pass")	5000-6000 Hz @30 dB HL	

Figure 13–2. Acoustics of Learning to Listen Sounds Chart

Some *Learning to Listen Sounds*, when spoken, contain acoustic properties that are rich in suprasegmentals that match those found in the child's native language. AV practitioners, therefore, guide parents to use infant-/child-directed speech that includes *Learning to Listen Sounds* so that spoken language sounds appealing appealing (Shultz & Vouloumanos, 2010), and is easy to attend to (Vouloumanos & Werker, 2007), and learn (Reschke, 2002).

Learning to Listen Sounds vary in frequency, number of syllables (e.g., "bu bu bu" for the bus and "ahhh" for the airplane), and tempo (e.g., "wow!" vs. "ah"). When used in various combinations in playful scenarios, in meaningful parent-child interactions, and when listening to stories, the *Learning to Listen Sounds* help the child to discriminate, and associate spoken language to objects and meaningful experiences. For example, adult-directed speech varies in tempo across speakers and dialects, but on average consists of seven sounds per second (Krause & Braida, 2004). Parentese or infant-directed speech has a slower tempo; *Learning to Listen Sounds* typically consist of one to three sounds per second when presented in isolation. The slower tempo of infant-/child-directed speech and the presentation of the *Learning to Listen Sounds* facilitate the discrimination of sounds (Goldstein & Schwade, 2008). Furthermore, changes in pitch and tone help gain and maintain the child's attention and facilitate auditory memory, and the understanding of the emotional content in language that promotes linguistic

and social development (Kaplan, Jung, Ryther, & Zarlengo-Strouse, 1996). Therefore, *Learning to Listen Sounds* are not only easy to hear, but easy to process auditorily, enjoyable to listen to, and easy to learn (Estabrooks, 2006).

Many *Learning to Listen Sounds* are those that children typically begin producing within the first two years of life and are easy for children to say and sing (Estabrooks, 2006). For example, infants pick up the vocal cues of infant-/child-directed speech and will often pattern their own babbling after it (Goldstein & Schwade, 2008). From 12 months of age onward, children produce approximations of many of the *Learning to Listen Sounds* and phrases heard throughout their daily routines and activities, and begin to use novel combinations of *Learning to Listen Sounds* followed by words to communicate their observations, wants, and needs.

When a young child understands a variety of *Learning to Listen Sounds*, the AV practitioner and parent will say the words without using the *Learning to Listen Sounds*. The transition, therefore, to real words is often spontaneous, especially if the child has had rich auditory experiences in a variety of playful scenarios and everyday experiences with these *Learning to Listen Sounds*. AV practitioners guide and coach parents to present *Learning to Listen Sounds* in creative and systematic ways, using a number of strategies described in Chapters 10 and 11, and move forward to the development of conversations as quickly and efficiently as possible.

LEARNING TO LISTEN SOUNDS AND SONGS (ENGLISH)

Sound	Activity/Toy	Song
ahh	airplane	The Airplane
oo	train	The Train
bu, bu, bu	bubbles or bus	Bubbles or The Bus
brr, beep, beep	car, truck	The Car
p, p, p	boat, popping toys	The Boat
t, t, t	clock	The Clock
ow/ouch	fall down, cut	Ouch!
ow, ow, ow	ambulance, fire truck	The Ambulance
wow	any surprise	WOW!
hee, hee, hee	monkey	Monkey in a Tree
Ha, ha, ha	clown, laughter	Funny Little Clown
g/go	running	Running, Running
Ya hoo!	cowboy	The Cowboy
Whee, whee!	slide or Chinese yoyo	The Slide or My Blue Yoyo
Mama	baby doll	Baby Doll
Hi!	mirror	The Mirror
meow	cat	Kitty Cat
ruff, ruff or bow wow	dog	The Dog
baa, oink	sheep, pig	Living on the Farm
moo, neigh	cow, horse	The Farm
quack	duck	Six Little Ducks
tongue clack	horse	Clip, Clop
hoo, hoo	owl	Mr. Owl
hop, hop	rabbit	The Rabbit
whistle	birdie	The Birds
cock-a-doodle-doo	rooster	The Rooster

Sound	Activity/Toy	Song
caw, caw	crow	Big Black Crow
round and round and round	windmill, top, wheels	The Windmill, The Spinning Top, and Wheels
mmmm	any good thing	Mmmm Good
n	"no"	No No!
d	toy shovel	Dig Dig
s	snake	The Snake
sh	sleeping games	Someone's Sleeping
La, la, la, la, la	rocking the baby	Rock the Baby
u, u, up	any "up" activity	Pick Me Up

REFERENCES

Bredin, H. (1996). Onomatopoeia as a figure and a linguistic principle. *New Literary History, 27*(3), 555–569. Johns Hopkins University Press. Retrieved February 2, 2016, from Project MUSE database.

Estabrooks, W. (1994). *Auditory-Verbal Therapy for parents and professionals.* Washington, DC: Alexander Graham Bell Association for the Deaf and Hard of Hearing.

Estabrooks, W. (2006). *Auditory-Verbal Therapy and practice.* Washington, DC: Alexander Graham Bell Association for the Deaf and Hard of Hearing.

Estabrooks, W., & Marlowe, J. (2000). *The baby is listening.* Washington, DC: Alexander Graham Bell Association for the Deaf and Hard of Hearing.

Goldstein, M. H., & J. A. Schwade. (2008). Social feedback to infants' babbling facilitates rapid phonological learning. *Psychological Science, 19*(5), 515–523.

Kaplan, P., Jung, P., Ryther, J., & Zarlengo-Strouse, P. (1996). Infant-directed versus adult-directed speech as signals for face. *Developmental Psychology, 32*(5), 880–891.

Krause, J. C., & Braida, L. D. (2004). Acoustic properties of naturally produced clear speech at normal speaking rates. *Journal of the Acoustical Society of America, 115*(1), 362.

Literary Devices Editors. (2016). *Onomatopoeias.* Retrieved February 2, 2016, from http://literarydevices.net/onomatopoeias/

Onomatopoeia. (n.d.). Dictionary.com Unabridged. Retrieved February 2, 2016, from from Dictionary.com website: http://dictionary.reference.com/browse/onomatopoeia

Reschke, K. L. (2002). Ohio State University, "Baby talk." Archived August 22, 2007, at the Wayback Machine.

Shultz, S., & Vouloumanos, A. (2010). Three-month-olds prefer speech to other naturally occurring signals. *Language Learning and Development, 6,* 241–257.

Singh, L., Nestor, S., Parikh, C., & Yull, A. (2009). Influences of infant-directed speech on early word recognition. *Infancy, 14*(6), 654–666.

Vouloumanos, A., & Werker, J. F. (2007). Listening to language at birth: Evidence for a bias for speech in neonates. *Developmental Science, 10*(2), 159–164.

14

CHILDREN WITH COMPLEX HEARING ISSUES AND AUDITORY-VERBAL THERAPY

Stacey R. Lim and Karen MacIver-Lux

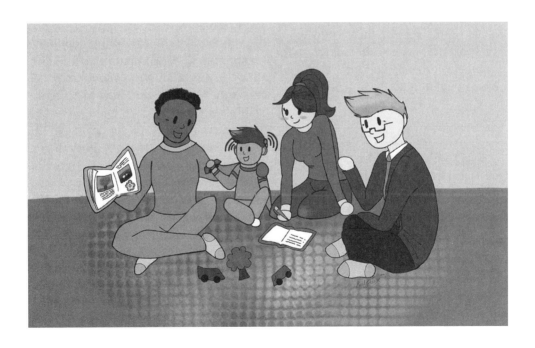

INTRODUCTION

In most cases, when early identified infants have auditory access to all sounds of the speech spectrum at soft conversational levels, they are able to take advantage of the critical period to develop spoken language primarily through listening. At various stages in some children's lives, however, a variety of complex hearing issues may arise, potentially affecting the child's auditory access or auditory functioning causing a negative impact on spoken communication. Thus, the AV practitioner needs to modify the auditory-verbal treatment plan, refer the child to appropriate allied health professionals, and/or develop a transition plan to another communication approach. This chapter provides an outline of some complex hearing issues, their impact on the development of listening and spoken language skills, and steps for management to help children reach their highest communication potential.

DETERMINING AUDITORY FUNCTIONING OF CHILDREN WITH COMPLEX HEARING ISSUES

AVT is always diagnostic. Consequently, the AV practitioner uses a number of ways to monitor progress in receptive and expressive language, and in particular, the child's auditory access and functioning in the AVT session.

The *Ling Six-Sound Test* and the *Learning to Listen Sounds* (see Appendix 13–1) are helpful *diagnostic* tools. By using them, the AV practitioner and the parent can do the following:

- Detect changes in hearing levels due to middle ear dysfunction or progressive hearing loss.
- Detect changes in function of hearing aids and/or cochlear implant.
- Detect reduced response to hearing aids and/or cochlear implant technology due to physiological changes.
- Determine the effects of distance from the speaker on audibility of speech features.

The *Ling Six-Sound Test*, a detection task of six speech sounds *(oo, a(r), ee, m, sh, and s)*, is presented at normal conversational level and provides valuable insight about the child's ability to perceive various speech sounds (Glista, Scollie, Moodie, & Easwar, 2014).

In addition to observing the child's responses and/or imitation of the *Ling Six-Sounds*, and the *Learning to Listen Sounds*, the AV practitioner listens to the child's speech and/or expressive language as children typically say what they hear. The AV practitioner, audiologist, and parents(s) work together to distinguish speech and/or language errors that are oral-motor related and/or de-velopmental, from those caused by inadequate access due to problems with any aspect of the child's hearing device(s).

The AV practitioner and the parent determine the child's auditory functioning based on

- consistency and nature of child's auditory responses;
- child's localization abilities to all sounds of the speech spectrum and environmental sounds;

- child's distance hearing for all sounds, especially conversational speech;
- conditions when the child did or did not detect or identify environmental or speech stimuli; and
- child's ability to comprehend spoken language in quiet, at a distance and in nonideal listening environments.

Finally, audiologists rely on reports from therapists and parent(s) about the child's progress in developing listening and spoken language. These reports provide additional evidence when evaluating the effectiveness of the child's hearing devices. Therefore, every 3 months, the AV practitioner administers assessments that evaluate several aspects of the child's listening and spoken language development and shares the results with the audiologist. Although complete assessments (tests) are administered no more frequently than once every 6 months, the AV practitioner can administer different assessments at different times. For example, an AV practitioner may administer the Preschool Language Scales, Fifth Edition (PLS™-5) at one time, and then 3 months later, administer the Clinical Evaluation of Language Fundamentals®-Preschool-2 (CELF®-Preschool-2), and so on.

The AV practitioner uses the different observations and assessments described above, when determining listening and spoken language progress in the children they see, including those who have complex listening needs. Although there are a number of challenges that can be present in children with hearing loss, this chapter focuses on four of them:

- unilateral hearing loss/single sided deafness (SSD),

- hard or soft cochlear implant failure,
- auditory neuropathy spectrum disorder (ANSD), and
- cochlear nerve deficiency/underdeveloped auditory nerve.

UNILATERAL HEARING LOSS/ SINGLE-SIDED DEAFNESS

Unilateral hearing loss, which has also been described as single-sided deafness (SSD), affects up to 5% of school-aged children and is present in 3.4% of infants identified with congenital hearing loss (Lieu et al., 2013). Although individuals with unilateral hearing loss have normal hearing function in one ear, they may still have compromised auditory abilities, due to the lack of information derived from the contralateral ear. For example, good hearing in two ears (the "adding up" of sounds arriving to both ears known as binaural summation) is required for optimal localization (knowing who is speaking at the dinner table), and speech understanding in quiet and noisy situations (interviews, classrooms, cafeterias) (Kerber & Seeber, 2012; Litovsky, Parkinson, Arcaroli, & Sammeth, 2006; Nittrouer et al., 2013). Untreated unilateral hearing loss can lead to poorer academic performance due to diminished access to auditory information (Lieu, Tye-Murray, Karzan, & Piccirillo, 2010). Despite this, a significant number of medical and educational communities do not consider unilateral hearing loss to be a problem (Lieu, 2010). Sometimes, parents and professionals adopt a "wait and see" philosophy to determine whether or not the child may require hearing technology. If they do this, it is of paramount importance that there be consistent, ongoing, and timely evaluations of auditory and language development and academic progress (McKay, Gravel, & Tharpe, 2008).

Since auditory brain development requires consistent, high-quality auditory access to language (Chapter 2), the same is true for those who have unilateral hearing loss. If there is a lack of auditory access in one ear, the brain structures will develop neural pathways for the good ear, and the ear without hearing will have an incomplete auditory pathway to the brain (Kral, Hubka, Heid, & Tillein, 2012). Furthermore, unilateral hearing loss has been associated with differences in executive functioning and cognition (Lieu, 2013). To develop the most complete auditory neural networks, it is critical to provide stimulation to the ear without hearing.

There are various options for providing auditory access to children with unilateral hearing loss (Chapters 5 and 6). The hearing technology selected needs to be determined by the type and degree of hearing loss, family support, and consideration of existing peripheral auditory structures, including that of a complete auditory system. Appropriately, the AV practitioner and parent(s) collaborate and provide information to the audiologist, regarding the child's hearing health and daily auditory functioning at home and school. The audiologist can then select and fit the appropriate hearing device.

One option is a hearing aid (HA). For some children, traditional amplification provides the needed auditory access to language. Parental reports suggest that children with unilateral hearing loss, who have been fitted with a conventional hearing aid, have greater ease of listening in noise and in quiet (Davis et al., 2001); children with uni-

lateral hearing loss who receive amplification at a *younger* age demonstrate better localization skills than those who receive a hearing aid later (Johnstone, Nabelek, & Robertson, 2010). During weekly AVT sessions, the AV practitioner monitors the child's progress in the development of auditory skills in the aided ear, and the integration of the two auditory signals (amplified ear and ear with typical hearing) for the purpose of developing bilateral listening skills critical for competency in spoken language, and the advancement of social-emotional and academic skills.

Another option is an *auditory osseointegrated implant system* (AOIS), which is available from various hearing aid and cochlear implant manufacturers which are designed for individuals with conductive/mixed hearing losses or unilateral hearing loss. Results in this population using AOIS have been excellent. In some pediatric populations, there have been significant improvements in speech understanding in quiet and in noise (Christensen, Richter, & Dornhoffer, 2010), and also in localization abilities (Saliba, Woods, & Caron, 2010). In addition to carefully monitoring the child's auditory functioning with the AOIS and working in tandem with the audiologist to ensure sufficient auditory access for learning to talk, the AV practitioner and parent(s) are vigilant about irritations at the site where the device is placed or implanted.

Some children with unilateral hearing loss receive a cochlear implant on the ear with hearing loss (Hassepass et al., 2013). Professionals engaged in working with children who receive implantable technology more commonly refer to children with unilateral hearing loss as children with single-sided deafness (SSD). The results from cochlear implantation in children with SSD are promising, as they demonstrate and perceive improved speech understanding in noise and quiet, localization (Hassepass et al., 2013). Although this option is just emerging, AV practitioners and parents need to be aware of the benefits of cochlear implantation in helping children with SSD establish bilateral hearing and listening skills.

Implications of Unilateral Hearing Loss/Single-Sided Deafness

Children with unilateral hearing loss who have experienced a period of auditory deprivation in one ear likely have morphological changes within the brain (Cardon & Sharma, 2013). When they are fitted with an appropriate hearing device, and are bathed in meaningful auditory experiences, the ear with the hearing device has the potential to develop auditory skills that will better match those of the contralateral ear. Auditory stimulation and auditory skills training can result in other morphological changes within the central auditory nervous system facilitating improvement in bilateral auditory processing skills. (Chermak & Musiek, 2007).

Sample AV Session Outline for a Child With Unilateral Hearing Loss

The AV practitioner works to develop listening skills through the ear that has received the hearing device. There are several parts to the AVT session to help the child integrate two different audi-tory signals for the purpose of developing spoken language.

Part I Beginning the Session With Both Ears

The practitioner begins the session with a conversation or an activity during which the child wears his or her hearing device (HA and AOIS) and leaves the ear with typical hearing unoccluded. The practitioner observes the child's hearing and listening behaviors and notes how he or she engages in conversation to determine how the child is integrating the two auditory signals.

Part II Listening With the Hearing Device Only

Depending on the child's level of auditory functioning with the hearing device, the AV practitioner presents a variety of activities that focus on auditory skill development *with the hearing device only*. The ear with typical hearing is occluded with an earmold or an earplug so that the AV practitioner can gain information about how the child is hearing with the hearing aid or cochlear implant and plans meaningful experiences to optimize auditory development.

Children who wear an AOIS receive auditory stimulation to both cochleae (via bone conduction). Thus, it is difficult for the AV practitioner to isolate the ear with AOIS to develop and/or enhance auditory skills. When measuring auditory functioning in the ear with the AOIS, the audiologist administers *speech perception tests with masking noise*. For these reasons, the AV practitioner plans and carries out therapy sessions for children with AOIS similarly to those for children who wear bilateral hearing devices.

Part III Listening With Both Ears

When the child's level of auditory functioning with the hearing device is similar to that of the ear with typical hearing, it is appropriate to begin using activities that stimulate the development of auditory skills that are supported by bilateral hearing. A variety of tasks are then presented to facilitate refinement of binaural interaction skills (e.g., localization skills, understanding of speech-in-noise, etc.), speech sound discrimination skills (e.g., speech perception), temporal processing skills (e.g., discrimination of prosodic features of speech (intent of messages), perception of music, etc.), and/or dichotic listening skills (e.g., ability to understand two competing messages presented at the same time (binaural integration) and ignore messages while concentrating on a message of importance (binaural separation), etc.).

Part IV Parent Guidance

As in all AV sessions, parents are active participants. At the end of each session, the practitioner and parents discuss the outcomes and exchange ideas of ways to incorporate the short-term objectives into the child's daily life.

Part V Child Guidance

The child needs to become an "active listener," so it is important to encourage the child to repair communication breakdowns that are caused by "mishearing" and to use self-advocacy

strategies to control the listening environment so successful communication exchanges take place.

HARD OR SOFT FAILURES IN COCHLEAR IMPLANT(S)

Over a lifetime, a cochlear implant recipient may require one or more cochlear implant revision surgeries, due to device failure, suspected device malfunction, medical or surgical problems, and the desire for device upgrades (Cullen, Fayad, Luxford, & Buchan, 2008). If a cochlear implant stops working entirely despite an adequately functioning processor, and results of integrity tests suggest a failed device, then it is considered to be a *hard failure*. When there is a suspicion that a cochlear implant is failing or has failed, yet results of integrity testing suggests otherwise, it is considered to be a *soft failure*. The AV practitioner and parent(s) document any changes in the child's auditory functioning and report these to the audiologist.

Estimates of cochlear implant device failures in children have been cited anywhere from 9% (Parisier et al., 1996) to 11.7% (Cullen et al., 2008). Hard failures make up 46% of the failures (Cullen et al., 2008) and are easier to recognize. In these situations, the child typically will not respond to auditory stimuli and may refuse to wear the cochlear implant processor. Soft failures, on the other hand, are more difficult to recognize and may be confused with malfunctioning cochlear implant processors and/or changes in T and C levels (see Chapter 6).

Implications of Hard or Soft Failures of CIs for AVT

Through weekly AVT sessions, parent(s) learn to become astute observers of their child's overall development and especially of his or her auditory functioning. In most cases, it is either the parent(s) or the AV practitioner who are first aware of any problems with the cochlear implant, when the child

- refuses to wear the cochlear implant processor or turns the cochlear implant processor off;
- has "good" hearing days and "bad" hearing days, with the "bad" hearing days outnumbering the "good" hearing days over time;
- demonstrates improved auditory performance after programming of cochlear implant(s), followed by performance decline following subsequent programming sessions;
- makes unusual errors involving the omission of previously produced speech sounds (e.g., "ka" for cats) or addition of sounds to words that were previously produced correctly (e.g., "airt" for air) and upon further examination by a speech-language pathologist, speech disorders unrelated to hearing loss or hearing age (e.g. phonological processes, apraxia, dysarthria, etc.) have been ruled out.
- becomes quiet, withdrawn, and/ or more difficult to engage in

conversation or becomes louder with displays of frustration;
- demonstrates a decrease in overall auditory functioning, particularly in detection, discrimination, identification, and auditory attention;
- demonstrates eye twitching or complains of pain;
- reports funny sounds such as "popping," "buzzing," "static," and "whistles";
- experiences regression or lack of progress in receptive and expressive language skills/ development;
- has fluctuating hearing performance, or worsening of sound quality;
- experiences pain or physical sensation in the ear canal, middle ear, throat, forehead, eyebrows, area surrounding the coil, and/or the mastoid in response to auditory stimulation (facial nerve stimulation), which are reliably reproduced when individual electrodes are stimulated during MAPping sessions. If five or more electrodes are deactivated, this may suggest an impending device failure (Zeitler et al., 2009);
- needs frequent programming sessions;
- experiences gradual changes in the primary goal of programming sessions, which go from "improving speech reception/quality" to "finding a comfortable and stable listening program";
- experiences increased difficulty understanding speech in quiet

and in noisy situations despite adjustments made in programming; or

- regresses steadily in overall auditory functioning and performance over time.

The decision for re-implantation is made in conjunction with the surgeon, audiologist, and/or other members of the cochlear implant team. When required, cochlear revision surgery needs to takes place as quickly as possible to avoid cross-modal reorganization (Peele, Troaiani, Grossman, & Wingfield, 2011; Sharma & Cardon, 2014). In most cases, revision cochlear implant surgeries are successful and one expects the child to return to, or to surpass the listening and spoken communication skills that he or she had, with the previously functioning cochlear implant (Cullen et al., 2008; Lassig et al., 2005). The child and/or family need to be counseled that a return to previous levels of functioning may take time.

When the child has a revision CI surgery, the AV practitioner may do a period of therapy and will follow the same session blueprint as used with children who have unilateral losses (see above). The practitioner and parent help the child learn to adjust to the signal from the new implant by doing therapy with the *new cochlear implant only*. The other cochlear implant processor is turned off for a portion of the session. Then both implants are used for the remainder of the AVT session. When the level of auditory functioning of the ear with the new cochlear implant closely matches that of the other ear, then the entire session is done with both hearing devices on.

CHILDREN WITH AUDITORY NEUROPATHY SPECTRUM DISORDER (ANSD)

Although the precise prevalence of ANSD is unknown, it is estimated that one in ten children with hearing loss has auditory-neuropathy spectrum disorder (ANSD) (Kirkim et al., 2008; Mittal et al., 2012; Sanyelbhaa Talaat et al., 2009). Due to the variations of presentations of speech perception and listening and spoken language outcomes in children with ANSD (Berlin et al., 2010; Praveena & Prakesh, 2014), outcomes with hearing aids (Berlin et al., 2010; Rance, Barker, Mok, et al., 2007), and the presence of additional challenges/disabilities or medical conditions (Buchman, Roush, Teagle, & Zdanski, 2009), audiologists and parents face challenges in making decisions regarding audiologic management (Roush, Frymark, et al., 2011), especially when the child is very young and has unaided thresholds in the mild to moderate hearing loss range (Ching et al., 2013).

General guidelines for the identification of ANSD and appropriate amplification of children when reliable behavioral thresholds can be found in Chapter 5 and cochlear implant candidacy considerations in Chapter 6. The child's auditory abilities and progress in the development of receptive and expressive language greatly influence the audiologic management, the selection, fitting and management of hearing devices, and the appropriateness of the early intervention approach implemented (Berlin et al., 2010). If listening and spoken language development is poorer than expected after a period of hearing aid use and AVT, cochlear implantation needs to be considered, even if unaided or aided thresholds are in the mild hearing loss or normal hearing range (Berlin et al., 2010; Estabrooks, MacIver-Lux, & Houston, 2014).

Auditory Capacities of Children With ANSD

ANSD results from disruptions in the neural synchrony of the inner hair cells or the auditory neural pathways, while outer hair cell function generally remains normal, affecting the temporal aspects of speech (Roush, 2008). This dys-synchrony can affect speech understanding because

- voice onset time may not be transmitted making it difficult to distinguish between voiced and unvoiced consonants (Rance, 2005;
- pitch discrimination in the lower frequencies is affected making it difficult to localize sounds/speakers (Zeng et al., 2005); and
- there is poorer integrity of interaural timing cues and temporal resolution (Rance, & Barker, 2007; Wang et al., 2015), especially in the low frequencies.

If the degree of neural disruption is significant, the child's speech recognition abilities will be poorer than suggested by behavioral results, particularly in noise. Predictions cannot be made about the degree of disruption and speech understanding based only on the pure tone audiogram (Berlin et al., 2010). Because ANSD has variable degrees of disruption, there is a range of speech perception abilities and spoken language progress. Six possible presentations of ANSD and their impact on the development of listening and spoken communication are presented in Table 14–1.

Implications of ANSD for Auditory-Verbal Therapy

Some AV practitioners offer two types of intervention that focus on listening and spoken language development for children with ANSD: *Auditory-Verbal Therapy* (AVT) (Estabrooks et al., 2014; Praveena, Prakash, & Rukmangathan, 2014) and *Auditory and Language Enrichment* (ALE) (Estabrooks et al., 2014). AVT is offered to those children with ANSD who are fitted with hearing technology and is based on all *Ten Principles of Auditory-Verbal Therapy (See Chapter 1)*. ALE follows nine of the Ten Principles and was designed by Estabrooks and MacIver-Lux in 2007 and does not incorporate the principle related to the use of hearing devices. Therefore, ALE is offered to children with ANSD who do *not* use hearing device(s).

The AV practitioner and the audiologist monitor the child's listening and spoken language communication development closely to ensure that the hearing technology and intervention are appropriate. The child may also be referred to other practitioners such as a pediatric neurologist (Chandan et al., 2015; Mohammadi, Walker, & Gardner-Berry, 2015), geneticist (Lepcha et al., 2015; Zong et al., 2015), physiotherapist/occupational therapist (Nash et al., 2014), and/or speech-language pathologist (Estabrooks et al., 2014).

Table 14–1. Various Presentations of ANSD in Children

	PRESENTATION I	PRESENTATION II	PRESENTATION III
BEHAVIORAL PURE TONE AUDIOGRAM	Can vary from mild to profound Reverse slope common Can also • fluctuate • be progressive	Can vary from mild to profound Reverse slope common Can also • fluctuate • be progressive	Can vary from mild to profound Reverse slope common Can also • fluctuate • be progressive
AUDITORY FUNCTIONING IN QUIET	Poorer than what audiogram would suggest to no response	As expected given the audiogram (similar to children with sensorineural hearing loss)	Better than expected given the audiogram
AUDITORY FUNCTIONING IN NOISE	Significant difficulty	Significant to mild difficulty	Mild to significant difficulty
SPEECH AND LANGUAGE	Delayed, considering developmental, chronological and/or hearing age. (Praveena & Prakesh, 2014; Raveh, Buller, Badrana, & Attias, 2007)	Approaching, or at expected levels considering developmental, chronological, and/or hearing age. (Rance et al., 2007; Raveh et al., 2007)	At expected levels considering developmental, chronological and/or hearing age (Berlin et al., 2010)

PRESENTATION IV	PRESENTATION V	PRESENTATION VI
Normal hearing sensitivity range	Hearing thresholds "recover" or improve significantly (e.g., transient ANSD) from previously obtained thresholds that were in hearing loss range Reverse slope common	Can vary from mild to profound Reverse slope common Can also • fluctuate • be progressive
Good	As expected given the audiogram and then either: • Improves • Remains the same	Can fluctuate upon changes in body temperature (temperature-sensitive ANSD)
Mild to significant difficulty	Mild to significant difficulty	Mild to significant difficulty
At expected levels considering developmental and/or chronological age (Berlin et al., 2010; Raveh et al., 2007)	Delayed, or at expected levels considering developmental, chronological, and/or hearing age (Psarommatis et al., 2006)	Delayed, or at expected levels considering developmental, chronological and/or hearing age. (Varga et al., 2006)

In both AVT and ALE, the parent(s) are actively involved in every session, and the AV practitioner ensures that parent(s) receive accurate and current information on ANSD and its impact on their child's listening and spoken language development. Parents need to have a clear understanding of the long-term goals and short-term objectives that have been set for a specific time frame. All practitioners on child and family's intervention team need to be consistent when presenting information about ANSD and the management required; conflicting expert opinions have been identified as a barrier to early and appropriate management (Uus & Young, 2015).

In both AVT and ALE, the AV practitioner will do the following:

- Observe the child's auditory functioning if the child is not wearing hearing technology.
- Check the child's hearing health if auditory functioning is poor and progress is limited.
- Consider hearing aids if hearing health is good.
- Observe auditory performance with hearing aids and without hearing aids. If the child performs better with hearing aid(s), then the continued use of hearing aids is monitored.
- Watch for behaviors such as pulling out hearing aids and fluctuating auditory functioning, that is associated with body temperature-sensitive ANSD (Varga et al., 2006) and transient ANSD (Eom, Min, Lee, & Lee, 2013; Psarommatis et al., 2006).

- Recommend regular follow-up visits with the audiologist to monitor hearing abilities (Chandan & Prabhu, 2015).
- Consider cochlear implant candidacy evaluation if there is limited progress in listening and spoken language skills and if there is poor aided speech perception with appropriately fit hearing aids.
- Refer the child and his/her family to an intervention approach that uses visual cues or sign language if CI(s) are not an option or if the child who is implanted makes limited progress.

When CI candidacy is being evaluated, the AV practitioner and audiologist on the CI team consider the child's auditory functioning in quiet and in noise, the child's ability to develop spoken language through listening at a suitable rate, and the impact of ANSD on the child's overall listening, communication, and daily living skills. The AV practitioner's report on the child's current skills in areas of audition, speech, language, cognition, and communication carries significant weight when determining the child's candidacy for cochlear implantation. (See Chapter 6.)

Outcomes for Children With ANSD

Hearing aids and cochlear implants are options for children with ANSD. Hearing aids have been beneficial for 30% (Berlin et al., 2010) to 50% (Rance, Cone-Wesson, Wunderlich, & Dowell, 2002) of this population. Cochlear implants can be considered if children with ANSD do not receive adequate benefit from appropriately fitted hearing aids (Fernandes et al., 2015; Kontorinis et al., 2014; Liu et al., 2014). The expected outcomes of early cochlear implantation (Cardon & Sharma, 2013; Liu et al., 2010) for children with ANSD, excluding children with cochlear nerve deficiency, are similar to children with sensorineural hearing loss who do not have ANSD (Breneman et al., 2012; Rance & Barker, 2009; Teagle et al., 2010). During the last decade, AVT has gained wider acceptance as a viable option for children with ANSD if listening and spoken language is the desired outcome (Estabrooks et al., 2014; Praveena & Prakesh, 2014).

COCHLEAR NERVE DEFICIENCY/ UNDERDEVELOPED AUDITORY NERVE

Sound transmitted to the middle ear is transformed into energy by the ossicles (bones) in the middle ear and sent to the fluid-filled cochlea, which houses the inner and outer hair cells. With the movement of the fluid in the cochlea, the stereocilia on top of the hair cells bend (shear) briefly, changing the electrochemical composition of the hair cells. This change signals a neural response to the auditory neurons that form the auditory nerve and continues to send neural impulses to the brainstem (Musiek & Baran, 2007).

Children with cochlear nerve deficiency, or an underdeveloped or absent auditory nerve, however, may not have the same type of neural transmission as children with typical hearing. Magnetic resonance imaging studies (MRIs) have shown that cochlear nerve deficiency is associated with a narrower opening in the internal auditory canal (a bony tunnel through which the auditory nerve travels) that creates a narrow space for the auditory nerve to develop (Glastonbury et al., 2002). Cochlear nerve deficiency can be unilateral or bilateral. In fact, the most common etiology of congenital unilateral single-sided deafness is cochlear nerve deficiency (Clemmens, Germiller, & Cohn, 2012; Glastonbury et al., 2002). Cochlear implantation and hearing aid technology have been options for some of these children, but the auditory and spoken language outcomes can be variable because there are fewer neural fibers transmitting information to the brain and thus there is variable auditory preservation (Colletti, Colletti, Mandalà, & Colletti, 2014; Zhang et al., 2012) which affects overall speech perception.

Auditory brain implants (ABI) are also used by these children. The electrode array for the ABI is placed on the cochlear nuclei a cluster of neurons in the brainstem (Schwartz, Otto, Shannon, Hitselberger, & Brackmann, 2008). Approximately 6 to 8 weeks following this surgery, the external devices are programmed in a manner that is similar to that of cochlear implants (Schwartz et al., 2008). The auditory outcomes of wearers of ABIs have shown variability in open-set recognition (Fayad, Otto, Shannon, & Brackmann, 2008), but open-set conversational skills have been observed in pediatric ABI recipients. Colletti, Shannon, and Colletti (2014) found that the highest performing children in their study sample were able to converse on the telephone, and that all the children continued to make progress in auditory skills over the duration of their project, although the amount of progress made was also variable.

Implications of Cochlear Nerve Deficiency/ Underdeveloped Nerve for Auditory-Verbal Therapy

Children with cochlear nerve deficiency/ underdeveloped auditory nerves are at risk for having additional challenges/ disabilities and medical conditions (e.g., CHARGE, Goldenhar syndrome, VATER syndrome, etc.) (Adunka, Jewells, & Buchman, 2007), which may affect learning and/or interfere with their ability to develop spoken communication. Therefore, it is important that the AV practitioner work together with the parent(s) to facilitate timely referrals and collaboration with other allied health professionals to address these challenges so that learning opportunities are maximized.

AV practitioners who work with the child with insufficient auditory nerve and his or her family need to be cautious about predicting outcomes in listening and spoken language development because the research shows that outcomes are uncertain for this particular group of children. Recognizing that there is a critical period for the development of communication for social and academic success (Cardon & Sharma, 2014; Liu et al., 2014), the CI team may

recommend that the family also receive sign language instruction in addition to *auditory-based intervention*. In these cases, the AV practitioner would provide Auditory Skills Training (AST). AST is the application of techniques, strategies, conditions, and procedures that promote the optimal acquisition of listening skills so that the child's auditory potential with hearing technology can be maximized. Through active participation in each therapy session, the parent(s) learns to help his or her child develop skills in audition only. This type of intervention is typically offered (by one of the authors) to children who who are learning to use sign-language as a mode of communication and who wish to maximize their newly acquired auditory potential.

If a child with cochlear nerve deficiency/underdeveloped auditory nerve is receiving AVT or AST, it is critical that the AV practitioner collaborate closely with parent(s) and the CI team in setting clear goals and determining what would be an appropriate diagnostic period to determine whether AVT or AST is meeting the needs of the child and family. Continuing AVT or AST when the child is making limited gains in the development of listening and/or spoken language skills, in the absence of sign language or any other visual mode of communication, is unethical. Therefore, the AV practitioner typically engages in conversation with the family about the potential need to transition to another intervention program that focuses on additional visual and/or tactile cues or sign language, so that the child can reach his or her highest communication potential.

CONCLUSION

Most children with complex hearing issues can develop spoken language with the guidance of the AV practitioner. Continued knowledge and research focusing on the areas of single-sided deafness, underdeveloped auditory nerve, ANSD, and cochlear implant revision surgery provide the AV practitioner and families with the understanding of *how* children who present with one of these conditions, perceive and develop understanding of spoken language. Because of the unique complexities of the four different challenges described here, there are a variety of ways the AV practitioner can guide families toward the best possible outcomes.

REFERENCES

Adunka, O.A., Jewells, V., & Buchman, C.A. (2007). Value of computed tomography in the evaluation of children with cochlear nerve deficiency. *Otology and Neurotology, 28*, 597–604.

Berlin, C., Conc-Wesson, B., Roush, P., Rance, G., Shallop, J., Sinninger, Y., & Starr, A. (2008). Presentations and panel discussions at NHS Newborn Hearing Screening Conference, Lake Como, Italy —AN/AD Guideline Developments.

Berlin, C., Hood, L. J., Theirry, M., Wiensky, D., Li, L., Matingly, K. R., . . . Frisch, S. A. (2010). Multi-site diagnosis and management of 260 patients with Auditory Neuropathy/Dys-synchrony (Auditory Neuropathy Spectrum Disorder). *International Journal of Audiology, 49*(1), 30–43.

Breneman, A., Gifford, R., & DeJong, M. (2012). Cochlear implantation in children with auditory neuropathy spectrum disorder: Long-term outcomes. *Journal of the American Academy of Audiology, 23*(1), 5–17.

Buchman, C. A., Roush, P. A., Teagle, H. F. B., & Zdanski, C. (2009). Clinical management of children with auditory neuropathy. In L. S. Eisenberg (Ed.), *Clinical management of children with cochlear implants*. San Diego, CA: Plural.

Cardon, G., Campbell, J., & Sharma, A. (2012). Plasticity in the developing auditory cortex: Evidence from children with sensorineural hearing loss and auditory neuropathy spectrum disorder. *Journal of the American Academy of Audiology, 23*(6), 396-411.

Cardon, G., & Sharma, A. (2013). Central auditory maturation and behavioral outcome in children with auditory neuropathy spectrum disorder who use cochlear implants. *International Journal of Audiology, 52*(9), 577–586.

Chandan, H. S., & Prabhu, P. (2015). Audiological changes over time in adolescents and young adults with auditory neuropathy spectrum disorder. *European Archives of Oto-Rhino-Laryngology, 272*(7), 1801–1807.

Chermak, G., & Musiek, F. (2007). *Handbook of (central) auditory processing disorder: Comprehensive intervention* (Vol. II). San Diego, CA: Plural.

Ching, T. Y., Day, J., Dillon, H., Gardner-Berry, K., Hou, S., Seeto, M., & Zhang, V. (2013). Impact of the presence of auditory neuropathy spectrum disorder (ANSD) on outcomes of children at three years of age. *International Journal of Audiology, 52*(S2).

Christensen, L., Richter, G. T., & Dornhoffer, J. L. (2010). Update on bone-anchored hearing aids in pediatric patients with profound unilateral sensorineural hearing loss. *Archives of Otolaryngology-Head and Neck Surgery, 136*(2), 175.

Chung, D., Kim, A. H., Parisier, S., Linstrom, C., Alexiades, G., Hoffman, R., & Kohan, D. (2010). Revision cochlear implant surgery in patients with suspected soft failures. *Otology & Neurotology, 31*(8), 1194–1198.

Clark, J. H., & Stewart, C. M. (2014). Osseointegration and its role in management of hearing loss. *Operative Techniques in Otolaryngology-Head and Neck Surgery, 25*(4), 333–337.

Clemmens, C. S., Germiller, J. A., & Cohn, S. (2012). Cochlear nerve deficiency: Prevalence and audiologic features. *Otolaryngology-Head and Neck Surgery, 147*(Suppl. 2).

Colletti, L., Colletti, G., Mandala, M., & Colletti, V. (2014). The therapeutic dilemma of cochlear nerve deficiency: Cochlear or brainstem implantation? Otolaryngology-Head and Neck Surgery, 151(2), 308–314.

Colletti, L., Shannon, R. V., & Colletti, V. (2014). The development of auditory perception in children after auditory brainstem implantation. *Audiology and Neurotology, 19*(6), 386–394.

Cullen, R. D., Fayad, J. N., Luxford, W. M., & Buchman, C. A. (2008). Revision cochlear implant surgery in children. *Otology & Neurotology, 29*(2), 214–220.

Davis, A., Reeve, K., Hind, S., Bamford, J., Seewald, R., & Gravel, J. (2001). Children with mild and unilateral hearing impairment. *A Sound Foundation Through Early Amplification, 4*, 179–186.

Eom, J. H., Min, H. J., Lee, S. H., & Lee, H. K. (2013). A case of auditory neuropathy with recovery of normal hearing. *Korean Journal of Audiology, 17*(3), 138.

Estabrooks, W., MacIver-Lux, K., & Houston, K. T. (2014). In S. Waltzman & T. Roland (Eds.), *Therapeutic approaches following cochlear implantation in cochlear implants* (3rd ed.). New York, NY: Thieme.

Fayad, J. N., Otto, S. R., Shannon, R. V., & Brackmann, D. E. (2008). Cochlear and brainstem auditory prostheses. Neural interface for hearing restoration: Cochlear and brain stem implants. *Proceedings-IEEE, 96*(7), 1085.

Glastonbury, C. M., Davidson, H. C., Harnsberger, H. R., Butler, J., Kertesz, T. R., & Shelton, C. (2002). Imaging findings of cochlear nerve deficiency. *American Journal of Neuroradiology, 23*(4), 635–643.

Glista, D., Scollie, S., Moodie, S., & Easwar, V. (2014). The Ling 6 (HL) Test: Typical pediatric performance data and clinical use evaluation. *Journal of the American Academy of Audiology, 25*(10), 1008–1021.

Hassepass, F., Aschendorff, A., Wesarg, T., Kröger, S., Laszig, R., Beck, R. L., & Arndt, S. (2013). Unilateral deafness in children: Audiologic and subjective assessment of hearing ability after cochlear implantation. *Otology and Neurotology, 34*(1), 53–60.

Hayes, D., & Sininger, Y. (n.d.). *Auditory neuropathy spectrum disorder (ANSD) guidelines*. Retrieved April 23, 2009, from http://www.thechildrenshospital.or/conditions/speech/danielscenter/ANSD-Guidelines.aspx

Johnstone, P. M., Náblek, A. K., & Robertson, V. S. (2010). Sound localization acuity in children with unilateral hearing loss who wear a hearing aid in the impaired ear. *Journal of the American Academy of Audiology, 21*(8), 522–534.

Kerber, I. S., & Seeber, I. B. U. (2012). Sound localization in noise by normal-hearing listeners and cochlear implant users. *Ear and Hearing, 33*(4), 445.

Kirkim, G., Serbetcioglu, B., Erdag, T. K., & Ceryan, K. (2008). The frequency of auditory neuropathy detected by universal newborn hearing screening program. *International Journal of Pediatric Otorhinolaryngology, 72*(10), 1461–1469.

Kontorinis, G., Lloyd, S. K., Henderson, L., Jayewardene-Aston, D., Milward, K., Bruce, I. A., . . . Freeman, S. R. (2014). Cochlear implantation in children with auditory neuropathy spectrum disorders. *Cochlear Implants International, 15*(S1).

Kral, A., Hubka, P., Heid, S., & Tillein, J. (2012). Single-sided deafness leads to unilateral aural preference within an early sensitive period. *Brain.* http://dx .doi.org/10.1093/brain/aws305

Lassig, A. A., Zwolan, T. A., & Telian, S. A. (2005). Cochlear implant failures and revision. *Otology & Neurotology 26,* 624–634.

Lepcha, A., Chandran, R. K., Alexander, M., Agustine, A. M., Thenmozhi, K., & Balraj, A. (2015). Neurological associations in auditory neuropathy spectrum disorder: Results from a tertiary hospital in South India. *Annals of Indian Academy of Neurology, 18*(2), 171–180.

Lieu, J. E. C. (2004). Speech-language and educational consequences of unilateral hearing loss in children. *Archives of Otolaryngology-Head and Neck Surgery, 130*(5), 524–530.

Lieu, J. E. C. (2013). Unilateral hearing loss in children: Speech-language and school performance. *B-ENT,* (Suppl. 21), 107–115.

Lieu, J. E., Tye-Murray, N., Karzon, R. K., & Piccirillo, J. F. (2010). Unilateral hearing loss is associated with worse speech-language scores in children. *Pediatrics, 125*(6), e1348–e1355.

Ling, D. (2012). The Six-Sounds Test and why is it so important in auditory-verbal therapy and education? In W. Estabrooks (Ed.), *101 FAQs about auditory-verbal practice.* Washington, DC: A.G. Bell Association for the Deaf.

Litovsky, R., Parkinson, A., Arcaroli, J., & Sammeth, C. (2006). Simultaneous bilateral cochlear implantation in adults: A multicenter clinical study. *Ear and Hearing, 27*(6), 714–731.

Liu, Y., Dong, R., Li, Y., Xu, T., Li, Y., Chen, X., & Gong, S. (2014). Effective of age on auditory and speech development of children with auditory neuropathy disorder. *Auris Nasus Larynx, 41*(6), 502–506.

Madden, C., Rutter, M., Hilbert, L., Greinwald, J. H., & Choo, D. I. (2002). Clinical and audiological features in auditory neuropathy. *Archives of Otolaryngology-Head and Neck Surgery, 128*(9), 1026–1030.

McKay, S., Gravel, J. S., & Tharpe, A. M. (2008). Amplification considerations for children with minimal or mild bilateral hearing loss and unilateral hearing loss. *Trends in Amplification, 12*(1), 43–54.

Mittal, R., Ramesh, A., Panwar, S., Nilkanthan, A., Nair, S., & Mehra, P. R. (2012). Auditory neuropathy spectrum disorder: Its prevalence and audiological characteristics in an Indian tertiary care hospital. *International Journal of Pediatric Otorhinolaryngology, 76*(9), 1351–1354.

Mohammadi, A., Walker, P., & Gardner-Berry, K. (2014). Unilateral auditory neuropathy spectrum disorder: Retrocochlear lesion in disguise? *The Journal of Laryngology & Otology, 129*(S1).

Musiek, F. E., & Baran, J. A. (2007). *The auditory system: Anatomy, physiology and clinical correlates.* Boston, MA: Pearson.

Nash, R., Veness, J., Wyatt, M., Raglan, E., & Rajput, K. (2014). Vestibular function in children with auditory neuropathy spectrum disorder. *International Journal of Pediatric Otorhinolaryngology, 78*(8), 1269–1273.

Nittrouer, S., Caldwell-Tarr, A., Tarr, E., Lowenstein, J. H., Rice, C., & Moberly, A. C. (2013). Improving speech-in-noise recognition for children with hearing loss: Potential effects of language abilities, binaural summation, and head shadow. *International Journal of Audiology, 52*(8), 513–525.

Parisier, S. C., Chute, P. M., Popp, A. L., & Suh, G. D. (2001). Outcome analysis of cochlear implant reimplantation in children. *Laryngoscope, 111*(1), 26–32.

Peele, J. E., Troaiani, V., Grossman, M., & Wingfield, A. (2011). Hearing loss in older adults affects neural systems supporting speech comprehension. *Journal of Neuroscience, 31*(35), 12638–12643.

Praveena, J., Prakash, H., & Rukmangathan, T. M. (2014). Original research. *The Hearing Journal, 67*(11), 29.

Psarommatis, J., Riga, M., Douros, K., Koltsidopoulos, P., Douniadakis, D., Kapetanakis, J., & Apostolopoulos, N. (2006). Transient infantile auditory neuropathy and its clinical implications. *International Journal of Pediatric Otorhinolaryngology, 72,* 121–126.

Rance. G. (2005). Auditory neuropathy/dys-synchrony and its perceptual consequences. *Trends in Amplification, 9*(1), 1–43.

Rance, G., & Barker, E. J. (2007). Speech perception in children with auditory neuropathy/dyssynchrony managed with either hearing aids or cochlear implants. *Otology and Neurotology. 29*(2), 179–182.

Rance, G., Barker, E., Mok, M., Dowell, R., Rincon, A., & Garratt, R. (2007). Speech perception in noise for children with auditory neuropathy/dys-synchrony type hearing loss. *Ear and Hearing, 3,* 351–360.

Rance, G., Cone-Wesson, B., Wunderlich, J., & Dowell, R. (2002). Speech perception and cortical event related potentials in children with auditory neuropathy. *Ear and Hearing, 23*(3), 239–253.

Raveh, E., Buller, N., Badrana, O., & Attias, J. (2007). Auditory neuropathy: Clinical characteristics and therapeutic approach. *American Journal of Otolaryngology, 28*(5), 302–308.

Roush, P. (2008) Auditory neuropathy spectrum disorder: Evaluation and management. *Pediatric Amplification Hearing Journal, 61*(11), 38–41.

Roush, P., Frymark, T., Venediktov, R., & Wang, B. (2011). Audiologic management of auditory neuropathy spectrum disorder in children: A systematic review of the literature. *American Journal of Audiology, 20*(2), 159–170.

Saliba, I., Woods, O., & Caron, C. (2010). BAHA results in children at one year follow-up: A prospective longitudinal study. *International Journal of Pediatric Otorhinolaryngology, 74*(9), 1058–1062.

Schwartz, M. S., Otto, S. R., Shannon, R. V., Hitselberger, W. E., & Brackmann, D. E. (2008). Auditory brainstem implants. *Neurotherapeutics, 5*(1), 128–136.

Sharma, A., & Cardon, G. (2014). Developmental Plasticity of the Central Auditory System. *Development of Auditory and Vestibular Systems,* 315-337.

Talaat, H. S., Kabel, A. H., Samy, H., & Elbadry, M. (2009). Prevalence of auditory neuropathy (AN) among infants and young children with severe to profound hearing loss. *International Journal of Pediatric Otorhinolaryngology, 73*(7), 937–939.

Teagle, H.F.B., Rousch, P.A., Woodard, J.S., Hatch, D.R., Zdanski, Charloton J., . . . Buchman, C.A. (2010). Cochlear implantation in children with auditory nueropathy spectrum disorder. *Ear and Hearing, 31*(3), 325–335.

Uus, K., Young, A., & Day, M. (2015). Parents' perspectives on the dilemmas with intervention for infants with auditory neuropathy spectrum disorder: A qualitative study. *International Journal of Audiology, 54*(8), 552–558.

Varga, R. A., Kelley, M. R., Keats, B. J., Berlin, C. I., Hood, L. J., Morlet, T. G., . . . Kimberling, W. J. (2006). OTOF mutations revealed by genetic analysis of hearing loss families including a potential temperature sensitive auditory neuropathy allele. *Journal of Medical Genetics, 43,* 576–581.

Wang, S., Dong, R., Liu, D., Wang, Y., Liu, B., Zhang, L., & Xu, L. (2015). The role of temporal envelope and fine structure in mandarin lexical tone perception in auditory neuropathy spectrum disorder. *PLoS ONE, 10*(6), e0129710.

Wiig, E. H., & Semel, E. M., & Secord, W. (2006). *CELF preschool 2 Australian* (2nd ed. Australian standardised ed.). Sydney, NSW: Pearson.

Zeitler, D.M., Budenz, C. L. & Roland, J.T. Jr. (2009). Revision cochlear implantation. *Otolaryngology-Head and Neck Surgery, 15*(5), 334–338.

Zeng, F. G., & Liu, S. (2006). Speech perception in individuals with auditory neuropathy. *Journal of Speech, Language, and Hearing Research, 49*, 367–380.

Zhang, Z., Li, Y., Hu, L., Wang, Z., Huang, Q., & Wu, H. (2012). Cochlear implantation in children with cochlear nerve deficiency: A report of nine cases. *International Journal of Pediatric Otorhinolaryngology, 76*(8), 1188–1195.

Zimmerman, I. L., Pond, R. E., Steiner, V. G., Pearson Education, Inc., & Psych-Corp (Firm). (2013). *PLS-5: Preschool Language Scales: Screening test.*

Zong, L., Guan, J., Ealy, M., Zhang, Q., Wang, D., Wang, H., . . . Wang, Q. (2015). Mutations in apoptosis-inducing factor cause X-linked recessive auditory neuropathy spectrum disorder. *Journal of Medical Genetics, 52*(8), 523-531.

15

INCLUSION AT SCHOOL AND AUDITORY-VERBAL THERAPY

Ellen A. Rhoades, Karen MacIver-Lux,
and Stacey R. Lim

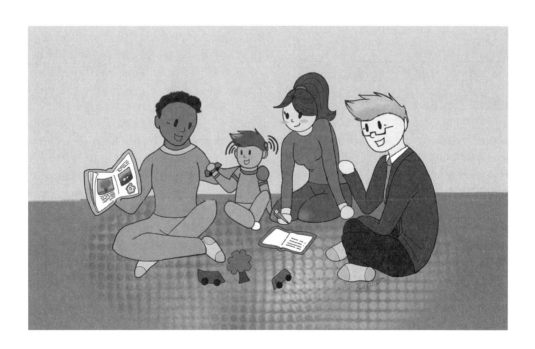

INTRODUCTION

Children with hearing loss can achieve impressive educational outcomes in large part because of early identification and hearing technology coupled with the Auditory-Verbal Therapy (AVT). As one of ten guiding principles of listening and spoken language specialist (LSLS) AVT, education in regular schools, beginning at the preschool level with typically developing peers distinguishes AV practice from other early intervention models for children with hearing loss and their families. The overwhelming majority of preschool children who "graduate" from AVT tend to be educated in regular elementary and secondary schools (Goldberg & Flexer, 2001).

FROM MAINSTREAMING TO INCLUSION

Mainstreaming usually refers to the physical placement of a child with special needs in regular classrooms with typically developing children. A change in terminology cultivated the widespread use of "inclusion" to replace mainstreaming. *Inclusion* is a broader term referring to a more complex process that involves the implementation of accommodations for adapting to each child's needs within the regular classroom (Armstrong, Armstrong, & Spandagou, 2011). The intent of *full inclusion* is to ensure that children with hearing loss become full and active participants in regular classrooms, in general school environments, and in the larger societal system.

EVIDENCE FOR EARLY AND FULL INCLUSION

Research findings show that (a) children in full-day preschools make faster rates of progress in spoken language, reading, and math than do those in half-day programs (Chang & Singh, 2008; Reynolds et al., 2014); (b) children enrolled in day care programs seem to benefit from a wider variety of social and communicative situations relative to children who do not attend day care programs (Stolk, Hunnius, & Bekkering, 2013); (c) young children with communication delays (irrespective of hearing status) can benefit more from full inclusion classrooms than do those in special groups for children with communication delays or hearing loss (Laws, Bates, Feuerstein, Mason-Apps, & White, 2012); and (d) early placement in regular preschool classrooms is one of many predictors of good auditory performance among school-aged children with hearing loss (Wang, Liu, Liu, Huang, & Kuo, 2011). Since the advent of Universal Newborn Hearing Screening, children who are identified with hearing loss and who are enrolled in family-centered early intervention programs show good progress across all developmental domains, including auditory and language development.

High-quality regular preschools positively support children's developmental outcomes (Weiland & Yoshikawa, 2013). It is therefore necessary that parents and AV practitioners recognize some of the high-quality preschools summarized as follows:

Classroom Materials:

- Variety of well-organized high-interest children's books

- Variety of writing implements
- Variety of games and toys, e.g., puzzles, blocks
- Above materials are easily accessible to children
- Variety of printed items on walls, e.g., calendars, posters

Classroom Structure and Composition:

- Established daily routines
- Time-based schedule
- Low child-to-staff ratios

Classrooms with fewer children are associated with more attention given to students and more rapid student learning (Brühwiler & Blatchford, 2010; Galton & Pell, 2012). Regardless of hearing status, young children can learn simply by watching and listening to people around them; they show an intuitive understanding of mathematical probability, engaging in statistical learning and pattern-making (Waismeyer, Meltzoff, & Gopnik, 2015). The importance of young children participating in AVT while simultaneously benefiting from play groups, daycare, or preschool programs with typically hearing peers cannot be underestimated.

SOCIAL INCLUSION AND FULL INCLUSION

Social inclusion, sometimes referred to as social connectedness, is the social dimension of full inclusion (Koster, Nakken, Pijl, & van Houten 2009). This occurs when children with hearing loss fully participate in both classroom and general school environment. It is critical that children with hearing loss have a sense of belonging with typically hearing peers. Interpersonal skills that

children are expected to learn while preschoolers are as follows:

- Listens to others, engaging in conversational turn-taking
- Engages in social reciprocity such as turn-taking, sharing, cooperative play
- Appropriately asks and answers questions of interest to peers
- Stays on topic when the subject is of interest to peers
- Demonstrates verbal negotiation and clarification skills
- Begins to use some conversational repair strategies

The better the child's language skills, the more likely social inclusion will occur (Most, Ingber, & Heled-Ariam, 2012). It is helpful when parents, teachers, and AV practitioners can offer children with hearing loss a comprehensive and systematic intervention program to address issues relevant to peer-related social competence.

Social skills may need to be explicitly taught in conjunction with listening and spoken language instruction, and opportunities for social interactions with peers should be provided during the preschool years. For example, the AV practitioner and the parent may model effective social interactions during role-play with toy props, or parents may enroll their children in preschool, play, art, dance, or sport programs with typically hearing peers.

By the time children usually enter first grade, they have a sense of self-esteem comparable in strength to that of adults (Cvencek, Greenwald, & Meltzoff, 2016). How they feel about themselves is a fundamental mindset that tends to be fairly stable across the life span (Orth & Robins, 2014). High self-esteem is a predictor of success in learning, relationships, work, and health (Orth & Robins, 2014). The practitioner, therefore, strives to promote and strengthen the social skills of children with hearing loss (Warner-Czyz, Loy, Evans, Wetsel, & Tobey, 2015). High self-esteem and age-appropriate social skills supported by listening and spoken language skills are imperative for successful social inclusion in regular schools (Martin, Bat-Chava, Lalwani, & Waltzman, 2011).

PREPARING FOR FULL INCLUSION

Although requisite skills differ according to age range (see Chapter 8) and grade level, there are certain conditions that facilitate full inclusion across preschool and grade school. All of the following factors are considered important contributors to successful inclusion.

The Teacher's Attitudes

Just as children and their families affect teacher expectations (deBoer, Bosker, & van der Werf, 2010), the teacher's set of beliefs affects the inclusion process and long-term child outcomes (Jussim & Harber, 2005). A teacher's attitude is the most critical factor in successful inclusion (Ben Yehuda, Leyser, & Last, 2010). Beyond attitude, other teacher characteristics that facilitate learning for children with hearing loss are as follows:

- speaks at appropriate volume and enunciates clearly;

- uses varied and increasingly complex vocabulary;
- has frequent conversations with children;
- asks open-ended questions and waits for children to respond;
- provides positive feedback to children;
- demonstrates an attitude that is motivating, even when mistakes are made;
- effectively manages children's behaviors;
- encourages children to share and engage in cooperative play;
- encourages children to problem solve; and
- maintains an open communicative relationship with parents.

Parents and AV practitioners, prior to placing a child in the classroom, informally evaluate the teacher's willingness, motivation, flexibility, and sensitivity in facilitating learning opportunities for children with hearing loss (Sari, 2007). AV practitioners recognize that teachers need informational support regarding hearing loss as well as instructional and environmental accommodations to facilitate optimal learning for the child with hearing loss.

The Child's Readiness Skills

School readiness begins with skills that are acquired across the first two to three years of life, particularly during play-based activities and daily routines. It is essential that caregivers, playgroups, and child care programs for infants and toddlers provide nurturing and active learning environments (Gray et al., 2015). Throughout early childhood, children are encouraged to participate in activities with typically developing peers. Acquisition of foundational readiness skills will increase children's academic success as they transition from one educational environment to the next.

It is helpful when parents and AV practitioners know the expected social skills for preschool, kindergarten, and first grade. Language-based math skills often expected by first grade teachers (Kritzer, 2009) include the ability to:

- solve simple story problems in real-world contexts;
- rote and skip count (counting by twos, threes, etc.);
- make number comparisons;
- read and write two- to three-digit numbers;
- add and subtract numbers;
- label, compare, define, and classify characteristics (shapes, sizes, etc.);
- recognize quantitative relationships (part-whole, patterns, etc.); and
- understand that routines tend to occur at certain times.

Social skills often expected by first grade teachers (Lane, Pierson, Stang, & Carter, 2010) include the following:

- uses time appropriately while waiting for help from teacher,
- controls temper in conflict situations with teacher and peers,
- follows and complies with teacher directions,
- attends to teacher instructions and arrives to class on time,
- exerts self-control when pushed or hit by peers,

- asserts self to make instructional needs known,
- ignores peer distractions when doing class work,
- easily makes transition from one classroom activity to another, and
- gets along with people who are different.

These skills are above and beyond the basic self-help skills expected by all kindergarten teachers, such as removing and storing clothes or preparing and serving snacks. The skills in these two lists do not include either literacy skills or spoken language skills because those skills are presented in Chapter 8.

The Child's Linguistic Competence

Linguistic competence is attained when the child demonstrates knowledge of formal language patterns and there is requisite grammatical knowledge for day-to-day communication (see Chapter 8). Linguistic competence is one of many factors that plays a critical role in academic success and social inclusion (Brown, Bortoli, Remine, & Othman, 2008) and is considered one of the important long-term goals of AV practitioners and parents of young children with hearing loss. Ideally, linguistic competence is attained prior to entering first grade, so that the child can follow the teacher's directions, keep up with peer conversations, and understand the printed language during the process of learning how to read. The foundations of linguistic competence are developed prior to school entry, but additional factors in the school environment are critical for the child's continued academic, language, social, and linguistic growth. These factors include the child's auditory access, a good listening environment, effective classroom management, as well as others described in the following sections.

The Child's Auditory Access

Auditory access refers to the child's ability to clearly hear spoken language (see Chapter 2). For children with hearing loss, acoustic accessibility occurs primarily with hearing technology and environmental accommodations. If children are unable to access the verbal message, learning is negatively impacted (DeConde Johnson et al., 2014). Therefore, the AV practitioner and parent secure the support of the child's audiologist and/or educational audiologist so that optimal access to auditory information across all learning environments is provided.

Roles and Responsibilities

The culture of inclusion entails consultation, cooperation, and collaboration between parents, AV practitioners, preschool, kindergarten, and general classroom teachers, administrators, hearing resource teachers, educational audiologists, and other appropriate school personnel. Innovation and flexibility among all involved adults are key ingredients within a successful inclusive environment. Every effort is made to support each child with hearing loss and teacher. See Chapter 16 for a more detailed description of the partnerships that are formed with vari-

ous members of the early intervention and early education team to maximize the child's listening, spoken language, and academic potential.

Parents

Parents are the key stakeholders in their children's future, so they typically act as liaison between teachers and other members of the intervention and educational support team. Parents ensure that open communication is consistent so that they can monitor and manage their child's hearing and educational access in the classroom and address any queries the teacher may have.

AV Practitioner

The AV practitioner provides the teacher with a report of the child's skills in areas of audition, speech, receptive and expressive language, and academic readiness. This information will assist the teacher in creating an Individual Family Service Plan (IFSP) or Individualized Education Plan (IEP) and in identifying which instructional accommodations may be necessary for the child with hearing loss. An IFSP (0–3 years) and an IEP (elementary through secondary grade students) refers to a written treatment plan for special services developed by parents and practitioners as well as other school personnel.

Hearing Resource Teacher

Hearing resource teachers, sometimes referred to as itinerant or peripatetic teachers, have received additional training in the education of children with hearing loss. Their services may or may not be used during the child's preschool and primary grade years. Hearing resource teachers provide support, as needed, in the development of auditory, speech, language, academic, and social skills. They also maintain the child's hearing technology, serving as liaison between teachers, AV practitioners, and other school support personnel as well as parents. Depending on the child's current skills, needs, and preferences, the hearing resource teacher may employ a "push-in" (provision of support to the child with hearing loss within the classroom) or a "pull-out" (provision of support to the child outside the classroom) model.

Educational Audiologist

The educational audiologist attempts to ensure that the child with hearing loss has optimal and consistent auditory access in the school. Aside from acoustic accommodations, the educational audiologist selects, fits, monitors, and maintains the child's hearing assistive technology (see Chapter 7). The educational audiologist also collaborates with the teacher, AV practitioner, and parents in developing an IFSP or IEP.

Challenges to Inclusion

Not all children are ready for kindergarten or first grade at the same time. The children "not yet ready" for full inclusion tend to be those not yet demonstrating linguistic or social competence. Linguistic competence plays a critical role in academic success and social inclusion (Brown et al., 2008). AV practitioners may advise parents to postpone entry to grade school if their

child does not demonstrate either linguistic competency or age-appropriate social skills (Mühlenweg, Blomeyer, Stichnoth, & Laucht, 2012).

Among the many factors to be considered are maturational or developmental levels, ages of identification and acoustic access, and learning differences. Just as each child is unique, so their challenges may also be unique. For different reasons, some children may benefit more from partially inclusive classrooms that include children with hearing loss as well as children with typical hearing (Wauters & Knoor, 2008). The AV practitioner is flexible in identifying and managing those challenges.

The Child With Additional Special Needs

AV practitioners are often uniquely able to tease out auditory learning due to peripheral hearing loss from other learning challenges. When a child with hearing loss is suspected of having difficulties in demonstrating goal-directed problem solving skills, referral for a developmental or neuropsychological assessment is appropriate.

Some children with hearing loss are identified as having sensory motor differences (Cushing, Chia, James, Papsin, & Gordon, 2008). Auditory deprivation has been identified as a cause of delays in the development of specific motor and language skills (Horn, Fagan, Dillon, Pisoni, & Miyamoto, 2007), thus referrals to appropriate pediatric occupational therapists and/or physical therapists for sensory motor dysfunction may be in order. Based on assessment findings, AV practitioners modify AVT objectives and strategies as needed, sharing suggestions with teachers.

The Child Who Is Identified Late With Hearing Loss

Some children with hearing loss are identified late for various reasons. These include lack of follow-up after a non-pass result on newborn hearing screening, a progressive or fluctuating hearing loss, and the late identification and management of auditory neuropathy spectrum disorder (ANSD). For obvious reasons, children who are later identified experience greater delays in development of listening and spoken language skills. See Chapter 13 for learning issues pertaining to complex hearing issues that challenge speech perception abilities.

The Child With Late Access to Auditory Information

Late accessibility to appropriate hearing technology that provides access to all the frequencies of soft and conversational level speech or clearer access to temporal aspects of speech (e.g., ANSD), regardless of reason, usually results in delayed language acquisition. For some children, additional support services or accommodations to the curriculum may be required. For other children, partial inclusion or full placement in self-contained classrooms for students with hearing loss may be recommended.

The Child With Developmental Immaturity

In general, children must be 5 years old to be eligible for enrollment in kindergarten. However, developmental differences between a kindergartner who barely qualifies for the state-mandated age requirement, compared to a child nearly a year older, may have negative implications for the younger child (NICHD Early Child Care Research Network, 2007). Age-related achievement gaps, also known as "the birthday effect," are present by the time a child enters kindergarten. Specifically, children who are young for their grade level are at a greater risk of repeating a grade. The youngest kindergarteners are five times more likely to be retained, or held back, compared to the oldest students. Requiring children to repeat a grade can affect their self-esteem and their ability to properly adjust as their peers' progress to the next grade (Huang, 2014). Consequently, it is sometimes suggested to parents that the child with hearing loss and delays in either language or social skills, not enter kindergarten until at least 6 years of age. In the meantime, the practitioner continues to work with parents and/or preschool teacher(s) in providing strategies and conditions that meet the child needs and strengthen the child's communication and social skills across different settings.

MANAGING THE ACOUSTICS OF THE CLASSROOM

Classrooms are noisy environments and present listening challenges for *all* children. Full maturation of the central auditory nervous system is not achieved until children reach late adolescence, and so immature auditory processing skills coupled with poor acoustics in the classroom may cause children to have difficulty attending to the teacher's voice. Children with hearing loss need to expend more energy to understand what was said; otherwise, there is an increased likelihood that some information will be missed. Consequently, some children with hearing loss require some classroom accommodations.

Background Noise

Unoccupied classroom noise has repeatedly been recorded at levels higher than the 30 dBA noise level recommended by the American National Standards Institute (Knecht, Nelson, Whitelaw, & Feth, 2002). Higher levels of background noise can mask critical components of speech, thus degrading speech understanding (Smaldino & Flexer, 2014). Children with hearing loss perform more poorly in noise than children with typical hearing (Lee, Ali, Ziaei, Hansen, & Tobey, 2015). Noise generally comes from children's movements, from traffic outside the room, from other students' voices, and from operational equipment.

Decreasing background noise is one way to provide greater acoustic access. One way to dampen this extraneous noise may include putting tennis balls on the chair and desk legs. Other adaptations include turning off any equipment that is not currently being used, closing windows and doors, or turning off noisy heating, ventilation, air conditioning systems during instructional time or test administration.

Signal-to-Noise Ratio

Signal-to-noise ratio is the relationship between the signal (speaker's voice) and background noise (Smaldino &

Flexer, 2014). Essentially, the more intense or louder the speaker's voice is, when compared to the level of the background noise, the clearer the auditory signal. When the background noise levels are high, the speaker's voice becomes masked by noise, making it harder for the listener to separate the noise from the signal.

Increasing the signal-to-noise ratio involves using such hearing technology such as a wireless remote microphone system that can be used in conjunction with the child's hearing device (see Chapter 7). The teacher wears a transmitter and the receiver is coupled to the child's hearing devices. As the teacher moves around the room, her voice is transmitted directly into the child's microphone at approximately 10 to 15 dB above the level of the noise.

Reverberation

Reverberation is the persistence of sound energy (similar to echo), even when the speaker has ceased speaking, such as what would occur in a gymnasium. Because the sound energy persists and reflects off hard surfaces in the room, the speech signals overlap and interact with each other. Reverberation time refers to the length of time it takes for the reflected sounds to fade away (Klatte, Lachmann, & Meis, 2010). The longer the reverberation time, the higher is the likelihood the teacher's voice will be masked by reverberated speech.

Reducing reverberation time involves modifying the surfaces and layout of the room. This includes putting absorbent materials on hard, reflective surfaces. For example, acoustic tiles can be placed on ceilings, rugs put on linoleum floors, drapes hung over windows, posters and corkboards placed on walls, and books put on shelves.

Distance

Speaker-to-listener distance refers to how far sound energy must travel from the speaker's mouth to the listener's ears. With a greater distance, the intensity (loudness) of speech decreases, due to the loss of speech energy. As a result, some aspects of speech are lost, resulting in poorer speech understanding (Smaldino & Flexer, 2014).

Reducing speaker-to-listener distance often involves arranging classroom seating so the child with hearing loss is seated relatively close to the area where the teacher will do most of his or her speaking and teaching. It may be feasible to offer the child with hearing loss the option of moving around the room for different situations, so that the child's proximity to the primary sound signal is improved. A wireless remote microphone can also be used to reduce speaker-to-listener distance (see Chapter 7).

STRATEGIES FOR INSTRUCTION

When teachers learn as much as they can about hearing loss and spend individual time with the child to gauge the child's listening and spoken communication competence, learning styles and interests, they are better able to incorporate suggested accommodations and strategies that enhance the child's learning opportunities.

Preparatory Strategies

Preparatory strategies involve implementing activities to facilitate peer knowledge and acceptance of the child with hearing loss. These strategies include reading books about children who have hearing loss, encouraging a group project to explore perceptions of hearing loss and simulate degrees of hearing loss with attendant misunderstandings, implementing a buddy system to help peers improve their social skills (Hughett, Kohler, & Raschke, 2011), asking children to speak one at a time and to avoid interrupting each other, referring to visual information prior to having verbal discussions, and reminding children to avoid obstructing their lips or face when talking.

Teaching Strategies

Teaching strategies that enhance auditory access to learning opportunities include consistently using hearing assistive technology every day, ensuring that necklaces are not touching the microphone of the hearing assistive technology, and performing daily listening checks with the hearing assistive technology. Additionally, teachers are advised that the following strategies benefit *all* students in the classroom: repeating or rephrasing questions or answers that peers provide, asking students to repeat instructions, repeating or rephrasing classroom PA announcements, providing lyrics or explaining the lyrics of songs before the song is played or sung, ensuring that movies are open captioned and, if they are not, providing a description of what was heard, ensuring that the teacher is positioned under light or facing the light, permitting the child with hearing loss the flexibility of being seated for optimal acoustic access (e.g., having the teacher's speech accessing the child's better ear/hearing technology), ensuring that the teacher's voice is at a natural volume level and not too loud as it will distort what the child hears, gaining the child's visual attention before speaking, ensuring that the teacher refrains from talking while his or her back is turned to the classroom, repeating new words and phrases often, writing out instructions or preparing outlines to help the child anticipate what's coming next, and asking, "What did you hear?" when checking whether instructions or information was heard correctly.

Some of these strategies may be implemented by the parent or hearing resource teacher (e.g., performing listening checks on hearing assistive technology) and others by the child with hearing loss (e.g., reminding the teacher to wear the microphone of the hearing assistive technology or asking students for repetition). It is essential that the parent, AV practitioner, and teacher encourage the child to take increasingly greater responsibility for his or her auditory access within all listening situations. For example, by grade school entry, it is expected that students will be responsible for carrying their own batteries and for changing the batteries on their own hearing devices.

Self-Advocacy Strategies

Prior to imparting self-advocacy strategies to young children with hearing loss, it is imperative that the AV practitioner and parent help the child embrace basic self-affirmation principles for everyday well-being. The following 10 "rules for everyday living" (Rhoades, 2003) to be shared with young children are

- I am loved.
- I will always help others.
- I am different; different is good.
- Nobody is perfect; nothing is perfect.
- Most people are kind and want to help.
- I will try to learn something new every day.
- When I don't understand, I will ask for help.
- Mistakes are important; they help me to learn.
- If I work hard, I can do anything I want to do.
- Tomorrow will be better; tomorrow belongs to me.

The child must first become secure with the self before learning what to do and what not to do regarding hearing loss.

Beyond self-security, the goal of self-determination is important. The child who is self-determined has a set of attitudes and skills that translate to goal-directed problem solving behavior, otherwise known as executive functioning. Self-determined children with hearing loss who do well in the regular academic environment are those who recognize their own strengths and limitations, and they take control of their own lives (Luckner & Muir, 2002). The process toward self-determination begins in early childhood (Wehmeyer, 2015).

Self-advocacy strategies facilitate self-awareness and self-appraisal of listening and communication skills as well as positive self-perceptions. The

AV practitioner and parent systematically ask questions as to what the child did or did not understand and why the child might have had difficulty following directions or performing tasks. Rather than telling the child what to say or do in difficult situations, the AV practitioner and parent encourage the child to problem solve. By the time children enter first grade, they are expected to manage their own hearing devices, including replacing batteries; they report problems to teachers, parents, and AV practitioner. First-graders are also responsible for reminding teachers to use, as needed, any appropriate hearing assistive and access technology.

MEETING THE CHALLENGES FOR FULL INCLUSION

Children with hearing loss reflect great heterogeneity. Depending on each child's strengths and needs, strategies vary across situations. Some strategies focus on modifying the school or classroom environment, and others focus on improving teacher interactions with children. The greatest challenges have to do with meeting the child's communication needs through AV intervention, and with enabling the child to have best acoustic accessibility across all learning conditions.

The AV practitioner and parent can facilitate progress toward these goals by developing a *strong partnership* with the child's teachers—one that encourages *flexibility* and *creativity* in meeting the child's needs. As the child matures and communication skills are improved, the best strategies for optimizing learning are those that facilitate self-determination. In the 21st century, the AV practitioner-parent partnership is well positioned to take advantage of the full range of inclusion opportunities in order to meet the many individual needs of young children with hearing loss.

REFERENCES

Armstrong, D., Armstrong, A. C., & Spandagou, I. (2011). Inclusion: By choice or by chance? *International Journal of Inclusive Education, 1,* 29–39.

Ben Yehuda, S., Leyser, Y., & Last, U. (2010). Teacher educational beliefs and sociometric status of special educational needs (SEN) students in inclusive classrooms. *International Journal of Inclusive Education, 14,* 17–34.

Brown, P. M., Bortoli, A., Remine, M. D., & Othman, B. (2008). Social engagement, attention and competence of preschoolers with hearing loss. *Journal of Research in Special Educational Needs, 8,* 19–26.

Brühwiler. C., & Blatchford, P. (2010). Effects of class size and adaptive teaching competency on classroom processes and academic outcome. *Learning and Instruction, 21,* 95–108.

Chang, M., & Singh, K. (2008). Is all-day kindergarten better for children's academic performance? *Australian Journal of Early Childhood, 33,* 35–42.

Cushing, S. L., Chia, R., James, A. L., Papsin, B. C., & Gordon, K. A. (2008). A test of static and dynamic balance function in children with cochlear implants. *Archives of Otolaryngology-Head and Neck Surgery, 134,* 34–38.

Cvencek, D., Greenwald, A. G., & Meltzoff, A. N. (2016). Implicit measures for preschool children confirm self-esteem's role in maintaining a balanced identity.

Journal of Experimental Social Psychology, 62, 50–57.

deBoer, H., Bosker, R. J., & van der Werf, M. P. C. (2010). Sustainability of teacher expectation bias effects on long-term student performance. *Journal of Educational Psychology, 102,* 168–179.

DeConde Johnson, C., Cannon, L., Oyler, A., Seaton, J., Smiley, D.. & Spangler, C. (2014). Shift happens: Evolving practices in school-based audiology. *Journal of Educational Audiology, 20,* 1–15.

Galton, M., & Pell, T. (2012). Do class size reductions make a difference to classroom practice? The case of Hong Kong primary schools. *International Journal of Educational Research, 53,* 22–31.

Goldberg, D. M., & Flexer, C. (2001). Auditory-verbal graduates: Outcome survey of clinical efficacy. *Journal of American Academy of Audiology, 12,* 406–414.

Gray, C., Gibbons, R., Larouche, R., Sandseter, E. B. H., Bienenstock, A., Brussoni, M., . . . Tremblay, M. S. (2015). What is the relationship between outdoor time and physical activity, sedentary behaviour, and physical fitness in children? A systematic review. *International Journal of Environmental Research and Public Health, 12,* 6455–6474.

Horn, D. L., Fagan, M. K., Dillon, C. M., Pisoni, D. B., & Miyamoto, R. T. (2007). Visual-motor integration skills of prelingually deaf children: Implications for pediatric cochlear implant. *Laryngoscope, 117,* 2017–2025.

Huang, F. L. (2014). Further understanding factors associated with grade retention: Birthday effects and socioemotional skills. *Journal of Applied Developmental Psychology, 35,* 79–93.

Hughett, K., Kohler, F. W., & Raschke, D. (2011). The effects of a buddy skills package on preschool children's social interactions and play. *Topics in Early Childhood Special Education, 32,* 246–254.

Jussim, L., & Harber, K. D. (2005). Teacher expectations and self-fulfilling prophecies: Knowns and unknowns, resolved and unresolved controversies. *Personality and Social Psychology Review, 9,* 131–155.

Klatte, M., Lachmann, T., & Meis, M. (2010). Effects of noise and reverberation on speech perception and listening comprehension of children and adults in a classroom setting. *Noise Health, 12,* 270–282.

Knecht, H. A., Nelson, P. B., Whitelaw, G. M., & Feth, L. L. (2002). Background noise levels and reverberation times in unoccupied classrooms: Predictions and measurements. *American Journal of Audiology, 11,* 65–71.

Koster, M., Nakken, H., & Pijl, S. J., & van Houten, E. (2009). Being part of the peer group: A literature study focusing on the social dimension of inclusion in education. *International Journal of Inclusive Education, 13,* 117–140.

Kritzer, K. L. (2009). Barely started and already left behind: A descriptive analysis of the mathematics ability demonstrated by young deaf children. *Journal of Deaf Studies and Deaf Education, 14,* 409–421.

Lane, K. L., Pierson, M. R., Stang, K. K., & Carter, E. W. (2010). Teacher expectations of students' classroom behavior: Do expectations vary as a function of school risk? *Remedial and Special Education, 31,* 163–174.

Laws, G., Bates, G., Feuerstein, M., Mason-Apps, E., & White, C. (2012). Peer acceptance of children with language and communication impairments in a mainstream primary school: Associations with type of language difficulty, problem behaviours and a change in placement organization. *Child Language Teaching and Therapy, 28,* 73–86.

Lee. J., Ali, H., Ziaei, A., Hansen, J. H. L., & Tobey, E, (2015, July 12–17). *Impact analysis of naturalistic environmental noise type on speech production for cochlear implant users versus normal hearing listeners.* 2015 Conference on

Implantable Auditory Prostheses. Lake Tahoe, CA.

Luckner, J. L., & Muir, S. (2002). Suggestions for helping students who are deaf succeed in general education settings. *Communication Disorders Quarterly*, *24*, 23–30.

Martin, D., Bat-Chava, Y., Lalwani, A., & Waltzman, S. (2010). Peer relationships of deaf children with cochlear implants: Predictors of peer entry and peer interaction success. *Journal of Deaf Studies and Deaf Education*, *16*, 108–120.

Most, T., Ingber, S., & Heled-Ariam, E. (2012). Social competence, sense of loneliness, and speech intelligibility of young children with hearing loss in individual inclusion and group inclusion. *Journal of Deaf Studies and Deaf Education*, *17*, 259–272.

Mühlenweg, A., Blomeyer, D., Stichnoth, H., & Laucht, M. (2012). Effects of age at school entry (ASE) on the development of non-cognitive skills: Evidence from psychometric data. *Economics of Education Review*, *31*, 68–76.

NICHD Early Child Care Research Network. (2007). Age of entry to kindergarten and children's academic achievement and socioemotional development. *Early Education and Development*, *18*, 337–368.

Orth, U., & Robins, R. W. (2014). The development of self-esteem. *Current Directions in Psychological Science*, *23*, 381–387.

Reynolds, A. J., Richardson, B. A., Hayakawa, M., Lease, E. M., Warner-Richter, M., Englund, M. M., Ou, S-R., & Sullivan, M. (2014). Association of a full-day versus part-day preschool intervention with school readiness, attendance, and parent involvement. *JAMA*, *312*, 2126–2134.

Rhoades, E. A. (2003). *Ten rules for everyday living*. Auditory-verbal intervention for preschoolers. Workshop in Minneapolis, MN.

Sari, H. (2007). The influence of an in-service teacher training (INSET) programme on attitudes towards inclusion by regular classroom teachers who teach deaf students in primary schools in Turkey. *Deafness and Educational International*, *9*, 131–146.

Smaldino, J., & Flexer, C. (2014). Acoustic accessibility room acoustics and remote microphone use in home and school environments. In J. R. Madell & C. Flexer (Eds.), *Pediatric audiology: Diagnosis, technology, and management* (2nd ed., pp. 255–267).). New York, NY: Thieme.

Stolk, A., Hunnius, S., & Bekkering, I. T. (2013). Early social experience predicts referential communicative adjustments in five-year-old children. *PLoS ONE*, *8*(8), e72667.

Waismeyer, A., Meltzoff, A. N., & Gopnik, A. (2015). Causal learning from probabilistic events in 24-month-olds: An action measure. *Developmental Science*, *18*, 175–182.

Wang, N-M., Liu, C-J., Liu, S-Y., Huang, K-Y., & Kuo, Y-C. (2011). Predicted factors related to auditory performance of school-aged children with cochlear implants. *Cochlear Implants International*, *12*, S92–S95.

Warner-Czyz, A. D., Loy, B. A., Evans, C., Wetsel, A., & Tobey, E. A. (2015). Self-esteem in children and adolescents with hearing loss. *Trends in Hearing*, *19*, 1–12.

Wauters, L. N., & Knoor, H. (2008). Social integration of deaf children in inclusive settings. *Journal of Deaf Studies and Deaf Education*, *13*, 21–36.

Wehmeyer, M. L. (2015). Framing the future: Self-determination. *Remedial and Special Education*, *36*, 20–23.

Weiland, C., & Yoshikawa, H. (2013). Impacts of a pre-kindergarten program on children's mathematics, language, literacy, executive function, and emotional skills. *Child Development*, *84*, 2112–2130.

16

PROFESSIONAL PARTNERSHIPS AND AUDITORY-VERBAL THERAPY

Karen MacIver-Lux, Warren Estabrooks,
Stacey R. Lim, Rebecca A. Siomra,
Wendy D. Visser, Jennifer K. Sansom,
Ellen Yack, Ariella Blum Samson,
and Dale V. Atkins,

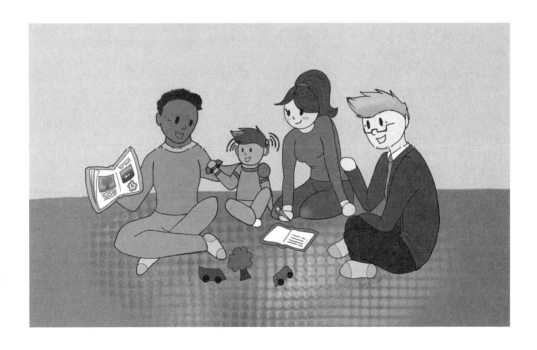

INTRODUCTION

Current knowledge about hearing loss, hearing technology, and related health and educational issues, makes collaboration and partnerships essential and vitally important in Auditory-Verbal Therapy (AVT). Each member of the family's team brings a unique set of skills. The fostering and maintenance of the interprofessional relationships on the team helps families to achieve the positive outcomes they want, as efficiently as possible.

Comprehensive AVT relies on accurate information about the child's hearing loss, auditory, speech and language skills, learning abilities, social-emotional and cognitive growth, personal and mental health development. All this information needs to be known by all team members, especially by the parents.

Conservative estimates by the Annual Survey of Deaf and Hard of Hearing Children and Youth suggest that 43% of children with hearing loss present with additional challenges such as low vision (4.4%), legal blindness (1.2%), developmental delay (8.5%), learning disability (12.4 %), orthopedic impairment (4.3 %), attention deficit disorder (ADD) (7.2%), traumatic brain injury (0.3 %), mental retardation (7.7 %), emotional disturbance (3.2 %), autism (1.9 %), Usher syndrome (0.1 %), and other health impairments (4.1 %) and conditions (8.0 %) (Gallaudet Research Institute, 2011).

When the AV practitioner and the parent have complete information about the child's additional challenges and about strategies and modifications that can facilitate ease of hearing, listening, talking, and learning, they can implement the latter into the AV session and into daily life. Conversely, other members of the team can use strategies that facilitate listening and spoken language development into their treatment sessions. Working together, these core members of the child's team provide the richest listening and spoken language learning opportunities possible.

Practitioners on any team also have unique temperaments and personalities. Some teams *gel* more easily than others. Team members do not have to be *friends* to be effective. What they *do* need, however, is a commitment to communicate respectfully, listen attentively, ask constructive questions, encourage perspectives from others, and a maintain solid commitment to the success of the child and the family.

THE PARTNERSHIP OF THE AUDIOLOGIST, AV PRACTITIONER, AND PARENT

The audiologist fulfills the roles set forth in the profession's Scope of Practice (e.g., AAA, 2004; ASHA, 2004) by providing audiologic assessments and treatments (hearing aids, cochlear implants, wireless remote microphone systems) to individuals with hearing loss. Pediatric audiologists are usually the first professionals who identify and confirm the presence of a hearing loss in very young children, and subsequently, provide management to ensure consistent auditory access to the sounds of life.

Parents enter a close and often long-term partnership with the pediatric audiologist the moment they receive the news that their child has a hearing loss that interferes with auditory information reaching their child's brain (see Chapter 2). Pediatric audiologists explain that the ears are the doorway to the auditory brain (Cole & Flexer, 2016) and they recommend and fit the most appropriate hearing aid(s) so that child has access to an *open* doorway to sounds of speech and the environment. Pediatric audiologists need to strike a critical balance of providing information about hearing and brain development so that informed decisions regarding the comprehensive management of the child's global development can be made. At the same time, pediatric audiologists are responsive to the parents' uncertainties and fears for their child's future, and help parents identify the desired outcomes they have for their child. If the parents require additional support, the pediatric audiologist provides referrals to other support providers and professionals in the community.

Although earlier is better, the goal is for the child to receive appropriately selected and programmed hearing technology (that directs clear auditory information to their child's brain) and to be enrolled in an early intervention program by 6 months of age (Joint Committee on Infant Hearing, 2007). In doing so, the pediatric audiologist lays down a solid technological foundation that allows the child optimal access to auditory information that will activate and stimulate the development of the child's auditory brain.

After the first set of appointments, the pediatric audiologist will have spent time with the parents reviewing the results of audiologic tests obtained on their child such as the auditory brainstem response (Click and Tone Burst) (ABR), otoacoustic emissions (OAEs), immittance audiometry (e.g., tympanograms, middle ear muscle reflexes), and behav-

ioral audiometry (audiogram). Additionally, the child's hearing technology will have been selected and appropriately fitted, and options of the various options of communication approaches and the early intervention programs in the family's community will have been shared in a nonbiased manner.

When parents choose the AV model of intervention, the AV practitioner is added to the team. Then, the pediatric audiologist, AV practitioner, and parent(s) work collaboratively for the duration of the time the child is receiving AVT. Their joint goal is to ensure that the best access of auditory information is available to the child's brain in order to develop and cement neurological connections for growth of spoken language, literacy, and social/communication skills (Richburg & Knickelbein, 2011).

The audiologist provides both the parents and AV practitioner with the most up-to-date audiological information on a regular basis. Information about the child's hearing technology, such as printouts of the child's cochlear implant maps or hearing aid output settings, are also shared with the AV practitioner and parents. This information indicates what auditory information (e.g., frequencies) is accessible to the child. After reviewing these results, the AV practitioner uses this information to plan, design, and/or adjust the AV treatment plan for the *child's individual listening profile*. The parent(s) ensure that the child wears the hearing technology during all waking moments, and that the hearing technology is in good working order by performing daily listening checks. The pediatric audiologist engages in dialogue with the AV practitioner and parents, keeping lines of communication open. In this way, there is an open discussion about the child's hearing, listening, and spoken language progress, and that goals are shared and implemented in a collaborative fashion.

To ensure that the child receives maximum auditory access, the audiologist not only uses information that he or she obtains through behavioral measures and verification, but also uses information given by the parents and AV practitioner. Because the AV practitioner sees the child on a weekly basis while the child's audiologist may only see the child several times a year, the AV practitioner provides information about the child's auditory functioning and listening and spoken language progress with hearing technology. This information provided by the AV practitioner helps the audiologist to determine what steps need to be taken to ensure continued access to sound. For example, the AV Practitioner may complete the Ling Six-Sounds at the beginning of every session. Over a course of several weeks, the AV practitioner notices that a child with a cochlear implant is no longer responding to /s/ and /sh/, and that the child is omitting word endings and speech productions are not as clear as they used to be. The parents also observe that the child is misunderstanding them at home. Based on the AV practitioner's and parents' observations, the audiologist evaluates the child's cochlear implant thresholds and re-maps the child's cochlear implant after determining there are no issues with the internal or external components.

Although the AV practitioner and parents can provide the audiologist with information in advance of appointments, the pediatric audiologist can monitor the development of discrete auditory processing skills. He or she monitors these skills using a battery of tests, such as electrophysiological tests (e.g., CAEP) or different types of speech perception tests in quiet variety of listening conditions (e.g., quiet vs. noise; increasing levels of background noise). Should the pediatric audiologist determine that the child is making limited progress with hearing aids, he or she can refer the parent to a cochlear implant audiologist. The cochlear implant audiologist will evaluate the child to determine cochlear implant candidacy, and when the child receives cochlear implant(s), the cochlear implant audiologist will continue to map the child's devices.

Some children with hearing loss have additional issues that may or may not be related to the hearing loss. The audiologist, AV practitioner and the parent will work collaboratively to ensure that all other areas of development are meeting milestones in a timely manner. When there are concerns, the child's otolaryngologist and/or pediatrician will be consulted to discuss the appropriateness of referrals to medical professionals who specialize in child development, genetics, neurology, vision, gross and fine motor skills, mental health, craniofacial issues, and so on.

In some hospitals or health clinics, there are pediatric audiologists who have training and experience in the assessment and treatment of childhood balance and vestibular disorders. A good number of children with hearing loss also experience balance issues associated with hearing loss. An example of this is meningitis, which can affect the structures of the auditory and vestibular (balance) systems in the inner ear. The information a vestibular audiologist provides may include information about what anatomical region is causing the balance disorder (e.g., inner ear or brain). This information would be shared with the child's PT/OT and the AV practitioner, who can then develop an appropriate intervention plan (e.g., movement and seating during sessions) (see PT/OT partnership for more information).

As audiologists work in close collaboration with AV practitioners and parent(s) they provide the family with information that extends well beyond the audiology clinic, into the home. With the AV practitioner's assistance, the listening environments and needs of families and the child in the home are evaluated, and audiologists keep parents informed of assistive listening devices or alerting devices such as personal wireless remote microphone systems, amplified telephones, vibrating alarm clocks, or flashing fire alarms, all of which will help the child prepare for independent living.

Audiologists and AV practitioners work collaboratively to provide support to the family as the child enters school (see Chapter 14). This is critical, because not all school districts have access to an educational audiologist. It may well be that the child's primary audiologist is the audiologist that works with the parents and school. This audiologist may provide in-services or IEP consultations to the school, ensure that FM technology is appropriately set with the child's hearing aids, and provide any other needed support as the child goes to school. If the child has an educational audiologist, the child's primary audiologist may also share information about the child's hearing and hearing technology with him or her.

The pediatric audiologist, AV practitioner, and the parent work continu-ously to ensure that the child with hearing loss has every opportunity to reach his/her highest listening, spoken communication and academic potential. The collaborative partnership between the audiologist, AV practitioner and the parent is a significant ingredient in laying the foundation contributes to the child's success in becoming an effective and independent member of society.

Case Study

Jenna is a 2.5-year-old who was identified with a mild sloping to moderate sensorineural hearing loss in both ears shortly after birth. The cause of her hearing loss was unknown, and her parents did not report any family history of hearing loss. She was fitted with binaural amplification at 7 months of age and was enrolled in AV therapy at 9 months of age.

According to her mother, Jenna is a consistent user of hearing aids, and asks for them first thing in the morning. She does not like to take her hearing aids out at bath time or bedtime, and often falls asleep with them on. Jenna's receptive language skills are similar to her peers with typical hearing, but she is lagging behind slightly in expressive language skills. The AV practitioner and parents have been working diligently to provide Jenna with the opportunities to express herself and help her to increase the frequency and length of her utterances.

Jenna's parents noticed a change in her behavior at home during the week prior to her most recent AV session. She had been taking her hearing aids out several times during the day. Even though they performed listening checks and changed the batteries, they did not perceive any change in the sound quality of Jenna's hearing aids. Jenna had also been responding to her name less frequently and her voice seemed "louder."

During the AV session, Jenna's AV practitioner noted that although Jenna previously identified all sounds of the Ling Six-Sound Test within 3 feet, her responses during the session were not as they used to be. She also noticed that there was a slight change in the quality of Jenna's speech as she sounded slightly slushy or muddled. During a play activity that provided numerous opportunities to discriminate plurals vs. singulars, Jenna often heard and repeated the singular form instead of the plural (e.g., cat vs. cats).

After Jenna's mother shared her concerns regarding Jenna's behavior and speech at home, the AV practitioner suggested that a complete audiological evaluation of hearing aids be completed. The AV practitioner shared her observations with the audiologist, and Jenna's mother arranged for an appointment the next day.

The audiologist reviewed the information provided by the AV practitioner and spoke at length with Jenna's parents to learn more about what has been happening at home. It was revealed that while playing, Jenna had bumped her head after which her parents noticed a change in her listening behaviors. Following a thorough audiological assessment, the results of the behavioral audiogram showed that Jenna's hearing thresholds were now in the moderate to severe hearing loss range. Because her last audiological appointment was only 2 months prior, the audiologist also recommended a follow-up with an otolaryngologist to determine if there was a medical cause

for this change in hearing. The otolaryngologist's recommendations included a CT scan that subsequently showed Jenna had enlarged vestibular aqueduct syndrome (EVAS), which is commonly associated with sudden, fluctuating, or progressive hearing loss.

The audiologist reprogrammed Jenna's hearing aids. With the new knowledge, the audiologist, AV practitioner, and parent formulated a plan to monitor Jenna's hearing status more closely. In addition to scheduling more frequent appointments, the audiologist requested that the AV practitioner send information related to Jenna's progress on a more frequent basis.

Within 2 months, it was jointly decided by the audiologist, AV practitioner, and parent(s) that a referral to the Cochlear Implant Team would be appropriate based on the Jenna's progress, and the fact that another drop in hearing thresholds occurred. Jenna received a cochlear implant 2 months later, and very shortly after activation of her cochlear implant, the AV practitioner and Jenna's mother observed significant improvement in her behavior and her listening and spoken communication skills.

THE PARTNERSHIP OF THE SPEECH-LANGUAGE PATHOLOGIST, AV PRACTITIONER, AND PARENT

Access to appropriate early intervention programs and early access to appropriately fitted hearing technology is known to have positive outcomes for young children, with hearing loss (Fricke, Bowyer-Crane, Haley, Hulme, &

Snowling, 2013; Meinzen-Derr, Wiley & Choo, 2011; Vohr et al., 2011). Delays in identification, access to intervention and/or fitting of appropriately programmed hearing technology can delay a child's development in listening, speech, language, socioemotional competence, and literacy (Yoshinaga-Itano, 2003).

Approximately 7% of all children exhibit speech and/or language delays; this includes children with hearing loss.

Communication is complex and greatly impacted by auditory development, social skills, verbal and non-verbal interactions, motor speech skills, the production of fluent speech, voice-quality, the ability to understand spoken messages, and the ability to organize thoughts into a message that can be understood by others. The partnership of an AV practitioner, family, and speech-language pathologist (SLP), therefore, is unique since each member brings their own perspective about how to most effectively help the child with hearing loss reach their communication potential (Hlady-MacDonald, 2012).

When the AV practitioner has any concern about a child's speech, language or communication development *that is unrelated to their hearing loss*, with the family's knowledge and support, they need to initiate a referral to an SLP. An SLP has the clinical skills to assess and confirm delays/disorders in these areas and knows when to refer on to a medical professional for further diagnostic support. Families are counseled to enlist the services of an SLP *with experience in the specific area of concern*. Due to the broad nature of speech-language pathology, practitioners often focus their practice on a specific population (e.g., children or adults), or area of disorder (e.g., artic-

ulation or social communication). The SLP is able to assess the concerns, set goals and create a treatment plan. In addition, he or she can evaluate progress critically and know when to ask for advice from the family, or from other professionals on the team.

Auditory-verbal practitioners have varied educational backgrounds, and may also be SLP's. In such cases, it is that professional's responsibility to be open with the family, to recognize if they have the appropriate skill set to address the noted concern effectively, and to refer to another SLP if needed.

Some concerns that require the specific clinical expertise of the SLP are as follows:

- articulation and phonology delays;
- motor speech delays/disorders, including childhood apraxia of speech;
- swallowing and/or chewing difficulties;
- social communication delays/ disorders, including autism spectrum disorder;
- word-finding difficulties;
- various types of stuttering, including repetitions, prolongations, and blocks;
- voice disorders such as pitch control, hoarseness, or vocal strain;
- resonance disorders such as hyper- or hyponasality;
- sentence-formulation challenges, including word order and grammar; and
- story-telling or recall difficulties.

When an SLP works with a child who is receiving AVT, he or she should collaborate with the AV practitioner to plan, discuss and share strategies that facilitate the development of listening and spoken communication skills. Parents need to be fully informed about the various strategies used by both practitioners. For example, while the AV practitioner focuses primarily on the development of listening first, the SLP may focus on providing visual and tactile cues to help a client who has childhood apraxia of speech, to plan motor movements necessary for producing clear speech. There are, however, some targets and strategies that may be used in both therapy sessions. For example, for a child who stutters, the SLP may suggest repeating the child's message back in an easy manner or by limiting the number of questions used as *fluency-enhancing strategies*, and the AV practitioner may suggest arranging seating/activities to encourage listening first and to minimize visual cues.

If the SLP is also the AV practitioner the above can and does occur within the *same session*. He or she needs to respect the guidelines of auditory-verbal therapy, be clear with the family about when, and why, any visual cues are used. If a therapy program requires mostly visual input (e.g., a picture communication system), or cues, the family needs to know that, while strategies used in AVT may continue to be incorporated, the therapy is not AVT. When the parents, SLP and AV practitioner keep communication open and fluid they can work together to provide the most highly consistent support.

Case Study

Ryan is an easy-going 3-year-old. His mother reported that there was nothing unexpected with her pregnancy (her third—Ryan has two older sisters), or his birth. She added that he did not pass the newborn hearing screening prior to being discharged from the local hospital.

Ryan was identified with a severe-to-profound bilateral sensorineural hearing loss at 3 months of age, which surprised his parents as no one in their family had a hearing loss. One of his sisters had chronic ear infections and had pressure equalization (PE) tubes inserted bilaterally at the age of 2 years, without any permanent hearing loss. Other than communication development, Ryan reportedly met all of his developmental milestones as expected and thoroughly enjoys playing with his friends at preschool. His family had some experience working with an Early Childhood Specialist and an SLP as their eldest daughter received a diagnosis of a high-level social communication disorder two years earlier, at the age of five years. Since then, the parents watched Ryan's peer interactions closely.

With their audiologist's support and guidance, Ryan and his parents started auditory-verbal therapy with an auditory-verbal practitioner, who is also a teacher of the deaf and hard of hearing, shortly after the hearing loss was confirmed. Ryan received bilateral cochlear implants with no complications at 13 months of age.

Recently, one of the preschool teachers reported to his father that Ryan talks much more now, participates appropriately in the classroom and is well-liked by his peers. His teachers, however, have more difficulty understanding him, compared to other children in his class. At their next AV session, Ryan's father discussed the teacher's concern with the AV practitioner. The AV practitioner agreed that Ryan's speech was challenging to understand, and that she also planned to discuss this concern with them. She explained that Ryan was really progressing well in his auditory development, general communication, comprehension, vocabulary, and sentence complexity. She echoed the teacher's concerns that his speech production was not advancing as she anticipated, given his hearing age. She was confident that he has good auditory access to the full speech spectrum, but when he tries to imitate her words he appears to struggle to produce the right sounds. The AV practitioner clarified that since she didn't believe the speech difficulty was related to Ryan's hearing loss or auditory development, she needed to suggest he be referred to an SLP for additional support.

Subsequently, Ryan's parents were referred to a community agency that specialized in working with toddlers and preschoolers with speech and language disorders and delays. They forwarded Ryan's most recent progress report from the auditory-verbal practitioner, and also shared information about their older child. During the SLP's first visit with Ryan, she evaluated his speech, language, and social communication development. She was pleased to find that he had excellent receptive language (comprehension) skills, and strong social communication and play skills for his age. She also noted that Ryan's expressive language was a little delayed but more specifically, he had difficulty producing sounds with the tip of his tongue (i.e., /t, d, n/), as well as the vowel sounds (e.g., "oo," "oh") some of the earliest sounds to develop. The SLP asked questions about Ryan's

cochlear implants and how he was hearing, and she wondered how the cochlear implants (CIs) impacted his speech development.

Ryan's parents were very happy to learn that the SLP was willing to talk with the auditory-verbal practitioner about his communication development. They were quietly concerned about how they would be able to follow communication therapy plans from two practitioners. Together, they discussed hearing age, auditory access and his progress in expressive language and motor speech production. Both professionals agreed that in setting short-term objectives and long term goals for his speech development, balanced expectations were needed between his hearing and chronological ages. With help from Ryan's parents, the SLP created a treatment plan and they shared it with the auditory-verbal practitioner. In doing so, both professionals were able to focus on their own area of expertise, support each other's goals, and coordinate specific objectives to simplify the family's *homework* and help them to help Ryan maximize the expertise of both service providers.

PARTNERSHIP OF THE ITINERANT TEACHER, AV PRACTITIONER, AND PARENTS

The itinerant teacher provides a plethora of services to a child with hearing loss throughout his or her school life. If a family has progressed through AVT, the parents have been the primary teachers throughout the listening and spoken language journey. Once the child is in school, the itinerant teacher plays an important role that may not engage the parents in the same kind of relationship the parents are accustomed to (Robertson, 2010). In addition to teaching the child, the itinerant teacher acts as a liaison between parents, audiologist, AV practitioner, and the school team that may include the classroom teacher, occupational therapist, additional support staff, and administration. The role of the itinerant teacher may include consultant, negotiator, collaborator, teacher, and listener depending on the situation (Bullard, 2002, p. 2).

Developing a trusting relationship and clear communication is essential as parents move from individualized therapy to helping their child in a classroom of children with typical hearing. The daunting reality of *letting go* is especially hard for parents with children who have any special needs, including those hearing loss. Robertson (2010, p. 370) suggests that parents need to be appreciated like "Caregivers as Colleagues," with the end result ensuring respect of their beliefs and goals for their children.

Common questions such as, will my child hear the teacher well?; will he or she understand?; what will happen if the batteries stop working?; will other children make fun of his CIs or hearing aids?; will we be consulted to make sure the best possible plan is established for my child? The AV practitioner will typically begin to counsel the parent about these concerns long before the child enters school, but certainly during the 6 months before school entrance. Some such counseling may have taken place as the child transitioned to preschool.

During the late winter and early spring of the year the child starts school, a great deal of information is gathered from observations, test results, and other diagnostic findings, and the transition to placement at school begins. Placement discussions include reviewing the child's listening and communication skills, social-cognitive progress, and the child's abilities to work and play in a group. Safety concerns, such as visual fire alarms, fenced-in yards, and types of play structures are considered along with the need for the types of educational support required for success. Meetings may be established so that the itinerant teacher might observe the child in a therapy session and/or a nursery school and with the parents. In the late spring, the itinerant teacher may welcome the parent and the AV practitioner to the new school. At this time, the AV practitioner most likely has completed the current assessments on the child and forwarded them to the itinerant teacher who will use the results in determining the first set of Individualized Educational Placement (IEP) goals and the level of direct support needed for the child. Typically, today, most children, if they have been diagnosed very early and in an AVT program from a young age, are discharged from AVT by the time this transition occurs. But, some families may continue on in AVT for various reasons.

An effective itinerant teacher needs to be be flexible, patient, and able to draw from his or her past experiences quickly, especially at the beginning of any school year when parents are often anxious about their child's transition back to school and who will be their teacher. The itinerant teacher may facilitate this transition by meeting with the school staff, in the early days of school. Whether it be in a group or individually, the adults working with the child will receive specific information about the child's hearing loss, cochlear implants or hearing aids and assistive hearing devices. The itinerant teacher provides suggestions and tips for working with a child to everyone and she or he may even do this in tandem with the parents and/or the AV practitioner. Parents will want to know how much time the itinerant teacher will be directly working with their child, when and where. They may want to know exactly what they will be doing and what the role of the parent is to be.

Educating the other students in the classroom about hearing loss and the accommodations required for the child is typically the responsibility of the itinerant teacher. Parents, of course, are often concerned about their child being viewed as different and about *how they will fit in*. Naturally, other children are very curious and usually they are very accepting of differences and embrace them in their peer group. With care and respect, the itinerant teacher explains that children want to know what the "things" are in their child's ears (HAs) or on their head (CIs). Once the peers learn the reasons for the hearing devices they often forget about them. However, when a child who has a hearing loss, is playing out in the yard and does not hear his or her friends calling, the child might be perceived as rude or antisocial, so the earlier the peers develop some simple communication strategies, the better. The itinerant teacher keeps the discussion going about how everyone is unique and to be embraced and often this is done jointly by the parent and the itinerant teacher, by the itinerant teacher and the AV practitioner, or by a combination of all three.

Hearing in noise is a great challenge for a child with hearing loss. From the moment the child enters a large classroom with concrete walls, high ceilings and desks and chairs on tile floors, his or her ability to listen changes immediately. The itinerant teacher is the main advocate and contact for implementing FM systems in the classroom, upon recommendation from the audiologist, and he or she ensures that the selected sound-field or personal FM system is supplied and *working to specifications* in the classroom. The use of FM systems can sometimes be challenging and the itinerant teacher endeavors *to get everyone on board*. At first, many teachers do not understand the need for such systems as they say they speak loudly, the child is sitting right in front of them or the child hears just fine without it. The itinerant teacher is almost always educating and encouraging school staff and parents about the need of this equipment for a child, *even with a mild hearing loss*. He or she needs to remind everyone that speech is best heard within 3 to 4 feet of the speaker. Within a classroom of children, even at its quietest moment, the speech energy reduces by 6 dB every 3 feet, resulting in the fact that someone talking in the back of a classroom is virtually inaudible to a child with any hearing loss (Souza, 2015).

If the child requires additional support in language development or speech, the itinerant teacher will work directly one on one with the child or in a small group including peers. Ideally, the itinerant teacher continues to use auditory-verbal strategies. Parents are encouraged to follow up and practice at home, as they are still regarded as the primary teachers of the child (see Chapter 1). Goals at school increase in difficulty as the curriculum does and in the higher grades, the itinerant teacher spends time helping the child with self-advocacy, social skills and understanding their own hearing loss which are all essential in becoming independent individuals.

Case Study

Anna is a 4-year-old girl who was identified with CHARGE syndrome. She has a profound conductive loss in her left ear, due to the malformation of the ossicles (Charge Syndrome Foundation, 2015). She is unable to wear a hearing aid due to the missing lobe. Anna wears a hearing aid on her right ear to amplify her moderate to moderately severe sensorial neural hearing loss. She has issues with balance and wears glasses. She began junior kindergarten in September with an educational assistant and a team of professionals, including the classroom teacher, who have come to understand her needs.

The success of Anna's entry into school started in late January, when her parents registered her for school and informed their AV practitioner of the upcoming transition. When the AV practitioner contacted the itinerant teacher for Anna's school, a meeting was set up to observe an AV session. The itinerant teacher and the AV practitioner also observed in Anna's daycare. Subsequently, in a feedback meeting with the parents, the daycare staff the AV practitioner and the itinerant teacher, a recommendation was made that Anna receive additional support in the classroom due to her balance and concerns about safety. The itinerant teacher also contacted the audiologist to talk about an FM system and obtain a recommendation to order a system in the fall.

In the first week of school the itinerant teacher and the school team had another meeting with the family to learn of progress achieved over the summer. With the staggered kindergarten entry and support of an educational assistant (EA), Anna was able to attend full days by the end of the first week. The itinerant teacher met with the children of the class to read them a short story about an animal with hearing loss. It explained the importance of facing someone when you are speaking to them as well as what happens when a child's ears do not work as well as they should. The parents are comfortable with the daily communication book from the teacher and EA. Daily listening checks are done by the EA to ensure the hearing aid and FM are working. The itinerant teacher visits Anna three times per week. *Homework* consists of games and activities and centered on weekly goals. Although the parents are not present at every school session, many strategies used in AVT are still used. This transition was only possible due to the partnership of the itinerant teacher, the AV practitioner and the parent. Through this partnership, Anna will have a successful start to the school year and the seeds to success have been planted.

THE PARTNERSHIP OF THE PHYSICAL THERAPIST, AV PRACTITIONER, AND PARENT

Hearing loss in infancy and early childhood is typically accompanied by delays in motor skill acquisition. However, delays in motor skill acquisition often do not become clinically relevant until infants or children fail to achieve motor milestones as anticipated. Thus, formation of a transdisciplinary team involving the child and family, supported by rehabilitation professionals, is central to optimizing opportunities for both communication and motor skill success. One of the allied rehabilitation professionals who may be included on this team to address a child's concurrent challenges in achieving and performing motor skills is a physical therapist. Physical therapists (PT) are uniquely qualified to diagnose and treat individuals with challenges and/or conditions that limit movement and performance of functional activities (APTA, n.d.).

Because AVT helps infants and children develop hearing as an active sense, listening and hearing become an integral part of everyday communication through speech, promoting interactions and socialization. However, if an infant or child who has hearing loss also has concurrent motor skill delays, it may result in difficulties effectively performing activities requiring balance, such as sitting, standing, walking, running, jumping, and so on. These balance difficulties can contribute to a child experiencing social isolation due to the inherent risk of increased injury during participation in physical activities. Therefore, to optimize a child's opportunities for successful communication and motor skill performance, it is imperative that the support and communication strategies of the AV practitioner be integrated into the child's sessions with physical therapy as well as the strategies to facilitate development of motor skills and control be incorporated into AV sessions.

From birth, auditory stimulation helps direct and intensify visual orientation behaviors. An infant's earliest response to an auditory stimulus includes visual-motor behaviors, typically involving movement of the head and/or eyes to localize sound. Because of this close relationship between audition and movement, the lack of early auditory input may contribute to delays in motor skill acquisition in children with hearing loss (Rajendran & Roy, 2011; Savelsberg, Netelenbos, & Whiting, 1991). There is growing evidence that children with hearing loss who have experienced long periods of auditory deprivation often demonstrate more delays in motor development than those who have experienced shorter periods of limited auditory input (Gheysen, Loots, & Van Waelvelde, 2008). Additionally, although early cochlear implantation to facilitate auditory stimulation typically promotes development of listening and spoken language, many of these children demonstrate increased challenges with balance compared to children with typical hearing and children with hearing loss who do not have a cochlear implant, increasing their risk of injury and/or social isolation (Gheysen et al., 2008; Kleinpeter, Wright, Lander, & Tucker, 2001; Miyamoto, Houston, Kirk, Perdew, & Svirsky, 2003; Robbins, Svirsky, & Kirk, 1997; Svirsky, Robbins, Kirk, Pisoni, & Miyamoto, 2000). Since PTs treat movement and activity limitations, they are thus ideally suited to help families address these motor delays and balance impairments.

Fortunately, early hearing screens have become common practice, facilitating prompt interventions to improve communication outcomes. Unfortunately, motor control and balance assessments are not routine parts of the screening procedure for infants and children with hearing loss. Subsequently many children with a range of motor and balance deficits go undiagnosed and untreated. To successfully address these limitations, it is imperative for the AV practitioner, PT, other allied rehabilitation professionals, and families to collaborate in order to accurately diagnose, formulate, and execute a treatment plan that adequately addresses auditory and *motor impairments* (Baker, Haines, Yost, DiClaudio, Braun, & Holt, 2012; Houston & Perigoe, 2011).

Case Study

Rianne is a 14-month-old infant referred for physical therapy (PT) services due to difficulty walking. She lost most of her hearing due to meningitis, which was treated with gentamicin. Rianne had cochlear implant (CI) surgery on her left ear shortly following the diagnosis and the CI was activated five weeks later.

Prior to meningitis, Rianne had been walking independently without problems for 3 months. However, since her recovery from meningitis and subsequent CI surgery, she has a widened base of support between her feet, her arms are held up and out to her sides, her steps are very short, and path of progression deviates significantly to the left, resulting in repeated falls and bumping into objects. All of these factors indicated to her parents and pediatrician that Rianne was having difficulty maintaining her balance when walking. Six weeks after the CI surgery, the pediatrician referred Rianne to

PT for an evaluation and subsequent services.

Because Rianne is just learning how to perceive and produce spoken language, collaboration among the parents, CI audiologist, AV practitioner, and PT is vital. The AV practitioner provides the PT with information about Rianne's gross motor skills with and without use of the cochlear implant processor. The CI audiologist advised the PT that Rianne may find the gym noisy and may take the implant off and then provided the PT with suggestions about how to manage the noise levels and, if necessary, gently replace the CI back on her head and behind her ear if it came off. Finally, because of the active nature of PT sessions, the CI audiologist gave suggestions about how the CI processor could be secured to her head so it did not fall off.

The AV practitioner indicates that because Rianne had only been listening with her CI for one week, and her brain not yet adjusted to the electrical signal, spoken language will be difficult for her to understand. When giving directions, the PT needs to make sure that Rianne was hearing, listening, and *watching* the PT's face. It is also helpful to *show* Rianne what to do if she appears not to understand. The AV practitioner suggests frequent positioning of the PT on Rianne's left side because it is the ear with better hearing.

The PT makes sure that Rianne's appointments are during quiet times in the clinic to minimize noise. Rianne wears a head wrap specifically designed to keep the CI process in place during tumbling. The PT focuses on challenging Rianne's balance during various play activities to help her re-learn how to walk without falling or deviating to the left; concurrently the PT coaches her parents in play activities they can do at home. This information is shared with the AV practitioner to incorporate into the AV sessions and into the family's at-home weekly plan.

The AV practitioner and the audiologist work with the PT on how to provide good auditory learning in the PT session, including how to provide instructions using clear speech and how to determine if Rianne is hearing the instructions correctly. All PT play activities are verbally directed face-to-face and require a verbal confirmation from Rianne. For example, the PT instructs Rianne to get a ball from the toy box and bring it to her father along a specified walking path. Rianne practices walking to the toy box and retrieving the object. The PT then asks her to say the name of *the ball*.

To facilitate Rianne's progress in PT, the PT works with the AV practitioner to incorporate activities that challenged her static and dynamic balance during the AV sessions. These activities include placement of desired objects just outside her limits of stability in sitting or standing so Rianne has to develop adaptive balance strategies to prevent falling. Additionally, the PT asks the AV practitioner to perform activities similar to those she does in PT but with the focus shifted to perception and production of sounds associated with actions instead of physical performance (e.g., Rianne says "Boom" when the AV practitioner tells her to knock down a tower of blocks just barely within her reach). During all activities, the AV therapist closely observes Rianne to ensure she does not move physically closer to the desired object(s), but rather challenges her to push the limits of her stability in standing and/or sitting.

Rianne progressed rapidly in PT and was discharged 3 weeks later. She no longer walks with an abnormally widened base of support between her feet nor deviates to the left. Consequently, she bumps into fewer objects and has fewer falls. By incorporating the principles of communication of AVT into Rianne's PT treatments and home program, the family was able to achieve the functional balance goals more rapidly and successfully while providing more opportunities for successful listening and spoken language.

THE PARTNERSHIP OF THE OCCUPATIONAL THERAPIST, AV PRACTITIONER, AND PARENT

The occupational therapist (OT) is a vital member of interdisciplinary teams that provide services to children with hearing loss and their families. Occupational therapy is a health profession that focuses on maximizing a child's ability to participate in and perform daily occupations that include self-care routines, play and school related tasks. Occupational therapists maintain a holistic view of the child with their knowledge of sensory integration and the development of balance and postural reactions, motor skills, visual perception, visual motor integration, self-regulation and social behavior. The OT's knowledge of sensory integration and its impact on motor development are particularly relevant for children with hearing loss. There is a growing body of research suggesting that children with hearing loss have challenges related to impaired sensory processing (Bharadwaj, Damiel, & Matzke, 2009; Bharadwaj, Matzke, & Daniel, 2012; Koster et al., 2014), and there is evidence that suggests that they have more challenges with motor skills and balance reactions than their peers (Engel-Yege & Weissman, 2009; Gheyson et al., 2008).

What Is Sensory Integration

Sensory integration is a neurological process that allows the brain to take in, sort out and organize sensory information from the body and the environment. Sensory modulation plays a key role in this process and involves registration, orientation, and interpretation of sensory inputs, allowing suppression of irrelevant input to allow focus on relevant inputs. Problems with sensory modulation can lead to over or under-responsiveness to sensory input and can contribute to challenges maintaining appropriate arousal and activity levels. The efficient processing of sensory information contributes to normal development and quality of life. For example, sensory input received from the skin, muscles, joints, and gravitational forces, need to be properly registered and integrated to allow the toddler to conquer gravity and walk independently. If the child is over-responsive to changes in gravitational demands, they may be fearful to take their first steps and if they have inefficient feedback from their muscles, they may have trouble initiating taking a foot off the ground.

The theory of sensory integration was first proposed by occupational therapist, A. Jean Ayres (1972, 1979) and has evolved and expanded (Bundy, Lane, & Murray, 2002; Mailloux & Miller-Kuhanek, 2014). Sensory integration theory assumes that impaired sensory processing can be inferred from behavioural responses and motor output and can improve with controlled sensory input provided through meaningful activities (Ayres, 1972, 1979). Although all sensory systems are addressed by this theory, there is heightened interest in the functions of the tactile system (provides information about light touch, pressure, temperature, pain, texture), proprioceptive system (provides information from muscles, tendons and ligaments), and the vestibular system (provides information about movement, gravity, and changing head positions). Sensory integration dysfunction was originally used to describe impairment in this area but the term *sensory processing disorder* has been proposed to differentiate from the theory and is increasingly used in the literature (Miller et al., 2007). Sensory processing disorder includes problems with sensory modulation, sensory discrimination, and sensory-motor based problems including poor motor planning and immature balance and postural reactions.

The knowledge of sensory integration theory and sensory processing disorders can assist AV practitioners and parents by providing

■ knowledge to analyze and interpret unusual responses to sensory input and atypical motor development;
■ an alternative perspective for understanding behavior;
■ solutions to improve challenging behavior; and

▪ practical strategies to increase attention, motivation, communication, and social engagement.

Sensory Processing Disorders and Children With Hearing Loss

Physical challenges that are consistent with vestibular impairment have frequently been identified in children with hearing loss (Rajendran, Roy, & Jeevanantham, 2012). More specifically, vestibular dysfunction, particularly hyporesponsivity to vestibular input has been identified in children with cochlear implants (Jerome, Kannan, Lakhani, & Palekar, 2013. Possible embryological connections between the vestibular and cochlear structures may be causing this dysfunction (Bharadwaj, Daniel, & Matzke, 2012) or problems can result from or be exacerbated by procedures during cochlear implant surgery (Todt, Basta, & Ernst, 2009). Atypical processing of tactile, visual, and oral input has also been identified in children with cochlear implants (Bharadwaj, Matzke, & Daniel, 2009). The motor deficits related to sensory processing disorders include challenges with balance reactions, postural control, praxis (motor planning), and delays in fine and gross motor development.

Inefficient sensory processing can contribute to problems with self-regulation. Self-regulation includes the ability to attain, maintain, or change arousal states required for specific events or activities. A calm, alert state is required for optimum learning. Sensory processing disorders can interfere with self-regulation and disrupt learning potential by contributing to over- or underarousal, reducing attention to tasks, increasing distractibility, and reducing frustration tolerance.

Signs of Sensory Processing Disorder

The following are motor and behavioral signs that the AV practitioner needs to be aware of that may suggest a child is experiencing some form of sensory processing disorder:

▪ avoidance of balance-related activities;
▪ unusual fear of falling or heights;
▪ difficulty walking on uneven surfaces;
▪ dislike of having head upside down;
▪ discomfort with movement-related activities, such as swings, merry-go-rounds;
▪ distress with self-care routines including hair washing and brushing, teeth brushing, face washing;
▪ avoidance of light touch, especially unexpected touch;
▪ dislike and avoidance of messy play or being barefoot, especially in sand and grass;
▪ discomfort with certain clothing items or textures and food textures;
▪ a fright-flight-fight response to unpredictable sensory input;
▪ poor body awareness;
▪ difficulty imitating postures and completing action sequences;
▪ delayed gross motor skills and/or fine motor skills, with particular difficulty learning new motor tasks;

- an excessive amount of energy and concentration to complete motor tasks;
- difficulty judging physical space, such as being unable to walk down center of hall;
- floppy or awkward appearance; and
- fatigue with physical activity.

The following are indicators that a child has poor self-regulation:

- easily distracted/startled,
- difficulty attending to tasks,
- high or low activity levels,
- problems with transitions,
- emotional outbursts not commensurate with the situation,
- problems calming self following emotional outbursts, and
- engagement in sensory seeking behaviors to calm or alert the nervous system.

Occupational Therapy Services

An occupational therapy assessment can help identify if a child is experiencing any sensory processing challenges or immaturities in development of motor, play, social, or self-care skills. The assessment may also provide the AV practitioner and parents important information about why a child may not be fully benefiting from AV therapy sessions. Efficient modulation of sensory input and good self-regulation are necessary for children to optimally attend to the AV practitioner, the parents, and the activities, and to respond to the strategies used in the AV sessions (see

Chapter 11). Regardless of whether a child has a sensory processing problem or not, sensory motor strategies can help children achieve a calm, alert state necessary for participation in AV sessions and in daily life.

Management strategies for home and preschool can also be provided to enhance quality of life and skill development in all settings. Depending on the nature and severity of the challenge, the occupational therapist may recommend individualized treatment sessions or may only provide consultation to the AV practitioner, parents, teachers, and/ or other health care providers.

Sample Strategies

1. Light touch excites any individual and can be particularly uncomfortable for a child who is tactile defensive. When touching such a child during AV sessions, light touch needs to be avoided to allow for enhanced concentration on tasks.
2. When a child is very excited, physically restless, having difficulty concentrating, deep touch pressure on the head or shoulders can help to relax the nervous system. Wearing a weighted belt, vest, or neck collar may also provide calming and helps organize input. Deep pressure input and engaging in resistance activities assists with calming and organizing the nervous system.
3. Frequent movement breaks during AV therapy sessions may improve attention to tasks
4. When seated to work at a table, the child needs to be well supported, with feet firmly on the floor or resting on a stool.

sort

5. A desensitization program around the ear areas may be required during introduction of hearing aid/cochlear implant wear.

Case Study

Sarah is a 4-year-old girl who was born following a normal pregnancy and delivery. Hearing loss was suspected as a young infant as she did not respond to or orient to sounds. A severe-to-profound bilateral hearing loss was confirmed at 4 months. Sarah and her parents began working with an AV practitioner at 8 months and received bilateral cochlear implants at 15 months of age. Along with delays in speech and language development, Sarah was slow to walk and crawl and had difficulty imitating simple actions. She was described as an irritable baby and toddler. She had difficulty transitioning from breast to bottle feedings and was slow to accept pureed and/or table foods. She continues to be a picky eater and does not like foods with mixed textures or seeds. She prefers soft clothing and primarily wears loose sweat pants and t-shirts. Labels need to be removed from her clothing and she will only wear socks without seams. She never liked a baby swing and avoids swings and climbing equipment on the playground.

Sarah's kindergarten teacher noted that she avoided messy play materials and was uncertain walking on uneven pavement. Sarah's AV practitioner noted that she was easily distracted during therapy sessions and withdrew from light touch. The practitioner was concerned that she was not making the expected progress. The AV practitioner, the teacher, and Sarah's mother consulted at the beginning of the school year and agreed that a referral to an occupational therapist was indicated.

The OT conducted an assessment that revealed that Sarah was overresponsive to tactile and vestibular input and reacted to these with a fright-flight-fight response. This sensory defensive response contributed to her irritability, poor attending behaviors, and fearfulness in a variety of settings. She also had impaired motor planning abilities as a result of atypical processing of tactile and vestibular input. Individualized OT treatment sessions were recommended to reduce her responsiveness and enhance her motor planning abilities. A therapeutic brushing protocol (developed by Patricia Wilbarger, OT, it involves brushing the arms, legs, and back followed by joint compressions several times per day) was implemented to reduce her sensory defensive responses.

Sarah is now less reactive to tactile and vestibular input. She has gained confidence in her motor skills, her imitation skills have improved, and she is better able to complete unfamiliar motor tasks.

The OT collaborated with Sarah's AV practitioner, teacher, and mother to identify barriers to participation and learning. Recommendations were generated to support Sarah in a variety of settings. Environmental accommodations were recommended for school, home, and AV sessions. It is very important that Sarah have appropriate chair and table heights when doing her work, eating meals, or during therapy sessions to ensure that her balance reactions are not overly challenged. The OT informed the other adults to avoid light touch during sessions and begin to use deep touch pressure.

Sarah is now much more able to attend to structured tasks especially in AV sessions when she wears a weighted neck collar. Sarah also has a "tool kit" with items that she can use throughout the day that provide sensory motor input that helps to reduce her anxiety. These items include a spouted water bottle that allows for repetitive rhythmic sucking.

Summary: The Partnership of the Occupational Therapist, AV Practitioner, and Parent

The OT as a professional partner was instrumental in enhancing outcomes of AV therapy sessions. Sarah is now less anxious and more attentive across all sessions and in daily life and her progress in all areas is advancing more rapidly and with more ease. Sarah is calmer both at home and in school. Her parents report that their quality of life has improved greatly and that the entire family can engage in a wider range of activities at home and in the community.

BRIDGE TO PARTNERSHIP: A PARENT PERSPECTIVE*

Over the past four and a half decades, our family has come into regular contact with pediatricians, doctors, otolaryngologists, audiologists, hearing aid dispensers, hearing aid sales representatives, psychologists, social workers, school and medical administrators, educational specialists, itinerant teachers, school principals, a stream of classroom teachers, private tutors, numerous bureaucrats, and auditory-verbal practitioner.

Like most parents, we came into this experience having to make many adjustments. Most of our first year was spent learning to accept, to understand, and to cope with "the news of hearing loss" news. We secretly hoped to discover that it was all a big mistake, a common response of parents to give us time to recover from the diagnosis. Denial allows us the necessary time to heal, regroup, and eventually to keep on going. We take steps to seek alternatives and answers, and the act of the search itself facilitates our acceptance and adaptation and gives us a small sense of control over our lives. This initial pursuit, however, often puts parents and practitioners at odds with each other in the earliest contacts. Alternative medicine and second opinions are acceptable in most medical areas today, yet searching parents are sometimes unfairly perceived and labeled as capricious.

We, as parents, experience different stages of mourning and different degrees of guilt (Kurtzer-White & Luterman, 2003). The anger that we commonly feel towards the practitioner is often the anger that comes from our own helplessness and our need to feel more in charge. Unconsciously, we redirect this energy into obtaining the best possible service for our child.

---

*Published first in Auditory-Verbal Therapy and Practice, A. G. Bell: Washington, DC. 2006. © 2016 by Warren Estabrooks, all rights reserved.

We come into the field of hearing loss as total amateurs. Unlike the practitioner we don't choose this domain, but we are faced with the reality of a great deal to learn. The practitioner is able to walk away from the problem or situation or just see it as another appointment. He or she remains detached and, consequently, can bring fresh vibrancy and enthusiasm into the arena. But this is a luxury never afforded to us as parents (MacKean, Thurston, & Scott, 2005).

The practitioner, furthermore, may have only one client to deal with during a session or appointment (Fingerhut et al., 2013). The family, on the other hand, has a variety of problems and dynamics (Fingerhut et al., 2013). We must deal with all our children and our own mourning, as well as the different stages of grief and acceptance among our siblings, grandparents, relatives, friends, and neighbors. Finally, we find ourselves stuck with the newly created and unasked-for job of public awareness and public relations.

In these early years, many parents find it difficult to reach out and ask for help. Going to meetings or even lifting the telephone can be emotionally draining. We feel helpless and alone within the community and, occasionally, within our family. In our own way, however, and at our own individual pace, we slowly master the situation as our lives gradually, return to "normal." We are compelled to create a new and different way of life because of the hearing loss. In time, old routines find their way back into our lives. Some of us choose to go back to work or find new careers. Some of us stay at home with our child and, maybe, have another. As we feel more empowered,

we also feel more comfortable in the company of practitioners.

During those early months, whenever someone told me what our son could never do or attain (as they often did), my guard always went up, and I dismissed those harmful comments. In fact, those comments spurred me to prove the practitioner wrong. When the otolaryngologist delivered the initial diagnosis to us, he concluded that our son would probably "never learn to speak." Strangely, that prognosis was actually the most helpful one; it became the mechanism that helped us succeed. That same verdict, however, could also have had the opposite effect on our family. This is why practitioners need to be *very careful* with the prognosis they give to families.

Looking back, I perceive our initial contacts with practitioners as challenges. However, they can and ought to be alliances in which the practitioners become our colleagues and allies. The control that practitioners can wield is immense (MacKean et al., 2005). When we deal with them, our child might be just a commodity, another statistic, or another audiogram. Practitioners, like parents, need to separate the child from the hearing loss in order to appreciate the youngster as a child first, to see the cup as half full instead of half empty; and to focus on the abilities of the child and family.

Many practitioners' training and educational backgrounds directly center on children, with little emphasis on counseling families. Conflicts can emerge over differences between the parents' and practitioners assessments of the child's needs. Practitioners can help by making adjustments in their services to the families' real and current needs. Practitioners need to recognize the value and importance of the parents' perspectives (Crais, Roy, & Free, 2006; Trute & Hiebert-Murphy, 2007). Differences in values will always exist. Good practitioners encourage families to make their own choices, even though they might encounter priorities, outlooks, and values that differ greatly from their own.

It is the parents' responsibility also to act professionally. Some parents are guilty of poor attendance, being late for appointments, or not following through on a required action. Such behaviors can frustrate the practitioners. Good professionals do not bypass clashes. They acknowledge them and attempt a reconciliation by working together. The child cannot be treated in isolation from the family. Ultimately, both parents and practitioners want success for the child and the family.

Unfortunately, parents and practitioners sometimes fail to communicate effectively, resulting in misunderstanding over each other's definition of success. One practitioner's view of success may mean a child with a healthy self-esteem. To a parent of a young infant, self-esteem may still be an abstract concept at a time when all concentration is on teaching language in the hope that the child will eventually be understood by playmates. Since goals may be prioritized differently, we must discuss the services we need for our child and define our goals out loud (Fingerhut et al., 2013).

The responsibility for our child's education falls directly on us, the parents. We must negotiate effectively to get the services our child needs (Mac-

Kean et al., 2005). It is, therefore, up to us to acquire the knowledge to coordinate and monitor services (Simons, 1987). This is a time-consuming task, and some parents find it easier to do than others. One useful strategy is to think of it as our profession. When a task seems impossible, or we feel too embarrassed to ask, it helps to remember that it is our job to ask, to talk to the practitioners, and if necessary, to get them to talk to one another. Finally, I also remind myself that although they may know the programs and services better, I know my child better.

Few of us find our ongoing daily interactions with practitioners as gratifying as we would like them to be. Parents and professionals may make comments about each other such as:

"They don't answer our questions."

"They don't listen."

"They don't make time to help us."

"They talk to us in unusual ways."

"They keep information from us."

"They insist that we make the decisions."

"They don't think about child behavior the way we do."

"They don't ask our opinion"

(Niagara Children's Services Committee, 1990).

Looking back, I now see conflicts as inevitable and essential, but at that time, they were a constant source of pain. My husband and I, and the practitioners did not always realize that we were working with different agendas. Our goals often differed, our needs for services varied, and we often focused on a different aspect or definition of success. Nevertheless, there are many things that we, as parents, can do to make the relationship more productive, satisfying, and rewarding:

Good Communication

All parents can develop better communication skills. It is in our interest to invest time and effort in our relationship with practitioners; it may prevent antagonism. If we communicate positively and with respect, we can prevent a stalemate and make it easier for practitioners to give us what we need.

Learn to Listen

We need to learn to listen actively and be open minded. It is easy to complain. Talking and sharing information is a two-way exchange. Often, we are so busy waiting our turn to speak that we tune out others. If we don't listen to the practitioners, how can we expect them to listen to us? We need to assess new information and allow ourselves time to absorb it and then act. In time, we might come up with a fresh perspective.

Stand Up for Our Rights

We can learn to be assertive without being aggressive. We need to concentrate on the issue at hand, not on the individual. We can express opinions with firm conviction, not indignation. We can talk it out. We are part of a team! We want the practitioner to hear what we have to say, not back them into a corner.

Practitioners need to remember that parents are individuals too, with individual styles and personalities, and will present different mannerisms and skills.

Keep Records

If we have a particular concern, we can prepare notes on the situation in advance. This will help the practitioner to deal with it, and will help us document our concerns. We can compare notes with other parents. We often hit a plateau or feel depressed at our slow progress. It is hard always to be enthusiastic. As parents, we face a lifetime of challenge requiring tremendous physical and emotional stamina. These records plot our progress, which often goes unnoticed while we are going through it.

Be Prepared—Keep Informed

We need to get the most out of our appointments by doing our homework. If we make a list of questions before the meeting, we arrive prepared. We also expect that preparation from a practitioner. We, too, are practitioners, who "work" with our children, so we can use our pen and notebook, or mobile device to record questions, information, and terminology exchanged during appointments. If possible, we obtain permission to record the meetings with practitioners. This is a helpful tactic for nervous parents, especially in the early years. It is particularly useful for reviewing new information and technical terminology. We can keep our own files. We don't need to be afraid to ask questions or for explanations. We don't need to feel intimidated. We never need to proceed or to leave unless we understand what has been said (Moeller, Carr, Seaver, & Stredler-Brown, 2013).

Establish or Use Available Support Networks

Parents are often intimidated at the prospect of meeting a roomful of practitioners. Anxiety can cloud our thought processes as well as our memory. Most parents can relate to the experience of hearing something for the first time, only to be told by the practitioner that the issue had already been discussed. We might take along a recording device to a meeting, explain its presence, and ask for permission to use it, so we can later review the information. We might be amazed at how much we miss when we listen to the recording again at home, and we have the added advantage of sharing the information accurately with family.

We don't need to go alone to school or hospital meetings. We can bring a spouse, friend, therapist, or itinerant teacher. There is strength in numbers (Moeller et al., 2013; Yoshinaga-Itano, 2013) even if only one person does the talking. The tag-along friend can help replay the events of the meeting, and may have a more objective point of view.

Learn the Lingo

We need to learn to use the same terminology that the practitioners use. This takes time and effort, but knowledge is a powerful tool (Sørensen et al., 2012). We gain confidence and respect along the way.

Access Information

We can ask for all copies of reports, tests, and audiograms. We have a legal right to such information. By learning to be comfortable with the information we acquire, we will become more familiar with all the issues, learn to ask relevant questions, and research new areas (Fitzpatric, Angus, Durieux-Smith, Graham, & Coyle, 2008; Woods, Wilcox, Friedman, & Murch, 2011).

Stay on Track

We need to stay within the subject matter. It is even helpful to keep a mental or written agenda to prevent us from digressing during a scheduled appointment and, consequently, running out of time. By verbalizing all our concerns, we can help the practitioners see our own agenda as well as lead us through it. We must also understand the importance of selecting the right time for a particular discussion or confrontation. We will be better prepared at the next meeting if we have time to ponder and analyze the situation.

Stay Calm

We need to be level headed and in control. As parents, we tend to bring emotional baggage into the room. Most practitioners understand that most of the time. Still, being emotional can be counterproductive and may cost us our credibility, which undermines our efforts. Unleashing anger doesn't work. We have a right to talk about what is bothering us, but we have a much greater chance of being heard and getting some or all of what we want if we wait until the heat of anger passes. Some practitioners will ignore us and may even mentally dismiss us; the more rational we can remain, the more likely it is that they will listen. If being calm, cool, and collected is not part of our personality, it often helps to explain our shortcomings to the practitioner, who might be able to to defuse the situation with humor.

Trust Our Expertise

We have our own area of expertise—our child. It is up to us to share information. We see sides of our child that practitioners never see. We need to trust our instincts about what our child needs. Even though it is not easy to convey that kind of information, we need to be listened to and we deserve respect for our opinions. We need to remind ourselves frequently that we will remain the most consistent support for our child. A practitioner usually enters our lives for short periods of time, while we have the greatest investment in our child. We have to listen carefully to all opinions, but remember that opinions are all that they are. We are the ones who will have to live with the consequences of the decisions made. We need to get the best advice we can, and then determine as a family what course of action makes the most sense for us.

Be Objective

If a problem or a special need occurs, we need to remain objective. We need to be as realistic as possible and, if necessary, reevaluate our goals and objectives. We need not be afraid to take a risk or recognize a mistake. We need to set our own limits if necessary. Sometimes, we even have to compromise.

Be Assertive—Remain Polite

This is the backbone of stellar conduct. If we disagree, we need to speak up. If we are not sure or would like a second opinion, we need to say so. No one can read our mind! We need to learn to persuade, not antagonize. Disagreement is difficult for most of us to deal with and for practitioners to accept. We need to separate the issue from the person. Parents and practitioners both need to be courteous and respectful of one another.

Get a Second Opinion

Second opinions are common in the medical field. We are entitled to them. We can ask for more information or literature on the subject, we can ask if another practitioner might feel differently, and we can ask how the practitioner might deal with the situation if our child were his or her own child. We all accept the fact that auditory-verbal therapy is an ongoing diagnostic and ever-changing process. We need to accept no less from our relationship with any practitioner. Our joint goal is to form an alliance—a potential partnership. We, as parents, bear part of that responsibility. It is advantageous for a practitioner to work with parents who can advocate effectively, make decisions, and solve problems by themselves or in a partnership.

Express Appreciation

We all need to be appreciated and complimented. It is not easy for a practitioner to say, "I don't know" to a parent. Yet the practitioner who says, "Maybe I can help you find out or find someone who knows the answer" can inspire a greater degree of confidence and be reassuring and helpful. This atmosphere of freedom is conducive to working things out.

Keep Expectations Realistic

Schools or doctors may tell us that our expectations are unrealistic or too high. This is a common source of conflict between parents and practitioners. We must learn to trust our own intuition about what are realistic expectations for our family. Our backgrounds and value systems may differ; what is realistic for one family may not necessarily work for another.

Trust Our Instincts

Sometimes a school system or practitioner perceives itself as the expert (Bruder, 2000). Such an attitude can shake our confidence and lead us to question what is best for our child. These practitioners may spend more time focusing on past failures than reflecting on future potential and see the proverbial half-empty cup! School personnel work with hundreds of children, whereas we are working with just one. They may look at what is wrong instead of what is right. They may tell us what our child cannot do instead of what our child can do. Most of us can set goals for our children better than anyone else. Even though some practitioners don't want to expose the child to failure or put too many stresses or demands on the family, there is dignity in risk. We have a right to try, a right to succeed, and the right to fail.

If parents and practitioners cannot agree on a course of action, we must at least establish the proper protocol for resolving our differences. The parent needs to move up the ladder of authority only as required. If we work with the practitioners instead of antagonizing them, our disagreements can often be resolved. Sometimes, no matter how well prepared we are, we run into a brick wall in the form of a practitioner. All parents have a list of such encounters; if we are lucky, the list is short. These are times when we get stuck and feel that there is no way out but to shoot them. There are, however, alternatives!

- *Reevaluate the situation.* There are always alternatives, and we can always learn new ways of dealing with problems.
- *Renegotiate whenever possible.* Sometimes, one of the most important things we can do is to get a second, or even a third, opinion. It is also our right.
- *Recognize the bright side of every situation.* We keep growing.

When our son had an inadequate itinerant teacher, I told myself that I was responsible for the work, and we would have a new teacher next year—and we did!

The practitioner needs to create an atmosphere of exchange (Crais, Roy, & Free, 2006; Woods, Wilcox, Friedman, & Murch, 2011). By facilitating parent participation in the entire process, the child remains the focus. He or she must recognize the specific requirements of every parent in receiving information, to refrain from using excessive "professional jargon" (Stableford & Mettger, 2007), and to furnish necessary information while remaining sensitive to the grieving process. Practitioners have to provide opportunities for parents to experience success while remaining cautious about positive reinforcement. The parents' and practitioners' concept of "doing great" may differ and may cause conflict. By using active listening skills, the practitioner can demonstrate willingness to implement a parent's plan of action instead of his or her own if it is possible and he or she need to provide legitimate program options while remaining focused on the process and the outcome, which is where most parents are focused (Luterman, 1991; Raver, 1991).

Conclusion: Bridge To Partnership: A Parent Perspective

There are many rewards to a true partnership between parents and practitioners. What began as a rather negative and difficult impact on our family slowly became positive. If necessity is the mother of invention, our family unit grew in a way we could not have predicted. We became self-reliant, closer, and stronger, and learned new skills and problem-solving techniques. People are resilient and, as parents, we can and do learn to cope in a variety of difficult situations. Whether out of practice or necessity, we become more adaptable and better able to meet the next challenge—more than we ever thought possible.

The role of a good parent is to eventually do oneself out of a job. The goal that we work towards is achieving independence for our child so that we are no longer needed. Having a child with a hearing loss certainly intensifies that role. It is thrust upon us. As our son's primary agents, we learned to advocate effectively, make the necessary decisions along the way, and solve problems for him and our family. We taught the teenager the skills of managing his own life; and as a young adult, he absorbed these lessons and learned to work in a respectful and effective partnership.

In order to establish a successful and caring program for a child who has a hearing loss, it is important that a genuine alliance be formed between the parents and the practitioners. Parents need to be respected as the primary players on the team, because we have the ultimate responsibility for our child's future. Even though a communication gap exists between some practitioners and some parents, it is more a gap of style than of intent. By planning initiatives together, the gap can be bridged and lines of communication can be opened.

A positive parent–professional relationship can be achieved only by responsible sharing of information, feelings, attitudes, and values. Trust, integrity, creativity, innovation, the respect of individual differences, acceptance of responsibility, and accountability, are essential for the making of such a relationship. A successful relationship between parents and practitioners is always changing and always maturing.

Parents and practitioners both want success for the child and for the family. For parents, success affirms parenting skills, and for practitioners, success justifies their careers. Our family crossed the bridge and formed many partnerships. Today, some of my best friends are indeed the practitioners who have entered and enriched our lives.

THE PARTNERSHIP OF THE PSYCHOLOGIST, AV PRACTITIONER, AND PARENT

Practitioners join the child's team with experience, expertise, and a responsibility to meet the needs of a diverse group of children and families. The parents join the team naked. They are desperate for gifted, compassionate practitioners to show up who are as committed to the welfare of their child as they are. The vulnerability and fear parents feel can contribute to misunderstandings between family members and practioners. Conversely, some practioners may have rigid boundaries and a brusque demeanor out of their own deep needs for self-protection due to personal and professional reasons; no one else knows the inner struggles that the practitioner is experiencing. Parents only see the outer behavior and feel angry, hurt, and resentful when it is directed at them. Psychologists can play a critical role as compassionate listeners who help parents and practitioners deal with their fears and inner struggles. They can also help them to develop effective communication strategies so that optimal outcomes for the child can be realized.

Vulnerabilities of Parents

Practitioners and families enter the team from radically different positions. Practitioners chose to develop expertise in service to the world of those with hearing loss. The scientific data, theories of hearing loss and treatment, advances on the horizon, the range of possibilities and limitations, and the technical language implicit in all these areas are familiar terrain. Not so for families. Families become part of the world of those with hearing loss. No one asks if this is a world into which they would like to enter. They wake up one day and realize it is the reality in which they now live. When we are thrown into an unexpected situation that threatens the well-being of a loved one, most of us experience significant fear and anxiety. What is this going to mean for their child? Will they be able to help their child flourish in the world in light of this new information? In addition, parents may find information on the Internet that may lead them to feel overwhelmed and defeated with the explosion of new words and issues. *The psychologist may be able to guide the parents in how to access and keep track of relevant information that will help them with their child's situation, and assist the parent(s) in mak-*

ing decisions that are consistent with their desires and needs, in spite of all the uncertainty and stress.

Vulnerabilities of Practitioners

Many practitioners are very aware of the vulnerabilities and fear with which the parents are grappling. They may recognize challenges in the family in regard to other health issues, the needs of other siblings, financial burdens, job losses, strain in the parents' marriage, etc. Practitioners hold in information about this child as well as all the other children they serve. This can create stress and anxiety because they are not able to meet all the needs that these children and parents bring with them. Although practitioners may be very gifted at what they do, knowledgeable, self-confident, and respected, when under stress, they may behave with indifference in order to cope, unaware that parents or others perceive them as arrogant, rude, and dismissive.

Role of the Psychologist

Psychologists can help practitioners and family members collaborate as an effective team. When they have different styles of communication, the psychologist may serve as a sounding board and coach by helping them develop effective ways of working together. The psychologist can help the practitioners understand what parents are experiencing, and the additional challenges parents may be facing beyond the child with the hearing loss. Through feedback and advice from a psychologist, practi-

tioners may come to realize that their communication style is impeding the very goals to which they are committed.

Psychologists can help parents feel more confident in contributing to the team for the child's benefit, rather than undermining the medical and scientific data that are relevant to their child's future. They can also help the practitioners communicate medical information about possible assessments, and various treatment options in ways that do not overwhelm the parents with technical jargon. In addition to providing individual professional help to a team member, psychologists can also serve as a bridge person to help practitioners and family members clarify misunderstandings. The psychologist may provide relevant developmental or personal information about a child and the child's family, including differences in cultural norms that may be impeding communication.

The psychologist can play a critical role in helping practitioners deal constructively with stress. A psychologist who recognizes the signs of unrelieved stress can help a practitioner realize what is happening to them physically, mentally, and emotionally. He or she can be empathetic, compassionate listeners and coach other team members to develop effective approaches to managing stress in healthy ways that make sense. In a private consultation with a psychologist, a practitioner may share what is happening and receive support and help. This help can be directed at both the personal issues and the ways in which the practitioner can interact more effectively as a team member, despite their internal struggles.

It is critical that those in the helping professions take care of themselves consistently through self-awareness of rising stress and wise choices for stress reduction, such as regular exercise, time with friends, laughter, meditation, healthy eating, sufficient sleep, and immersion in nature. When stress is not managed in healthy ways, it leads to health problems for the practitioners themselves and decreases their ability to flourish in both their personal and professional lives. The practitioner who incorporates healthy stress management in daily life is able to model for other team members and families some effective ways of managing stress. If team members help each other deal with the stress inherent in the helping professions, it will contribute to making the team more effective on behalf of each child they seek to help.

Case Study

Gina, age 4, received a cochlear implant after a nearly 2-year debate between her parents about whether she *should* get one. As older parents, deeply concerned about the well-being of their only child, Joe and Linda had strong, but divergent feelings about what would be best for Gina.

Gina's sensorineural loss was severe to profound in both ears. Based on information from practitioners and their own research about CIs, Linda felt they should proceed with the cochlear implant immediately to maximize the language learning during this crucial time in Gina's brain development. In contrast, Joe focused on the great strides Gina made with hearing aids. He wanted to give her more time to mature. Although he didn't speak of it directly, he was also experiencing significant fear of putting his daughter through such major surgery.

Joe was a stay-at-home dad who would be the primary person participating in and overseeing Gina's AVT. He had strong feelings of anxiety about his competence in providing the level of care Gina would need.

Gina's ENT doctor, audiologist, and auditory-verbal practitioner agreed that Gina was a good candidate for a CI, but both parents needed to support the decision. The auditory-verbal practitioner, Suzanne, was anxious about what she perceived to be an ever-narrowing window of *workable language time*. She felt Joe would eventually come around, but she was frustrated because *he just doesn't get the importance of this language learning time.*

Having both parents fully integrated into Gina's *team* as she moved through this process was essential for her long-term success. As is often the case, Joe's resistance was fueled by his fear, not uncommon for one or both parents. Given the potential consequences of prolonged delay, and the difficulty of enlisting Joe's support, Suzanne asked me to see the parents and I met with them.

I also talked with Suzanne about her investment in Gina and all of the children with whom she worked. A long-time and respected practitioner, she rose to all sorts of issues with *her children*, many of whom had multiple challenges. When parents did not take her advice, however, she became visibly frustrated and short-tempered. She felt that she was the expert and could not understand how this loving father would deny his daughter a chance to soar. Her frustration and disappointment were becoming evident in their interactions.

If this was going to be a successful partnership, Suzanne would need to let go of her negative assessment of Joe. She felt she was allied with Linda in a battle for Gina. Through our work together, Suzanne was able to see how her mindset and negative perceptions were keeping her from having compassion for Joe. She began to focus on imagining the fear and the huge weight of responsibility on Joe's shoulders regarding the surgery, and his anxiety about his competence to fill the role of the primary teacher at home.

It was important for me to help her see and then emphasize the benefits of having Joe become her trusted and engaged partner. Her success with Gina depended on this collaboration. Joe was just not ready and he felt very alone. What did she think it would take to help him be ready? As a natural problem solver, she put herself in Joe's shoes, and without judgment, began to imagine what he might need to feel safer in what he experienced as an unsympathetic and risky atmosphere.

Simultaneously, in my sessions with Joe and Linda, Linda began to listen to Joe differently. She no longer saw him as an obstacle that she needed to move out of the way, but allowed him to share the deeper reasons behind his reluctance to proceed with Gina's surgery. As Linda became less hostile and more accepting, he shared the roots of his trepidation about Gina having surgery and how responsible he would feel if it did not go well. We talked about how certain decisions that parents make for their children were a combination of

advice, information and gut feeling. Would this be the right decision? One could only hope. Were there other alternatives? Of course there were. What would he need to feel more comfortable? How could Linda help him? How could the Cochlear Implant Team be more responsive?

Over time, Joe's anxiety lessened and he allowed himself to move into a space of exploration. Was he eager? Not really. Although refusing to meet them before, he agreed to speak with two other fathers who, like him, had significant trepidation before their children's surgeries. Joe also recognized that he needed to learn more about what he would do with his daughter after the surgery. With the parents' permission, he observed Suzanne work with other children and their parents.

In our own daily lives, our timetable is just that—ours. We cannot predict the time it will take for others to adapt to changes in their lives that we are expecting of them and helping them with. What we can do is be present in ways that will help them on their journey. An important aspect of that is to *observe ourselves and notice what it means to us to have them do what we know is best for them and what it means to us when they do not.*

Tips for Strengthening Partnerships

Partnerships are critical in AVT. While working within the limitations of our realms of influence and expertise, it is important that practitioners remember how critical it is for the child to have a stable, reliable, interested person in their life who focuses on them during their sessions. This reminds us of the value of staying in the present and focusing on what we are able to deliver to the child instead of worrying about what we are unable to provide. The possibility of creating and sustaining strong, effective partnerships is enhanced when partners communicate respect for one another and an unflagging commitment to the success of the child.

Cultivating an Environment of Respect

Respect for another is communicated primarily through nonverbal behaviors such as gestures, facial expression, eye contact, use of space, and time. No matter what words we speak, if people feel disrespected, it creates tension and negativity. Although we cannot control how another interprets our nonverbal behaviors, it is important to be aware of and take responsibility for the many ways we communicate to other practitioners without saying a word.

Nonverbal communication is also critical when meeting with children and their parents. By giving parents our full attention by listening carefully and patiently when they speak allows us to create a welcoming, supportive environment in which we are fully present with the family. If the practitioner delivers difficult messages with a tone of voice, facial expression, and body posture that communicates compassion and respect, it is more likely that the parents will be able to hear the recommendations and recognize that the practitioner does have the best interest

of their child as the ultimate goal. These all contribute to the family's confidence in our respect for them and our commitment to the child's success.

Creating Openness Between Partners

When practitioners skillfully combine their respective areas of expertise, they maximize the potential for finding creative and effective solutions that benefit a particular youngster and family. With this in mind, practitioners need to approach new team partners with a sense of curiosity and an open mind. Openness to each new person helps us see the unique strengths, skills, and needs of the individual with whom we are working.

When team members are meeting for the first time, it is advisable to make the time and space to meet in person to maximize the potential for good rapport. If a personal meeting is not possible, we need to consider Skype, FaceTime, or a phone conversation. Staying connected through e-mail and text works, but meeting in person initially enhances the potential for a productive partnership. When establishing a strong partnership with parents, practitioners need to keep in mind the degree to which fear and anxiety may influence the ways parents communicate. If a practitioner observes behaviors in the child, which suggest the need for further testing or a referral to another practitioner, the parents may feel threatened. Their first response may be to blame any problems on the practitioner who is working with the child because they may not see the behavior as a red flag. A parent may also perceive a suggestion for more testing or referral as a concern that there may be additional issues as *giving up on the child or family.* The parents may feel abandoned at the very point when they most need to feel they are part of a committed team. Practitioners who do not take the parents' blame, defensiveness, or anger personally, are more likely to listen carefully to them and assure them that the goal of gathering more information comes from a deep commitment to meet the needs of their child.

It may also be wise to engage a psychologist to help parents work through their fears and concerns. He or she may be very useful as a bri*dge person.* The psychologist may be able to give professionals additional insight into what is going on with a child and the parents, and help resolve misunderstandings and conflict among other members of the team and between them and the family.

Playing to the Strengths of the Team

The needs of an individual child and family can be overwhelming. It is critical that the practitioners focus *on what is possible within the realm of AVT. A successful relationship with an AV practitioner can motivate the family to rise to the challenge of helping their child learn to listen and talk.* Working effectively in tandem involves establishing clear goals. What are we trying to accomplish today? This week? This month? This year? Given all the opportunities and obstacles, which ones can be reasonably incorporated, and which

ones do we need to deal with, overcome or adapt to?

Although practitioners do not have identical styles or approaches, if they incorporate compatible styles and work together respectfully toward common goals, they increase their ability to meet the needs of the child and the family.

If one member of the team has a particularly strong relationship with the parents, it may be wise to have that practitioner deliver recommendations for more tests or referrals when they are needed. In each situation it is helpful to recognize existing strengths in various partnerships and build on them. This same principle may apply if there are challenges with one of the practitioners on the team. Who is in the best position to talk with that person individually and try to work through the difficulties that interfere with healthy team functioning?

AV practitioners are not in a position to *fix* the child, the family, or a situation. They are in a position to help people learn to live with the situation they are in as healthfully as possible. Through healthy partnerships, we maximize our ability to help the family be more successful in making the changes necessary to live enriched lives.

CONCLUSION

It cannot be assumed that just because well-trained practitioners are involved that they will form an effective team with one another and the family on behalf of the child. Constructive partnerships that lead to the emergence of an effective team are organic, intentionally developed, and sustained over time. This requires self-awareness and effort on the part of each team member. Arriving at the most complete understanding of a child's situation and the best treatment plan at a given time may require working through strong differences of opinion held by highly capable practitioners. Constructive conflict may be essential in arriving at the most complete picture of a child's hearing, communication, physical, psychological, and social needs. Clinical insights are advanced when practitioners advocate for the best interests of the child as viewed through the lens of their discipline and these may produce heated exchanges. If team members advocate strongly, putting forth their evidence and listening carefully to those who disagree, the fire created may illuminate a plan that serves the child far better than would have otherwise been the case. The commitment this requires is strengthened when each team member is focused on one common goal: to serve the needs of the individual child.

REFERENCES

American Academy of Audiology. (2004). *Scope of practice*. Retrieved from http://www.audiology.org/resources/documentlibrary/Pages/ScopeofPractice.aspx

American Speech-Language-Hearing Association. (2004). *Scope of practice in audiology*. Retrieved from http://www.asha.org/policy

American Physical Therapy Association (APTA). (n.d.). Retrieved August 9, 2015, from http://www.apta.org/PTCareers/RoleofaPT/

Ayres, A. J. (1972). *Sensory integration and learning disabilities*. Los Angeles, CA: Western Psychological Services.

Baker, T., Haines, S., Yost, J., DiClaudio, S., Braun, C., & Holt, S. (2012). The role of family-centered therapy when used with physical or occupational therapy in children with congenital or acquired disorders. *Physical Therapy Reviews, 17*(1), 29–36.

Bharadwaj, S., Daniel, L., & Matzke, P. (2009). Sensory processing disorder in children with cochlear implants. *American Journal of Occupational Therapy, 63*, 208–213.

Bharadwaj, S., & Matzke, P. L., & Daniel, L. (2012). Multisensory processing in children with cochlear implants. *International Journal of Pediatric Otorhinolaryngology, 76*, 890–895.

Bruder, M. B. (2000). Family-centered early intervention clarifying our values for the new millennium. *Topics in Early Childhood Special Education, 20*(2), 105–115.

Bullard, C. (2002). *The itinerant teacher's handbook*. Hillsboro, OR: Butte.

Bundy, A., Lane, S., & Murray, E. (2002). *Sensory integration theory and practice*. Philadelphia, PA: F. A. Davis.

Charge Syndrome Foundation. (2015). Retrieved from http://www.chargesyndrome.org/about-charge.asp

Cole, E. B., & Flexer, C. (2016). *Children with hearing loss: Developing listening and talking birth to six* (3rd ed.). San Diego, CA: Plural.

Crais, E. R., Roy, V. P., & Free, K. (2006). Parents' and professionals' perceptions of the implementation of family-centered practices in child assessments. *American Journal of Speech-Language Pathology, 15*(4), 365–377.

Eisler, R. T., & Potter, T. M. (n.d.). *Transforming interprofessional partnerships: A new framework for nursing and partnership-based health care*.

Engel-Yeger, B., & Weissman, D. (2009). A comparison of motor abilities and perceived self-efficacy between children with hearing impairments and normal hearing children. *Disability and Rehabilitation, 31,* 352–358.

Engum, S. A., & Jeffries, P. R. (2012). Interdisciplinary collisions: Bringing healthcare professionals together. *Collegian, 19*(3), 145–151.

Fingerhut, P. E., Piro, J., Sutton, A., Campbell, R., Lewis, C., Lawji, D., & Martinez, N. (2013). Family-centered principles implemented in home-based, clinic-based, and school-based pediatric settings. *American Journal of Occupational Therapy, 67*(2), 228–235.

Fitzpatrick, E., Angus, D., Durieux-Smith, A., Graham, I. D., & Coyle, D. (2008). Parents' needs following identification of childhood hearing loss. *American Journal of Audiology, 17*(1), 38–49.

Gallaudet Research Institute. (2011) *Regional and National Summary report of data from the 2009-2010 Annual Survey of Deaf and Hard of Hearing Children and Youth.* Washington, DC: GRI, Gallaudet University.

Gheysen, F., Loots, G., & Van Waelvelde, H. (2008). Motor development of deaf children with and without cochlear implants. *Journal of Deaf Studies and Deaf Education, 13*(2), 215–224.

Houston, K. T., & Perigoe, C. (2011). Future directions in professional preparation and development. *Volta Review, 110*(2), 339–340.

Jacot, E., Abbcclc, T. V., Dcbrc, H. R., & Wiener-Vacher, S. R. (2009). Vestibular impairments pre- and post-cochlear implant in children. *International Journal of Pediatric Otorhinolaryngology, 73*(2), 209–217.

Jerome, A., Kannan, L., Lakhani, H., & Palekar, T. (2013). Prevalence of vestibular dysfunction in hearing impaired children. *International Journal of Pharmaceutical Science and Health Care, 3,* 1–6.

Joint Committee on Infant Hearing. (2007). Year 2007 position statement: Principles and guidelines for early hearing detection and intervention programs. *Pediatrics, 120*(4), 898–921.

Kleinpeter, R. D., Wright, L., Lander, J., & Tucker, D. (2001). *The effects of cochlear implant stimulation on the balance skills of children with sensorineural hearing impairment.* Poster presented at the annual Combined Sections Meeting of the American Physical Therapy Association, San Antonio, Texas.

Kurtzer-White, E., & Luterman, D. (2003). Families and children with hearing loss: Grief and coping. *Mental Retardation and Developmental Disabilities Research Reviews, 9*(4), 232–235.

Luterman, D. (1991). *When your child is deaf.* Timonium, MD: York Press.

MacKean, G. L., Thurston, W. E., & Scott, C. M. (2005). Bridging the divide between families and health professionals' perspectives on family-centred care. *Health Expectations, 8*(1), 74–85.

Mailloux, Z., & Miller-Kuhaneck, H, (2014). Evolution of a theory: How measurement has shaped Ayres Sensory Integration. *American Journal of Occupational Therapy, 68,* 495–499.

Miyamoto, R. T., Houston, D. M., Kirk, K. I., Perdew, A. E., & Svirsky, M. A. (2003). Language development in deaf infants following cochlear implantation. *Acta Otolaryngologica, 123,* 241–244.

Moeller, M. P., Carr, G., Seaver, L., Stredler-Brown, A., & Holzinger, D. (2013). Best practices in family-centered early intervention for children who are deaf or hard of hearing: An international consensus statement. *Journal of Deaf Studies and Deaf Education, 18*(4), 429–445.

Niagara Children's Services Committee. (1990). *Parents in case management.* Thorold, ON.

Pinborough-Zimmerman, J., Satterfield, R., Miller, J., Bilder, D., Hossain, S., & Mcmahon, W. (2007). Communication disorders: Prevalence and comorbid intellectual disability, autism, and emotional/behavioral disorders. *American Journal of Speech-Language Pathology16*(4), 359.

Pollack, D. Consumer Subcommittee. (1970, 1985). *Educational Audiology for the Limited-Hearing Infant and Pre-schooler.*

Rajendran, V., & Roy, F. G. (2011). An overview of motor skill performance and balance in hearing impaired children. *Italian Journal of Pediatrics, 37*, 33–37.

Rajendran, V., Roy, F. G., & Jeevanantham, D. (2012). A preliminary randomized controlled study on the effectiveness of vestibular-specific neuromuscular training in children with hearing impairment. *Clinical Rehabilitation, 27*(5), 459–467.

Rajendran, V., Roy, F., & Jeevanantham, D. (2013). Effect of exercise intervention on vestibular related impairments in hearing-impaired children. *Alexandria Journal of Medicine, 49*, 7–12.

Raver, S. A. (1991). Effective family-centered services: Supporting family choices and rights. *Infant–Toddler Intervention, 1*, 169–176.

Rhoades, E. A., & Duncan, J. (2010). *Auditory-verbal practice toward a family-centered approach.* Springfield, IL: Charles C Thomas.

Richburg, C. M., & Knickelbein, B. A. (2011). Educational audiologists: Their access, benefit, and collaborative assistance to speech-language pathologists in schools. *Language, Speech, and Hearing Services in Schools, 42*(4), 444–460.

Robbins, A. M., Svirsky, M., & Kirk, K. I. (1997). Children with implants can speak, but can they communicate? *Otolaryngology-Head and Neck Surgery, 117*, 155–160.

Robertson, L. (2014). *Literacy and deafness. Listening and spoken language* (2nd ed.). San Diego, CA: Plural.

Savelsbergh, G. J. P., Netelenbos, J. B., & Whiting, H. T. A. (1991). Auditory perception and the control of spatially coordinated action of deaf and hearing impaired children. *Journal of Child Psychology and Psychiatry, 32*, 489–500.

Simon, A. (1997). A follow-up study of 35 young stutterers: Parents' reactions to counseling. *Journal of Fluency Disorders, 22*(2), 101.

Simons, R. (1987). *After the tears: Parents talk about raising a child with a disability.* San Diego, CA: Harcourt Brace Jovanovich.

Sørensen, K., Van den Broucke, S., Fullam, J., Doyle, G., Pelikan, J., Slonska, Z., & Brand, H. (2012). Health literacy and public health: A systematic review and integration of definitions and models. *BMC Public Health, 12*(1), 80.

Souza, P. (n.d.) *Improving audibility: The foundation for speech understanding.* Retrieved from http://www.listeningand spokenlanguage.org/ImprovingAudi bility/

Stableford, S., & Mettger, W. (2007). Plain language: A strategic response to the health literacy challenge. *Journal of Public Health Policy, 28*(1), 71–93.

Svirsky, M. A., Robbins, A. M., Kirk, K. I., Pisoni, D. B., & Miyamoto, R. T. (2000). Language development in profoundly deaf children with cochlear implants. *Psychological Science, 11*, 153–158.

The AG Bell Academy for Listening and Spoken Language Knowledge. (2007). *Principles of LSLS.* Retrieved from http://www.listeningandspokenlanguage.org/AcademyDocument.aspx?id=563

Todt, I., Basta, D., & Ernst, A. (2008). Does the surgical approach in cochlear implantation influence the occurrence of postoperative vertigo? *Otolaryngology-Head and Neck Surgery, 138*, 8–12.

Trute, B., & Hiebert-Murphy, D. (2007). The implications of "working alliance" for the measurement and evaluation of family-centered practice in childhood disability services. *Infants and Young Children, 20*(2), 109–119.

Wilcox, M. J., & Woods, J. (2011). Participation as a basis for developing early intervention outcomes. *Language Speech and Hearing Services in Schools, 42*(3), 365.

Woods, J. J., Wilcox, M. J., Friedman, M., & Murch, T. (2011). Collaborative consultation in natural environments: Strategies to enhance family-centered supports and services. *Language, Speech, and Hearing Services in Schools, 42*(3), 379–392.

Yoshinaga-Itano, C. (2013). Principles and guidelines for early intervention after confirmation that a child is deaf or hard of hearing. *Journal of Deaf Studies and Deaf Education, 19*(2), 143–175.

17

FAMILY JOURNEYS IN AUDITORY-VERBAL THERAPY: STORIES FROM TWELVE COUNTRIES

Parents of Children with Hearing Loss

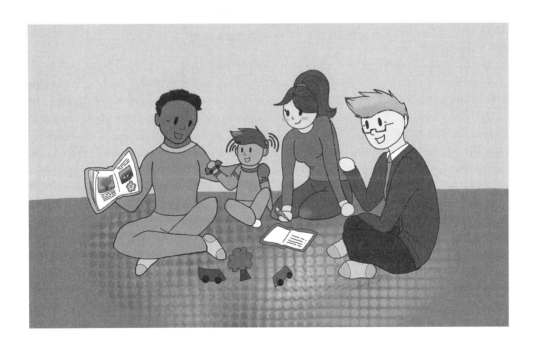

INTRODUCTION

Today's hearing technologies and Auditory-Verbal Therapy (AVT) can help many children with hearing loss achieve the expected outcomes in listening and spoken language that their parents have for them. From the Middle East to Australia, from North America to South America, and from Europe to Asia, interest in this intervention model continues to find its way into the hearts and minds of practitioners and parents.

In this chapter, 12 families from 12 countries share their personal journeys from the birth of their child to the diagnosis of hearing loss, from their active participation in therapy, to the successes they and their children enjoy today. All families chose AVT when their child was young and were coached and guided by a LSLS Cert. AVT. These families no longer attend auditory-verbal sessions.

Parents have written anonymously and make no references to particular practitioners or programs. These individual and private journeys continue today and provide hope and encouragement sought by many families around the world. Journeys from the following countries are presented in alphabetical order: Argentina, Australia, Canada, Germany, Hong Kong, India, Israel, Mexico, Spain, United Arab Emirates (UAE), United Kingdom (UK), and United States (US).

ARGENTINA

The Story of Enzo*

In February 2004, we learned with great joy that I was expecting twin boys, Enzo and Mateo who would join our family with two daughters we already had. They were born at 6 months gestation, and unfortunately, they had to go to intensive care, and that brought lots of moments of despair. One day, at the nursery, I realized Enzo was purple, and had stopped breathing. He immediately received CPR and from then on, everything was hard for Enzo. One afternoon, I felt deeply anguished so I called the intensive care unit and the doctor told me, "Enzo is not well." He had sepsis. The pediatrician told me the worst thing a mother can hear: "He has only a few hours left." "No!" I shouted desperately. "I have two sons, and I want them both, no matter how." I don't know where I found strength but I carried on with my prayers. Miracles happen, of course, and Enzo gradually got better.

Diagnosis

At 5 months, Enzo was happy during the day but I noticed he was different at night when he cried a lot. We feared he might be autistic or deaf, but the pediatrician told us he was perfect. But we weren't satisfied so we saw an otorhinolaryngologist. He listened to us and understood our worries. He ordered some other tests and gave us the diagnosis of profound hearing loss. We didn't know what that meant, but suddenly the world seemed to crumble when the doctor told us about cochlear implants and we started our journey in a new direction. And we became familiar with words such as electrodes, speech processors, surgery, etc. We searched the Internet and found out about AVT.

When Enzo was 9 months old we contacted a practitioner in Buenos Aires who told us about AVT and she showed us videos of various children who spoke very well. We both said, "This is what we want!" In the meantime, we never stopped talking to our son and we stimulated him with different sounds. Enzo was implanted on August 18, 2005, in his right ear, the day of his first birthday.

A month later the implant was activated. We had looked forward to that moment which was very moving, hard to explain, marvelous. The moment our son heard for the first time was wonderful. Then we had to work hard to make lots of progress in listening and language development.

We traveled to Buenos Aires where I learned to help my son learn to listen with the AV practitioner. Every session started with a greeting song. Next, the practitioner showed us the objectives she had planned for the session and the strategies we should use. I would do the Ling Six-Sound Test to check that the implant was working well and we would start. We played fun games, role played everyday routines that we repeated at home in real life, we told stories and sang a lot. Everything was presented through audition first and then we would show him the object which made the sound or the action. While he played, we narrated what he did and we paused regularly for him to be able to process all the information. I wrote down the objectives to achieve for the next session, together with the strategies. The AV practitioner taught me three pillars of stimulation: routines, stories, and songs. I learnt from her to play the clown, to be dramatic and to model naturally all day long. A day in Enzo's life was wonderful: he would wake up, put on his implant, do the Ling Six-Sound Tests, and then start

listening and learning as we played. His twin brother was a great playmate.

All the family members read books to Enzo. I think about 10 a day! Through reading, Enzo's vocabulary and imagination grew. We had a song for every routine and object we played with. When I talked to him I tried to speak with lots of intonation so that Enzo paid more attention but I never raised my voice and just talked naturally. As days went by, Enzo started to understand directions and expressions, and he started to vocalize, play with sounds, and imitate the sounds he heard.

Then the big day arrived. It was unforgettable. We were on holiday at the beach and my husband, my daughters and I ran toward the sea. When the twins saw us leaving, they started calling us, and suddenly I said, "Wait, that was Enzo!" He said, " Mom! Dad!" We got him to repeat it 100 times!!! From that moment, he started talking. It was music to my ears.

Enzo loved his implant from the first day. His progress was steady. We took advantage of every waking moment by playing in the "imaginary park" we set up at home. We went to the gym to practice *up, down, backward, forward.* We played with concrete objects, such as chairs, we would move them up, down, in front, behind and on the side. When we went in the car, we practiced riddles and played "I Spy with My Little Eye." At the petrol station, we got out of the car and I described everything there: pump, hose, petrol, wheels, and I taught him about *danger*! We described the world for him, but mostly we just loved him.

Enzo started kindergarten in a regular school, the same as his brother and sisters. School helped him to socialize. He learned how to explain about the cochlear implant and what it was for. All his classmates were curious, and many wanted to have an implant like Enzo's. Years went by and every time we visited our AV practitioner, we would tell her everything. She answered all our questions and helped us reinforce what was necessary or teach us something new. At the hearing age of 3, after several evaluations, our practitioner said that Enzo had graduated!

Some months later, the practitioner started talking to us about a second implant. Confronted with our fears, we spoke to our otorhinolaryngologist and we were on board, convinced it was the best for Enzo.

Enzo received the second implant in his left ear at the age of 5. The experience was totally different because Enzo took part in the decision-making process. I believe it was he who gave us the strength to go on.

Once the surgery and activation were over, we returned to AVT for a couple of months to help Enzo learn how to listen with his new implant. During these sessions Enzo would only use his new implant and I would take objectives home to achieve during the week. I put them into practice through daily routines, only using the new implant. Enzo achieved the same hearing level as with his first implant fairly quickly. He finished kindergarten with both implants and was ready to start primary school.

Enzo started first grade being able to read and write. He never had any difficulty at school and he was just one of the gang. When he didn't understand something I suggested he ask his teacher. This fostered independence. We try not to pamper and overprotect him but we are always working on that.

Enzo is a very sociable boy. He is good, helpful, and mischievous and he has a strong personality. He is able to manage in a regular school where he does well in all subjects. He is learning English, is a member of the drama club, loves music, expresses himself creatively though his art, and he loves to read.

Today Enzo is in fifth grade and making steady progress. I believe he has all the tools he needs to manage in life and most importantly, to be happy. We are still in touch with our AV practitioner who has left her mark on each of us.

I have always said Enzo came into to this world to teach me how to be a mom in a different way, and he succeeded. He made me laugh, play, and experiment with things I had never expected to do. He made me see things in a simpler way, and not to be too demanding with my other children. I devoted time to my child and worked along with my AV practitioner and I gained a lot of confidence. As parents, we knew that we were not alone.

We feel the same way as many parents everywhere and we have the same dreams for Enzo as most parents have for their children. It is a journey and it is sometimes hard, but in the end, it is really something special and beautiful, like my son, and really, like all my children.

*Translated from Spanish

AUSTRALIA

The Story of Lewis

Before the birth of Lewis, our first child, I used to love seeing friends' babies do the "startle reflex." So when Lewis was born on the eighth of May 1996, it was something I waited for him to do. And I waited and waited. By about 6 weeks of age, he still hadn't done it despite being in situations where a loud noise should have woken him. I mentioned this to my husband, and later that day he deliberately dropped an empty plastic juice bottle on the wooden floor next to where Lewis was lying. I wasn't expecting the sudden loud noise, and I got a huge shock. Unfortunately, Lewis gave no reaction.

It was a profound moment for both of us, because after that very crude "hearing test," we knew there was something wrong with our beautiful, healthy baby boy. It began a process of desperately trying to prove that he could hear, while increasingly we grieved for the "perfect" baby we thought we had. I feel terrible now for thinking he was anything other than perfect, but I suspect that's a common reaction for parents who suddenly learn that their child has a hearing loss.

Over the next few months, Lewis underwent testing. By around 5 months of age, he had been formally diagnosed with a bilateral severe-to-profound sensorineural hearing loss. He was fitted with powerful hearing aids, which looked enormous on his bald, little head. We were aware of the importance of early detection and intervention and wanted to quickly make choices after getting the best advice we could find. We were open to doing what would give Lewis the most options for future relationships and education, but we knew we wanted him to listen and talk. We were fortunate to live in Sydney, because we had a choice of early intervention programs. We chose to investigate one that was close to home and offered AVT.

Our first appointment was just before Christmas in 1996. I was very anxious about attending that appointment. It meant acknowledging that Lewis had a hearing loss, and we were to be part of a community of other families with children like our boy. Again, I'm ashamed of that now, but I was reluctant to accept that's who we were: parents of a child with *special needs*. Thinking of Lewis this way made me feel sick every morning when I woke up. It terrified me that he wouldn't learn to talk, wouldn't hear our voices, wouldn't be able to communicate with his cousins, wouldn't understand our family's silly jokes, wouldn't have regular friends, or wouldn't attend our local school. I was overwhelmed by the thought that Lewis would never be able to fully participate in the life my husband and I had planned for our family.

So, we went to that first appointment, and we met two AV practitioners. We spent time talking, and they played with Lewis and listened to him laugh and babble. Afterward they gave us hope that Lewis would learn to listen and talk. "How did they know?" I wondered.

We started AVT, and Lewis' first AV session was a great surprise. We spent most of it switching a light on and off, while we said, "light on, light off," which fascinated him. Immediately he attempted to repeat our words. It was as much a session for me as it was for him. That is the way AVT works. We learned that everything he and I did together was an opportunity to get him listening and talking. It was fun and rewarding, and it quickly became our natural way of doing things. Every nappy change, every car trip, and every book we read was a chance to encourage him to listen and talk. It was a great success, and it amazed us. We also had a very supportive family, and Lewis' grandparents and aunty often came along to his sessions so they could also learn how to help him listen and talk when he was with them. He didn't realize it, but every day was a real life AV session. By the age of 2, his speech was age appropriate.

While Lewis made wonderful progress, it was clear that he was struggling to hear high-frequency sounds in everyday life. Our AV practitioner suggested we consider a cochlear implant to help him access all speech sounds more easily. Subsequently, we decided on a cochlear implant for his ear with the profound loss just before his third birthday. The activation of the CI was a bit rocky, and Lewis cried for his "buzzies" (hearing aids). I wondered if we'd done the right thing, but over the weeks and months that followed, he learned to love his implant and how much easier it was to hear speech.

At age 3½, Lewis began attending our local preschool. He was the only child with hearing loss they had ever taught. The AV practitioner met regularly with the preschool director to help Lewis adjust to his new environment and always offered help with anything they might require. The staff of the school went out of their way to provide the best listening and learning environment possible for Lewis. The director even wrote a page of notes every day about what Lewis said and did and what we needed to work on at home. Lewis made friends quickly in that lovely preschool, and he was soon socializing with them outside of preschool. Some of these children

are still friends today. It was clear that my fear for him never making friends was unnecessary.

At the age of 5½, Lewis started at the same primary school his father had attended, and the AV practitioner helped again with that transition. Lewis was assigned an itinerant teacher who visited him at school 5 hours a week and was a huge help in assisting Lewis' teachers who had no experience with children with hearing loss. Lewis didn't like being taken out of class for these lessons or other help, so she would often work with him and a small group inside the classroom. The other students came to love being chosen to work with her, and Lewis didn't feel the stigma of being excluded from the classroom. The itinerant teacher connected with the rest of the teachers and requested that Lewis always get the most appropriate teacher every year.

We have always valued our community, and we were keen to help Lewis be involved in church, sports, and other extracurricular activities. We loved seeing other families genuinely want Lewis to fit in, communicate well, succeed, and make friends.

Lewis' school years were filled with happy and successful times. He excelled academically, and from year 3, he was included in the school's extension program for gifted and talented students. He played soccer with the local club, played cricket, and learned to surf.

When Lewis was 12, he received a cochlear implant in his other ear. He had greater access to speech in noisy environments, could localize sounds more easily, and had a new appreciation for music, a wonderful thing as he entered his teenage years.

Lewis had had an FM system at primary school, but at high school, he didn't feel the need to use it. We chose a relatively small nongovernment coeducational high school, which meant he no longer had an itinerant teacher. It was a wonderful nurturing environment. He only had one friend there when he started, but he made new friends quickly and joined the school's cadet program and soccer team. Lewis knew to sit close to the front of the classroom, and his teachers were impressed by his willingness to ask questions when he wasn't sure about something. They wished other students would do the same thing. We can honestly say that in his 6 years at high school, he was never teased!

Today, Lewis communicates so well that we go for long periods when we forget he has any challenges at all, and his friends feel the same. From a technology viewpoint, there has never been a better time in history to have a hearing loss. Hearing technology, social media, vibrating clocks, close-caption TV, and direct iPod/technology connections are fantastic.

Lewis performed extremely well in his final school exams and is now at university studying chemical engineering and loves being there. He achieved excellent distinctions in his first semester exams. He currently works part-time at our local supermarket where he communicates easily with colleagues and the public, and he has friends and great community connections. All of that is due to many factors, including AVT and to Lewis himself.

Not all parents are fortunate to have access to AV practitioners, but it would be good if all parents did. Parents everywhere, however, do need access to strong early intervention practitioners whom they can trust over the years. We are extremely proud of Lewis and his achievements, and we feel very optimistic about his future.

CANADA

The Story of Leah

Leah, our second child and our first daughter, was born in 2000. Her arrival meant a playmate for our son. A sister was his second choice, after a dog. In those days, hearing tests were not given to newborns, and so we left the hospital with our smiling baby, no wiser about her hearing capabilities. I went back to work after 6 months, and Leah went to day care, just as her brother had done. She seemed to be a happy child. I remember Leah cooing and gurgling at 6 months. We visited our pediatrician and were content that she was meeting her developmental milestones as expected. We had raised our first child successfully and were confident we could manage a second just as easily!

One Friday afternoon, when my husband picked Leah up from day care, he noticed that she did not respond excitedly to his arrival as she usually did. She was not facing him and did not seem to react to his voice at all. He raced her directly to the pediatrician. The two adults spent the next 10 minutes setting off their cell phones behind her, but she was totally unresponsive. We spent that weekend totally devastated, sad and crying, thinking our daughter would be isolated from her family, our community, and the joy of sound by her hearing loss.

We ruled out a cold and had tubes inserted into her ears but to no avail. It took a long time to get an appointment at the hospital. We could not determine the cause of hearing loss and do not know it to this day. Leah got hearing aids, but they were not very effective.

We were lucky to be associated with a children's hospital in a large urban Canadian center that had a cochlear implant program. We were waitlisted for an implant and researched all we could about the cochlear implant. We even subscribed to a mail list to follow others' experiences, which we still use today. We also spoke to other parents whose children had cochlear implants, and they reassured that there were better days ahead. We were sorry, however, that it took so long to get the implant, because Leah had stopped cooing and gurgling. I wondered if I would ever hear her say "mama."

Our research indicated that receiving the cochlear implant was only part of the equation. It needed to be followed up with AVT for Leah to be able to integrate fully into our lives, and the original life we had hoped for her. We met with the director of a well-respected agency that provided AVT. He lent us a video of another family in therapy, and although the child with hearing loss did not have perfect speech, he was communicating verbally and responding through listening. My husband and I were elated at the thought that Leah might achieve this too. We were keen to begin!

We understood that this therapy would require commitment and family participation, but the effort would

pay off. One month prior to Leah's first cochlear implant, we arrived for our first of many weekly sessions of AVT. We were happy to meet our friendly practitioner who was very committed to her clients: our child, Leah, and us. Leah was perched in her high chair, dressed in a pretty yellow dress, and sat attentively engaged with the variety of age-appropriate games. Our AV practitioner became an informal addition to our family over the next few years as a variety of family members accompanied Leah to therapy. She holds a special place in our hearts.

One month later, Leah received her first cochlear implant. Although she came out of surgery with her whole head wrapped in bandages, her surgeon reassured us that all had gone according to plan. Leah was activated 1 month later, and her auditory-verbal life really began.

Leah continued at day care and subsequently transferred to the nursery school her brother had attended, and we continued our weekly AVT sessions. I was lucky to work at a company that was willing to accommodate me with shorter days for much of our first year of AVT, so we could work at "playing" together at home to master the goals of the week. We were also eligible for some regional support and had a teacher who visited us at our home, at Leah's grandparents' home, or at day care. I would say, however, that Leah's biggest inspiration came from her brother and her desire to communicate with him and for him to communicate with her.

We spent a lot of the early days of therapy pointing to our ears and helping Leah become aware of all the sounds of life, such as the beep of the microwave, the hissing of a boiling kettle, or the thunder of a flushing toilet. Soon the vocalizations of the learning to listen sounds came along, and we inched forward. I remember how excited we were when she said *ahhhh* at the sight of an airplane.

Leah made rapid progress, and we were about to be discharged from therapy after 3 years when a second cochlear implant was offered to her. We were nervous again but having seen what one implant could provide, we agreed, after research and discussion with another family whose daughter had received bilateral implants, that Leah should receive another.

As a person who works with computers, I was keen for Leah to have a disaster recovery (DR) system, a second cochlear implant to depend on in case one failed. At times, when her cochlear implant had malfunctioned, she felt isolated. So at four, she received her second implant, and we extended her AVT to train her "new ear." We were finally discharged just before she entered kindergarten. I felt very nervous about being *set free*, but it was time.

We have always partnered with Leah's teachers so that they were aware of her cochlear implants. In junior high school, this entailed introducing the teachers to Leah prior to school starting. We explained her equipment, settings and batteries, even though Leah had become fairly adept at managing her equipment independently. At the end of elementary school, Leah did try using an FM system, but it was not a positive experience. She once did a presentation to her class about her cochlear implants in an attempt to familiarize other children about them, but she never felt it benefitted her and refused to do it again.

Leah coerced me into sending her for swimming lessons when she was five. I was worried about how she would manage, but she told me that all her friends were doing it and she needed to, too. Sadly, she was not introduced to cochlear swimming hearing equipment until her teenage years, and she never liked using it. Sometimes, she received instruction before swimming, and at other times she relied on physical guidance and gestures during class. She learned to swim well.

Leah also played piano for several years, and it improved her musicality. I think one of the hardest things for her is the limited ability to hold a tune, but neither her father nor I can hold much of a tune, and we can't blame that on any hearing issues.

Fortunately, today's technological world provides great support to compensate for hearing loss; mobile phones connect via Bluetooth to cochlear implants; music and lyrics are easily available on the Internet, and texting is the most common form of teenage communication.

Leah has completed the first year of high school while participating in a multilanguage program without any additional support. She has done well and integrated into a new bigger school and made new friends.

Much to my chagrin, Leah refused to set up an Individualized Educational Plan (IEP) going into high school. In her first year of high school, I secretly sent a note to all of her teachers informing them of her reliance on cochlear implants, the need for preferential seating, sound reduction, difficulties in the noisy spaces, etc. Leah was livid with me for breeching her confidentiality, but I felt it was necessary for the teachers to be aware of her challenges.

Entering second year, she and her guidance teacher agreed that she would tell her teachers independently about her hearing challenges, and that she would request closed captioning on movies and videos as required. I am happy she can advocate for herself.

Leah wears her long hair down, so people do not know that she has cochlear implants. High school can be a very judgmental time when all one wants to do is "fit in." Today, Leah likes to think of herself as an independent, playful, artistic, TV-addicted, chocolate-craving, music-loving 15-year-old, who lives a full social, academic, and family life, and happens to have a hearing loss!

We are amazed at how Leah continues to manage, and we know that she is not limited by her hearing loss. We look forward to seeing what her future holds.

GERMANY

The Story of Ella*

We're just a normal, ordinary family: mother, father, one son and one daughter. We live on the outskirts of a major city in a semi-detached house that has a small garden. My husband works full time, and I've had a part-time job since my son was born in February 2005. When our second planned child, our daughter, came into the world on December 11, 2006, we felt that our family was complete. We were overwhelmed with joy.

Even though it was not mandatory at the time, the maternity hospital where both of our children were born already performed newborn hearing screenings as a standard procedure. From a present-day perspective, I can see what a great chance this was for us and for our daughter.

After the screening, the pediatrician told us that the findings were conspicuous—for both ears—but that this could also have other reasons. It didn't necessarily indicate any problem. He asked us to come back after eight weeks for further examinations. At first, we weren't worried at all. All of us could hear perfectly fine, so why should it be any different for our daughter? We did, however, pay some extra attention: Could she hear us? Did she react when we entered the room? But to us, everything seemed normal. We thought that everything was fine.

When, 8 weeks later, we went back to the hospital, the scheduled examinations revealed that we'd been wrong: The physician told us gently but firmly that our daughter was moderately hearing impaired. She told us that there was a range of things we could do—acoustic instruments, cochlear implants—but I couldn't really listen; it felt as if there was a glass wall between us. She gave us a letter for the hearing instrument specialist and further information.

Back home, thousands of thoughts and thousands of questions were running through our heads: Would our daughter ever find a husband? Would she ever be able to attend a school and find a job? Would she understand us? Would she learn how to speak? Could she ever pin up her hair?—One would see the hearing instruments! And would we have to learn how to use sign language? Should we even sing to and speak to our baby if she could not hear us? How would our life go on from now?

We were rather upset but wanted to take action immediately. We contacted the hearing instrument specialist. Three weeks later, our daughter got two hearing aids that she accepted from the start. But her hearing response was far from ideal, and soon afterward, her diagnosis was changed from "moderate" to "profound" hearing impairment.

We kept gathering information. We read books and talked with parents who shared our fate: How well did their children learn how to speak? What were their fears; what were their sorrows? Which of them would stay at home; which of them would go to work? We met other families in our hospital and the local school for children with hearing loss. We got to know a girl whose hearing loss was very similar to that of our daughter, and indeed, she could speak very well even though she "only" used hearing aids.

After consulting the hospital's cochlear implant experts, we decided for an implant on the left side and for AVT to start soon after. We wanted our daughter to be best equipped for a life with spoken language and living amid hearing people, so that someday she would be able to decide for herself what her life would be like. It was a terrible feeling to leave a 10-month-old baby behind—without anything to do except wait for the operation to be over. Would everything be fine? Would she be able to hear?

The operation and the healing process all went very well. Then came the great moment: the processor was switched on for the first time. Our auditory-verbal practitioner and an engineer were sitting in front of our daughter, examining her reactions: a twinkle, a twitch, or a facial expression—very often, the first

reactions are tiny. But even if I couldn't make out anything, our practitioner was convinced that our daughter had heard something.

What followed then was a weekly therapy session in our hospital where our daughter was to learn the first learning-to-listen sounds and to learn to associate certain sounds with certain objects. The whole family was included in the therapy. Our practitioner kept trying to strengthen the trust in ourselves as supporting parents. We were told to follow our intuition, to sing with our baby, to tell her stories, to visualize our speech acts (e.g., to point at myself when I used the word "mom"), and to lead a life as normal as possible. It was about a year after the operation that our daughter began to speak her first words. It was an incredible, immense relief.

In addition to the weekly therapy, we took our daughter to an ordinary regular playgroup, to baby swimming, and to the playground. From the age of two and a half years, our daughter attended an integrated kindergarten. For this she got—as advised by our therapist—an FM system that would later, at school, become absolutely indispensable. Moreover, she received speech therapy and, since her diagnosis, weekly training with a special education teacher at the school for the deaf.

These were a lot of appointments, and it was good to have so many wonderful people around who helped us —after all, we also had a son who needed us, too. But with the help of our parents, our brothers and sisters, close friends and neighbors, it all went very well and our daughter made progress almost every day. It did not take long until she pronounced her first two-word sentences. She didn't have any trouble understanding us and her surroundings. In the kindergarten, she was well integrated, was often invited to birthday parties, and frequently met her friends at home.

At the hospital, we regularly met children who also lived with cochlear implants or hearing aids. This has always been an important part of our daughter's life and has, through exchanges with their parents, also been very helpful for us. From our point of view, our daughter benefited a lot from the early provision of hearing aids, and we think that she grew up just as well as her hearing friends.

We still had regular appointments at the hospital but less frequently. The practitioner and the engineer regularly checked the cochlear implant and the hearing aid and performed fine adjustments. They examined whether our daughter could hear all sounds, how well she understood speech, and how advanced her vocabulary was—all with a lot of trust, calmness, love, and patience. Our daughter made progress in an atmosphere that, in spite of the seriousness of the situation, put emphasis on the fun side of learning—with rubber animals and puzzles. Even today, our daughter likes going to the hospital.

As she grew older, we wondered which type of school would be best for her. Since the summer of 2013, our daughter has attended an integrated primary school. We chose it, because of the good experiences we had with the integrated kindergarten. We also saw that our daughter's progress had advanced so much. She shares a class with 23 other children and has two teachers, one of whom is a special education teacher. Furthermore, the school gets support from a teacher from the school for the deaf. She is there to explain the specific problems that people with hearing loss typically have, such as difficulties with word endings and the general noise level. She also gives practical advice, such as our daughter should always sit in front or that the microphone should be used as often as possible.

We had been worrying so much, but our daughter proves to us every day that everything is just fine. She had learned how to swim before she attended school, so she doesn't even have any problems in the swimming lessons. She also attends a sports club and loves to play soccer with her brother and her friends. She feels just like a typical child! It will always be a little more difficult for her to concentrate fully on everything, but with love, with the best technical equipment, and with a supportive environment, she will find her way and will definitely be able to lead an independent life. We have always been very open about her hearing loss and that has proven to be very positive.

We're often asked: "Really? Your daughter is deaf? We wouldn't have noticed if you hadn't told us!" Dear parents, could there be any greater success? Do trust in your decisions and remember that you are not alone! And trust in your child!

*Translated from German

HONG KONG

The Story of Hugo

My wife and I live with our teenage twin boys in Hong Kong. I am Chinese and, of course, I pinned my hopes on carrying on the family bloodline. Therefore, many years ago, the news of my wife expecting twin boys brought exceptional happiness to the whole family. We expected the boys to be healthy, smart, and good looking. When we learned that the younger twin, Hugo, had a hearing loss, we were so devastated that the whole world seemed to have shaken.

Hugo's hearing loss was initially suspected when, 1 month after birth, we took the baby boys to attend the health check offered by the public health care system. Hugo showed no reaction when the nurse rang a sounding device at the back of his ears while his brother turned to the sound sources. Hugo was scheduled to go through a hearing screening by an audiologist 1 week later.

I swallowed the fear and all alone I took Hugo to the screening. Upon arriving at the auditory lab, we were ushered into a tiny soundproof room where there was a chair and a window facing the audiologist's control suite. Hugo was wearing a pair of disproportionately large headsets and some "measuring buds" were attached to his forehead, upper head, on both sides. The screening took about 30 minutes and ended with two loud thuds and a lasting beep from the headsets. This signaled an ominous verdict to Hugo's hearing as he was not disturbed in his nap. I had a very bad time that afternoon and could not concentrate on my work. The pain was so unbearable that I hid in the washroom and let out my anger and dismay in tears. I'm glad that I did.

It was arranged that we would see the audiologist for a detailed briefing on the report and be offered a series of follow-up dates at the hospital and later at the Education Department. We first got started at a center for "Hard of Hearing" kids, and at the same time, we had sessions with the AV practitioner who had an office at the hearing aid company. Hugo wore an analog hearing aid (from the public health department) on one ear for a few months from age 2 months until we bought him two digital hearing aids when he was around 6 months old.

We knew nothing about AV therapy beforehand but immediately "bought into" the idea. Hugo had two sessions every week, each lasting for almost 2 hours. Both my wife and I attended the sessions acting as playmates. Generally, the practitioner arranged the session into several parts, including vowel and consonant sound development, auditory memory training, and listening to verbal instructions and dialogue. The depth and difficulty of the content increased as Hugo grew.

After each session, the practitioner would fax us the lesson review of what Hugo could and couldn't do plus suggested activities at home. We would follow the suggestions and try the activities as many times as we could before the next session. I remember some activities prominently such as taking Hugo to many places during which I took photos and later arranged them in a sequence of three for each place in order to teach him the sequence of events; giving him instructions in his bedroom so that he had to go to the sitting room and find a number objects to train his auditory memory; and regularly reading stories so that he could model the words and learn to enjoy print.

We continued AV therapy and at the age of 2, Hugo received a cochlear implant. But, for some unknown auditory nerve issues, the implant didn't work for him. It took a whole year to ascertain the strategy forward and finally the implant was "tweaked to the maximum signal output" which, I was told, reduced the capabilities of it. Against this background, we dared to not slow the therapy down.

The activities went along the same route as Hugo was going in the earlier years, but now the content was much more complicated: the therapist would ask him to solve a riddle or let him take the teacher's role to lead an activity in the session. The therapist also asked us to encourage Hugo to take the lead more in activities at home so that he could practice more conversations. The twin boys liked "playing truck drivers" using the sofa as an imaginary vehicle, and it was a great time when they communicated verbally during the "driving."

Hugo was as outspoken as his twin brother around the age of 3. The regular testing at the hospital even confirmed that the pool of his receptive vocabulary was 9 months *ahead* of his peers. Around the age of 3, we often took him to museums to enrich his general knowledge of the world. Another special activity we did was to write journals with Hugo using lots of photos. We also placed key photos of the day's activities on a calendar to teach him the concepts of time and space.

One of the benefits of AV therapy is that by the age of 3, Hugo was able to respond more naturally using colloquial terms in a casual conversation. One prominent point is that Hugo also uttered the right interjections at just the right time in conversations. By the time Hugo was 4, the sessions intensified in the training of articulation and word intonations, since our mother tongue, Cantonese, is a tonal language.

The AV practitioner also placed more emphasis on teaching Hugo relationships between people. So, we would bring photos of family members to the sessions, and then later on, we brought photos of friends for sharing stories and to act out dialogues using the photos and practice conversations. In fact, most of the AV activities integrated elements of conversation among all the participants, of course including Hugo. At home, we spent hours in conversations and learned from the practitioner as she did more problem-solving activities to prepare him for the regular primary school, where he would need those skills.

Hugo entered primary school at the age of 6. We prepared some written materials to brief the school about his hearing loss, what we expected, and the cochlear implant. Before the first school year started, an education officer arranged some meetings between the school management and us to discuss Hugo's case. We first refrained from making too much noise and let Hugo connect with others at school on his own. As he had his twin brother at the same school, we did not have to press the school for details we might have otherwise missed. We had our own "spy." We let Hugo take "dictation," and oral and music examinations just like all the other children. We told him that he could always try. The dictation was the most difficult part, but my wife did the dictation with him at home to give him enough preparation. The oral and music examinations were actually exempted for him, but the teachers were kind enough to do them with him regardless, just to instill in him the idea that he could always try. That was the message we constantly and confidently communicated to the school. To reinforce the message to Hugo, I encouraged him to learn piano, swimming, and drawing, and he even took part in the annual interschool music and poem recitation competitions. He did them right alongside his twin brother. This positive do-not-make-a-fuss attitude was important for the school, as well as Hugo, to be open to the idea of giving children with hearing loss equal opportunities.

Hugo received the second implant at the age of 8, and it did not work well either. Now a teenager, Hugo doesn't receive AV therapy anymore, but he still has a monthly appointment with a speech therapist to monitor his speech articulation. Studying in middle school is different from the primary school in terms of the demand on self-learning. One setback of his hearing loss is that he misses much more of the teaching in class than before because the content is presented in a much more complex way. For Hugo and our family, the greatest benefit of AVT is that it has fostered the notion that he can try what any other person can try, go where they can go, and do what they can do. That said, Hugo is not afraid to argue. Well, we wanted him to talk like everyone else, and that is what we got from applying the principles of AVT.

In Hong Kong, we had some choices, and we chose AVT because it made sense to us as a family. Fortunately, it paid off for us and especially for our son. Hugo will tell the rest of this story in the years to come.

INDIA

The Story of Manas

We live in Mumbai, India, the city of dreams, where life runs by the clock and where amidst our very busy existence, we decided to have a child. On September 24, 2008, I gave birth to a baby boy whom we named "Manas," which means *mind*. Our lives changed forever.

Manas was born through C-section and, fortunately, there were no complications at birth. At the first follow-up appointment with the pediatrician, however, he was diagnosed with patent ductus arteriosus, an abnormal flow between arteries. Although he had no symptoms, the pediatric cardiologist advised us to avoid any risk of infection that could lead to complications. I wouldn't go back to work. At the age of 6 months, Manas was diagnosed with low muscle tone. He had not achieved his first milestone of holding his head up. He was prescribed physiotherapy three times a week. At the first physiotherapy appointment, when he was just 7 months old , he was crying uncontrollably. The therapist, however, remained extremely calm and unfazed by his behavior and continued with the exercises. She never doubted that Manas would walk and she propelled us to do whatever it took to make everything work for Manas. He was fitted with prescription eye glasses at 8 months of age, and there were concerns about his overall neurological development.

I had started to suspect that Manas was not responding to sound since he was 5 months old, but my family wouldn't believe it. Later, at 10 months of age, he was diagnosed with severe-profound hearing loss, and after a series of investigations, he was diagnosed with congenital rubella syndrome.

Our lives were shaken! But, our parents, Manas' grandparents, supported us through all these years. While we attended therapy sessions and consultations with many specialists, they took care of the house. At 11 months of age, Manas was fitted with hearing aids, and we started speech therapy. Almost 5 months into this, I realized that it was not of much benefit to Manas or to our family. Fortunately, we were guided to the place that eventually became our early intervention center for services. Manas underwent a battery of audiological tests, and his hearing aids were reprogrammed. We embarked on our journey into AVT.

Both my husband and I are fluent in English, but as a family, we speak Marathi at home. With reprogrammed hearing aids, we assumed that our baby would learn both Marathi and English, just as we had, and go on to an education in English. We soon learned that given his hearing loss, Manas needed to hear as much of the language of his education (i.e., English), throughout all his waking hours from infancy.

As we started our therapy sessions, we quickly realized that our baby had to be taught to listen, and he was expected to pay attention! So, we invested in a high chair, one of the wisest early decisions, since we could talk and play with him as he ate his meals and participated in family life. We were able to be close to the microphone of his hearing aids, and we learned to keep him entertained.

With all the different therapies that Manas needed, we also realized that consistency and discipline would make life a lot easier! We managed our household routines in such a manner that we had sufficient time every day to follow-up on our therapy goals with Manas when he was alert and wanting to play. My husband began work earlier in the day, so that he could return home early and allow me some "time off" without depriving Manas of valuable listening and language learning time. We all benefitted greatly. We followed the therapy goals diligently through life at home and came to realize how the most progress was made doing daily things that were natural. We also realized how much we supported one another and how we had adapted to raising our son with his many needs.

In India, "playing" with children is not a big part of our culture; we just expect them to grow up and learn on their own. We, however, learned to interact differently with Manas by opening many conversations through play. These playful conversations helped Manas to learn new skills and strengthened our bond with him. Although Manas had started responding to speech, we were guided to understand that despite our best efforts, he did not hear spoken language clearly enough to talk fluently and intelligibly. Manas needed a cochlear implant, which he received at the age of 2 years and 1 month. Once implanted, AVT began again and every small response from him gave us mountains of hope. When Manas uttered his first words, "I heard that," at one of the audiology mapping sessions, we were overjoyed!

AVT became a part of our lives. We found opportunities to stimulate

Manas in every activity we did at home and wherever we went. We created in Manas the need to communicate. We waited for verbal responses. We helped Manas make sense of the world around him through pretend play. Our apprehension at having to visit the barber or doctor turned into wonderful learning experiences. We took our young son with us everywhere, and as we did so, he soaked up all of the rich language we gave him. Our routine activities were filled with conversations. I had always wanted to instill the habit of reading in Manas. Therapy sessions and workshops gave us a lot of insight into how to read to babies from infancy, and I religiously followed up on all the guidance. We started "reading" picture books and slowly but surely increased the level of complexity. We wove toys and books into the fabric of our family life, and today Manas is an avid reader, one of the top in his class.

We didn't want Manas just to hear and talk but to have high-level spoken language. We worked on creating opportunities for conversation and expanding those with humor. Early on in therapy, we learned the importance of using correct vocabulary rather than simplifying our language too much Some years later, Manas' kindergarten teacher told us in amazement how Manas had talked about getting "a prescription" when the class had been asked to talk about a visit to the doctor. Slowly but steadily Manas' vocabulary began to grow. After 1 year of therapy sessions following cochlear implantation, it was time to go to school. Our dream for Manas to be mainstreamed was becoming a reality.

We met the school principal and the supervisor and presented the background of Manas' medical history and hearing loss. The school, fortunately, had a policy of inclusive education, but the people in management were apprehensive about Manas, and I was asked to attend school with Manas until he was "settled." On Day 3 of school, Manas' nursery class teacher was confident enough to handle him, and at the first parents' meeting she told us that Manas was an asset to the class!

We did our therapy sessions in the mornings, and Manas went to school in the afternoons. Soon, he was participating in skits and dance performances in front of live audiences, and at the end of his pre-primary year, he became the "little gentleman" of the class.

Four years after we embarked on this journey, Manas' annual evaluation showed that he was on par with his hearing peers. At graduation, we were proud parents!

Today, Manas attends primary school along with typical children his age. AVT has played a huge role in Manas's overall development. Through play, conversations, and reading, we have fostered a strong closeness with Manas. We love our child's company, and he loves ours. Indians love a celebration, and socializing is an integral part of our lives. We prepared Manas to socialize, and he was never shy to participate in any social gathering. Our families love Manas, and at any occasion, he is easily the center of attention. Manas' growing passive listening skills are evident as he teaches himself Marathi.

What blew us away was our son's insistence on learning Classical Indian music. We tried to discourage him for a month, but he wore us down with his persistence. Eventually, very skeptical, my husband took Manas to his first singing class. When he returned, I asked him how he had enjoyed it. I will never forget his whispered awe-struck reply, as he said "Superb!"

Our journey so far has been an enriching experience. Manas has taught us more than we could ever have imagined. We never underestimate him or ourselves. The journey continues.

ISRAEL

The Story of Dana and Tamar

Dana and Tamar were born in March 1990, younger sisters to Michal and Noa, then 5 and 3 years old. I remember proudly strolling down the street with my four beautiful daughters in tow thinking, "I have the "perfect" family." Being so close in age, I imagined my four daughters going to school together and growing up as a "team" of friends.

We live in Jerusalem. I had moved to Israel in 1980 after college and married Eli, an Israeli born filmmaker. By the time Dana and Tamar were born, I was no longer a high school teacher but was working as a partner with Eli in our family film business. Keeping up with four little girls under the age of 5 was challenging but hardly as challenging as what was to come! By the age of 2, I noticed that Dana and Tamar had not developed any language. We were told that it was because we were a bilingual household speaking both Hebrew and English. There were a number of hints in their first two years that could have helped us make an earlier diagnosis, but hearing loss was totally unfamiliar to me. I had seen hearing aids up close only on my grandmother when she was over 90 years old!

One afternoon, I took only one of the twins to the grocery store. As we were checking out, she started walking away with our groceries. I called out to her, "Tamar, wait for me!" She kept going. I thought maybe she doesn't really understand English, so I called out in Hebrew. She kept walking. Finally, I thought maybe she doesn't know which twin she is so I called, "Dana and Tamar, wait for me." When she did not respond to that either, I grabbed her shoulder, caught my breath, and realized that we were into some new territory.

Eli was going to the pediatrician with one of the other girls, and I told him to ask for a referral for a hearing test. On the referral form, the doctor wrote skeptically the following: "Mother concerned about hearing. Speaks two languages at home." Dana and Tamar were diagnosed with profound hearing loss, and our journey began. It was also then that I realized and later knew for a fact: Mothers always know!

In 1992, the year of Dana and Tamar's diagnosis, services in Israel for children diagnosed with hearing loss were centered in special education programs where the kids attended preschool and received their habilitation services. I went to visit the program. After experiencing the deadly silence in a room full of children, I thought to myself while watching the teacher as she highlighted her lips while over articulating words like *banana*, "this cannot be the only way!"

Fortunately, my sister, a physician in Canada, checked out the departments in her hospital. The practitioner who worked there with children with hearing loss connected her with Auditory-Verbal International, a global organization that supported AVT. I began to meet some of its members who were in Israel. Contacts from my hometown connected me with another Toronto family who had moved to Israel with their three children, two of whom were graduates of AVT. I remember going to visit their home with my family on a Friday afternoon. We sat around just talking to the children with hearing loss and when we were leaving, my eldest said, "You said we were going to be meeting deaf children! Where were they?" It was clear to my husband and I that this is what we wanted for our girls.

The challenge for us was to bring AVT to Israel so that Dana and Tamar could learn to listen and talk. Luckily, we found a local speech therapist interested in learning about this new approach. My husband and I sent to her to train with an experienced auditory-verbal practitioner in Canada, and upon her return, we began our foray into this new world.

We began to work with Dana and Tamar regularly. I was present in each session, and feverishly wrote down the "homework assignments." I drew word cards and made games well into the night. The practitioner worked closely with us and guided us in how to maximize the listening experience. Our home became a language laboratory with vocabulary lists on the fridge, so all of our friends and guests knew what we were working on and could participate. We put stickers on every item in the house with the word on them—*picture, door, clock*—long before the girls could read. But, we were starting from

scratch trying to help them understand that everything had a name.

After 6 months of hard work, the girls plateaued in their learning, and we were stuck. Our professional contact from abroad helped us to see that Dana and Tamar's hearing was insufficient for learning speech and language through AVT and suggested that we investigate the cochlear implant. The girls had their first implant in 1993 when the benefits of the implant for language learning were still fuzzy, but we understood that if we wanted them to learn to talk, we had to take the plunge. And so we did. By the age of 3.5, Dana and Tamar had undergone cochlear implant surgery in the United States and the next chapter began.

We were all feeling Dana and Tamar's frustration at not having language. There were many tears and not only theirs! The implant gave them more hearing, and we could now really maximize learning through the techniques and strategies used in AVT. Slowly but surely, we witnessed them respond to sound, learn their names, say Ima and Abba, learn their sister's names, the names of their kindergarten teachers, and gather new words to help navigate the world.

Dana and Tamar attended the same programs as their older sisters had done, the same preschool, and the same elementary school. When they began first grade at the age of 6, they had limited expressive vocabulary, but they understood a lot. But, they were nowhere close to their classmates in terms of their language abilities. And yet, we took the leap of faith and followed our understanding of the auditory-verbal principle of mainstreaming for achieving normative behavior and language modeling. It was not an easy time for them at school. We made sure that their classroom was treated for acoustic access. They received a couple of hours a week of remedial help and continued with speech therapy. We worked hard at home to enrich, expand, and deepen their language learning. We had a music teacher at home to help them with listening, and they began to learn to play the piano. We enriched daily life with experiences that would help them learn meaningful language. We would travel on the weekends to gather experiences that I would put into an experience book, and later they would write in a special notebook. We expanded the horizons of all our children this way.

Dana and Tamar are extremely friendly and charismatic young women. They have never had a problem making friends. Perhaps having each other gave them added confidence. They have someone close who understands what they are going through. I also think that we accepted their hearing loss from the beginning, and we embraced the technology. We understood that we had no time to postpone action. We were not ashamed to tell people about hearing loss when they noticed their purple and blue hearing aids with colorful earmolds. Every year, my husband and I, and later with Dana and Tamar, would give an informative presentation to the class about hearing, the need to speak clearly and not yell, the FM system, and strategic placement in the classroom to maximize their access to the teacher's voice. I was in constant contact with their teachers trying to preteach materials, so they would be ready for class. It was important to make sure the teachers felt that we were all a team. We volunteered for school committees and activities to show that we were prepared to give back to the school for what they were doing for our kids. At the end of elementary school, the school administration thanked us for teaching the children with typical hearing about our children. It was a socialization process for learning about others that was welcomed and regarded as critical for the development of good citizens of the world.

Dana and Tamar are now 25 years old. They have had bilateral cochlear implants since the age of 14. They completed their high school matriculation at a renowned School for the Arts, did a 2-year army service, a year of agricultural work, and then traveled to the Far East just like other young Israelis. They are now in college working towards a Bachelor's degree in the arts, one in Visual Communication and the other in Photography. They advocate for themselves, and they are successful getting the hours of assistance they need, sitting strategically to hear lectures, and interfacing with the authorities. I have seen them share their hearing challenges through their artistic media with openness and confidence that make me proud. They are both working in their fields of interest and living independently. They would not consider themselves as "deaf artists" rather as "artists" with a hearing loss.

Dana and Tamar were born at the beginning of the revolution for children with hearing loss. Technology and AVT made it possible for them to live fully integrated and independent lives. We were fortunate to be introduced to this amazing world in its early days. To parents of children diagnosed with hearing loss born today, I can truly see the future filled with all the sounds of life and personal fulfillment.

MEXICO

The Story of Felipe*

Felipe was born in January 2013. His father and I are Colombian, but we had emigrated to Mexico 7 years before we knew Felipe was on his way. We spend part of our year in Miami where Felipe was born. Those few months in Miami waiting for Felipe's birth was a good time. We had time for ourselves, and we spent most of it getting organized for his arrival. Away from work and the stresses of everyday life, we planned how our lives would be when our brand new little one was with us.

The pregnancy was easy, the delivery uneventful, and Felipe arrived as a healthy baby boy. Nurses took Felipe for his hearing screening and when they returned very calmly told us that he did not pass. They gave us vague directions on how to proceed. I was unable to imagine the impact this would have on our lives. He was my first child, and I was full of the fears common of a new mother. I did not even know how to take care of a baby.

A few hours later our doctor arrived to sign the discharge for us. We asked about the failed screening and he told us that it was common for newborns with typical hearing to fail! He explained that we needed to return in 15 days to retest, and that the liquid in Felipe's ears would have cleared. He would likely pass the screening then. But, Felipe failed the test again. My heart was in knots and my anxiety was out of control. Our pediatrician referred us to an ENT doctor, and after hitting a tuning fork near Felipe´s ear said that he could hear. The doctor advised that we were worrying too much.

Somehow we made our way to an audiologist, hoping for some final say on what the problem might be. We got an appointment for an Auditory Brainstem Response (ABR) test on the same day. I remember that Friday perfectly; that day would completely change our lives forever. Felipe was only 20 days old, and we already had a diagnosis that would forever define him and us as a family. We would not be an ordinary family.

Felipe's father and I were proactive. My only experience with hearing loss was growing up with a girl from my neighborhood. Everyone close to her had learned some sign language. We tried to include her in our games with only a handful of signs. Fifteen years later, I saw her at university where we shared a class. I was amazed to see her success using a cochlear implant and thought that this technology might offer the same opportunities for my baby.

By the time we arrived at the cochlear implant center, I had read all of the information available on current cochlear implant technology and candidacy criteria. I had also viewed many videos in an attempt to determine what I could expect. I saw that some of the children had very promising outcomes and others less so. Our whole family was prepared to do everything possible to give Felipe the opportunity to hear, listen, and talk.

Felipe was 2 months old and already had hearing aids, but they did not help him hear enough. We understood that at least they allowed him to hear some sounds, and that this was enough for us to get started while we waited for his first implant surgery.

We met the CI surgeon who had a lot of experience. We trusted him. He gave us the tranquility we needed to proceed. So we began the journey to sound and talking. We had some sessions with an AV practitioner, and we had a very vague idea what we needed to find in terms of therapy back home in Mexico.

All his follow-up appointments were in Miami, and the task to find an AV therapist in Mexico seemed impossible. We traveled every 2 or 3 weeks to Miami, and we waited for Felipe to reach 6 months of age, which was that center's requirement for cochlear implant surgery.

I had decided before Felipe was born that I wanted to continue working. I loved my job, but our reality was no longer the same. I felt someone had to be very invested in stimulating Felipe's language and listening throughout the day. I needed to rethink how things could be ideal. But I thought that to stop working was not the best option. I needed to prepare for the cost of surgery and all of the subsequent treatment for my son. So, I needed to ask for help. My parents had traveled to be with me for a few days. On that visit, I dared to ask my parents to move from Colombia to Mexico to help support me. Remarkably, in an act of pure love, they said yes. My father, mother, brother, and sister all moved from their home to Mexico to help us. We made the best team I could imagine for dealing with what was ahead.

We were lucky to find an AV practitioner in Mexico to help us, and we began sessions once a week but there were no major quick results. We were often upset, but we reminded ourselves that gains could only be made when Felipe had better access to sound. We focused on learning the skills we would need when he could hear through the cochlear implant.

Finally, he had the surgery on his right ear at 6 months of age. With the cochlear implant mapped and ready to go, AVT was now the intervention of our choice. Of the many success stories we had seen in the course of our research, one factor to make success possible was early implantation and the second was the involvement of the entire family. We certainly had that, too.

Then the hard work began. My husband and I requested permission to be absent from work, and everyone in the family attended auditory-verbal sessions, including Felipe's grandmother who would help to incorporate the goals and strategies at home. Our house seemed like a scene from a musical. There were songs for everything: for waking him up, for saying "hello," for bathing, for dressing, and for breakfast. And our house was full of books. Felipe used his cochlear implant from morning till night.

In time, our efforts began to pay off. Felipe began to understand certain words and phrases. His progress was our best incentive to keep working. I remember when Felipe was only 13 months old, he could point assertively to pictures of animals after listening to their names. He pointed successfully to over 30 different animals! I thought that was amazing for any baby of that age.

At 15 months of age, Felipe underwent surgery for his second implant, this time on his left ear. We noticed right away that bilateral hearing was very useful to him. He heard much better in noise and seemed to excel in conversations outside the home. We enrolled Felipe in extra activities, because we wanted to expand his learning opportunities. He attended music classes, swimming lessons, and has recently added English classes.

Today, Felipe is 3 and a half years old and his receptive and expressive language is well above expectation for a boy of his age. After a successful year of day care, we decided to enter his application to a competitive school that offers programs in English. Our goal is that Felipe will become bilingual, speaking English as well his mother tongue of Spanish. As part of the application process, he successfully passed all of the entrance tests that allow him entrance to the first year of preschool. The road is still long, but he has already started on the journey in life that we had dreamed of when he was born. He never stops talking and never ceases to amaze us about what a good listener he is. Listening is something completely natural for him.

Felipe is our greatest pride and our greatest example of joy. We have learned so much from him. No doubt his presence in our lives has redefined us as a family. This life is not as I imagined it would be, but I think it may actually be better. He has helped us to become more caring and connected people. He has taught us the true value of "I love you," of simple songs and of sound. He is very sure of himself, and he is so positive that he captivates everyone he meets. His life has provided countless lessons and no matter which direction he takes, our mission is to provide him all the tools he may need. Today, Felipe

shines for himself and his whole family. If he decides to become a carpenter, a blacksmith, an architect, a doctor, or an engineer, he will be the best he can be.

*Translated from Spanish

SPAIN

The Story of Nicolás

We were very excited by the arrival of Nicolás into our lives. He was our very wanted first child, the first grandchild for both families, and a dream fulfilled when we finally held him in our arms on March 7 and kissed him. The most important project of our lives was bringing our baby to the world and giving him all our love and affection while growing up. We had talked a lot about how he would be, even before his birth. We liked to imagine if he would look like mom or dad, if he'd like to sing like his father, or dance like his mother, and if he would play football or basketball. We also wondered about his studies and what he would be as a professional. But, finally, my wife always said that, basically, the one important thing was that he would be happy and a good person.

When we left the hospital with our baby, 3 days after his birth, we knew that something was not going well: his neonatal hearing screening had not gone well. For 2 weeks, until they repeated the tests, we did not give it too much importance. We just waited for everything to turn out well, but it did not turn out that way. We just knew that *his ears were not working properly*. In 1 month, after an Auditory Brainstem Response Test, Nicolás was diagnosed with bilateral profound deafness.

Silence fell over us, and suddenly we were in a dark street where we were alone in a nightmare.

Then, we started visiting medical specialists. In one of those visits, I remember holding a cochlear implant in my hands. I remember all those moments in the third person, as if they were happening to another person, like a movie where we didn't want to be the actors. My wife got to work right away, she took charge *leading the team:* by contacting doctors, the government, parent support associations, and institutions for rehabilitation. Meanwhile, I started to do my research online. I needed to understand what was happening inside the ears and mind of Nicolás, what the most modern hearing technology was, and how a cochlear implant worked. I read and read in the hope of finding solutions, and I didn't really get any. One night, I was watching how Paralympic sports were organized, and I imagined that my son would win thousands of medals and I would go with him. I envisioned that as an opportunity to have a great experience. Time went by so slowly. We went to an early intervention program three or four times in a week, but Nicolás did not hear anything; he just felt vibrations.

Finally Nicolás got his first implant at 12 months and gradually started to say his first sounds and words. At 24 months, he received a second implant. Everything was going slowly around us, and everyone told us that we shouldn't be in such a hurry. They said he would eventually start talking in sentences, and that we needed to give him time. Future expectations from professionals in our city were never too high. They just based everything on long hours of speech therapy, and that maybe, just maybe with a lot of effort, he might even go on to higher education.

There was something within us that made us rebel against low expectations. We wanted Nicolás to be a child like the others, to play in the park, go to school, take part in everything at home. We did not know what to do, but we thought about it all the time.

One night at the computer, I decided to apply for a course for Spanish-speaking parents on the west coast of the United States. The reason was that if we had to learn something new then, the sooner, the better. And if it did not help us, we would at least enjoy a good vacation at Disneyland.

That trip changed our lives. The bitterness and weight that had accompanied us in everyday life was changed by a special strength to fight. There, some great professionals helped us to have very high expectations, to fight for everything we wanted. We learned about AVT and the commitment required by parents who work along with an AV practitioner.

In the United States, we met an AV practitioner, who, at that time, lived in Madrid. We were fortunate to find her, and she has been our coach and guide since then. We had sessions every 15 days, so we needed to travel to Madrid twice a month. It took 4 hours to get there, and 4 hours to return, and we had just a 1 hour session.

I remember the first day. I had to read Nicolás a story. I did not really know how to do it, and I felt ashamed. I suddenly realized that all the spotlight was on me. I had a goal in therapy. The AV practitioner guided us: she instructed us on how to read a story and how to capture his attention verbally. She coached us to talk him about life, about what he was doing, and about everything around him. She asked us to take notes in a notebook, and for the next 2 weeks, we would integrate these natural strategies and routines with our child at home. We talked about clothes and narrated every step while doing the laundry. We told him about what we were buying at the supermarket. I remember assembling a bookshelf with him and explaining what everything was: a screw, a washer, a nut, a screwdriver, and a hammer. Every day while we were playing, Nicolás learned a lot of language, and we discovered many possibilities. The AV practitioner encouraged us to raise the level of vocabulary and to say more complex sentences in every session. We left the sessions with activities we thought would be impossible for Nicolás, and noticed that after a few days of practice, he just did them. At the beginning of every session, she asked about our concerns and our expectations. We knew Nicolás's level, and the AV practitioner continually checked him, even when we didn't realize it. She defined objectives and planned ahead, so that we could reach for a new target. When Nicolás succeeded, we moved on to the next one. Our goal was to close the gap between his hearing age and his chronological age. Each day we felt stronger than the day before.

The choice of school was difficult! Nicolás was 4 years, and we had to choose either a mainstream class or some kind of *special education*. The professionals in our city did not see a regular school as a good choice, because there were few resources. With the support of the AV practitioner, who always encouraged us to make our own decisions, we took the steps

to a regular school, and we obtained the cooperation of all the teachers. We must make our own decisions. If we do not try, how will we ever know if it was worth it or not? There is always fear and uncertainty, but it's worth the challenge.

During the 3 years of early childhood education, the gap reduced. By the end of his preschool education, Nicolas had higher results than many of his peers. At this stage, we realized Nicolás began to "fly alone." He didn't need much outside help or teacher support, using only an FM system in class and studying just the same way as other children his own age.

This year, Nicolás finished first grade in primary school, and his grades were excellent. He obtained one of the best qualification marks in his grade. As his parents, we feel very proud, because we are convinced Nicolás is a fully competent little boy with a bright future.

It has been 4 years of diligent work since we started working with the AV practitioner, and we know how important our role is in Nicolás's progress and in his life. The AV practitioner helped us find the tools, and we found the strength to help Nicolás become the self-sufficient boy he is today. He is not limited by his hearing loss! We are convinced that Nicolás is on the same level as he would have been if he not had a hearing loss. We have no doubt he is ready to face the future with the same expectations as any other child his age.

Nicolás can participate in life and all it offers and maybe even take his own place in the Olympic Games, competing with larger, higher, and stronger people. To do it, we all need to have one clear goal: the "Gold Medal," achieved by Nicolas and a team of people who love him: his family, his AV practitioner, his friends, and himself. With all of this he can go "to infinity and beyond."

UNITED ARAB EMIRATES

The Story of Thomas

Thomas was born in London at the height of spring, 2009. The city was in bloom. Like most mothers coming face-to-face with my newborn child, I experienced a honeymoon of emotions. The world seemed complete, with everything in its place. I felt the deepest love, I was fully alive, and I had a powerful sense of purpose. Thomas was my first child, and a much-anticipated grandchild. We celebrated his arrival with tea and toast in the recovery room of a hospital on the edge of Regent's Park.

I was already a long way from home, as I grew up in the northern suburbs of Chicago. My mother is an investor who taught me by example about hard work, determination, and focus. My father was a professor of English and a musician who raised me with a deep love of literature and music. So at only a few hours old, Thomas had already inherited a culture and tradition of learning, expression, and communication through a world of spoken language and sound.

Problems with Thomas' hearing were first identified when he failed a newborn hearing screen. The nurse tried to reassure us that all was well and listed all the reasons to not worry. We had no family history of hearing loss. My pregnancy was uneventful. The delivery was routine, and Thomas had no difficulties afterward. But, I remember feeling a chill as the nurse took my hand and told me that the odds of any serious hearing problem were very, very, slim. "Only one in a thousand," she said.

It took several months and multiple tests to accurately diagnose Thomas' hearing loss. We encountered broken machines, inexperienced clinicians, and doctors dismissing Thomas' hearing loss as "developmental." Finally, we found an interdisciplinary team who took us through the steps of testing, counseling, and early intervention planning. They confirmed what we had feared. Thomas was born with profound bilateral sensorineural hearing loss.

I waited more than 6 months before telling our family. How could I tell my father that his first eagerly awaited grandchild was profoundly deaf? How could I explain that Thomas might not ever experience the beauty of the music and language that my father loved so much? Every time I imagined having that conversation, I cried. I cried for Thomas. I cried for myself.

It was a time of desperation, cursing, and making deals with God. I resolved to do everything in my power to support this small person who suddenly needed me so much.

Months before Thomas was born, we had planned to move to Abu Dhabi. But Thomas' diagnosis made us think twice. By moving here, we would forgo the public services and professional networks available to us in the United States and face the challenge of raising Thomas in a country unprepared to support him. I made a promise to myself. If we couldn't find the right therapy support in Abu Dhabi, I would become the "practitioner" that Thomas needed. AVT was our way forward.

We were introduced to AVT during the cochlear implant candidacy process. We chose AVT, because it matched our values, our family's culture, and our desire to maximize Thomas' capacity to listen and develop spoken language using his CIs. We believed that AVT gave Thomas the best opportunity to learn and communicate through listening and spoken language and to be fully integrated into our family and community.

Importantly, AVT empowered me and gave me the confidence to raise Thomas far away from our support system in the United States. It allowed me to keep the promise to myself by putting me in the driver's seat and giving me the tools to be Thomas' principal language teacher. AVT is teachable. AVT is portable. Guided by our practitioners, we learned, practiced, and carried AVT everywhere we went.

When we arrived in 2009, the UAE itself was only 38 years old, and the capital of Abu Dhabi was still a developing city. It bustled with growth and potential, but the support and healthcare that Thomas needed was either under construction or still in the plans. So, we traveled from Abu Dhabi, to London, Washington D.C., and Baltimore, to undergo testing and evaluation for cochlear implant candidacy, and to build a brain trust of experts we fondly refer to as "Team Thomas."

Thomas received bilateral cochlear implants in Baltimore in the spring of 2010, and we remained in the United States for the rest of the year to begin AVT. Our sessions started on a warm April day just before Thomas' first birthday. The room was a large, open space, full of daylight and toys. Guided by our practitioner, we played and sang songs.

Our activities were cleverly designed to help Thomas detect sounds, discriminate them, and, with time and practice, comprehend them. At home, we applied what we had learned. To my surprise, therapy was fun. We followed Thomas' lead, responded to his vocalizations, and gave him language by narrating our activities throughout the day.

When we returned to the UAE in 2011, we took the environment of AVT with us. We packed extra suitcases with books and materials to create a rich language learning world at home in Abu Dhabi. But, we still had to travel to access resources for Thomas. The only practitioner in the country was in Dubai, about an hour's drive from our home. We made weekly trips to Dubai for therapy and spent our summers at schools in St. Louis in 2010 and Los Angeles in 2011. Each experience brought us new insights, new skills, and new members of "Team Thomas."

After our practitioner left Dubai in 2012, we found a British speech-language pathologist who was experienced in treating children with language delays. By that time, I felt confident in my skills as an "auditory-verbal parent," and what I didn't know, our speech-language pathologist (SLP) and I learned together. When Thomas was 4 years old, his language was nearly on par with his hearing peers. In therapy, we worked on gaps in grammar, vocabulary, and complex sentence structure. But, in terms of listening and spoken language, Thomas was ready for school.

There are no schools or programs for children with hearing loss in Abu Dhabi. Our only option was to enroll Thomas in the regular school. So off he went, from the start of his preschool years. But, grade schools for expatriate children in the UAE are private and admission is by application only. These schools do not have the experience or resources to support children like Thomas, and they are not obligated to include them. After several rejections, Thomas was accepted to only one of the many schools we applied to.

The first year, Thomas was welcomed. He was popular, nurtured, and successful. But, over time, we had to fight to justify Thomas' place in the classroom. The second year, Thomas' teacher was less flexible, less supportive, and unwilling to make small accommodations. Gradually, Thomas lost interest in school and his morale broke down. He became negative and despondent. As parents, that was our breaking point. When school no longer offered Thomas a positive learning environment, we withdrew him and enrolled him in homeschool.

For 6 years, we have waited for Thomas to reach a point of inertia and continue learning on his own. We asked ourselves, are we there yet? Have we done enough? While Thomas' graduation from "therapy" is just around the corner, I realize that AVT has become part of all of us. We live it. We breathe it. For us, graduation marks only the end of formal therapy. AVT will continue as part of our lifestyle, our culture, our way of teaching, learning and communicating. Always.

Today, Thomas is the joyful, outgoing, curious, creative, six-year-old we had always hoped he would be. He has learned how to listen, and he is listening to learn. Every day brings new surprises as Thomas learns to play the piano, ice skate, ride a bicycle, and read. Someday, Thomas will read this.

I hope he will reflect on it and be proud of the strength we have had as a family, the challenges we have overcome, and how much we have learned together.

Parenthood changes everything. Becoming Thomas' mother altered the course of my life, my career, and my way of thinking. I found strength I did not know I had, and accomplished things I did not know that I could do. Life with Thomas has taught me that we do not change the world by playing a small part in a large organization, hoping *our* voice will be heard. We change the world by playing a big part in the life of a small person, knowing that one day *his* voice will be heard.

Thomas has found his voice.

UNITED KINGDOM

The Story of Alice

We are a fairly boring family, born and bred in the South of England, fairly close to London. We are currently a family of five, and our AVT story starts back in 2007. Our second child, Alice, was born at the end of March of that year. Alice had an uneventful birth and a fairly uneventful early life. She was born at 39 weeks by elective caesarean, and she had APGAR scores of 9 and 10 with no jaundice or any other problems. She had an Otoacoustic Emissions Test (OAE) shortly after arriving in the world that was quite normal. Alice was blonde and cute and reached all of her early milestones with ease. She preferred rolling to walking places and loved her special cuddly toy. By and large, Alice was just what we were expecting!

As Alice passed her first birthday, it became apparent to that she was not talking and seemed to only intermittently respond to sounds and prompts. We played games that involved slamming doors and banging drums, and she seemed to respond sometimes. I wondered if she was just stubborn or if there was something else. After more time than we care to remember passed by (certainly several months) and arguing with health professionals that she wasn't just *slower than her brother,* we finally got a referral for hearing tests in July 2008. In the behavioral tests, Alice provided inconsistent results and was then referred for further OAE and auditory brainstem response (ABR) tests. Alice was a patient child, but she just didn't understand doing these tests. Alice's OAE was, again, normal, but she had an absent ABR up to 90 dB.

The audiologist, in three short sentences, dashed all our hopes and dreams and talked about Alice never being able to communicate, except through a language neither of us knew, and told us to start thinking about low expectations and difficult outcomes. To say we were devastated would be an understatement. My husband and I both cried, but we did so privately, so that Alice, as cute as ever, would never see our pain.

She was then referred to a bigger hospital in London, which had a proper specialized audiology department and a cochlear implant center. In between times, we chose to seek the advice of a private Ear, Nose and Throat surgeon, who also runs a cochlear implant center for the National Health Service (NHS). It was the first time we had heard the word "dis-synchrony," and then we started to hear about what we now know as Auditory Neuropathy Spectrum Disorder (ANSD). Even though it was only 6 years ago, it was clear that most professionals dealing with young children had barely heard of ANSD.

For her second birthday, Alice received a cochlear implant on her right ear and shortly after her fourth birthday she received one on the left side. Or, as we described it to her 4-year-old brother, the doctor has put a new battery for Alice's ears under her hair.

AVT is rarely provided in the United Kingdom, something that many other countries find baffling. In fact, when we first received Alice's diagnosis, we were bombarded with both useful and useless advice, and it was clear we would to have to find our own way through the minefield.

At the time, many professionals considered AVT to be *strict* and generally were negative towards it. But, we kept reading blogs and chat rooms that demonstrated wonderful achievements of children with hearing loss, and the common theme was this early intervention model called AVT. The teacher of the deaf (TOD) who visited us had heard of it, our speech and language therapist had seen a presentation about it, but no one seemed to know very much. It was only our constant search for the *right thing*, and the support of one SLT that we decided to try it. We booked an initial appointment. Alice was two and had been implanted for a few weeks. Everyone seemed happy with her progress, but we waited for the *tangible proof.*

We were scared parents at that first meeting, and we prayed that we had done the right thing putting our child through surgery and that our hopes and dreams could be resurrected. We still have the DVD of that appointment, and we both looked terrified. We are so scared of even daring to hope that we stared at the floor and barely spoke.

The AV practitioner asked us to tell her about Alice. She's deaf, and we don't know anything anymore. Then the practitioner asked, "What are your hopes?" Dear God, I thought, I hope she may one day say, "I love you mummy." Then the most interesting of all the questions, "What's she thinking?" I may have gotten to the stage where I am so worried, I don't think she has any thoughts at all.

Then we started to play a game. It was the simplest game in the world, but one that I will never forget. The penguins went up the stairs and down the slide, but in order to do that, we had to tell them to go "up." That was not easy for a child who had never used her voice for anything meaningful. But, by the end, we had earned an approximation for "up" from Alice, tears from us, and a firm family commitment to AVT. The AV practitioner opened the door to our and hopes, and she understood our fears. We always ran overtime in our sessions by asking questions and sharing worries. We felt we had a friend in the practitioner.

Therapy goes in waves. We actually have two children with hearing loss now, and our youngest, Oliver, sits firmly in the early part of his hearing journey. Both children are fundamentally different, but both follow some similar patterns. I have lost count of the number of times we've said to ourselves, "Improvements are not linear." Sometimes we could go months plugging away at a particular goal, then all of a sudden, Alice would wake up and make it look easy. We had to always remember *not to talk down to her*. In

the early years, we modeled our language to find a way that she could understand quickly and then one day we took a step back and realized we needed to raise our expectations, again.

I think one of the key aspects for us was our ability to change our thinking. We don't see that AVT leads us to a different way of talking to our children, but it did lead us *to a more thoughtful way*. We look for the best opportunities in our everyday life rather than constantly creating artificial situations. Equally, we've noticed that the children learn best from each other, rather than us. Oliver's use of verbs increased exponentially when Alice decided to play a game that involved marching, sitting, jumping, spinning, and goodness knows what else. It was better than any game I could have created.

Alice started nursery school at 2 and a half. She only had 30 words. We spent hours showing the staff how an implant worked, and the AV practitioner offered training courses and a school visit. Two years later, Alice had age appropriate language. It was a team effort. The staff had high expectations for her learning, used her FM system, and designed the listening environment to make the sounds of speech accessible. Alice *graduated* from her AVT program at age 5.

Today Alice is in year 4 and has a reading age about 2 years above that. The vocabulary gaps are filling in by reading books by Enid Blyton and Roald Dahl. Alice loves to learn. She is confident in her school environment and has the tools to make that environment work. She still has the odd challenge when the hearing technology fails, or the batteries or cables don't work. Alice does have the confidence to tell her teacher that she can't hear or didn't catch something. These are soft skills that AVT has given her. She also has amazing self-reliance and drive. Her teachers often comment that she is a diligent worker, which reminds me of all those hours we spent sitting at a table. I still remember those parents of children with CIs who told us that mainstreaming would never work.

Our AV practitioners coached us to say our dreams out loud, so we said, "We want Alice to talk." She said, " No, what are your real dreams, the ones that have nothing to do with hearing loss!" "Oh, we want her to be whatever she was always going to be, before we knew she didn't hear well." I now know that will be her reality.

When Oliver was diagnosed at around 18 hours old, we told our family, we hugged each other, and then we phoned our AV practitioner who said, "All right then, you'll need some homework, so come and see us." We have no regrets.

UNITED STATES

The Story of Blake

We had only been dating a few months when the name for our first-born son was determined. After much discussion, we agreed upon Blake Evans. Two years later, we found out we were expecting on the Friday before Mother's Day, 2002. We learned that we were indeed expecting a boy. I had a very normal pregnancy, right up until the week before Christmas. At my doctor's appointment, I learned of the concern about my blood pressure. After a stress test and a protein test revealed preeclampsia, I was admitted to the hospital and closely monitored. Unable to control the blood pressure, things happened quickly, and the doctors induced the delivery of our 34-week-old son.

Blake Evans let the world know that after an emergency C-section, he was not happy to be evicted from his safe home. There were three pediatricians standing by to check him and much to our relief, they proudly announced that although he was small, our bundle of joy was breathing on his own, had a great heartbeat, and appeared to be doing just fine out of the womb. Our strong-willed son was perfect. Or at least that is what we thought. A hospital volunteer came to do his newborn hearing screening. Blake was in the nursery for quite some time, but finally the volunteer returned him to the room with a bit of a wrinkle on her brow. "Your son did not pass his hearing screening."

So at 2 days of age, Blake failed his first, of many, newborn hearing screenings. We were told that the "refer" could be due to his prematurity, his delivery, equipment challenges, or perhaps he wasn't cooperating. Over the next 6 weeks, we took him in to repeat the testing with different equipment. Because the results were all the same, they finally referred us to a clinic an hour from home. The nurse who made the appointment told us nothing and didn't ask for any information about our son. She simply gave us a time, date, and address along with instructions to keep him awake and hungry until we arrived. We had no idea what was happening, but we watched the audiologist and the machine as if we understood what it was telling us. Even before the

ABR was finished, we were told that Blake had a profound loss in both ears. Without explanation, we were told to come back in a week for hearing aids, but that they wouldn't provide much help. The professional told us to start learning sign language, because Blake would never learn to listen and talk. I cried all the way home. My husband said, "If they told us he had cancer, we'd get a second opinion, right?" I agreed and called our pediatrician.

Blake was the first baby with hearing loss in her practice. She encouraged us to get a second opinion, and I told her that we didn't care where or what it would cost, but that we wanted the BEST opinion available. Two days later, after our own research, the pediatrician called and told us about a clinic where there were leaders in pediatric audiology, CI surgeons and AV practitioners.

In my head, I was calculating plane fares and the logistics of traveling with a new baby when she finished with, "I have an appointment for you next week—in a city an hour from your home." This appointment was completely different from our first. We met with an otologist, had a comprehensive ABR, and met with an auditory-verbal practitioner for the first time. The auditory-verbal practitioner asked what we dreamed of for our son, and we both agreed that what we wanted for him was no different than what we dreamed of for him before we learned he had a hearing loss. They explained the audiogram in great detail, and we understood what a profound bilateral loss meant. With only a minimal response to a 105 dB stimulus, we learned that cochlear implants would be necessary to give our son access to sound. The team explained options for communication, from total communication, to AV therapy. We left with hope.

A road map was provided. We needed to get the best hearing aids on Blake as soon as possible to keep his auditory nerve stimulated. The auditory-verbal practitioner and the audiologist emphasized that every decibel counted, and therefore we needed numerous sets of earmolds as Blake grew. We started AV therapy immediately. We were excited, bewildered, and amazed at every visit to the clinic, especially when we heard the toddlers and children with profound hearing loss in the waiting room, talking to their parents and to each other! They were talking! I could hear them, understand them, and they could understand me! THAT is what I wanted for my child. SO we jumped in full force. We were all in.

From 2 to 9 months, we met with the AV practitioner once every 2 weeks to learn how to create a "listening home." She coached us in how to practice listening strategies, and we found ourselves becoming "shade-tree" speech therapists all the time. Every night we read and read and learned to pour as much language into our little sponge as we could. One day, during one of our book readings, Blake mimicked the sound, "bok bok bok" of a chicken! We were thrilled. It was often hard to tell if Blake heard sounds, but we talked to him as if he heard every word. Finally, at nine months, Blake was determined to be a candidate for CI surgery, but our insurance company did not approve it until 12 months of age. Fortunately, his first birthday fell just in time to get the surgery done before the end of the calendar year. So, for his first birthday, Blake received the gift of hearing. His activation day was full of happy tears.

The next 2 years were full of listening games and lots of learning. When he was 2 years and 5 months, we elected to have a second cochlear implant in his opposite ear. From the moment we activated the second ear, Blake's development went from one-word utterances, such as mama, cup, yummy, pish (fish) to full sentences such as, "Mommy, I want more chocolate milk!" in a matter of months. Learning was fun and full of lots of sound.

The entire family joined in when it came to teaching Blake to listen and talk. We bought books, toys that corresponded with lessons, toys that made sounds, and used every opportunity to teach him how to listen. We worked with his preschool teachers to learn the songs, routines and games that they taught so he could participate and practice at home. We treated every opportunity as a "lesson in listening and learning," and Blake blossomed. He had a love for Thomas the Train, and we used that love to discover new sounds and listening strategies. Our auditory-verbal practitioner helped us in learning how to use everyday life as a listening and learning experience.

When Blake was 3 years and 6 months, weekly therapy was no longer needed. He had the vocabulary of a much older child and was ready to transition into the public school program. Although the early childhood program that he would attend was for 4 year olds, Blake was accepted a few months early.

While he loved school, we found that group time was a challenge for him. Together, our team worked to make listening in a group easier through the use of an FM and sound-field systems. When he entered first grade, Blake was reading slightly below grade level. His teacher was very patient and worked with him as we continued to read to-gether at home every chance we got. Sometime mid-year, the "reading bug" finally bit and by May, he was reading at a second-grade reading level. His vocabulary just exploded and by fourth grade, he was reading at a very high level. He qualified for the gifted and talented program. Blake has always been very analytical, and even in those early years demonstrated an interest in engineering and for figuring out complex machines.

Today, Blake is entering the seventh grade, is taking high-level language arts and mathematics, and enjoys building model cars with his father. He is an active Boy Scout, loves hiking, camping, and computer programming. He plays a drum in the school band and is an outstanding student. When he is asked about which college he would like to attend, his answer is the Massachusetts Institute of Technology (MIT). Life as I imagined for my son is unfolding. I know it holds many challenges for Blake, but I don't believe any will be greatly related to his hearing loss. Fortunately, we formed a team dedicated to AVT, and it has been a success for our family.

*The editors are very grateful to the parents from around the world who have shared these personal, courageous, and encouraging journeys. Any reader who wishes to communicate with one of the parents may contact Warren Estabrooks at **we.listen.international@rogers.com***

EPILOGUE

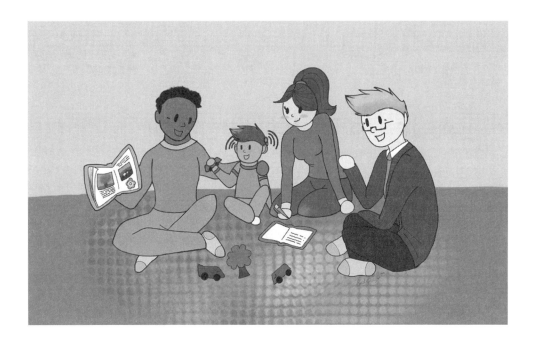

Epilogue

Learning to Listen

Warren Estabrooks

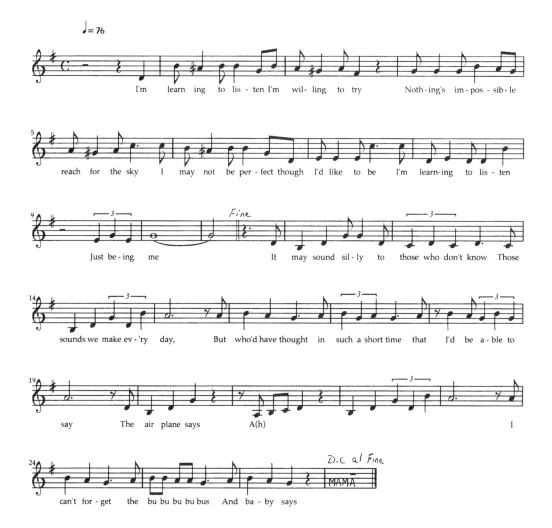

CHORUS
I'm learning to listen
I'm willing to try
Nothing's impossible
Reach for the sky
I may not be perfect
Though I'd like to be
I'm learning to listen
Just being me

VERSE 1
It may sound silly to those who don't
    know
Those sounds we make every day
But who'd have thought in such a short
    time
I'd be able to say:
The airplane says a(h) . . .
I can't forget the bu – bu – bu – bus
And baby says "mama."

VERSE 2
Blowing bubbles and spinning a top,
Is it work, or is it play?
Mommy and Daddy, working so hard
Am I turning them gray?
The clock says "t, t, t, t, tick tock, tick tock"
The cowboy shouts "ya - hoo"
Is that a bell? I hear that!
The owl sings "hoo hoo!"

VERSE 3
Later on, I was feeling so good,
All those sounds that were mine,
If I could only say a few words
For Mommy and Daddy, I'd shine
"Roll that ball, tie my shoe,
Hear that knock on the door?
Round and round, up and down,
Look, all gone, no more."

VERSE 4
Boy, was I happy with what I could say
Mommy started to cry
Daddy beamed and gave me a kiss
I felt like I could fly
Then came phrases like "reading a book,"
"Walking home," "Kicking a ball,"
"Making a snow man," "Playing with
    blocks,"
Who could remember them all

VERSE 5
I went to those lessons week after
    week
Always in the same chair!
Blowing at windmills, beating the drum
Getting so mad I could swear!
Then came sentences, stories I'd tell
Words I'd make up myself
Puzzles and books and puppets and
    dolls
And all those other toys on the shelf

VERSE 6
They think I'm ready to try it at school
But I admit I'm afraid
All those kids who talk very fast
And me with two hearing aids
I hope I can make it, it may take some
    time
And there is no guarantee
With those lessons from Mommy and
    Dad
How unlucky I'd be

VERSE 7
I'm growing up quickly and making
    new friends
Finding that I can survive
With Mommy and Daddy helping me
    talk
I'm happy just being alive
I still have lessons, a regular thing
Listening skills to maintain
My speech ain't perfect, but I talk real
    good*
Except that "s," it's a pain.

VERSE 8
It wasn't easy, but it was worthwhile
Just low far I have come
From sounds and stories and speaking
    to friends
'Cause of teacher and Daddy and Mum
I can't stop now, things are going too
    well
I'm learning to sign a new song
The melody's mine, the lyrics my own
My listening helps me be strong!

INDEX

Note: Page numbers in **bold** reference non-text material